An

Search for the Causes of Schizophrenia

Volume V

Edited by
W. F. Gattaz and H. Häfner

With 61 Figures and 54 Tables

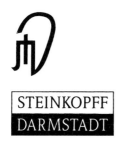

STEINKOPFF
DARMSTADT

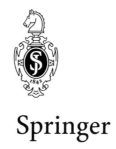

Springer

Wagner F. Gattaz, M.D.
Full Professor of Psychiatry &
Director of the Laboratory of Neuroscience
Department and Institute of Psychiatry – Faculty of Medicine
University of São Paulo, P.O. Box 3671
05403-010 São Paulo – SP – Brazil
e-mail: gattaz@usp.br

Dr. med. Dr. phil. Dr. h.c. mult. Heinz Häfner
Prof. em. of Psychiatry, University of Heidelberg
Director em. of Central Institute of Mental Health
Head, Schizophrenia Research Unit
P.O. Box 122120, 68072 Mannheim, Germany
e-mail: hhaefner@as200.zi-mannheim.de

Volumes I to III were published under the same title by Springer Berlin, Heidelberg, New York

---

ISBN 3-7985-1451-8 Steinkopff Verlag Darmstadt

Cataloging-in-Publication Data applied for
A catalog record for this book is available from the Library of Congress. Bibliographic information published by Die Deutsche Bibliothek. Die Deutsche Bibliothek lists this publication in the Deutsche Nationalbibliografie; detailed bibliographic data is available in the Internet at <http://dnb.ddb.de>.

Steinkopff Verlag Darmstadt
is a part of Springer Science+Business Media

www.steinkopff.springer.de

© Steinkopff Verlag Darmstadt 2004
   Printed in Germany

Medical Editor: Sabine Ibkendanz
Production: Klemens Schwind
Cover Design: Erich Kirchner, Heidelberg
Typesetter: K+V Fotosatz GmbH, Beerfelden

SPIN 10975336   85/7231-5 4 3 2 1 0 – Printed on acid-free paper

▊ Preface

This volume is a compilation of the presentations and discussions, arranged in a systematic manner, of the fifth symposium on the Search for the Causes of Schizophrenia, held in Guaruja/Brazil in April, 2003. The meetings look back on a great tradition. The first symposium, held in 1986 on the occasion of the 600th anniversary of the University of Heidelberg, was our first effort to assemble successful schizophrenia researchers to present and discuss research results in a spirit overcoming methodological boundaries and disciplines. The result was one of the most interesting and exciting meetings and a proceedings volume published in 1987. Like the present volume it contained the presentations and discussions of the meeting conveying an excellent picture of what was going on in schizophrenia research at that time and outlining the main future perspectives. Four further symposia followed at an interval of 2 to 3 years each. They were guided by the same principle and characterised by illustrious contributors and a highly stimulating atmosphere. The proceedings volumes, all entitled "Search for the causes of schizophrenia" and looking alike, were published by the same publisher. They reflect the considerable progress made in schizophrenia research since 1986 and have been widely used as a source for information on the most promising research lines and results and as a reference for comprehensive reviews.

The 5th symposium, too, met the standards set by the previous meetings in the range of topics covered, the quality of the contributions and the pleasantness of atmosphere. Again, leading schizophrenia researchers presented their latest results and discussed the future perspectives of their fields. The topics include epidemiology with special reference to aetiologically relevant risk factors predisposing to or precipitating the disorder as well as explanatory models of course and outcome. The section on the precursors of schizophrenia deals with early (childhood) and later (adolescence) indicators of risk and causally relevant triggers. The third section looks into pathophysiological mechanisms: associations between genetic liability, brain structure and formation of symptoms with special reference to the hippocampus. One of the contributions deals with sex differences in schizophrenia and their explanation by the protective effect of oestrogen. Advances in the genetic field are given special focus. With the topics ranging from family studies to different phenotypes on the schizophrenia dimension to the prospects offered by human genome research a wide spectrum of aspects is covered. In section 5 "Controversies in schizophrenia" results such as elevated crime rates of people with schizophrenia, contradictory explanatory models and traditional versus novel views are discussed, some in a controversial, others in a consensual manner. The key issues are the aetiological hypothesis of a psychosis continuum, progressive brain changes in the course of the disorder and Kraepelin's model of schizophrenia as a deteriorating illness. The final section, on treatment, outlines the psychological techniques and evaluates the overall therapy arsenal. The promising, but ethically sensitive field of early intervention at the prepsychotic prodromal stage is also discussed in detail.

We hope that like its predecessors the present volume will help the reader to see how far the search for the causes of schizophrenia has progressed and what still remains to be done, issues to which the sixth symposium will be dedicated.

In the name of all participants of the meeting, we would like to express our gratitude to Eli Lilly, Indianapolis and Eli Lilly do Brasil for the sole sponsoring of the meeting and of the publication of this volume.

São Paulo, Mannheim, Spring 2004   W. F. Gattaz

H. Häfner

▌ List of Contents

Section 3 – Pathophysiological mechanisms

Section 4 – Genetics

Section 5 – Controversies in schizophrenia

Section 6 – Treatment

List of Authors

BAHN, SABINE, Dr.
University of Cambridge
and Babraham Institute
Cambridge CB2 4AT, UK
sabine.bahn@bbsrc.ac.uk

CROW, T. J., Dr.
SANE POWIC
Warneford Hospital,
Oxford OX3 7JX, UK
timc@gwmail.jr2.ox.ac.uk

DELISI, LYNN, Dr.
Department of Psychiatry
New York University
650 First Avenue
New York 10016, USA
Lynn.DeLisi@med.nyu.edu

DIAS NETO, EMMANUEL, PhD
Laboratory of Neuroscience
Department and Institute
of Psychiatry
University of Sao Paulo
P.O. Box 3671
05403-010 Sao Paulo-SP, Brasil
emmanuel@usp.br

DONE, D. JOHN, Dr.
Department of Psychology
University of Herfordshire
Hatfield, Herts AL10 9AB, UK
D.J.Done@herts.ac.uk

EATON, WILLIAM, Dr.
Department of Mental Health
John Hopkins University
624 North Broadway
Baltimore, MD 21205, USA
weaton@jhsph.edu

FALKAI, PETER, Prof. Dr.
Clinic for Psychiatry
and Psychotherapy
Saarland University
66421 Homburg/Saar, Germany
Peter.Falkai@uniklinik-saarland.de

GAEBEL, WOLFGANG, Prof. Dr.
Clinic for Psychiatry
and Psychotherapy
University of Bonn
Bergische Landstr. 2
40629 Düsseldorf, Germany
wolfgang.gaebel@uni-duesseldorf.de

GATTAZ, WAGNER F., Prof. Dr.
Laboratory of Neuroscience
Department and Institute
of Psychiatry
University of Sao Paulo
P.O. Box 3671
05403-010 Sao Paulo-SP, Brasil
gattaz@usp.br

HÄFNER, H., Prof. Dr. Dr.
Dr. h. c. mult.
Schizophrenia Research Unit
Central Institute of Mental Health
P.O. Box 122 120
68072 Mannheim, Germany
hhaefner@as200.zi-mannheim.de

HARRISON, GLYNN, Prof. Dr.
Division of Psychiatry,
University of Bristol
Cotham House, Cotham Hill
Bristol BS6 6JL, UK
G.Harrison@bristol.ac.uk

HECKERS, STEPHAN, Dr.
Schizophrenia and Bipolar Disorder
Program
McLean Hospital, AB320
115 Mill Street
Belmont, MA 02478, USA
heckers@psych.mgh.harvard.edu

HODGINS, SHEILAGH, Prof. Dr.
University of London
Institute of Psychiatry
Department of
Forensic Mental Health Sciences
De Crespigny Park
London SE5 8AF, UK
s.hodgins@iop.kcl.ac.uk

LEWIS, SHÔN, Prof. Dr.
School of Psychiatry
and Behavioural Sciences
Wythenshawe Hospital
Southmoor Road
Wythenshawe, Manchester M23 9LT,
UK
shon.lewis@man.ac.uk

MAIER, W., Prof. Dr.
Clinic for Psychiatry
and Psychotherapy
University of Bonn
Sigmund-Freud-Str. 25
53105 Bonn, Germany
Wolfgang.Maier@ukb.uni-bonn.de

McGLASHAN, THOMAS H., Dr.
Yale University School of Medicine
301 Cedar Street
New Haven, CT 06519, USA
thomas.mcglashan@yale.edu

McGORRY, PATRICK DENNISTOUN,
Prof. Dr.
Department of Psychiatry
Mental Health Service for Kids
and Youth
PACE Clinic and Early Psychosis
Prevention and Intervention Centre
University of Melbourne
Locked Bag 10, 3052
Parkville, Victoria, Australia
mcgorry@ariel.unimelb.edu.au

McGUIRE, PHILIP, Dr.
Section of Neuroimaging,
Lambeth Early Onset Service,
Institute of Psychiatry & GKT School
of Medicine
London, SE5 8AF, UK
p.mcguire@iop.kcl.ac.uk

McINTOSH, ANDREW, Dr.
Division of Psychiatry
Kennedy Tower
Royal Edinburgh Hospital
Edinburgh, EH10 5HF, UK
andrew.mcintosh@ed.ac.uk

MORTENSEN, PREBEN BO, Prof. Dr.
National Centre for
Register-based Research
University of Aarhus
Tåsingegade 1
8000 Aarhus C, Denmark
pbm@ncrr.au.dk

MYIN-GERMEYS, INEZ, Dr.
Department of Psychiatry
and Neuropsychology
University of Maastricht
P.O. Box 616 (PAR45)
6200 MD Maastricht
The Netherlands
i.germeys@sp.unimaas.nl

VAN OS, JIM, Prof. Dr.
Department of Psychiatry
and Neuropsychology
University of Maastricht
P.O. Box 616 (PAR45)
6200 MD Maastricht
The Netherlands
J.vanOs@SP.UNIMAAS.NL

PILOWSKY, LYNN, Dr.
University of London
Institute of Psychiatry
Department of Psychological Medicine
De Crespigny Park
London SE5 8AF, UK
l.pilowsky@iop.kcl.ac.uk

SELTEN, JEAN PAUL, Dr.
University Hospital
PO Box 85500 Ref.Nr A00.241
3508 GA Utrecht, The Netherlands
j.p.selten@azu.nl

SOARES-WEISER, KARLA, Dr.
Chaim Sheba Medical Center
Tel-Hashomer 52621, Israel
karla.soares-weiser@sheba.health.
gov.il

STEVENS, JANICE, Prof. Dr.
Oregon Health Sciences University
Department of Psychiatry
3181 Sam Jackson Park RD
Portland, OR 97201-3098, USA
stevenja@ohsu.edu

WADDINGTON, JOHN L., Prof. Dr.
Royal College of Surgeons in Ireland
St Stephen's Green
Dublin 2, Ireland
jwadding@rcsi.ie

WITTON, JOHN
University of London
Institute of Psychiatry
National Addiction Centre
4 Windsor Walk
London SE5 8AF, UK
j.witton@iop.kcl.ac.uk

WOODS, BRYAN T., Prof. Dr.
Texas A&M Health Science Center
Neurology Section
CTVA HCS, 1901 S 1st Street
Temple, Texas 76504, USA
Bryan.Woods@med.va.gov

Section 1
Epidemiology and environment

Schizophrenia and migration

Jean-Paul Selten[1] and Elizabeth Cantor-Graae[2]

[1] Dept of Psychiatry, Rudolf Magnus Institute of Neuroscience, University Medical Center, Utrecht, The Netherlands
[2] Dept of Community Medicine, Lund University, University Hospital UMAS, Malmö, Sweden

Introduction

Although a large number of factors have been proposed to play a role in the etiology of schizophrenia, no single environmental factor has yet been established with compelling certainty. Moreover, if phenomena such as monozygotic twin discordance for schizophrenia may be accounted for by random or epigenetic events, as some would even argue (McGuffin et al. 1994), there may be no room for environmental risk factors in current explanatory models. Nevertheless, much can be learned from migration studies, an area of research increasingly concerned with the influence of the environment.

Current researchers tend to overlook the rich body of literature on schizophrenia and migration that existed already in the first half of the 20th century, with the major contributions originating in the USA. The writings of the Norwegian psychiatrist Ødegaard are still regarded by many as influential, although his emphasis on selective migration as the explanation for the increased risk of schizophrenia characteristic of certain groups did act as a deterrent for further investigations in the field. An interest in the topic was rekindled by the alarming findings concerning first- and second-generation African-Caribbean immigrants to the UK (e.g., Harrison et al. 1988). This chapter summarizes briefly the older as well as the more recent literature on schizophrenia and migration, reviews the hypotheses that have been proposed to explain the findings, and attempts to formulate a model of schizophrenia that could incorporate the insights suggested by this type of research.

Review of main findings

USA, 1930–1965

Ødegaard (1932) examined data on first admissions to Rochester State Hospital in Minnesota, USA, and showed that the rates for immigrants from Norway were twice as high as those for Norwegians in Norway and those for individuals born in the USA. The majority of the Norwegian immigrants (94%) experienced their first psychotic episode while in the USA. Admission rates for mania or depression were, however, not increased. When Ødegaard examined the biographies of Norwegian immigrants who developed psychosis while in the USA, he became impressed by their histories of poor social adaptation in Norway and reasoned that these patients would have also developed the disorder had they stayed in their home country. "They roam around from one job to another, partly because nobody wants them, but also evidently because of an innate restlessness which is one of the fundamental elements in their schizoid personality, and which must be one of the deciding factors in their emigration to America" (p. 113). Ødegaard did not question the reliability of his assessment of premorbid social functioning and assumed that the findings on immigrants from Norway applied to all immigrant groups.

Malzberg published studies on a large variety of population groups in New York State. For this purpose he used information on first admissions during certain fiscal years (1929–1931, 1939–1941, 1949–1951, 1960–1961) and population denominators derived from the censuses for those years. He showed that *foreign-born* were often over-represented in the age groups with the highest risks for schizophrenia and that statistical correction for age reduced the differences between migrants and non-migrants. He also demonstrated that the risks for people resident in New York City were higher than for those living in the more rural areas of New York State and that adjustment for this urban factor further reduced the differences between migrants and non-migrants. Nonetheless, in the majority of studies the risks for migrants remained significantly increased even after appropriate adjustments were performed. The excess varied greatly among the different foreign-born populations, with the mean value of the relative risk ranging from 1.3 to 1.5 (Malzberg 1935a, 1955a, 1964a). The excess was not unique for the group of people diagnosed with "dementia praecox", but the findings were more consistent for this group and the excess was generally larger. The risks for second-generation immigrants were intermediate: lower than for the first generation and higher than for natives of native parents (Malzberg 1935a).

In his search for an explanation for these findings, Malzberg vacillated throughout his life between Ødegaard's selection hypothesis and explanations which emphasized the role of social stressors. Other prominent findings by Malzberg include the following:

▌ He demonstrated an increased risk for *internal migrants*, i.e., people who had been born in other US states and who had subsequently moved to New York State at some point in time (Malzberg 1936a,b, 1956, 1962a,b, 1965, 1967). It may be worthwhile to note that the Great Migration of African-Americans from the rural south to the cities in the north and east had occurred mainly between 1915 and 1960. This migration was of a massive scale, and on April 1, 1930, only 32% of the native African-Americans in New York State had been born in that state. Internal migrants were consistently shown to be at a higher risk than those born in New York State. This was true for each period of investigation (1929–1931, 1939–1941, 1949–1951, 1960–1961) and for both whites and non-whites. Malzberg (1964b) obtained similar results for internal migrants within Canada.

In New York State, the risks were highest for internal migrants first admitted during the period 1929–1931. While Malzberg did not have at his disposal completely adequate denominators for these analyses, i.e., denominators stratified by state of birth *and* by age, the crude relative risks obtained for this period were 4.2 for non-white internal migrants (predominantly rural-born African-Americans vs. African-Americans born in New York State) and 3.2 for white internal migrants (vs. whites born in New York State). The relative risk of 4.2 for black internal migrants was likely to be inflated, because the New York State-born population was significantly younger. The age-adjusted relative risks calculated during later investigations (1949–1951, 1960–1961) were significantly elevated and varied between 1.4 and 1.6. Malzberg (1936a) expressed as his firm belief that the higher risk for black internal migrants could not be the consequence of negative selection and should be ascribed to the "economic and social difficulties to which a migratory population is subjected".

▮ Malzberg reported that the hospitalization rates of African-Americans for most psychiatric disorders were in substantial excess over those for whites (Malzberg 1935b, 1940, 1962a, 1965). This was especially true for general paresis, the alcoholic psychoses, and dementia praecox. The rates for the psycho-neuroses and for manic-depressive psychosis were generally lower. Malzberg also observed, however, that the black-white difference for dementia praecox became somewhat smaller when it was adjusted for urbanicity and internal migration (most African-Americans resided in New York City and were more frequently internal migrants).

▮ Malzberg (1964c) demonstrated the impact of *ethnic minority status*. When French Canadians resided in areas where they formed a minority, they had higher first admission rates for dementia praecox than the English Canadians. Likewise, when the English Canadians resided in areas where they formed a minority, their rates were higher than those for the French Canadians. Also, the French Canadians in Ontario had higher rates than the French Canadians in Quebec, and the British living in Quebec had higher rates than those living in Ontario. These findings have been replicated many times, and the underlying hypothesis is known as the "*ethnic density hypothesis*" (e.g., Rabkin 1979; Boydell et al. 2001).

▮ Malzberg (1962a, 1965) compared the risks of mental disease for native- and *foreign-born blacks* in New York State and observed that almost all foreign-born blacks were immigrants from the British Caribbean. He found that the standardized first admission rates for dementia praecox in 1960 and 1961 were 30% *lower* for the foreign-born. It was significant, however, that this difference was entirely explained by the high rates for internal migrants, whose rates exceeded those of the foreign-born by 37%. The rates for blacks born in New York State were even slightly lower than those for the foreign-born. The same pattern had emerged for the period 1949–1951. Malzberg (1962a, pp. 143–144) wrote: "There is a marked social difference between American-born Negroes and those from the West Indies. In particular, the psychological consequences of race discrimination are not so potent in the development of the West Indian. The social results of greater freedom were made clearly evident by data presented by the United States Bureau of the Census for 1940. Greater social stability is seen in the fact that 64.1 per cent of foreign-born male Negroes were living as head of the household in a private household, compared with only 32.7 per cent of native male Negroes".

Thus, Malzberg was one of the first to explore the effects of internal and external migration, and many of his ideas continue to remain provocative. All in all, the above body of evidence provided the groundwork for the notion that migration, either to another country or to a different place within the same country, could be a significant risk factor for schizophrenia. It should be noted that the emphasis here has not primarily been upon a particular characteristic or aspect pertaining to the country of origin or the country of destination, as in research on somatic disorders such as multiple sclerosis, but rather upon the process of migration itself. We will see below that many of the issues raised by Ødegaard and Malzberg (the role of selective migration, the urban factor, internal migration, uprootedness, ethnic minority status, discrimination) return in the more recent discussions on immigrants to Western Europe.

Immigrants to Western Europe: risks for schizophrenia

The British economy flourished during the 1950s and 1960s and the country recruited many immigrants from the Caribbean and the Indian subcontinent. Since the possibilities for entry have become more restricted in later years, most subjects with a Caribbean, Indian, Pakistani or Bangladeshi background, who now present to the medical services, are of the second or the third generation. A number of studies conducted in the 1970s and 1980s attracted attention to the increased risks of schizophrenia for first- and second-generation African-Caribbeans. Indeed, all of the 15 population-based studies published to date reported significantly higher risks for African-Caribbeans than for "whites", "natives", "Europeans" or "others". The size of the relative risk, however, varied between 1.7 and 13.2 (see reviews by Jarvis 1998; Eaton and Harrison 2000; and Sharpley et al. 2001). There were also reports of an increased incidence among West-African immigrants to the UK (e.g., van Os et al. 1996 a), but the evidence for an excess among Asians was not conclusive. The King et al. study (1995) reported a five-fold elevated risk for this group, but the results of some other studies were negative or mixed (e.g., Cochrane and Bal 1987; Bhugra et al. 1997).

In response to these somewhat alarming findings, the British government funded a 2-year multi-center incidence study, from which preliminary results continue to suggest that African-Caribbeans are at a dramatically high risk for schizophrenia. An impressive excess, however, was also shown for members of other ethnic minority groups, including West-Africans, Indians and Pakistanis (Aesop Study Team 2002). It is likely, therefore, that the initial focus on African-Caribbeans should be enlarged to encompass ethnic minorities in general.

The findings in the UK were supported by similar findings in *the Netherlands*. The Dutch colony of Surinam became independent in 1975 and doubts about its future caused mass emigration to the Netherlands during the period 1971–1981. The two most important ethnic groups of the Surinamese population are the African-Surinamese (blacks and colored people) and Asians, whose ancestors emigrated at the end of the 19th century from the Indian subcontinent to work on Surinamese estates. The Netherlands have also received a significant number of immigrants from the Netherlands Antilles, Caribbean islands near the coast of Venezuela. The population of these islands is an ethnic mix and consists mainly of people of African descent. Finally, between 1965 and the present day there has been a steady increase in the numbers of immigrants from rural areas in Turkey and Morocco. Initially, the men from these countries came on their own, but at a later stage they received the opportunity to settle in the Netherlands with their families.

The population-based studies in the Netherlands showed a consistent picture: 3- to 5-fold increased rates for immigrants from Surinam and the Netherlands Antilles and for male immigrants from Morocco. No increase has been found for female immigrants from Morocco or for immigrants from Turkey, while there is no evidence that they avoid the psychiatric services (Selten and Sijben, 1994; Selten et al. 1997, 2001; Schrier et al. 2001; Dieperink et al. 2002).

The increased risk for the Surinamese concerned the Asian as well as the African-Surinamese sections of the population (Selten 2001). The single Dutch study which examined the risks for subjects of the second generation found an increased risk for the Surinamese (RR = 5.5; 2.5–11.9) and for the Moroccans (RR = 8.0; 2.6–24.5) (Selten et al. 2001). The same study also assessed the risks for immigrants from western or westernized countries (Western Europe, USA, Canada, Australia, New Zealand, Japan and Israel) and non-western countries (all other countries, except Surinam, the Antilles, Turkey and Morocco). The risks were found to be increased for immigrants from non-western countries (RR = 2.4; 1.3–4.7), but not for those from western or westernized countries. Most immigrants from non-western countries had been born in Africa.

A study from *Germany*, reporting normal rates for immigrants from Turkey (Weyerer and Häfner 1992), may be regarded as a confirmation of the above findings showing normal rates for the Turkish immigrants to the Netherlands.

Further evidence regarding migration has come from *Scandinavia*. A population-based study of hospital admissions (not solely first admissions) for schizophrenia-like psychoses to the single psychiatric hospital in Malmö, *Sweden*, showed that the rates were most increased for immigrants from Africa (mostly refugees from Somalia; RR=11.3; 6.4–19.9) and Asia (RR=3.0: 1.5–6.1), less so for immigrants from European countries (RR=1.9; 1.0–3.4) (Zolkowska et al. 2001).

Some rather unexpected findings emerged from a study using data from the Central Psychiatric Register in *Denmark* (Cantor-Graae et al. 2003). In order to minimize the impact of selective migration, the authors formed a cohort of people who were resident in Denmark by the age of 15 and examined, then, history of migration as a putative risk factor. The relative risk of developing schizophrenia was 2.5 (2.4–2.7) and 1.9 (1.7–2.1) among first- and second-generation immigrants, respectively. The authors observed that age at first residence and duration of residence in Denmark had no effect on risk. The relative risks differed significantly across regions of birth, with persons born in Africa and the Middle East at the upper end of the spectrum and those born in Scandinavia and Europe at the lower end, albeit risks for these latter groups were still significantly higher than for persons born in Denmark. However, quite unexpectedly, highest risks were obtained for persons born in Australia. Also notable were high risks for persons born in Greenland, a former colony of Denmark. Most of the Greenlanders included in the sample would be of Inuit ethnicity. Another surprising finding was a RR of 1.6 (1.3–2.1) for Danish-born subjects who had a history of foreign residence before the age of 15. Thus, a temporary stay abroad may have negative consequences even for persons of Danish ethnicity.

This notion is further supported by an observation made in another study utilizing data from the Danish registry. Mortensen et al. (1999) reported an increased risk for children born to Danish mothers in countries others than Denmark (RR = 3.5; 2.7–4.4) or in Greenland (RR = 3.7; 2.0–6.8). These children born to Danish mothers, while not strictly immigrants, would nevertheless, upon return or entry to Denmark, have been exposed to the experience of migration.

In summary, the findings in the UK, the Netherlands, Sweden and Denmark differed in some important aspects from the earlier observations made in the USA: the relative risks for certain immigrant groups in Europe were much higher than the risks for European immigrants to the USA, and this is also true for immigrants of the second generation. Generally speaking, the risks for immigrants with an African background were higher than the risks for those with an Asian background. The risks for the latter, in turn, appeared higher than the risks for people of European background.

The increased incidence among immigrants is not caused by a high risk shortly after arrival. Ødegaard (1932), for instance, reported that the interval between arrival and the first psychotic episode in Norwegian immigrants to the USA exceeded 5 years in 75% of cases. The Dutch first-contact incidence study found that immigrants to the Netherlands had been living there for an average of 13.5 years before they made a first contact for a psychotic disorder (Selten et al. 2001) and similar figures were reported by Haasen et al. (1998) and Zolkowska et al. (2001).

Furthermore, there is no definitive evidence for an earlier or later age at onset in immigrants (e. g., Cantor-Graae et al. 2003). Ødegaard (1932) found that the age difference between Norwegian- and US-born individuals was statistically not significant and used this as an argument for the selection hypothesis: "If immigrant life had any tendency to provoke schizophrenic reactions, then we might certainly expect to find an earlier onset of such reactions in Minnesota than in Norway, which is not the case" (p. 118).

Immigrants to Western Europe: risks for other psychiatric disorders

Despite the mounting evidence that immigrants are at increased risk for schizophrenia and schizophrenia-like psychoses, it may still be argued that immigrants are at a greater risk for psychiatric disorders in general. What is known about this topic? With regard to African-Caribbeans in the UK, evidence suggests that their risks for anxiety disorders or depressive disorders, if elevated at all, are *not as strongly* elevated as their risk for schizophrenia. A population survey in Manchester, for instance, found that depressive disorders were almost twice as common among African-Caribbean women than among white European women (19% vs. 11%) and that the difference between males (4% vs. 7%) was not significant. Anxiety disorders, in contrast, were significantly *less* common among African-Caribbeans of either gender (Shaw et al. 2001). Among Caribbeans in South-London, the rates of suicide or parasuicide were not increased (Neeleman et al. 1996, 1997). There is evidence, however, that African-Caribbeans in the UK are at an increased risk of developing mania, especially mania with psychotic features (e.g., van Os et al. 1996b; Harrison et al. 1997; Kirov and Murray 1999). While information from the Netherlands is solely hospital-based, a study of the Dutch registry showed that those ethnic groups which were known for their high schizophrenia risks were also at a higher admission risk for drug-induced psychosis or drug dependence. Again, for Turkish immigrants these rates were not increased (Selten and Sijben 1994). Another registry study found that the first admission rates for major depression were somewhat increased for male immigrants from Turkey and Morocco, but not for those from Surinam or the Antilles. For female immigrants these rates were significantly decreased. Contrary to the findings in the UK, the risks for mania were not significantly increased (Selten et al. submitted). In sum, the available information, although very limited in quality and not very consistent, does suggest some specificity for the psychotic disorders. The risks for the depressive disorders do not seem to be increased or are only moderately elevated.

Immigrants to Western Europe: risks for schizophrenia in country of origin

First-contact incidence studies in the Caribbean have consistently shown normal incidence rates for schizophrenia (Hickling and Rodgers-Johnson 1995; Bhugra et al. 1996; Mahy et al. 1999), similar to those for White Europeans in Europe. Hospital-based first admission rates in Surinam were also within the normal range (Hanoeman et al. 2002). Such findings are important in so far as they indicate that race or ethnicity per se cannot explain the findings in Europe and any further attempts at explanation must take into consideration the context within which such aspects appear. Nevertheless, incidence studies are still lacking concerning some of the countries thus far implicated: Morocco, Turkey, Somalia, Greenland. However, given the similar incidence rates of schizophrenia, narrowly defined, obtained by the WHO Ten-Country Study (Jablensky et al. 1992), it is highly unlikely that the high rates for immigrants from all of these areas are explained by a higher rate in the country of origin A significant gap in our knowledge concerns the incidence in the various parts of Africa.

Explanatory hypotheses

What are the variables under study?

While migration in and of itself does not likely cause schizophrenia, some aspect associated with migration does clearly increase one's risk, as shown by the increased risk for Danes who spent their early childhood residing outside of Denmark. Nevertheless, second-generation immigrants have not migrated themselves, and it is thus unclear what migration, even in the broadest sense of the concept (i.e., history of migration in the parents), represents in terms of an exposure variable. Since many immigrants suffer adverse social circumstances, one might suggest that "ethnic minority disadvantage" is the common denominator for the high-risk groups. For practical purposes, however, in the discussion that follows, we shall designate the subjects under study as "immigrants".

Bias

Studies using semi-structured diagnostic interviews have ruled out misdiagnosis as the explanation for the findings in the UK and the Netherlands (e.g., Harrison et al. 1997; van Os et al. 1996; Selten et al. 2001). Short- and long-term follow-up studies in both countries have done the same (e.g., Takei et al. 1999; Veen et al. in preparation). A lower threshold for hospital admission is also an unlikely explanation, because the first-contact studies subsumed the first contacts with outpatient services. In the UK some uncertainty may exist regarding the accuracy of population denominators, but it is difficult to conceive how errors in the denominator could account for five- to ten-fold elevated rates. Denominators in the Netherlands, Sweden and Denmark do not rely on household censuses and are highly reliable.

Selective migration

Although it may be premature to exclude some role for selection, after 70 years we can definitively reject Ødegaard's selection hypothesis as the *sole* explanation for the findings on immigrants. First, according to an authoritative textbook on epidemiology, a general assumption in migrant studies is that "the healthy and physically most able are most likely to migrate. These are features that may be strengthened by health-related restrictions or job opportunities in the host country" (MacMahon and Trichopoulos 1996). Thus, the selection hypothesis is not plausible given the nature of the prodromal phase of schizophrenia, which includes negative symptoms and frontal dysfunction. Moreover, weaknesses in the selection hypothesis are rather clearly demonstrated in the examples of large-scale migration provided by Ireland, Croatia and Surinam. In the 19th century and at the beginning of the 20th century the larger part of the Irish-born population emigrated to the USA, but this did not lead to a decreased frequency of the disorder in Ireland. The earlier reports of an increased prevalence of the disorder in Ireland have later been disputed, but no claims have been made for a decreased prevalence in this country (Kendler et al. 1993). Kendell (1987) wrote: "Certainly, one cannot at the same time attribute the high incidences of schizophrenia in Western Ireland to the selective emigration of the healthy and the high breakdown rate of Irish immigrants to the United States to a selective immigration of the pre-psychotic". In Croatia, the admission risks were found to be highest in those areas where the emigration rates were highest (Folnegovic and Folnegovic-Smalc 1992). Since the emigration from Surinam subsumed more than one third of the Surinamese-born population, the five-fold elevated risks for immigrants to the Netherlands are incompatible with the selection hypothesis (Selten et al. 2002 a). Also, if selective migration were to account for the findings concerning Surinamese immigrants to the Netherlands, one would also expect the disorder to have disappeared from Surinam, which is certainly not the case (Hanoeman et al. 2002). Moreover, selection cannot explain the findings in the above-mentioned study of the Danish psychiatric registry, showing an increased risk for people who had arrived in Denmark before their fifteenth birthday (Cantor-Graae et al. 2003). Likewise, the median ages of migration of the Surinamese- and Moroccan-born patients who participated in the first-contact study of incidence in the Netherlands were 9 and 15 years, respectively (Selten et al. 2001). Finally, and perhaps most importantly, the findings of extremely high risks for African-Caribbeans of the second generation are difficult to understand in terms of selective migration of their parents. Also, the study of the Danish registry found that the risk associated with second-generation immigrant status was actually lower in second-generation immigrants with a parental history of psychiatric disorder than in those without a parental history of psychiatric disorder (Cantor-Graae et al. 2003). Also pertinent in this regard, Rosenthal et al. (1974) compared the emigration rates for adopted children born to a biological parent with a schizophrenia spectrum disorder to the emigration rates for children born to non-schizophrenic parents and found that the rates for the first group were lower than those for the second.

"Biological" hypotheses

Increased risks for schizophrenia found in both first and second generation immigrants indicate by and large that *strictly biological* hypotheses are not parsimonious. One might speculate, for instance, that immigrants have an impaired immunity to a neurotropic virus in Europe, but this hypothesis does not explain the findings for those of the second generation, who grow up in the same physical environment as their European peers. Likewise, one could hypothesize that female immigrants, while pregnant, have a shortage of vitamin D and that this contributes to the higher risk in offspring (McGrath 2000), but this does not explain the higher risk in the first generation.

Given the association between cannabis and schizophrenia (e.g., van Os et al. 2002), the most important hypothesis to consider here would be that immigrants have higher rates of *illicit drug use*. It should be kept in mind that the ascertainment of drug use among the general population or among ethnic minority groups is fraught with methodological problems and that the validity of population surveys can be highly questioned. Laboratory analyses may provide more valid information, but only concerning recent drug usage. An epidemiological study using hair analysis was not successful, because too many patients, especially immigrants, refused to yield hair (Selten et al. 2002b). Another way to address this issue is to examine whether rates of drug-related disorders are also elevated among immigrants, as elevated rates could be interpreted as evidence of differentially greater substance abuse. Unfortunately, however, the available data is very limited. In the Netherlands, as outlined previously, those ethnic groups which were known for their increased risks for schizophrenia were also at a higher admission risk for drug psychoses and drug dependence (Selten and Sijben 1994). This pattern of findings is compatible with the substance-abuse hypothesis, but it could also indicate, of course, that those ethnic groups which are vulnerable for schizophrenia are also at an increased risk for drug abuse.

In any evaluation of the substance-abuse hypothesis one must keep in mind that the diagnoses in the various incidence and follow-up studies concerned schizophrenia or schizophrenia-like disorders and did not include drug-induced psychotic disorders. Whether drug abuse can give rise to the development of a chronic disorder like schizophrenia, a disorder that persists after the discontinuation of use, is at present uncertain. Second, the studies that examined illicit drug use in patients diagnosed with schizophrenia or schizophrenia-like disorders failed to find higher rates for African-Caribbeans in the UK (Cantwell et al. 1999) or immigrants to the Netherlands (Veen et al. 2002). Finally, the contribution of illicit substance usage towards the development of schizophrenia would be too small to fully account for the size of the migrant effect currently indicated in recent studies.

To our knowledge there have been two studies that tested *virological* hypotheses, in Surinamese immigrants to the Netherlands, and both were negative (Selten et al. 1998, 2000).

While increased rates of *obstetric complications* (OCs) have previously been considered as a possible explanation for increased incidence of schizophrenia among immigrants, this hypothesis has become increasingly unlikely. First, these complications are unlikely to constitute a very strong risk factor for the disorder (Cannon et al. 2002). Second, if a greater prevalence of OCs among, e.g., African-Caribbean immigrants than among White British was the explanation for their higher incidence of schizophrenia, it remains unclear why one does not find similarly high incidence rates in the Caribbean. Finally, a study of OCs in Caribbean schizophrenia patients resident in the UK found the frequency of these complications to be lower, not higher, than in their White counterparts (Hutchinson et al. 1996). *Increased paternal age* has recently been suggested to contribute to the etiology of schizophrenia, perhaps by producing a greater prevalence of mutations in sperm (Malaspina et al. 2001). Since the process of migration may lead to a higher age at reproduction, increased paternal age could be a factor of some importance for subjects of the second generation, but to date no study has addressed this question. Several other known risk factors for schizophrenia could be relevant here (for example, an increased frequency of head trauma or a change in diet, from high to low in polyunsaturated fatty acids), but their possible contribution to the immigrant phenomenon has not been examined. A change from a hot to a cold climate is an unlikely explanation, given the increased risk in Denmark for immigrants from Greenland.

Social adversity and psycho-social hypotheses

After a century of research there is still no firm evidence that social adversity contributes to the etiology of schizophrenia. Thus, while it might be appropriate to question the etiological relevance of socially adverse aspects of the migration process or membership in an ethnic minority group, it is important to keep in mind that social factors may well influence brain function and its anatomical substrates. Thus, psychosocial hypotheses may nevertheless merit closer examination.

People of lower socioeconomic status (SES) are more often exposed to certain risk factors for medical disorders than others. These risk factors may be biological (e.g., malnutrition, drug abuse) or psychosocial (e.g., stress). Since both schizophrenia patients and immigrants are more often of lower SES, one could hypothesize that some variables associated with socioeconomic deprivation explain their high risks. However, the negative association between SES and schizophrenia has been shown to be more due to social selection (downward mobility of the genetically predisposed) than to social causation (Dohrenwend et al. 1992). It is at present uncertain whether people born to parents in the lower social classes are at an increased risk, because some studies reported an association with higher SES of the parents (e.g., Jones et al. 1994; Makikyro et al. 1997; Mulvany et al. 2002) and others an association with lower SES (e.g., Harrison et al. 2001). It may be difficult to disentangle the effects of migration and socioeconomic deprivation, because they tend to be associated with the same phenomena: unemployment, poor housing, lower educational levels. In this regard, it may be particularly important to note the normal risks for Turkish immigrants to the Netherlands, as Turkish immigrants have always had lower income, lower educational levels and higher unemployment rates compared to immigrants from Surinam. Also, in the Dutch first-contact incidence study, adjustment of the relative risks for the SES of the patient's neighborhood had only a small effect on the relative risks (Selten et al. 2001). Consequently, low socioeconomic status by itself is an unlikely explanation for the findings in immigrants.

Murphy (1965) was one of the first to emphasize a role for psycho-social factors, with his hypothesis that the stress of particular *complex social tasks* was of central importance: "The theory, therefore, proposes that schizophrenia can be evoked in suitably predisposed people when they are repeatedly called upon to make decisions on relatively complex matters, which they perceive as important and on which they have received only confused or inadequate guidelines, without escape being possible" (Murphy 1965, p. 417). Murphy illustrated his ideas with several examples, one of which is the case of the Achinese, a people of warriors in Indonesia. The Achinese had always despised the maintenance of a peacetime economy and left it in the hands of the women.

After a 20-year period of war with the Dutch army, a large increase of schizophrenia was observed in the male, not in the female part of the population. The Dutch had defeated the Achinese and had forbidden them to wage war on their neighbors. In this new situation, the Achinese men had to find new social roles to perform, whereas the Achinese women could continue performing the tasks they had always done. Eaton and Harrison (2000) elaborated on Murphy's ideas, emphasizing that the planning of one's life is more difficult for members of ethnically disadvantaged groups and that the core problem is "*an inability to formulate the life plan*".

Janssen et al. (2003) on the other hand, suggested that *discrimination* gives rise to a paranoid attributional style, which places individuals at risk of developing a psychotic disorder. A prospective study provided some evidence in support of this hypothesis, but the numbers were small (see also Chakraborty and McKenzie 2002).

When one considers each of the proposed mechanisms, it is nevertheless difficult to distinguish between what might be regarded as "causal" and what might be regarded as "consequence". It is important to note, for instance, that the frontal-executive functions of schizophrenia patients and their relatives have been shown to be weaker (e.g., Cannon et al. 1994) and that an inability to formulate a life plan could therefore be a consequence of earlier events. Likewise, the discrimination hypothesis may be difficult to test, because it is often not easy to decide whether reports of discrimination precede a psychotic disorder or are already a symptom of it. By way of summary, we could say that none of these interesting hypotheses has been adequately tested. A more serious limitation is that none of them fully integrate aspects of brain function that may be pertinent both to schizophrenia and to the immigrants' experience.

Additional factors have been examined in other studies. A case-control study among African-Caribbeans in the UK found that a long period of separation from either or both parents was associated with a higher risk for schizophrenia (Mallett et al. 2002). It is possible, therefore, that *growing up in a single parent household* is a contributing factor in some immigrant groups. It is also evident, however, that these childhood circumstances are not a common denominator for all immigrants suggested to be at an increased risk. *Extreme duress under migration* cannot be the explanation, given the easy entries of people from former colonies (see also Zolkowska et al. 2001).

It may be helpful also to consider hypotheses concerning protective factors. According to the *ethnic density* hypothesis, immigrants living in areas where they constitute a larger proportion of the total population are at a lower risk (Malzberg 1964 c). This finding has been replicated so many times that it can be regarded as reliable (e.g., Murphy 1965; Rabkin 1979; Boydell et al. 2001). There is no evidence indicating that the association is explained by selection bias, in that people who choose to live in areas where they are more isolated from their own ethnic community could be more at risk (Rabkin 1979; Boydell et al. 2001). Although the precise mechanism is uncertain, it is likely that some form of social support is operating here. Strong social and family networks have been suggested as explanations for the relatively low rates for

Asian immigrants to the UK and for Turkish immigrants to the Netherlands, but this hypothesis, albeit attractive, is not supported by a great deal of empirical research. None the less, it is worthwhile to note that the crime rates for Turkish immigrants to the Netherlands are much lower than those for their Moroccan counterparts (Junger et al. 1992).

Cognitive vulnerability

Since low IQ has been shown to be an important predictor of risk for schizophrenia (Gunnell et al. 2002), it is of relevance that many immigrant groups known to be at an increased risk for schizophrenia show poorer levels of academic achievement than the European host populations. Nevertheless, it would perhaps be hazardous to conclude that the low levels of academic achievement among certain immigrant groups are causally related to their increased risks of schizophrenia. First, the validity of IQ differences among ethnic groups as well as the origins of these differences are highly controversial (Herrnstein and Murray 1996). Second, it is possible that the association between low IQ and schizophrenia is confounded by a third factor producing both low IQ and schizophrenia. However, it may be useful here to distinguish between intelligence and intellectual development. As many immigrants have had few opportunities to develop themselves intellectually, it would be premature to dismiss completely the possible role for a low level of education in the causal chain that leads to their higher risks. It is possible, for example, that the lower a person's intellectual development, the more difficult it may be for him to comprehend the complexities of social interaction, and this in turn could lead to feelings of paranoia and social withdrawal. It is also important to keep in mind that intellectual development is highly valued in western societies and that individuals who are illiterate or poorly educated are often ranked lowest in the social hierarchy.

Urbanicity

The association between urban residence and risk for schizophrenia has been described since the beginning of the 20th century: the larger the town, the higher the risk (e. g., Malzberg 1955 b). Many researchers believed that this association was explained by "drift" of genetically predisposed individuals who sought the anonymity of the urban environment, but the more recent studies have shown that it is urban birth or urban upbringing, rather than urban residence at the time of illness onset, which determines one's risk (e. g., Lewis et al. 1992; Marcelis et al. 1998; Mortensen et al. 1999). A sophisticated analysis of Danish registry data showed that the risk for schizophrenia depended on the level of urbanicity of the place of residence and on the numbers of years spent there before the 15th birthday (Pedersen and Mortensen 2001 a). For example, living in a higher degree of urbanicity at the 10th birthday than at the 5th birthday increased one's risk, while living in a lower degree of urbanicity decreased this risk. Urban birth turned out to be a proxy for urban upbringing and the data showed no indication of any particularly vulnerable ages.

The effect of urbanicity was not explained by a greater frequency of mental illness in the family members (Pedersen and Mortensen 2001 b).

The underlying risk components are unknown and might variously involve aspects of the physical environment (e. g., exposure to toxins, viruses, head trauma), the psycho-social environment (e. g., social isolation or stress) or a combination of both (e. g., use of illicit drugs). Since many immigrants to Western Europe have settled in urban areas, presumably due to the greater access to social networks, employment and housing opportunities, the question arises whether the higher risks for immigrants are mediated by their higher level of urbanicity. The Surinamese immigrants to the Netherlands, for instance, are more than twice as likely than the Dutch population as a whole to live in municipalities of 100 000 inhabitants or over. An evaluation of this hypothesis should take into consideration, *first*, that many immigrants of the first generation have grown up in rural areas and, *second*, that the European incidence studies have controlled for the urban factor by comparing immigrants to natives who were resident in the same town. One could argue that immigrants may be more intensively exposed to this urban factor or that they may be more sensitive to it, but this remains speculative until we know more about its nature. It is doubtful whether information on the small numbers of immigrants who have settled in rural areas is helpful, because the latter constitute a selected group. Data from the Dutch psychiatric registry indicate that the risks for Surinamese immigrants living in Amsterdam, Rotterdam or The Hague are no greater than the risks for those in smaller municipalities (unpublished data). Consequently, the immigrant phenomenon cannot be considered a manifestation of the urban effect without making the arbitrary assumptions that immigrants are more frequently exposed to the urban factor or are more sensitive to it.

▌ Uncertainty about social rank

A new hypothesis

We sought a common mechanism that could explain the salient findings described below:

1) increased incidence among first- and second-generation immigrants from non-western countries to Western Europe; 2) increased incidence among internal migrants; 3) protective effect of high ethnic density and social cohesion; 4) increased incidence among children born to Danish mothers in countries other than Denmark and among Danish-born subjects with a history of foreign residence before the age of 15; 5) increased incidence in urbanized areas.

As discussed previously, poverty or low SES is *not* a likely explanation for the increased risks among immigrants. Since many immigrants have the experience of being an outsider and thus must conquer a place for themselves in the social hierarchy, we propose that the common mechanism is *uncertainty about social rank or status*. This uncertainty concerns both one's membership of society and the level of one's position (high or low).

Contrary to hypotheses which focus on low SES, this hypothesis can also be applied to people of middle and upper social class who nevertheless may have "outsider" status and is therefore compatible with the observation that many migrants from Western and Eastern Africa, who developed psychosis in Europe, are well-educated. The concept also applies, of course, to second-generation immigrants, who may lack the sense of belonging that being born in a country usually confers upon its citizens. Uncertainty about social rank could account for the urban effect and the ethnic density phenomenon, because social competition would be greater in urban environments and because people would feel more uncertain in neighborhoods with few people of their own kind. Uncertainty about social rank could also explain the higher risks for white and black internal migrants in the USA. Note that it is difficult to conceive how misdiagnosis or racial discrimination could explain the higher risks for black internal migrants than for black people born in New York State, but that black internal migrants would have to secure a place for themselves within the existing black social hierarchy. As for Danes returning to Denmark, many of them may have felt uncertain about their new place in the social hierarchy. Since uncertainty about social rank is more stressful for male immigrants whose background culture places masculine pride into focus, the hypothesis could explain why in several studies the effect of migration is more prominent in males than in females (e. g., Harrison et al. 1997; Selten et al. 1997, 2001; Fossion et al. 2002). A greater effect of the urban environment on schizophrenia risk among males has been observed in the Netherlands (Marcelis et al. 1998), but not in Denmark (Pedersen and Mortensen 2001 a).

The uncertainty-about-social-rank hypothesis has a strong evolutionary perspective. The ability to sense where one stands in reference to others is a fundamental aspect of animals living in groups and has strong implications for the chances of survival and for the ability to reproduce.

Uncertainty about social rank differs from many other stressors in that it has particular relevance for the psycho-social well-being of children and adolescents. This is important, because the onset of psychosis is preceded by a decline in functioning over the course of many years. The adolescent period is the peak period during the human life cycle for the establishment of one's social status and there are few concerns which occupy adolescents more than their status in the peer group.

The uncertainty-about-social-rank hypothesis has several notions in common with hypotheses that focus on complex social tasks, the formulation of a lifeplan, and racial discrimination, but differs from them in that it specifies which social task is relevant (finding a place in the social hierarchy) and why it is difficult to make a life plan (uncertainty about social status). It recognizes that discrimination is damaging and stressful, but, contrary to the discrimination hypothesis, it can be applied to the more general notion of "outsider status", such as that which might occur when growing up in or moving to urban areas. As animal studies have shown that social dominance has a great impact on synaptic dopamine levels, we propose furthermore that uncertainty about social rank contributes to the etiology of schizophrenia by disturbing *brain dopaminergic function*. In the next section we will describe some animal experiments which may have relevance for our hypothesis.

Animal studies

A study of male *Cynomolgus macaques* demonstrated the impact of social dominance on brain dopaminergic function. In this experiment, the monkeys were first individually, and later, socially housed. Positron emission tomography imaging revealed no difference in dopaminergic function during individual housing, whereas social housing increased the amount or availability of dopamine D2 receptors in the dominant monkeys and produced no change in subordinate animals. Moreover, the subordinate monkeys consumed significantly more cocaine, which was available for self-administration, than the dominant monkeys did. The results indicated that the individually housed monkeys and the subordinate animals displayed *dopaminergic hyperactivity* and that cocaine functioned as a reinforcer in the subordinate, but not in the dominant monkeys (Morgan et al. 2002).

Another interesting model for *social defeat stress* is the *resident-intruder paradigm,* whereby a male rodent (the intruder) is put into the cage of another male (the resident). Control animals are usually placed in an empty, clean and novel cage. Within a few seconds the aggressive resident attacks the intruder and prompts him to display submissive behavior. In some experiments contact with the resident is maintained by placing the *defeated intruder* within a protective wire mesh cage inside the resident cage. These experiments showed that social defeat stress leads to elevated levels of dopamine in the nucleus accumbens and the prefrontal cortex, but not in the lateral striatum. The rise in dopamine was not explained by a increased locomotor activity and was synchronous with high levels of orienting toward the resident (Tidey et al. 1996). The rise in dopamine is probably mediated by endogenous opioids, because social defeat stress causes increased expression of μ_1-opioid receptors mRNA in the ventral tegmental area, not in the substantia nigra (Nikulina et al. 1999). Interestingly, the activation of mesolimbic dopamine transmission by cannabinoids and heroin is also mediated by a μ_1-opioid receptor mechanism (Tanda et al. 1997). The normal levels of μ-opioid receptors mRNA in the substantia nigra and the normal levels of dopamine in the striatum suggest that the dopaminergic system involved is not the nigrostriatal pathway, but the mesocorticolimbic dopaminergic pathway (Tidey et al. 1996; Nikulina et al. 1997). The common finding of these experiments on non-human primates and rats is that social defeat has a profound impact on brain dopaminergic function. It is important to note, however, that several other stressors can also lead to dopaminergic hyperactivity in the mesocorticolimbic pathways of rodents, for instance footshock, restraint or immobilization stress (e.g., Watanabe 1984; Cabib and Puglisi-Allegra 1996).

Another important phenomenon is *behavioral sensitization,* which is caused by a single dose of amphetamine or repeated doses over several days. Behavioral sensitization implies that the animals display an enhanced response to a variety of stressful challenges or to dopamine agonists. It can also be induced by stressful experiences, including social defeat (e.g., Sorg and Kalivas 1991). Covington and Miczek (2001), for example, demonstrated that repeated exposures to social defeat stress led to a greater locomotor response to a cocaine challenge and to an enhanced consumption of this substance. These findings regarding behavioral sensitization suggest that the experience of social defeat could make humans more vulnerable to the pathogenic effects of illicit drugs.

The results from the above experiments do not explain why uncertainty about social rank in humans should lead to schizophrenia, rather than depression or addiction, nor do they explain why other stressors, which have been demonstrated to cause dopaminergic hyperactivity in rodents, are unlikely to cause schizophrenia in humans. They do suggest a mechanism, however, whereby the experiences of migration and city-residence can lead to a disturbance of brain function.

Does the hypothesis explain other aspects of the epidemiology of schizophrenia?

Since uncertainty about social rank need not be the only risk factor involved in schizophrenia, one should not expect it to explain all epidemiological findings. The hypothesis is compatible, however, with some observations unrelated to migration.

The first detailed and recognizable descriptions of schizophrenia date from the period around the French Revolution, the very revolution that broke apart the fixed social hierarchy in Europe and menaced the status of those in the highest social classes. Subsequently, increasing industrialization and urbanization made all people less secure about their place in society. The claims of a rise in schizophrenia during the 18th and 19th century, therefore, are compatible with the uncertainty-about-social-rank hypothesis (Torrey and Miller 2001).

Second, uncertainty about social status may be one of the factors underlying the frequent onset of the disorder in early adulthood. Since males may feel more pressed to achieve a certain rank than females, it is possible that a higher degree of uncertainty in males contributes to their younger age at onset. Third, uncertainty about social rank could be one of the factors that account for the strong association between low IQ and schizophrenia.

One could argue that the emancipation of women during the 20th century, which caused an increasing role ambiguity and, conceivably, a greater uncertainty about social status, should have led to a rise in schizophrenia. It is possible, however, that this rise was prevented by the introduction of oral contraceptives, because estrogens may have a protective effect against schizophrenia (e.g., Häfner et al. 1993). It is also possible that the actual rise in social status had a protective effect or that females are less vulnerable to uncertainty about social status than males. Seemingly, it may be difficult to comprehend all the underlying mechanisms involved in these processes.

A model of schizophrenia

Antipsychotic drugs are D2 dopamine receptor-blockers and agents that trigger the release of dopamine can produce psychosis. Since neuroimaging studies have shown that schizophrenia patients, *when psychotic*, show a heightened synthesis of dopamine, a heightened dopamine release in response to an impulse, and a heightened level of synaptic dopamine, several models of schizophrenia include a final mesolimbic dopamine dysregulation (reviewed by Kapur 2003). Kapur hypothesized that this dysregulation leads to an aberrant assignment of salience to the elements of one's experience and to delusions and hallucinations. The causes of the dysregulation, however, remain unknown. It is proposed here that uncertainty about social status *contributes* to the etiology of schizophrenia, or to a certain subtype of the disorder, by dysregulating dopamine transmission in the brains of people with an *underlying biological vulnerability*.

This vulnerability, probably the result of genetic and early developmental influences, could be an inability to regulate dopaminergic systems (e.g., Breier et al. 1993), but this is uncertain. We do know, however, that this vulnerability is often manifest in early childhood as an *outsider status* (e.g., Jones et al. 1994). Socially adverse experiences during childhood and adolescence, perhaps mediated by dopamine, could lead to an avoidance of social interaction, to an arrest in the development of social skills and to an increasing uncertainty about social rank. The experiments on behavioral sensitization in rats suggest that these experiences could make individuals more vulnerable to the pathogenic effects of illicit drugs. These processes are much more likely to become a malignant condition in first- and second-generation immigrants, who are outsiders by definition. It is also worthwhile to note here that the ability to recognize facial expression, which plays a key role in establishing social hierarchy, seems to be impaired in schizophrenia (Edwards et al. 2002). If this impairment is also present in pre-schizophrenic individuals, it could contribute to their uncertainty about social status.

The development of higher resolution neuroimaging techniques will make it possible to test the hypothesis and to examine the dopaminergic function of migrants and city-dwellers. Studies of this kind will contribute to an integration of current neurobiological and psychosocial theorizing concerning the pathogenesis of schizophrenia.

▌ **Acknowledgment.** The authors thank Iris Sommer, M.D., for comments on the manuscript. Dr. E. Cantor-Graae is supported by the Stanley Medical Research Institute.

▌ References

Aesop Study Team (2002) Raised incidence of all psychoses in UK migrant populations. Schizophr Res 53:33

Bhugra D, Hilwig M, Hossein B, Marceau H, Neehall J, Leff J, Mallett R, Der G (1996) First-contact incidence rates of schizophrenia in Trinidad and one-year follow-up. Br J Psychiatry 169:587–592

Bhugra D, Leff J, Mallett R, Der G, Corridan B, Rudge S (1997) Incidence and outcome of schizophrenia in whites, African-Caribbeans and Asians in London. Psychol Med 27:791–798

Boydell J, van Os J, McKenzie K, Allardyce J, Goel R, McCreadie RG, Murray RM (2001) Incidence of schizophrenia in ethnic minorities in London: ecological study into interactions with environment. BMJ 323:1336–1338

Breier A, Davis OR, Buchanan RW, Moricle LA, Munson RC (1993) Effects of metabolic perturbation on plasma homovanillic acid in schizophrenia. Arch Gen Psychiatry 50:541–550

Cabib S, Puglisi-Allegra S (1996) Different effects of repeated stressful experiences on mesocortical and mesolimbic dopamine metabolism. Neuroscience 73:375–380

Cannon M, Jones PB, Murray RM (2002) Obstetric complications and schizophrenia: historical and meta-analytic review. Am J Psychiatry 159:1080–1092

Cantor-Graae E, Pedersen CB, McNeil TF, Mortensen PB (2003) Migration as a risk factor for schizophrenia. Br J Psychiatry 182:117–122

Cantwell R, Brewin J, Glazebrook C, Dalkin T, Fox R, Medley I, Harrison G (1998) Prevalence of substance misuse in first-episode psychosis. Br J Psychiatry 174:150–153

Chakraborty A, McKenzie K (2002) Does racial discrimination cause mental illness? Br J Psychiatry 180:475–477

Cochrane R, Bal S (1987) Migration and schizophrenia: an examination of five hypotheses. Soc Psychiatry 22:181–191

Covington HE, Miczek KA (2001) Repeated social-defeat stress, cocaine or morphine. Psychopharmacology 158:388–398

Dieperink C, Dijk van R, Wierdsma A (2002) GGZ voor allochtonen. MGV 57:87–97

Dohrenwend BP, Levav I, Shrout PE, Schwartz S, Naveh G, Link BG, Skodol AE, Stueve A (1992) Socioeconomic status and psychiatric disorders: the causation-selection issue. Science 255:946–952

Eaton W, Harrison G (2000) Ethnic disadvantage and schizophrenia. Acta Psychiatr Scand 102 (Suppl. 407):38–43

Edwards J, Jackson HJ, Pattison PE (2002) Emotion recognition via facial expression and affective prosody in schizophrenia: a methodological review. Clin Psychol Rev 22:789–832

Folnegovic Z, Folnegovic-Smalc V (1992) Schizophrenia in Croatia: interregional differences in prevalence and a comment on constant incidence. J Epidemiol Community Health 46:248–255

Fossion P, Ledoux Y, Valente F, Servais L, Staner L, Pelc I, Minner P (2002) Psychiatric disorders and social characteristics among second-generation Morroccan migrants in Belgium: An age- and gender-controlled study conducted in a psychiatric emergency department. Eur Psychiatry 17:443–450

Gunnell D, Harrison G, Rasmussen F, Fouskakis D, Tynelius P (2002) Associations between premorbid intellectual performance, early-life exposures and early-onset schizophrenia. Cohort study. Br J Psychiatry 181:298–305

Haasen C, Lambert M, Mass R, Krausz M (1998) Impact of ethnicity on the prevalence of psychiatric disorders among migrants in Germany. Ethn Health 3:159–165

Häfner H, Riecher-Rössler A, Heiden an der W, Maurer K, Fätkenheuer B, Löffler W (1993) Generating and testing a causal explanation of the gender difference in age at first onset of schizophrenia. Psychol Med 23:925–940

Hanoeman M, Selten JP, Kahn RS (2002) Incidence of schizophrenia in Surinam. Schizophr Res 54:219–221

Harrison G, Owens D, Holton A, Neilson D, Boot D (1988) A prospective study of severe mental disorder in Afro-Caribbean patients. Psychol Med 18:643–657

Harrison G, Glazebrook C, Brewin J, Cantwell R, Dalkin T, Fox R, Jones P, Medley I (1997) Increased incidence of psychotic disorders in migrants from the Caribbean to the United Kingdom. Psychol Med 27:799–806

Herrnstein RJ, Murray CM (1994) The bell curve. Intelligence and class structure in American life. Simon and Schuster, New York

Hickling F, Rodgers-Johnson P (1995) The incidence of first contact schizophrenia in Jamaica. Br J Psychiatry 167:193–196

Hutchinson G, Takei N, Bhugra D, Fahy TA, Gilvarry C, Mallett R, Moran P, Leff J, Murray RM (1997) Increased rate of psychosis among African-Caribbeans in Britain is not due to an excess of pregnancy and birth complications. Br J Psychiatry 171:145–147

Jablensky A, Sartorius N, Ernberg G, Anker M, Korten A, Cooper JE, Day R, Bertelsen A (1992) Schizophrenia: manifestations, incidence and course in different cultures. A WHO Ten-Country study. Psychol Med, Monograph Suppl 20

Janssen I, Hanssen M, Bak M, Bijl RV, Graaf de R, Vollebergh W, McKenzie K, van Os J (2003) Discrimination and delusional ideation. Br J Psychiatry 182:71–76

Jarvis E (1998) Schizophrenia in British immigrants: recent findings, issues and implications. Transcultural Psychiatry 35:39–74

Jones P, Rodgers B, Murray R, Marmot M (1994) Child developmental risk factors for adult schizophrenia in the British 1946 birth cohort. Lancet 344:1398–1402

Junger M, Polder W (1992) Some explanations of crime among four ethnic groups in the Netherlands. J Quant Criminol 8:51–77

Kapur S (2003) Psychosis as a state of aberrant salience: a framework linking biology, phenomenology and pharmacology in schizophrenia. Am J Psychiatry 160:13–23

Kendell RE (1988) Schizophrenia. In: Kendell RE, Zealley AK (eds) Companion to psychiatric studies. Churchill and Livingstone, Edinburgh, pp 310–334

Kendler KS, McGuire M, Gruenberg AM, O'Hare A, Spellman M, Walsh D (1993) The Roscommon family study. I. Methods, diagnosis of probands, and risk of schizophrenia in relatives. Arch Gen Psychiatry 50:527–540

King M, Coker E, Leavey G, Hoare A, Johnson-Sabine E (1994) Incidence of psychotic illness in London: comparison of ethnic groups. BMJ 309:1115–1119

Kirov G, Murray R (1999) Ethnic differences in the presentation of bipolar affective disorder. Eur Psychiatry 14:199–204

Lewis G, David A, Andreassón S, Allebeck P (1992) Schizophrenia and city life. Lancet 340, 137–140

MacMahon B, Trichopoulos D (1996) Epidemiology. Principles and Methods. Little, Brown and Co, Boston, pp 153–154

Mahy GE, Mallett R, Leff J, Bughra D (1999) First-contact incidence rate of schizophrenia on Barbados. Br J Psychiatry 175:28–33

Makikyro T, Isohanni M, Moring J, Oja H, Hakko H, Jones P, Rantakallio P (1997) Is a child's risk of early onset schizophrenia increased in the highest social class? Schizophr Res 28:245–252

Malaspina D, Harlap S, Fennig S, Heiman D, Nahon D, Feldman D, Susser ES (2001) Advancing paternal age and the risk of schizophrenia. Arch Gen Psychiatry 58:361–367

Mallet R, Leff J, Bhugra D, Pang D, Zhao JH (2002) Social environment, ethnicity and schizophrenia. Soc Psychiatry Psychiatr Epidemiol 37:329–335

Malzberg B (1935a) Mental disease in New York State, according to nativity and parentage. Mental Hygiene 19:635–660

Malzberg B (1935b) Mental disease among Negroes in New York State. Hum Biol 7:471–513

Malzberg B (1936a) Migration and mental disease among Negroes in New York State. Am J Phys Anthropol 21:107–113

Malzberg B (1936b) Rates of mental disease among certain population groups in New York State. J Am Stat Assn 31:545–548

Malzberg B (1940) Social and biological aspects of mental disease. State Hospitals Press, Utica

Malzberg B (1955a) Mental disease among the native and foreign-born population of New York State, 1939–1941. Mental Hygiene 39:545–563

Malzberg B (1955b) The distribution of mental disease in New York State, 1949–1951. Psychiatr Quarterly 29(Suppl 2):209–238

Malzberg B (1956) Migration and mental disease in New York State, 1939–1941. Hum Biol 28:350–364

Malzberg B (1962a) The mental health of the Negro. A study of first admissions to hospitals for mental disease in New York State, 1949–1951. Research Foundation for Mental Hygiene, Albany, NY

Malzberg B (1962b) Migration and mental disease among the white population of New York State, 1949–1951. Hum Biol 34:89–98

Malzberg B (1964a) Mental disease among native and foreign-born whites in New York State, 1949–1951. Mental Hygiene 48:478–499

Malzberg B (1964b) Internal migration and mental disease in Canada. Research Foundation for Mental Hygiene, Albany, NY

Malzberg B (1964c) Mental disease in Canada. A study of comparative incidence of mental disease among those of British and French origin. Research Foundation for Mental Hygiene, Albany, NY

Malzberg B (1965) New data on mental disease among Negroes in New York State, 1960–1961. Research Foundation for Mental Hygiene, Albany, NY

Malzberg B (1967) Internal migration and mental disease among the white population of New York State, 1960–1961. Int J Soc Psychiatry 13:184–191

Marcelis M, Navarro-Mateu F, Murray R, Selten JP, van Os J (1998) Urbanization and psychosis: a study of 1942–1978 birth cohorts in The Netherlands. Psychol Med 28:871–879

McGrath J (1999) Hypothesis: is low prenatal vitamin D a risk-modifying factor for schizophrenia? Schizophr Res 40:173–177

McGuffin P, Asherson P, Owen M, Farmer A (1994) The strength of the genetic effect. Is there room for an environmental influence in the aetiology of schizophrenia? Br J Psychiatry 164:593–599

Morgan D, Grant KA, Gage HD, Mach RH, Kaplan JR, Prioleau O, Nader SH, Buchheimer N, Ehrenkaufer RL, Nader MA (2002) Social dominance in monkeys: dopamine D2 receptors and cocaine self-administration. Nat Neurosci 5:169–174

Mortensen PB, Pedersen CB, Westergaard T, Wohlfahrt J, Ewald H, Mors O, Andersen PK, Melbye M (1999) Effects of family history and place and season of birth on the risk of schizophrenia. N Engl J Med 8:603–608

Mulvany F, O'Callaghan E, Takei N, Byrne M, Fearon P, Larkin C (2001) Effect of social class at birth on risk and presentation of schizophrenia: case-control study. BMJ 323:1398–1401

Murphy HBM (1972) The evocative role of complex social tasks. In: Kaplan AR (ed) Genetic factors in "schizophrenia". Thomas, Springfield, pp 407–422

Neeleman J, Jones P, van Os J, Murray RM (1996) Parasuicide in Camberwell. Ethnic differences. Soc Psychiatry Psychiatr Epidemiol 31:284–287

Neeleman J, Mak V, Wessely S (1997) Suicide by age, ethnic group, coroners' verdicts and country of birth. Br J Psychiatry 171:463–467

Nikulina EM, Hammer RP, Miczek KA, Kream RM (1999) Social defeat stress increases expression of μ-opioid receptor mRNA in rat ventral tegmental area. NeuroReport 10:3015–3019

Ødegaard Ø (1932) Emigration and insanity. Acta Psychiatr Neurol Scand Suppl.4:1–206

van Os J, Castle DJ, Takei N, Der G, Murray RM (1996 a) Psychotics illness in ethnic minorities: clarification from the 1991 census. Psychol Med 26:203–208

van Os J, Takei N, Castle DJ, Wessely S, Der G , MacDonald AM, Murray RM (1996 b) The incidence of mania: time trends in relation to gender and ethnicity. Soc Psychiatry Psychiatr Epidemiol 31:129–136

van Os J, Bak M, Hanssen M, Bijl RV, Graaf de R, Verdoux H (2002) Cannabis use and psychosis: a longitudinal population-based study. Am J Epidemiol 156:319–327

Pedersen CB, Mortensen PB (2001 a) Evidence of a dose-response relationship between urbanicity during upbringing and schizophrenia risk. Arch Gen Psychiatry 58:1039–1046

Pedersen CB, Mortensen PB (2001 b) Family history, place and season of birth as risk factors for schizophrenia in Denmark: a replication and reanalysis. Br J Psychiatry 179:46–52

Rabkin J (1979) Ethnic density and psychiatric hospitalization: hazards of minority status. Am J Psychiatry 136:1562–1566

Rosenthal D, Goldberg I, Jacobsen B, Wender PH, Kety SS, Schulsinger F, Eldred CA (1974) Migration, heredity, and schizophrenia. Psychiatry 37:321–339

Schrier AC, van de Wetering BJ, Mulder PG, Selten JP (2001) Point prevalence of schizophrenia in immigrant groups in Rotterdam: data from outpatient facilities. Eur Psychiatry 16:162–166

Selten JP, Sijben N (1994) First admission rates for schizophrenia in immigrants to the Netherlands. Soc Psychiatry Psychiatr Epidemiol 29:71–77

Selten JP, Slaets JPJ, Kahn RS (1997) Schizophrenia in Surinamese and Dutch Antillean immigrants to the Netherlands: evidence of an increased incidence. Psychol Med 27:807–811

Selten JP, Slaets JPJ, Kahn RS (1998) Prenatal exposure to influenza and schizophrenia in Surinamese and Dutch Antillean immigrants to the Netherlands. Schizophr Res 30:101–103

Selten JP, van Vliet K, Pleyte W, Herzog S, Hoek HW, van Loon AM (2000) Borna disease virus and schizophrenia in Surinamese immigrants to the Netherlands. Med Microbiol Immunol 189:55–57

Selten JP, Veen ND, Feller WG, Blom JD, Schols D, Camoenië W, Oolders J, van der Velden M, Hoek HW, Vladár Rivero VM, van der Graaf Y, Kahn RS (2001) Incidence of psychotic disorders in immigrant groups to the Netherlands. Br J Psychiatry 178:367–372

Selten JP (2001) Methodological rigour in cross-cultural research. Reply to Bhui and Bhugra. Br J Psychiatry 179:269

Selten JP, Cantor-Graae E, Slaets JPJ, Kahn RS (2002 a) Ødegaard's selection hypothesis revisited: schizophrenia in Surinamese immigrants to the Netherlands. Am J Psychiatry 159:669–671

Selten JP, Bosman IJ, Boer de D, Veen ND, van der Graaf Y, Maes RAA, Kahn RS (2002 b) Hair analysis for cannabinoids and amphetamines in a psychosis incidence study. Eur Neuropsychopharmacol 12:27–30

Sharpley MS, Hutchinson G, Murray RM, McKenzie K (2001) Understanding the excess of psychosis among the African-Caribbean population in England: review of current hypotheses. Br J Psychiatry 178:60s–68s

Shaw CM, Creed F, Tomenson B, Riste L, Cruickshank JK (1999) Prevalence of anxiety and depressive illness and help seeking behaviour in African Caribbeans and white Europeans: two phase general population survey. BMJ 318:302–305

Sorg BA, Kalivas PW (1991) Effects of cocaine and footshock stress on extracellular dopamine levels in the ventral striatum. Brain Res 559:29–36

Takei N, Persaud R, Woodruff P, Brockington I, Murray RM (1998) First episodes of psychosis in Afro-Caribbean and white people. An 18-year follow-up population-based study. Br J Psychiatry 172:147–153

Tanda G, Pontieri FE, di Chiara G (1997) Cannabinoid and heroin activation of mesolimbic dopamine transmission by a common mu opioid receptor mechanism. Science 276:2048–2050

Tidey JW, Miczek KA (1996) Social defeat stress selectively alters mesocorticolimbic dopamine release: an in vivo microdialysis study. Brain Res 721:140–149

Torrey EF, Miller J (2001) The invisible plague. The rise of mental illness from 1750 to the present. Rutgers University Press, New Brunswick

Veen ND, Selten JP, Hoek HW, Feller W, van der Graaf Y, Kahn RS (2002) Use of illicit substances in a psychosis incidence cohort: a comparison among different ethnic groups in the Netherlands. Acta Psychiatr Scand 105:440–443

Watanaba H (1984) Activation of dopamine synthesis in mesolimbic dopamine neurons by immobilization stress in the rat. Neuropharmacol 23:1335–1338

Weyerer S, Häfner H (1992) The high incidence of psychiatrically treated disorders in the inner city of Mannheim. Soc Psychiatry Psychiatr Epidemiol 27:142–146

Zolkowska K, Cantor-Graae E, McNeil TF (2001) Increased rates of psychosis among immigrants to Sweden: is migration a risk factor for psychosis? Psychol Med 31: 669–678

Childhood meningitis and adult schizophrenia

WAGNER F. GATTAZ, ANDRÉ L. ABRAHÃO, and ROBERTO FOCCACIA

Department of Psychiatry, Faculty of Medicine, University of São Paulo, Brazil,
e-mail: gattaz@usp.br

The fact that the rates of concordance for schizophrenia among monozygotic twins is far below 100% proves that non-genetic factors must be operant for the development or not of the disease. Such factors have frequently been discussed as related to the environment and were recently summarized elsewhere (Häfner 2002). They comprise obstetric complications, maternal psychopathology during pregnancy, intrauterine factors such as growth retardation, viruses, nutrition and low birth weight. Moreover, the risk of psychosis was also found to be influenced by factors such as urbanicity and migration respectively, two environmental factors that are complex because they comprise a series of elements such as culture, socioeconomics, infection and pollution.

In spite of the heterogeneity of these risk factors, most authors agree to give them a longitudinal mode of action emphasizing their interaction over time to increase the risk of psychosis. The environmental contribution is discussed as "something that acts continuously during most of the childhood rather than at some specific vulnerable period" (Mortensen and Pedersen 2002), whereas Harrison and Eaton (2002) proposed a "life-course model involving multiplicative effects of provocative and protective agents across the individual's life course". Thus, there is an obvious consensus that the development or not of psychosis, and more specifically of schizophrenia, depends upon the interaction between genetic and environmental factors during the development of the brain.

We will attempt to frame the contribution of the different risk factors within one model that considers schizophrenia as a disorder of brain maturation. For this, we would like to review first the concepts of synaptogenesis and synapse elimination, which are both crucial phenomena during the maturation of the brain. These data were brilliantly investigated by P.R. Huttenlocher and his collaborators (1982, 1984, 1987, and 1997) and will be summarized below.

Synaptogenesis and synapse elimination

Synaptogenesis in human neocortex occurs during the third trimester of gestation and during the two postnatal years. This period of intensive synaptic proliferation occurs concurrently with dendritic and axonal growth. It is then followed by a period of synapse elimination, during which synaptic density and number decrease to about 60% of the maximum. In humans synaptogenesis and synapse elimination are heterochronous in different cortical regions.

For instance maximum synaptic density in the auditory cortex is reached at age 3 months, whereas in the middle frontal gyrus at age 15 months. The end of synapse elimination in the auditory cortex is reached by age 12 years, but in the prefrontal cortex at midadolescence.

One decisive factor for the development and maintenance of synaptic connections is synaptic activity, which determines the competition for neurotrophic factors. As a simple rule, synapses that work tend to remain, those that do not, are eliminated. Thus, the input of environmental stimuli may influence the rates of synapse formation and elimination. The human brain is a product of genetic instructions, cellular interactions and influences of innate activity and external stimulation (Lagercrantz and Ringstedt 2001).

The effect of external stimulation upon activity-dependent synaptic modification has been investigated in animal experiments. O'Kusky (1985) reported that visually deprived (dark-reared) cats showed a twofold increase in synaptic elimination in the visual cortex compared to normally reared cats. Similarly, Meisami and Firoozi (1985) found that rats submitted to odor deprivation during the neonatal period showed in the olfactory bulb neuronal loss and permanent reduction of growth, total cell number and enzymes related to the metabolism of neurotransmitters.

These data show the profound modifications that environmental stimuli exert upon brain maturation. It is not unlikely that the interaction of the different environmental factors with the individual genetic constitution may increase the risk of schizophrenia through a disruption of the physiological process of synapse modification. Thus, it has been suggested that the risk of psychosis would depend upon the interaction of the different factors acting continuously, rather than at some specific vulnerable period, involving multiplicative effects of provocative and protective agents across the individual's life course (Mortensen and Pedersen 2002, Harrison and Eaton 2002). Figure 1 illustrates the effects of the different risk factors over time.

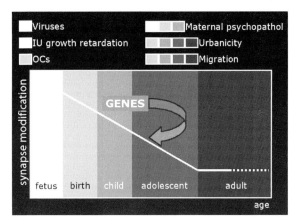

Fig. 1. Timing of environmental influences against the degree of synapse modification during the maturation of the brain. The result of the interaction between both is modulated by the genetic factors (*IU* intra-uterine; *OCs* obstetric complications)

▌ Childhood meningitis and adult schizophrenia

We would like to present now a preliminary evaluation of our data showing that a meningitis infection during childhood may increase the risk of psychosis in general, and of schizophrenia in especial during adulthood. The basis for our study was a meningitis epidemic that affected the population of São Paulo from 1971 until 1974, in which the infection rates increased from 2 cases to 170 cases per 100 000 inhabitants. Ninety percent of the infected individuals were committed to the Hospital Emilio Ribas, a 400 bed academic hospital linked to our Faculty of Medicine of the University of São Paulo.

The objectives of our study were to evaluate the lifetime psychiatric morbidity in adults infected by meningitis at an age between 0–4 years, and to compare this morbidity to a control group matched by genetic and environmental (cultural, socio-economic, etc.) backgrounds. For this purpose, we chose as a control group the siblings of our subjects who had not been infected by meningitis.

Our database was the microfilmed medical records from Hospital Emílio Ribas, which provided us with the individual data: name, birth date, name of the parents, age at meningitis, CSF exam and duration of hospitalization. With these data a team of psychiatrists and psychologists tried to locate the individuals or their relatives through an Internet telephone directory (*www. telefonica.net.br*) (mean: 150 calls to locate one subject).

When the subjects were located, the following script was said to them: "Here is Dr. X, from the University of São Paulo. We are doing a research about meningitis. We would like to interview personally you and one of your siblings, with the closest age to yours. Your collaboration will be important for our study. You will receive for this interview an honorarium of R$ 100 to cover part of your costs."

If patients accepted, *then* we would give him the address at the *Institute of Psychiatry*. This script was made to avoid the pre-selection of a sample with an overrepresentation of psychiatric morbidity, interested in receiving priority in psychiatric care at the University Department. This bias could be expected

Table 1. Sample description of adults infected by meningitis at age 4 years or less and their siblings without childhood meningitis infection

	Meningitis (n = 173)	Siblings (n = 141)
▌ Male	77 (44%)	50 (36%)
▌ Female	96 (56%)	91 (64%)
▌ Age (years)	29.1 ± 1.6	30.0 ± 5.9
▌ Years at school	11.6 ± 3.6	11.4 ± 4.0
▌ IQ (estimated)	89.1 ± 10.4	88.8 ± 12.6
▌ Income (R$/month)	938 ± 953	734 ± 806 *

*p < 0.05

in a city like São Paulo, in which there is a shortage of psychiatric facilities as compared to the existent need.

We found 4951 records of individuals who had a meningitis at age 4 or less. From these we searched for 1745 individuals, and we found and contacted 331; from these, 173 (52%) came to the interview, bringing with them 141 siblings without childhood meningitis. The samples were well matched regarding age, sex distribution, educational performance and IQ. The only significant difference was a higher income in the meningitis group (!) as compared to their siblings (Table 1).

All individuals underwent a semi-structured interview based on the ICD-10 Checklist (Janca and Hiller 1996), followed by a neurological exam and a neuropsychological test battery evaluating IQ, frontal function and logical memory (neuropsychological data will not be presented here).

In general, we found a similar prevalence of psychiatric disorders in the meningitis (62.2%) and the siblings (58.2%, n.s.) groups. This prevalence is higher than that observed in a representative sample of the population from São Paulo (Andrade et al. 1999). Individuals with childhood meningitis had a 5-fold higher prevalence of psychotic disorders in general than their siblings (20.8% vs. 4.3%, p<0.001). This difference was observed for each of the diagnoses schizophrenia, mood disorder with psychotic symptoms and 'other psychoses' (Fig. 2). No differences were found between both groups in the prevalence of the other psychiatric disorders (anxiety, personality disorder, alcohol and drugs abuse, mood disorder without psychotic symptoms).

As expected, individuals with childhood meningitis had a higher prevalence of neurological disorders (24.8% vs. 5.6% in their siblings, p<0.001), being the most frequent deafness (10.4%). Because there are some studies suggesting an association between deafness and psychoses, we analyzed the data separately in individuals with and without deafness. The increased prevalence of psychoses remained in the individuals with childhood meningitis (p<0.001), whereas no other difference regarding the remaining diagnoses arouse. Moreover, the asso-

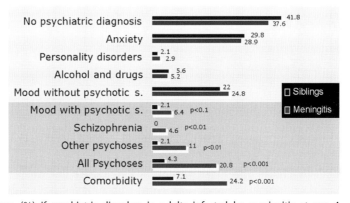

Fig. 2. Lifetime prevalence (%) if psychiatric disorders in adults infected by meningitis at age 4 years or less (n = 173) and their siblings without meningitis infection (n = 141)

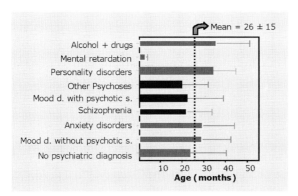

Fig. 3. Mean age at meningitis infection (in months) by diagnosis

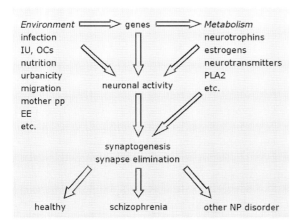

Fig. 4. Model for the effects of genetic and environmental factors on synapse modification during the maturation of the brain. Environmental factors may influence gene expression or directly neuronal activity disrupting synapse modification. Genes affect directly programmed neuronal activity or determine metabolic changes which, in turn, affect neuronal activity or synapse modification. Depending upon the degree (and probably location) of synapse changes, an individual can develop schizophrenia or other neuropsychiatric disorders. Conversely, the interaction of these factors can have a protective effect in an individual prone to develop psychosis (*IU*=Intra-uterine factors, *Ocs*=Obstetric complications, *EE*=Expressed emotions, *pp*=psychopathology, *PLA2*=phospholipase A2, *NP*=neuropsychiatric)

ciation between meningitis and psychoses remained significant ($p < 0.001$) when we excluded from the sample all individuals with neurological diagnoses.

The mean age at the time of the meningitis infection was 26 ± 15 months. No difference was found in the timing of the meningitis between individuals with psychosis and those without a psychiatric diagnosis (Fig. 3).

Taken together, the results from our prospective study suggest that childhood meningitis could enter the heterogeneous list of environmental factors that may increase the risk of adult psychosis (Fig. 4). All these factors may be operant at one or more levels, influencing gene expression, neuronal activity or directly synaptogenesis and synapse elimination, ending in some cases in schizophrenia. Besides the further identification of other potential risk factors, we think that our major challenge would be to identify the protective agents which, counteracting the genetic and environmental risks, would avoid or attenuate the suffering caused by a psychotic outburst.

▌ References

Andrade LHSG, Lólio CA, Gentil V, Laurenti R (1999) Epidemiologia dos transtornos mentais em uma área definida de captação da cidade de São Paulo, Brasil. Rev Psiq Clin 26:257–261; also available at *http://www.hcnet.usp.br/ipq/revista/r265/ artigo(257).htm*

Huttenlocher PR, de Courten C, Garey LJ, Van der Loos H (1982) Synaptogenesis in human visual cortex – evidence for synapse elimination during normal development. Neurosci Lett 33:247–252

Huttenlocher PR (1984) Synapse elimination and plasticity in developing human cerebral cortex. Am J Ment Defic 88:488–496

Huttenlocher PR, de Courten C (1987) The development of synapses in striate cortex of man. Hum Neurobiol 6:1–9

Huttenlocher PR, Dabholkar AS (1997) Regional differences in synaptogenesis in human cerebral cortex. J Comp Neurol 387:167–178

Janca A, Hiller W (1996) ICD-10 Checklists – A tool for clinicians use of the ICD-10 classification of mental and behavioral disorders. Comprehensive Psychiatry 37: 180–187

Lagercrantz H, Ringstedt T (2001) Organization of the neuronal circuits in the central nervous system during development. Acta Paediatr 90:707–715

O'Kusky JR (1985) Postnatal changes in the numerical density and total number of asymmetric and symmetric synapses in the hypoglossal nucleus of the rat. Brain Re Dev Brain Res 108:179–191

Meisami E, Firoozi M (1985) Acetylcholinesterase activity in the developing olfactory bulb: a biochemical study on normal maturation and the influence of peripheral and central connections. Brain Res 353:115–124

The course and outcome of schizophrenia: toward a new social biology of psychosis

GLYNN HARRISON

Head, Division of Psychiatry, University of Bristol, UK

In recent decades, those searching for the causes of schizophrenia have not been especially interested in the social and cultural environment of their subjects. To some extent this is understandable: the prospect of models of risk in which causal agents are embedded in the social environment, operating at micro-, mezzo-, and macro levels, with untold complexities of interaction, has not seemed overly attractive. Moreover, because much of the earlier research into the role of family and social factors in the genesis of schizophrenia was so seriously flawed and of poor methodological quality, we focused on 'harder' and more easily measured biological mechanisms. The emphasis shifted to schizophrenia as a 'brain disease' with arguments appearing to rest on the proposition that if a disease is biological in character, it follows that it is biological in causation. The need for scientific respectability, the seductions of emerging new technologies, and the skilful and highly resourced advocacy roles of pharmaceutical companies, all played their part in ensuring that theory development in schizophrenia largely ignored social models of causation. As a result, our conceptual approach to the social environment became relatively crude and dualistic, with a tendency to dismiss associations between the schizophrenia phenotype and its environment as 'fall out' from what is happening in the brain.

These simplistic polarities have not served us well. Over the same period a vast literature has emerged linking disease outcomes and social context. Drawing on the insights of sociologists such as Durkheim, epidemiologists researching the social patterning of a variety of chronic diseases have made tangible progress in their understanding of the interplay between biology and social context. My argument is that it is time for schizophrenia researchers to join them and to re-address the role of contextual factors in our models of causation. Indeed, I shall argue that accumulating evidence for an association between 'place' and the longitudinal patterning of the schizophrenia phenotype requires us to think in terms of a 'new social biology' of the disorder.

Social space and disease: the influence of Durkheim

To understand where schizophrenia fits into the broader body of work exploring relationships between health and social context, we shall briefly re-examine the development of these ideas over the last century. The work of Durkheim remains crucial to understanding the potential role of social and cultural environment in mental illness. Durkheim's primary aim, over a century ago, was to explain individual pathology as a function of social dynamics. Essentially, Durkheim argued that groups of individuals think, feel and act differently from what would happen if the individual members acted alone, or if their actions were simply added together. He illustrated his theory by addressing one of the most 'individualistic' and autonomous acts of human agency: suicide. Comparing suicide statistics across European countries, he demonstrated a relationship between rates of suicide and broader indicators of relational quality. The highest rates of suicide seemed to occur in societies characterised by the lowest rates of social cohesion and greatest levels of social disintegration. The nub of his argument was that the suicide rate in any given society seemed to remain relatively constant whereas individuals at risk of committing suicide came and, quite literally, 'went'. 'There is therefore for each people a collective force of a definite amount of energy, impelling men to self-destruction. The victim's act, which at first seems to express only his personal temperament, is really the supplement and prolongation of a social condition which they express externally'. Perhaps the most cogent summary of Durkheim's thesis is this: 'suicide varies inversely with the degree of integration of the social groups of which the individual forms a part' (Durkheim 1897, 1951, p. 209). It was Durkheim who made us think that it is the nature of human relationships, that is the degree to which an individual is interconnected and embedded in community, that is critical to his/her health and mental well-being.

In subsequent decades, Durkheim's work gave way to a diverse theoretical literature, as sociologists sought to identify and quantify the distinctive elements of constructs such as 'social integration' and social 'cohesion'. Whilst such terms role off the tongue relatively easily, what they actually mean in terms of observable and quantifiable experience and behaviour is less clear. One attempt to elucidate this was the development of the theory of social 'networks' (Barnes 1954). Here, attempts were made to think outside the envelope of traditional social groupings such as family, social class and residential areas; instead, researchers focused upon broader, transcending, patterns of social ties among individuals in any given social system. The argument was that the essence of community is its social structure, not its spatial or even its kinship structure. Thus, network theorists began to use structural network characteristics to explain social support, health behaviours and disease transmission (Morris 1994).

Although the work of sociologists such as Durkheim and Barnes laid the groundwork for modern clinical epidemiology, it was only in the 1970's that epidemiologists began seriously and systematically to explore associations between social relationships and health outcomes (Cassel 1976). Preliminary findings were exciting and revealing: a series of studies produced robust evidence of a relationship between measures of social 'connectedness', or 'embedded ness', and all cause mortality. Their work (reviewed by Greenwood et al. 1996; Anderson et al. 1996; Helgeson and Cohen 1996) began to uncover social patterning in chronic 'physical' diseases such as coronary heart disease and cancer. A new 'social biology' began to emerge allowing a more integrative interactive understanding of the relationship between an organism and its social as well as its physical environment.

▌ Social space and the aetiology of schizophrenia

Research into the relationship between schizophrenia and social space has been hampered by several methodological issues related to the slow and insidious onset of the disease (reviewed in detail by Eaton and Harrison 2001). The discovery of an association between the prevalence of schizophrenia and neighbourhood type, illustrated in the classic work of Faris and Dunham (1939), is a case in point. Because of the slow development of the disorder, and its chronic course in a proportion of individuals, it is difficult to interpret the role of social context because of the problem of reverse causality. Does social position at the individual level, or neighbourhood type at the contextual-level, contribute to the causation of schizophrenia, or does social decline in the early stages of the disorder cause these patterns of social segregation? Or is it a combination of both factors operating simultaneously? The matter appeared to be laid to rest by Goldberg and Morrison (1963), who showed a normal class distribution among fathers of a cohort of males with schizophrenia. They showed that the association between schizophrenia and low social position (as measured by individual occupational status) appears to be a product of the social decline in the early stages of the disorder, a finding given greater plausibility by evidence of cognitive impairment many years before onset of psychotic symptoms (Gunnell et al. 2002). But the literature has not been entirely consistent. Harrison et al. (2001), for example, examined a first-episode cohort in Nottingham, UK, using a case control methodology that extracted father's occupation and street of birth from birth certificates. This methodology, similar in design to that used earlier by Goldberg and Morrison (1963) found a trend toward *lower* social class occupation for fathers of subjects who would later develop schizophrenia. More importantly, there was a significant association (OR=2.7, CI 1.2–6.5) between broadly defined adult onset schizophrenia and the deprivation score of subjects' street of birth. Those with low social class fathers *and* birth in a deprived area were at greater risk still (OR=8.1, CI 2.7–23.9). Although the study was based upon relatively small numbers, and the authors could not eliminate all sources of selection bias in their case control design, their data contradicted those of Goldberg and Morrison. The picture is further confused by findings from birth cohort follow-up studies (reviewed by Eaton and Harrison 2001). On balance, these report an association between schizophrenia and *higher* paternal social class, indexed by occupation or educational status of father at the subject's birth. These findings are largely based upon early onset cases in the early period of disease risk, and may not hold for later onset cases. It is also important to note that birth cohort studies have only examined social position indexed by parental educational or employment status. None have explored (usually because of sample size and power considerations) the different components of social space based upon neighbourhood type, social networks or social cohesion. Many questions remain unanswered.

Social space and the outcome of schizophrenia

Although the literature is confused regarding the relationship between social space and the *causation* of schizophrenia, there appears to be greater consistency in studies that have investigated the relationship between social space and the *outcome* of the disorder. We have argued elsewhere (Harrison and Eaton 2002) that the distinction between 'onset' and 'outcome' grows increasingly questionable if schizophrenia is conceptualised as a life course phenotype: it is likely that multiple risk factors interact over the life course to modify a *pattern of outcomes* that develops through early and intermediary phenotypes, prodromal symptoms, positive psychotic symptoms and negative 'deficit' syndromes. But these conceptual issues aside, there is evidence (Pharoah et al. 2003) that treatments that attempt to manipulate the social environment at the micro-social level (altering levels of expressed emotion among family members) may favourably affect outcome, and that psychological approaches utilising cognitive techniques may also modify course in some cases (Cormac et al. 2003). These data have encouraged advocates in the 'recovery' movement, who argue that 'non-specific' social factors linked to social support have powerful effects upon the course and outcome of the disorder. However, the strongest evidence for the potential role of social context in recovery comes from observational studies of course and outcome carried out in different social and cultural settings.

Schizophrenia outcomes in different social and cultural settings

In 1967, WHO initiated what was to become a series of studies investigating the manifestation, consequences and course of schizophrenia and related disorders in different countries. Beginning with the International Pilot Study of Schizophrenia (WHO 1973), nearly 30 research sites in 19 countries eventually participated in this programme of studies. The International Pilot Study of Schizophrenia was seen as preparing the ground for in-depth international comparative studies of schizophrenia and related mental disorders, focussing on methodological issues of feasibility, questions of instrumentation, including reliability in different cultural settings, and the logistical problems of managing complex research networks. It is important to note that the IPSS was not a first episode study: cases were not sampled from clearly defined populations based upon geographic areas. Instead, screening criteria were constructed to identify all those patients 'in the early stages of schizophrenia disorder who were likely to participate in follow-up'. There was therefore a mixture of incident and prevalent cases, and there were several sources of sampling bias with unknown effects.

The first group of field centres participating in the IPSS were the following: Cali (Columbia), Taipei (China), Prague (Czech Republic), Aarhus (Denmark), Agra (India), Ibadan (Nigeria), Moscow (Russia), London (UK), and Washington (USA). In all, the study population consisted of 1202 patients subject to a number of standardised assessments of mental state and social functioning. The researchers successfully demonstrated the feasibility of international collaborative work, and they undertook ground-breaking work in the standardised assessments of psychotic disorders, leading to the further development of the Present State Examination (Wing, Cooper and Sartorius 1974).

A key finding emerged from the 2-year follow-up study. Variables describing patterns of relapse and social functioning revealed sharp differences between the participating centres (WHO 1979). Patients in 'developing' non-industrialised countries achieved consistently better outcomes. Subjects in Ibadan (Nigeria) showed the most favourable course and outcome, with 57% in the 'best' and only 5% in the 'worst' overall outcome group. Patients ascertained in Agra achieved the next 'best' outcomes. The 'worst' 2-year outcome scenarios were found in Aarhus, Denmark, where 50% were still in the episode of inclusion at the point of follow-up and only 6% fell into the 'best' group (see Table 1). These striking findings were sustained over a longer period of follow-up. Further, as Table 1 shows, a 5-year follow-up study of the

Table 1. WHO outcome studies – a synopsis (Hopper et al. 2000)

Study	Percentages "Best" vs. "Worst" outcomes[1]		
	Developed[2]	Developing	Odds ratio[3]
IPSS (1967-)			
2-yr follow-up	35 vs. 33	52 vs. 19	2.01
5-yr follow-up	23 vs. 24	38 vs. 14	2.05
DOSMeD (1976-)			
All subjects	33 vs. 17	49 vs. 11	1.95
ICD-9 SZ	32 vs. 19	49 vs. 13	2.04
ISoS 15-yr follow-up (incidence only), % never psychotic in last 2 yrs vs. continuously psychotic			
ICD-9 SZ	40 vs. 33	58 vs. 23	2.07
ICD-10 SZ	37 vs. 38	53 vs. 27	1.92
All psychoses	45 vs. 30	58 vs. 22	1.69

DOSMeD Determinants of Outcome of Severe Mental Disorders Study; *IPSS* International Pilot Study of Schizophrenia; *ISoS* International Study of Schizophrenia; *SZ* schizophrenia; *WHO* World Health Organization

[1] Various measures of patterns of course were used in the individual studies
[2] Assignment of centres to categories of developed vs. developing is as per individual studies
[3] These are the odds of good outcome in developing centres vs. the odds of good outcome in developed centres

IPSS cohorts carried out by Leff et al. (1987) revealed that these differences were sustained over the medium term.

In view of the significance of these findings, WHO undertook a second, more methodologically secure study, the Determinants of Outcome of Severe Mental Disorders (DOSMeD) study (Jablensky et al. 1992). Here, incidence cohorts were traced in geographically defined areas, using standardised methods of case finding and diagnosis. Although cases were still confined to those seeking some type of help, researchers extended case finding to include 'helping agencies' other than traditional psychiatric services (e.g. religious institutions and traditional healers). The total population included in this second study consisted of 1379 subjects. There was marked variation in the incidence of first episode psychoses, although this narrowed if the case definition for schizophrenia was based upon Schneider first-rank symptoms. Once again the 2-year follow-up study (Table 1) reported more favourable outcomes in developing countries: a significantly higher percentage of subjects (56%) in developing countries achieved 'mild' patterns of course, compared to their counterparts in developed countries (39%). Conversely, 40% of cases in so-called 'developed' countries had 'severe' patterns of course compared with only 24% in developing countries.

▌ Methodological objections

These findings provoked great interest and considerable scepticism (Hopper 1991; Jablensky et al. 1994; Edgerton and Cohen 1994). Inevitably, the question of diagnosis arose and the degree to which consistency was achieved across the different centres. Stevens (1987), for example, proposed that the excess of good outcome cases could be explained as a function of the increased prevalence of acute psychoses in developing countries. These might be considered to be analogous to culturally conditioned hysterical states or related to acute brain syndromes caused by infections and nutrition. There was support for this contention in a re-analysis of some of the DOSMeD centre data by Susser and Wanderling (1994) who showed a 10-fold difference in the incidence of non-affecting remitting psychosis between developing country and industrialised settings.

In addition to problems of diagnosis and case ascertainment, there were concerns about the extent to which recovery, say in terms of work functioning, could meaningfully be compared across cultures where opportunities for work and rehabilitation are so different. A third area of concern centred upon the conceptual adequacy of labels such as 'developed' and 'developing' (Edgerton and Cohen 1994) and the utility of lumping together such diverse cultural landscapes. Finally, even if these findings proved to be reliable, there was speculation about what precisely might be the recovery promoting benefits of living in a 'developing' country. This was by no means clear. Cultural expectations of recovery, therapeutic benefits of low demand work patterns, family-based social support, differential patterns of stigma, and 'self-exempting' modes of illness attribution were all proposed as explanatory mechanisms

(Cooper and Sartorius 1977; Kleinman 1988; WHO 1979; Warner 1985), but with little supporting evidence.

In the centres themselves, these issues remained relatively dormant and under-researched, apart from two sets of 'spin-off' studies from the DOSMeD programme. A comparison of components of expressed emotion among two samples of relatives of first contact patients were examined in Aarhus (Denmark) and Chandigarh (India) (Wig et al. 1987; Leff et al. 1987; Katz et al. 1988). The expressed emotion parameters were those identified and defined in earlier British studies. Danes were found to be similar to samples of British relatives, whereas relatives of patients in Chandigarh expressed significantly fewer critical and positive comments, and appeared less emotionally over-involved. There were differences, too, between the two samples from Chandigarh: city dwellers were more expressive than rural villagers in all expressed emotion components, except over-involvement. These authors attributed the better outcome at one year follow-up of first episode patients in rural Chandigarh, compared with those in London, to the significantly lower patterns of expressed emotion in relatives of the former. Over the next decade, these issues received little further attention until a 3rd study – the International Study of Schizophrenia (ISoS) – was developed and co-ordinated by the World Health Organisation.

▌ The International Study of Schizophrenia (ISoS)

The International Study of Schizophrenia (ISoS) (Harrison et al. 2001) was based upon a long-term follow-up study of some of the earlier IPSS and DOSMeD cohorts. In addition, first episode cohorts from a third WHO European study, the Assessment and Reduction of Psychiatric Disability (RAPyD; Wiersma 1996) were included. The cultural diversity of the sample was further enhanced by adding cohorts from 3 'invited' centres: 2 first episode groups from Chennai (India) and Hong Kong that had cohorts available that had been identified using broadly comparable methodology to DOSMeD and IPSS, and with similar periods of follow-up; and 1 prevalence case group from Beijing, China. These 4 sets of cohorts offered a unique opportunity to carry out a 15 (DOSMeD, RAPyD, invited centres) and 25 (IPSS) year follow-up study. In total, ISoS involved 14 culturally diverse first episode cohorts, and 4 prevalence cohorts, totalling 1633 subjects. For the purposes of this chapter, we shall exclude the prevalence cohorts because of greater attrition and heterogeneity of samples, and concentrate upon the treated incidence case groups comprising a total of 1171 subjects.

▌ The long-term outcome of schizophrenia in different countries

One of the key objectives of ISoS was to investigate the durability and robustness of earlier findings from IPSS and DOSMeD regarding significant 'centre' effects on the outcome of schizophrenia and related psychoses at 2- and 5-year follow-up and, specifically, to explore the apparent advantage of those cases found in 'developing' centres. The study design and methods are described in Sartorius et al. (1996) and Harrison et al. (2001). Data on attrition at follow-up, reliability and mortality are also reported in Harrison et al.

Table 2 reports aggregated outcomes for first episode cohorts, sub-categorised into schizophrenia and other non-schizophrenic psychoses (Harrison et al. 2001). These aggregate data reveal marked heterogeneity of outcome, with 56% of subjects found alive being rated 'recovered' on the Bleuler scale. Nearly one-half had been free of psychotic experiences in the past two years. Although these are global data, more detailed ratings of current symptomatology and functioning closely tracked the overall assessments. Outcomes for schizophrenia compared with other non-affective psychoses (baseline diagnoses were converted to ICD-10 using diagnostic 'cross-walk' algorithms) were less favourable for all domains, although there was still marked heterogeneity and surprising levels of global 'recovery'.

Raw outcome data for the different centres showed marked variation in patterns of course and cross sectional outcome. Harrison et al. (2001) report preliminary analyses carried out by, and to be reported more fully by Siegel et al.

Table 2. Symptoms and social disability at follow-up, percentages (range across centres) (Harrison et al. 2001)

	Schizophrenia only		Other psychoses	
	Incidence	Prevalence	Incidence	Prevalence
N	502	142	274	87
Male/Female	254/248	85/57	119/155	36/51
Bleuler recovered [1]	48.1 (14.3–75.7)	53.5 (37.9–77.8)	71.1 (47.1–100)	71.4 (64.0–75.8)
GAF-S [2]	54.0 (8.3–78.4)	56.7 (47.7–81.5)	70.7 (48.0–100.0)	77.1 (54.2–88.5)
DAS [3] ("Excellent"/"Good")	33.4 (8.3–66.7)	47.7 (25.0–60.0)	52.1 (12.5–81.8)	51.5 (16.7–62.5)
DAS [3] ("Fair")	22.6	30.2	29.4	28.8
GAF-D [4] (0.60)	50.7 (16.7–77.8)	60.3 (48.3–77.8)	62.1 (41.7–100)	74.7 (62.5–80.8)
Not psychotic in past 2 yrs	42.8 (16.7–67.6)	40.8 (31.8–63.0)	61.5 (37.5–75.0)	60.0 (44.0–71.4)

[1] 1–4 point scale, with 'recovered'=4
[2] 1–90 point scale, with >60=2 mild, minimal or absent symptoms
[3] 0–5 global scale, with 0=excellent, 1=good, 2=fair
[4] 1–90 point scale, with >60=mild, minimal or no difficulty in social functioning
DAS Disability Assessment Schedule; *GAF-D* Global Assessment of Functioning-Disability; *GAF-S* Global Assessment of Functioning-Symptoms

(in press), who investigated 'centre' effects and other associations between baseline/early course variables and longer-term outcome. These analyses were confined to the DOSMeD cohorts only (461 subjects), because these were the only subjects for whom a sufficiently consistent dataset existed for multivariate analyses. Of those with a baseline diagnosis of psychosis, 60.2% were found alive and assessed; 30.4% were lost to follow-up; and 9.4% had died. A separate examination (Drake et al. in press) used a propensity score method to assess the potential bias introduced by basing the analysis on the 'found alive' cases only, and found the effect to be negligible.

Multivariate analyses used two measures of outcome derived from the GAF scale (Symptoms and Disability) as dependent variables. Course of illness over the entire follow-up period was described in terms of patterns constructed from longitudinal data on symptom presence and strength obtained by a life chart schedule. Following the precedent of Jablensky et al. (1992) and Craig et al. (1997), the early (2 year) pattern of course was divided into 'complete' remission (no residual symptoms between episodes, return to premorbid functioning) and 'incomplete' remission (or continuing psychosis) to allow comparisons with earlier analyses of short-term outcome.

The complete set of variables chosen by Siegel et al. (in press) for the multivariate analysis was based on a conceptual framework linking environmental, predisposing and clinical factors to outcomes, and taking account of factors that may mediate their impact. These items included predictor variables for poor outcome in a prior analysis of the 2-year outcome data for DOSMeD (Craig et al. 1997). These comprised age at first contact, sex, marital status, level of social contact with friends, history of substance or alcohol misuse, type of onset and diagnosis at baseline. In addition, the analysis introduced negative symptoms from the PSE. Duration of untreated psychosis (DUP) (Larsen et al. 1996) could not be used because of insufficient reliable data.

The diagnosis was the baseline ICD9 clinical consensus diagnosis, converted to ICD10 and grouped into 5 categories: schizophrenia, schizo-affective disorder, acute schizophrenic disorder, bipolar disorder/depression and other psychoses. The short-term (2 year) outcome measure was 'percentage of time experiencing psychosis' and 'pattern of course'. Siegel et al. attempted to disentangle hypothesised 'centre' effects by constructing coarse-grained area-level mediating variables for: social stability, prevailing conventions of illness attribution, configuration and strength of kinship ties, and certain aspects of the treatment system (for example existence of national health insurance). These constructions were based upon qualitative data supplied in answer to open ended questions by key informants in each of the centres. A Delphi-like procedure, employing 5 independent raters, was used to arrive at composite scores.

A two part stepwise linear regression was applied: first, the variables most highly predictive of outcome were identified, followed by a second model fitted using only the variables distinguished in step one. In the first analysis, 'centre' was included as a categorical variable; in a second analysis 'centre' was replaced by the complete set of descriptive local variables described above.

For GAF-S and GAF-D, in all regression models, the most powerful predictor was the percentage of time experiencing psychotic symptoms in the first 2 years of illness after first contact (Table 3). For symptom scores, the only additional variable that entered the model in which 'centre' was included was the variable 'centre'. The same held for disability, except the diagnosis also entered, with baseline schizophrenia categories having significantly poorer scores. When 'centre' was excluded, and replaced by the coarse grained 'area variables', the only variable to enter the model was the presence of national

Table 3. Multiple regressions for GAF-S and GAF-D: analyses with centre in area variables excluded; centre out area variables included

Variable	Regression model			
	GAF-S; centre in area var.	GAF-S; centre out area var.	GAF-D; centre in area var.	GAF-D; centre out area var.
Percent time psychotic	* (1)	* (1)	* (1)	* (1)
Centre (Chandigarh Urban Contrast)	(2)		(2)	
❚ Chandigarh Rural				
❚ Dublin	*		*	
❚ Honolulu	*			
❚ Moscow				
❚ Nagasaki				
❚ Nottingham	*			
❚ Prague	*		*	
❚ Rochester	*		*	
Area variable				
❚ National health insurance				* (4)
Family involvement				* (6)
Drug use				* (5)
Diagnosis (Schizophrenia contrast)		(2)	(3)	(2)
❚ Schizoaffective			*	*
❚ Acute schizophrenia		*	*	*
❚ Bipolar disorders/depression		*	*	
❚ Other psychotic				
Age at study entry		* (3)		
Blunted affect				* (3)
R^2	0.25	0.22	0.26	0.25

* Indicates significance, p < 0.05; # in parentheses indicates order of entry in stepwise regression

health insurance which, interestingly, was associated with better disability scores.

Reviewing these data it is clear that, of all the variables thought to relate to long-term outcome, the strongest predictors were measures of early (2-year) illness course and 'centre'. Percentage of time spent experiencing psychotic symptoms in the 2 years following onset was the main predictor for all outcome measures. Other key predictive variables were: presenting diagnosis of schizophrenia; age; family involvement in treatment; history of drug use; and symptoms of blunted affect (although the predictors varied slightly depending on whether symptoms or social disability were used for 'outcome').

The regression model highlighted the role that 'centre' played in determining outcome. The 'Centre' variable entered the regression model for both symptoms and disability at the second step, indicating that rates of recovery do vary by location. Thus, living in certain areas appears to improve chances of recovery, even for subjects with unfavourable early illness course. The attempt to disaggregate 'centre' effects using the coarse grained local descriptors was largely disappointing: the association between national health insurance and poor outcome may only be approximating a developing country effect, since those without insurance were in large part those in the two Indian centres. This brings us to the question of types of 'centre' and specifically the differences in outcome of subjects followed in centres in 'developing' compared with those in 'developed' countries.

▍ Long-term outcome of schizophrenia in 'developing' versus 'developed' centres

The findings of differences between developing and developed countries in the earlier IPSS and DOSMeD studies are summarised in Table 1, which also reports the results of analyses of the 15 year follow-up data from the ISoS first episode cohorts (DOSMeD) plus the invited centres with comparable first episode cohorts (n = 809), carried out by Hopper and Wanderling (2000). These authors had a specific interest in the developing versus developed country hypothesis. The studies summarised in Table 1 demonstrate a consistent outcome differential in favour of 'developing' centres that is remarkably robust over short- (2 year), medium-term (5 year) and long-term (15 year) periods of follow-up, and this applies whether the subjects included are first episode or 'prevalence' cases.

Hopper and Wanderling (2000) showed that the earlier WHO studies' finding of more favourable outcomes in developing centre holds even when the make up of the 'developing' and 'developed' groupings changes between DOSMeD and ISoS with the inclusion of the 'invited' centres. The effect sizes also appear to be comparable. Moreover, the pattern was consistent for early illness course, across measures of symptoms over the entire illness course, the late illness course, and for disability and work performance. It held, too, whether a narrow (ICD10) or broad (spectrum) classification of schizophrenia was used, or if the diagnostic net was expanded to take in all psychoses. Hopper and Wanderling (2000) questioned whether Hong Kong (cases ascertained in 1980) should be included as a developing or a developed centre. Their data showed that the developing centre effect reduced somewhat when Hong Kong was re-classified with developed centres but still consistently favoured the developing group.

▮ Centre effects resulting from non-random sampling bias

Despite the consistency of these findings, such contextual differences may still be due to imprecisions of measurement, unmeasured individual characteristics or residual confounding, as we have noted above. The strength of Hopper and Wanderling's (2000) analysis of the ISoS data was that they were able to address several of these key methodological issues:

Diagnostic differences

We have noted that Stevens (1987) argued that apparent differences in the course of schizophrenia may be explained by a greater incidence of acute remitting psychoses in developing countries. Although the epidemiological evidence is somewhat thin, there is growing evidence of increased incidence of short-lived, fully remitting psychoses (NARP), in 'developing' countries (Susser and Wanderling 1994; Malhotra et al. 1998). The supposed advantage conferred by 'centre' on the outcome of schizophrenia could simply be due to the fact that these cases are not schizophrenia at all. There is some degree of tautology in the argument, however, because course is built into the definition of NARP. However, to test this assertion, Hopper and Wanderling calculated recovery rates within both the NARP group and the 'non-remitting psychoses' group (see Table 4). While NARP was found to be more common among cases diagnosed as schizophrenia in the developing world, the recovery rates of non-remitting subjects in the developing centres were still more favourable in developing centres: 52% compared with 38%. Hopper and Wanderling (2000) argued that, whilst it is clearly the case that NARP turns out to be more common among cases diagnosed as schizophrenia in the developing world, 'that selection advantage is countered by an interaction effect: the difference non-affective remitting psychosis makes in enhancing the chances of recovery is more profound in the developed world'. Hopper and Wanderling proceeded to exclude all subjects with a single episode psychosis from their analysis of the broad spectrum schizophrenia group and found that the differential outcome was still preserved in favour of developing and developed centres, although there was a definite narrowing to 49% and 40% respectively. Finally, they showed a 'two stage' effect in which there was a delayed secondary advantage in the developing centres with respect to subjects whose early course was unfavourable: 42% of them (compared with 33% in the developed centres) went on to gain significant levels of recovery. Overall, these authors felt able to discount the assertion that the developing country effect is simply a function of the higher prevalence of NARP in these centres.

Table 4. The effect of NARP (Hopper et al. 2000)

Centre grouping	% Recovered		"Effect" (recovery ratio: NARP/non-NARP)
	NARP	Non-NARP	
ICD-10 SZ; onset <1 week[1]			
▌ Developed	79	38	2.1
▌ Developing	71	52	1.4
SZ spectrum; onset <1 week[2]			
▌ Developed	83	42	2.0
▌ Developing	75	55	1.4

NARP non-affective remitting psychosis; *SZ* schizophrenia
[1] The percent NARP in developed centres is 9.8; in developing centres, it is 15.5
[2] This is ICD-10 schizophrenia, plus schizoaffective disorder and acute schizophrenia-like psychoses; the percent NARP in developed centres is 12.5; in developing centres, it is 27.2

Sex and differences in age at onset

Hopper and Wanderling (2000) did not carry out a multivariate analysis taking into account age effects but, on comparing raw data by centre, they found no evidence of a sex or age bias between developed and developing groups in any of the 'found alive' samples with respect to recovery rates or in subjects lost to follow-up. Indeed, with regard to age, subjects in developing centre were disproportionately younger. The finding that early age of onset predicted poor outcome overall would therefore tend to favour outcome in the *developed* world.

Differences in attrition at follow-up

Lost to follow-up rates were comparable for the two groups (25%) and mortality differences were small (11% vs. 8%). Furthermore, for both narrow and broader diagnostic classifications, the chances of those with favourable early (2 year) course of illness being identified in the long-term follow-up were *better* for those subjects in the developed world (87%) compared with those in developing centres (84%). This discounts the assertion that the developing centre effect can be explained by a differential follow-up of cases with poor 2 year outcomes, resulting in more early unfavourable outcomes being lost to follow-up in developed countries.

We shall consider one additional piece of data from a study conducted by Craig et al. (1997). These authors reanalysed the two year outcome data from the DOSMeD study in order to examine the role that 'centre' played in predicting course. A recursive partitioning or Classification and Regression Trees (CART) analysis was used, in which predictor variables are not pregrouped.

This confirmed earlier findings (Jablensky et al. 1992) that a strong predictor of pattern of course was a certain grouping of centres. However, in the CART analysis, that grouping, whilst resembling the 'developing/developed' dichotomy of the earlier WHO studies, was not entirely identical to it. Interestingly, subjects in Nottingham and Prague joined the 'developing' countries in forming a grouping with more favourable outcomes. This points to the relative courseness of arbitrary groupings such as 'developed' and 'developing', which have been rightly criticised as more bureaucratic convenience than robust analytic distinction.

Overall, these different analyses of the IPSS, DOSMeD and ISoS data present a coherent message. There are unresolved methodological difficulties centred upon unmeasured individual differences and residual confounding but, considered in the round, the different analytic approaches adopted by Jablensky et al. (1992), Craig et al. (1997), Harrison et al. (2001), Siegel et al. (in press), together with those by Hopper and Wanderling (2000), build a strong case in favour of different outcomes for schizophrenia-related syndromes in different parts of the world. The precise nature of these centre effects remains to be unravelled and represents a rather large 'black box' effect. Where do we go from here?

▌ Social space and the outcome of schizophrenia: a confusion of concepts and levels

We saw earlier that in recent years a vast literature has emerged linking differences in social space with differences in physical and mental health. Reviews have covered a broad array of disease outcomes including all-cause mortality, cardiovascular disease, stroke cancer and infectious disease (e.g. Greenwood et al. 1996; Anderson et al. 1996; Helgeson and Cohen 1996). In developing their thinking, however, social epidemiologists have needed to grapple with several conceptual and methodological issues, not least the much-vaunted 'ecological fallacy'. As these are relevant to the interpretation of contextual level effects in schizophrenia outcomes we shall consider some of them briefly.

The 'ecological fallacy'

The 'ecological fallacy' occurs when we assume that observations made at the level of the individual can be applied to those observed at an aggregate level, such as area or 'country', or vice-versa. For example, coronary heart disease can be shown to be associated with economic development at country level: more affluent countries may have higher rates of coronary heart disease. However, this does not hold at the individual level, where we find an association with low socio-economic status. This does not mean that one has to choose between a model of coronary heart disease as being either a disease of affluence or of poverty; it simply means that one has to be clear about the appropriate level of analysis and exercise caution in extrapolating from one level to another (McIntyre and Ellaway 2000). A raft of intermediary factors confound these relationships at these different levels.

This mistake continues to be made in the epidemiological literature. Schneider et al. (1997) for example found that those born in the south of the United States had higher mortality than those born in the mid-west, north-east or west. They suggest that childhood adversity linked to poverty and nutrition are likely to be related to mortality on the basis that 'southern blacks historically suffered from abject poverty with nutritional deprivation'. But there are many ways in which the south and north of the United States may differ and, without individual level data to control for childhood adversity, there is no way of knowing which risk factors, among those of poverty, nutrition, gene pool, climate, migration and employment opportunities, might be responsible for the excess mortality. Such differences identified by observational studies are important in pointing to the potential role of environmental factors and for our theorising about the exposures underpinning these differences, but we need to be cautious about applying population level differences to individual level data.

The individual in context

This kind of confusion led to a general disdain for ecological approaches that gave rise to an equally fallacious perspective: that the only important factors in health behaviour and health outcomes are those operating at the individual level. Schwartz (1994) argues that the notion that group level variables do not cause disease is itself 'the fallacy of the ecological fallacy'. This is associated with an unbalanced emphasis in which life-style and risk behaviours are conceptualised within a tightly defined individualistic, or atomised, framework that excludes the broader social context. Whilst such 'biomedicalisation' of behaviour allows for simpler and clearer hypothesis testing in carefully designed trials of psychosocial factors in health, for example those targeting highly specifiable behaviours such as smoking or diet, it fails to take into account the difficulties of changing behaviour viewed in isolation from the broader biopsychosocial context.

As we have noted, however, in recent years there has been a renewed focus on 'upstream' factors that determine the way larger social contexts effect individual ('downstream') behavioural and psychological factors. Thus, Duncan et al. (1996) identified 'smoking cultures' that develop in local neighbourhoods, whereby the co-presence of similarly behaving people influences the number of times people practice that behaviour, even when controlling for the individual characteristics of people in those areas. Similarly, a study of Finnish adolescents (Karvonen and Rimpela 1996), which linked individual data to information about socio-economic characteristics of areas (municipalities), found that alcohol consumption was related to *contextual* socio-economic factors as well as to the socio-economic background of the individual adolescents.

There has also been a renewed emphasis on theory development concerning how distinctive types of influence may be keyed to different phases of the development of illness, especially if we are attempting to develop psychosocial interventions. A case in point is the difference between the *structural* social ties that we call social networks and the *functional consequences* of those ties, namely social support. These different components of social context may be keyed to different phases of illness development, and outcome, and be sensitive to quite different types of interventions. Moreover, social support may have a direct effect on an outcome or, alternatively, may simply ameliorate the effects of another risk factor. This is of more than speculative interest as robust interventions require strong theory. The greater the level of theory-driven specification of a proposed intervention, the more likely the results will be capable of interpretation and generalisation.

Authors such as Berkman and Glass (2000) have therefore developed more highly specified models of how social context might impact might upon health. They have attempted to deconstruct the different components of 'social context' that could be operating in disease outcomes whilst, at the same time, integrating socio-cultural and biological factors. Their model envisions a cascading causal process beginning with *macro-level* social conditions, such as political culture, inequality and over-arching cultural norms and values. These are considered to condition the nature, shape and extent of social networks at the *'mezzo'* level, which in turn provide opportunities for *micro-level* psychosocial mechanisms, such as social support and social influence (peer support and constraining/enabling influences on health behaviours). At the final stage, the *individual* level, these are considered to impact on health behaviour, psychological and physiological pathways. The latter include biological outcomes such as effects upon the HPA axis and other hormonal regulatory systems, 'allostatic' load, and patterns of growth and maturation.

Social space and outcome trajectories of schizophrenia

Returning to the question of disease outcomes in schizophrenia, it is clear from our brief overview of the literature that the conceptual development and quality of empirical research falls well short of what has been achieved elsewhere. Data suggesting differences in course and outcome of schizophrenia in different countries is based on individual level measures in relatively small cohorts. Various authors have attempted to explain these differences in terms of the 'usual suspects': a disparate list of anthropological variables long hypothesised as likely factors in achieving recovery. These include factors such as kin-based stores of social capital, flexible and more accommodating work, alternative or 'self-exempting' attributions of illness and more socially integrated subjectivities (Cooper and Sartorius 1997; Warner 1985; Hopper 1991; Hopper and Wanderling 2002). However, in view of the methodological problems considered above, there are obvious difficulties in attributing differences in course and outcome to such broad-brush cultural integrities that we assume to be shared by all 'traditional' societies around the globe. Edgerton and Cohen (1994), among others, point to the conceptual inadequacy of such labels and Craig et al. (1997) showed in their CART analysis of the DOSMeD data that some industrialised centres, such as Nottingham in the United Kingdom, group more closely with developing centres on the basis of outcomes at 2-year follow-up.

Having conceded these difficulties, however, the relationship between outcome of schizophrenia and social space is clearly of great interest. Yet, surprisingly, there has been a remarkable dearth of studies exploring these issues further and very little new material has emerged from first episode cohorts in developing countries. This is perhaps not surprising given problems of resourcing and the difficulties of carrying out population-based research, but carefully designed studies are needed.

Next steps in research

Before suggesting potentially fruitful avenues of research, our brief overview of related literature in the field of social epidemiology suggests there is more work to be done in theory development. The differences between developed and developing countries need to be conceptualised in a more comprehensive framework than hitherto. To date, the arguments have tended toward polarisation, perpetuating old rivalries between biological and social causation in schizophrenia. We have also tended to assume that differences in outcome in different cultures must be due to differences in 'culture' that can only be articulated in broadly social terms. But as we noted earlier, we have no way of knowing, given present knowledge, which factors amongst those of poverty, nutrition, gene pool, migration, and employment opportunities may be responsible for these differences.

Using a similar framework to that described by Berkman and Glass (2000) a conceptual model of how schizophrenia outcomes might be related to different levels of social context is shown in Fig. 1. This kind of framework allows a more considered approach to hypothesis development and subverts the old dichotomy between biological and social. The model I have shown for schizophrenia encompasses three key principles. First, 'culture' and 'biology' are seen to be integrated within the same causal network, with the scope for both 'upstream' and 'downstream' interactions. Differences in the social biology of schizophrenia in different cultures are construed to be associated with different patterns of biological exposures that shape the life-course development of the schizophrenia phenotype. Such differences encompass the nature and quality of obstetric care, nutritional aspects of foetal growth, climatic differences affecting viral exposures and Vit D availability to the developing brain, and differential patterns of infant mortality. These biologically mediated exposures are as much a part of 'culture' in the sense of being sensitive to variations in patterns of maternal/family behaviours, childcare, and higher level cultural norms governing style and availability of health care, as are the usual candidates of 'self exempting modes of illness attribution'. Second, cultural differences are linked dynamically with micro-level psychosocial influences on course and outcome, such as expressed emotion and over-involvement. These, too, are embedded in wider cultural networks which exert protective (buffering) or accentuating effects of their own. In addition, the timing of these in-

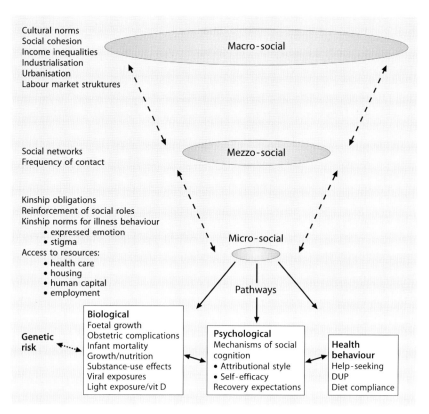

Fig. 1. The social biology of schizophrenia

fluences may be crucial: differential kinship-based patterns of response to early decline in schizophrenia (leading up to the first episode) may have a profound impact on longer term outcomes through the resulting duration of untreated psychosis. These same influences could have effects in the opposite direction if symptoms become entrenched and enduring. Third, at individual level, the nature and content of early personal psychotic experience is likely to be powerfully shaped by wider social influences which, given the critical period of early syndromal development, may effectively determine the 'malignancy' of the disorder over the next 10 years of its development. The model proposed in Fig. 1 does not reduce the complexity of the web of causation surrounding the life course phenotype of schizophrenia, but it at least attempts to embed cultural differences in patterns of recovery within an integrated social biology of the disorder.

Turning to more specific areas of investigation, two main pieces of work could begin to illuminate the relationship between social space and outcome. Hopper and Wanderling (2002) point out that, in the ISoS data, if one subtracts Hong Kong from the 'developing group' the remaining members are all Indian – Chennai and the two Chandigarh centres. Whilst they recognise that this restricts the generalisability of the finding of differential advantage, it may also help to simplify the cultural questions. They argue that we might legitimately enquire into salient cultural aspects of the Indian sub-continent and in particular the extraordinary engagement of India families in the course of treatment – 'one of the 'signature features' of psychiatry in that country' (Nunley 1998). Family involvement has been observed from the initial decision to seek help, to attending to basic needs and medication adherence during hospitalisation, to support afterward including monitoring medications and functioning. Styles of family interaction, for example focused on the early expressed emotion studies (Wig et al. 1997), are obvious candidates for more detailed outcome research in those centres. The role of the family in reducing duration of untreated psychosis (Davidson and McGlashan 1997) and in early detection of relapse is another area that lends itself to robust hypothesis development and testing. Finally, there is a need for qualitative research, exploring the micro-contexts of support in the lives of patients as the disorder develops and unfolds in their lives.

Conclusions

The series of studies we have considered in this article play an important part in relieving patients, carers and clinicians of the old chronicity paradigm which dominated thinking throughout much of the 20th Century. If the course of severe mental disorder depends upon the nature of the social space in which they emerge, there may be important recovery promoting factors in the environment waiting to be harnessed. If it were possible to achieve the outcomes seen in developing centres for industrialised countries, the burden of disease would be drastically reduced. It is depressing that with the pace of urbanisation and social fragmentation in 'developing' centres, the overall burden of disease may well begin to rise. For clinicians in all parts of the world, the challenge remains to open up further the 'black box' of "culture" and find ways of translating customary practices into interventions by design.

Acknowledgements. This paper is based on the data obtained in the International Study of Schizophrenia (ISoS), a project sponsored by the World Health Organization, the Laureate Foundation (United States of America) and the participating centres. The International Study of Schizophrenia, a transcultural investigation coordinated by WHO in 18 centres in 14 countries, was designed to examine patterns of long-term course and outcome of severe mental disorders in different cultures, to develop further methods for the study of characteristics of mental disorders and their course in different settings, and to strengthen the scientific basis for future international multidisciplinary research on schizophrenia and other psychiatric disorders seen in a public health perspective.

The chief collaborating investigators in the field research centres are: Aarhus: A. Bertelsen; Agra: K.C. Dube; Beijing: Y. Shen; Cali: C. Leon; Chandigarh: V. Varma and (since 1994) S. Malhotra; Dublin: D. Walsh; Groningen: R. Giel and (since 1994) D. Wiersma; Hong Kong: P.W.H. Lee; Honolulu: A.J. Marsella; Madras: R. Thara; Mannheim: H. Hafner and (since 1989) W. an der Heiden; Moscow: S.J. Tsirkin;

Nagasaki: Y. Nakane; Nottingham: G. Harrison; Prague: C. Skoda; Rochester: L. Wynne; and Sofia: K. Ganev. Coordination of the data collection, experimental design and data analysis were carried out by the WHO Collaborating Centre at the Nathan S. Kline Institute for Psychiatric Research under the direction of E. Laska. At WHO Headquarters, Geneva, the study has been coordinated by N. Sartorius (until August 1993), by W. Gulbinat (September 1993 – April 1996) and by A. Janca (since May 1996). The authors also gratefully acknowledge the contribution of Ezra Susser, Sarah Conover, and John Cooper to the early design and development of instruments for the ISoS.

▪ References

Anderson D, Deshais G, Jobin J (1996) Social support, social networks and coronary artery disease rehabilitation: a review. Canadian Journal of Cardiology 12:739–744

Barnes JA (1954) Class and committees in a Norwegian island parish. Hum Relations 7:39–58

Berkman LF, Glass T (2000) Social integration, social networks, social support, and health. In: Berkman LF, Kawachi I (eds) Social Epidemiology. Oxford University Press, pp 137–173

Casell J (1976) The contribution of the social environment to host resistance. American Journal of Epidemiology 104:107–123

Cooper J, Sartorius N (1977) Cultural and temporal variations in schizophrenia: a speculation on the importance of industrialization. British Journal of Psychiatry 130:50–55

Cormac I, Jones C, Campbell C, Silveira da Mota Neto J (2003) Cognitive behaviour therapy for schizophrenia (Cochrane Review). In: The Cochrane Library, Issue 4. Chichester, UK. John Wiley & Sons Ltd

Craig TJ, Siegel C, Hopper K et al (1997) Outcome in schizophrenia and related disorders compared between developing and developed countries. A recursive partitioning re-analysis of the WHO DOSMD data. British Journal of Psychiatry 170:229–233

Davidson L, McGlashen TH (1997) The varied outcomes of schizophrenia. Canadian Journal of Psychiatry 42:34–43

Drake C, Levine R, Laska E (in press) Identifying prognostic factors that predict recovery in the presence of loss to follow-up. In: Hopper K, Harrison G, Janca A, Sartorius N (eds) Prospects for Recovery from Schizophrenia – an International Investigation: Report from the WHO-Collaborative Project, The International Study of Schizophrenia. Psychosocial Press, Westport, CT

Duncan C, Jones K, Moon G (1996) Health related behaviour in context – a multilevel modelling approach. Soc Sci Med 42:817–830

Durkheim E (1897, 1951) Suicide: A study in sociology. Free Press, Glencoe, IL

Eaton W, Harrison G (2001) Life chances, life planning and schizophrenia: a review and interpretation of research on social deprivation. International Journal of Mental Health 30(1):58–81

Edgerton R, Cohen A (1994) Culture and schizophrenia: the DOSMeD challenge. British Journal of Psychiatry 164:222–231

Faris RE, Dunham W (1939) Mental disorders in urban areas. University of Chicago Press, Chicago

Goldberg EM, Morrison SL (1963) Schizophrenia and social class. British Journal of Psychiatry 109:785–802

Greenwood DC, Muir KR, Packham CJ, Madeley RJ (1996) Coronary heart disease: a review of the role of psychosocial stress and social support. Journal of Public Health Medicine 18:221–231

Gunnell D, Harrison G, Rasmussen F, Fouskakis D, Tynelius P (2002) Associations between premorbid intellectual performance, early-life exposures and early-onset schizophrenia. British Journal of Psychiatry 181:298–305

Harrison G, Eaton W (2002) Migration and the social epidemiology of schizophrenia. In: Häfner H (ed) Risk and Protective Factors in Schizophrenia. Steinkopff, Darmstadt, pp 113–122

Harrison G, Gunnell D, Glazebrook C, Page K, Kwiecinski R (2001) Association between schizophrenia and social inequality at birth: case-control study. British Journal of Psychiatry 179:346–350

Harrison G, Hopper K, Craig T, Laska E, Siegel C, Wanderling J, Dube KC, Ganev K, Giel R, An der Heiden W, Holmberg SK, Janca A, Lee PWH, Leon CA, Malhotra S, Marsella AJ, Nakane Y, Sartorius N, Shen Y, Skoda C, Thara R, Tsirkin SJ, Varma VK, Walsh D, Wiersma D (2001) Recovery from psychotic illness: a 15 and 25 year international follow-up study. British Journal of Psychiatry 178:506–517

Helgeson VS, Cohen S (1996) Social support and adjustment to cancer: reconciling descriptive, co-relational and intervention research. Health Psychology 15:135–148

Hopper K (1991) Some old questions for the new cross cultural psychiatry. Medical Anthropology Quarterly (New series) 5:299–330

Hopper K, Wanderling J (2000) Revisiting the developed versus developing country distinction in course and outcome in schizophrenia: results from ISoS, the WHO Collaborative Follow-up Project. Schizophrenia Bulletin 26(4):835–846

Jablensky A, Sartorius N, Cooper JE, Anker M, Corton A, Birtleson A (1994) Culture and schizophrenia: criticism of WHO studies are answered. British Journal of Psychiatry 165:434–436

Jablensky A, Sartorius N, Ernberg G et al (1992) Schizophrenia: manifestations, incidence and course in different cultures: a World Health Organisation 10-country study. Psychological Medicine (suppl) 20:1–97

Karvonen S, Rimpela A (1996) Socio-regional context as a determinant of adolescents' health behaviour in Finland. Soc Sci Med 43:1467–1474

Katz MM, Marsella A, Dube KC, Olatawura M, Takahashi R, Nakane Y, Wynne LC, Gift T, Brennan J, Sartorius N, Jablensky A (1988) On the expression of psychosis in different cultures: schizophrenia in an Indian and in a Nigerian community: a report from the World Health Organization Project on determinants of outcome of severe mental disorders. Culture, Medicine and Psychiatry 12:331–355

Kleinman A (1988) A Rethinking Psychiatry. Free Press, New York

Larsen TK, McGlashen TH, Moe LC (1996) First episode schizophrenia: 1. Early course parameters. Schizophrenia Bulletin 22:241–256

Leff J, Wig NN, Gosh A, Bedi H, Menon DK, Kuipers L, Nielsen JA, Thestrup Grethe, Korten A, Ernberg G, Day R, Sartorius N, Jablensky A (1987) Expressed emotion and schizophrenia in North India: III. Influence of relatives' expressed emotion on the course of schizophrenia in Chandigarh. British Journal of Psychiatry 151:166–173

Malhotra S, Varma VK, Misra AK, Das MK, Wig NN, Santosh PJ (1998) Onset of acute psychotic states in India: study of sociodemographic, seasonal and biological factors. Acta Psychiatrica Scandinavica 97:125–131

McIntyre S, Ellaway A (2000) Ecological approaches: rediscovering the role of the physical and social environment. In: Berkman L, Kawachi I (eds) Social Epidemiology. Oxford University Press, pp 332–348

Morris M (1994) Epidemiology and social networks: modelling structured diffusion. In: Wasserman S, Galaskiewicz J (eds) Advances in Social Network Analysis: Research in the Social and Behavioural Sciences. Sage, Thousand Oaks, CA, pp 26–52

Nunley M (1998) The involvement of families in Indian psychiatry. Culture, Medicine and Psychiatry 22:317–353

Pharoah FM, Rathbone J, Mari JJ, Streiner D (2003) Family intervention for Schizophrenia (Cochrane Review). In: The Cochrane Library, Issue 4. Chichester, UK. John Wiley & Sons Ltd

Sartorius N, Gulbinat W, Harrison G et al (1996) Long-term follow-up of schizophrenia in 16 countries. Social Psychiatry and Psychiatric Epidemiology 31:249–258

Schneider D, Greenberg MR, Lu LL (1997) Region of birth and mortality from circulatory diseases among black Americans. Am J Public Health 87:800–804

Schwartz S (1994) The fallacy of the ecological fallacy: the potential misuse of a concept and the consequences. Am J Public Health 84:819–824

Siegel C, Wanderling J, Shang L et al (in press) Predictors of long-term course and outcome for the DOSMeD cohort. In: Hopper K, Harrison G, Janca A et al (eds) Prospects of Recovery from Schizophrenia – An International Investigation. Psychosocial Press, Madison, CT

Stevens J (1987) Brief psychoses: do they contribute to the good prognosis and equal prevalence of schizophrenia in developing countries? British Journal of Psychiatry, 151:393–396

Susser E, Wanderling J (1994) Epidemiology of nonaffective acute remitting psychosis vs. schizophrenia: sex and sociocultural setting. Archives of General Psychiatry 51:294–301

Warner R (1985) Recovery from Schizophrenia. Routledge & Kegan Paul, New York

Wiersma D, Nienhuis FJ, Giel R et al (1996) Assessment of the need for care 15 years after onset of a Dutch cohort of schizophrenic patients and an international comparison. Social Psychiatry and Psychiatric Epidemiology 31:114–121

Wig NN, Menon DK, Bedi H, Ghosh A, Kuipers L, Leff J, Korten A, Day R, Sartorius N, Ernberg G, Jablensky A (1987) Expressed emotion and schizophrenia in North India: 1. Cross-cultural transfer of ratings of relatives' expressed emotion. British Journal of Psychiatry 151:156–160

Wing JK, Cooper JE, Sartorius N (1974) Present State Examination. Cambridge University Press, Cambridge

World Health Organisation (1973) The International Pilot Study of Schizophrenia. John Wiley & Son, New York

World Health Organisation (1979) Schizophrenia: An International follow-up study. John Wiley & Sons, New York

Psychotic features in the general population. Risk factors for what?

LYDIA KRABBENDAM[1], MANON HANSSEN[1], MAARTEN BAK[1], and JIM VAN OS[1,2]

[1] Dept. Psychiatry and Neuropsychology, European Graduate School of Neuroscience, Maastricht University, PO BOX 616; 6200 MD Maastricht, The Netherlands
[2] Division of Psychological Medicine, Institute of Psychiatry, De Crespigny Park, Denmark Hill, London SE5 8AF, UK

Introduction

For clinical purposes, psychosis is defined as a discrete entity that can be identified by applying certain criteria. This does not mean, however, that this condition exists as such in nature. Disease at the level of the general population generally exists as a continuum of severity rather than an all-or-none phenomenon (Rose and Barker 1978). Evidence that variation in the psychosis phenotype can be better represented by the concept of a continuum comes from studies measuring psychotic symptoms in the general population (Claridge et al. 1996; Peters et al. 1999; Tien, 1991; Van Os et al. 1999, 200; Verdoux et al. 1998). These studies have found that the positive symptoms of psychosis are prevalent in the general population and show a similar pattern of correlation with each other as their equivalents do in clinical psychotic disorder.

The majority of the individuals experiencing these "symptoms" are not in need of care. However, longitudinal studies indicate that they may nevertheless have an increased risk of developing a clinical disorder (Chapman et al. 1994; Kwapil et al. 1997; Poulton et al. 2000). This suggests that these attenuated psychosis-like experiences are a risk factor for more full-blown psychotic symptoms and that transitions over the continuum occur over time. This chapter will discuss two issues in relation to transitions over the psychosis continuum:

- would it be useful to identify individuals at high risk for psychotic disorder on the basis of self-reported psychotic experiences, and
- what are the psychological mechanisms that mediate transition from having one or two psychotic symptoms to becoming a patient with a psychotic disorder?

Self-reported psychotic experiences in the general population as a screening tool for psychotic disorders

Early detection and intervention of psychosis has become increasingly topical in mental health practice and research (McGorry et al. 2001; Verdoux 2001), with interest extending well into the prodromal phase of psychosis (Falloon 1992; Hafner et al. 1999; Yung et al. 1998). One of the key variables used to identify possible cases of psychosis in the early stages is the use of attenuated, brief or limited psychotic experiences as well as schizotypal signs and symptoms (Chapman et al. 1980; Larsen et al. 2001; McGorry et al. 1995). Longitudinal studies suggest that psychotic and psychosis-like symptoms indeed predict clinical disorder (Chapman et al. 1994; Kwapil et al. 1997; Poulton et al. 2000). However, the prevalence of such experiences is many times higher than that of psychotic disorders fulfilling DSM or ICD criteria (Eaton et al. 1991; Johns and van Os 2001; Van Os et al. 1999). This opens the possibility of unacceptably high rates of false positive diagnoses, with the exception of selected special groups with a very high baseline prevalence of psychotic disorder (Klosterkotter et al. 2001; Susser and Struening 1990). While the movement of early recognition and intervention, including intervention in the prodromal phases, is rapidly progressing to the stage of randomised controlled trials, there is little basic epidemiological work investigating the sensitivity, specificity and post-test probability (predictive value) of diagnostic procedures.

It is crucial to distinguish at what level along the different filters on the pathway to mental health care (Goldberg and Huxley 1980) early detection of psychosis is actually intended to take place (see Fig. 1). In the general population, psychotic disorders are rare, and individuals may not have developed illness- and/or help-seeking behaviour. At the level of mental health services and above, the prevalence of psychosis is higher and help-seeking behaviour the rule. Thus, risk of stigmatisation in false positives should be lowest at the level of mental health services whereas at this level violation of the right "not to know" (that one has an illness) in true positives should be absent.

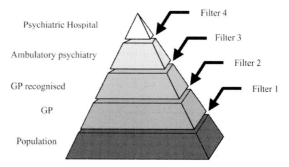

Fig. 1. The filter model of psychiatric morbidity. In order to reach the level of psychiatric care, individuals have to pass through a number of "filters". Thus, individuals in the general population with psychiatric morbidity have to develop illness behaviour (filter 1), resulting in (generally) a visit to their GP. The GP may subsequently recognise the psychiatric problems (filter 2), and may refer (filter 3) the patient to ambulatory psychiatric care. Finally, the ambulatory psychiatrists may refer (filter 4) on to the psychiatric hospital

▌ Study 1

Background

This study investigates *cross-sectionally* to what degree the presence of self-reported psychotic experiences in the general population may be used as an indicator of clinician-assessed psychotic *disorders* (the longitudinal predictive efficiency will be discussed in the section after) (Hanssen et al. 2002 b). This was investigated in two groups. The first group comprised a random cross-section of the general population, and the second comprised a random cross-section of individuals in the general population who had been in contact with mental health services (MHS). The aim of this study was to investigate the accuracy of self-reported psychotic experiences as a screening tool in 1) a general population sample and 2) a MHS sample, by calculating likelihood ratios, or how much more likely it is that a psychotic experience is seen in those with as opposed to those without a psychotic disorder, and post-test probabilities, or the likelihood of psychotic disorder given a psychotic experience.

Methods

The Netherlands Mental Health Survey and Incidence Study (NEMESIS) is a longitudinal study with three measurements points over 4 years (Bijl et al. 1998 a; Bijl et al. 1998 b). The current analysis is based on the baseline data. A multistage, stratified, random sampling procedure was used to first select ninety municipalities, then a sample of private households (addresses) was taken and finally a Dutch-speaking individual aged 18–64 years from each household. A total of 7076 subjects participated at baseline, representing a response rate of 69.7%. Of these, 1352 (19.1%) had been in contact with the mental health services during their lifetimes.

The Composite International Diagnostic Interview (CIDI) version 1.1 was used (WHO 1990). The CIDI psychosis section (G-section) consists of 17 core psychosis items on delusions (13 items) and hallucinations (4 items): items G1–G13, G15, G16, G20 and G21. These items correspond to classic psychotic experiences like persecution, thought interference, auditory hallucinations and passivity phenomena.

All these items can be rated in five ways:
1) no experience;
2) experience present but not clinically relevant (not bothered by it and not seeking help for it);
3) experience is the result of drug use or somatic disease;
4) experience is not a real symptom because there appears to be some plausible explanation for it;
5) true psychotic symptom.

Categories 2–5 will be denoted hereafter, respectively: NCR symptom (Not Clinically Relevant), secondary symptom, possible symptom and clinical symptom. Each time when possible or clinical symptoms were detected in the

NEMESIS study, a psychiatrist conducted clinical re-interviews over the telephone using questions from the Structured Clinical Interview for DSM-III-R (SCID) to validate the ratings (Spitzer et al. 1992). If a clinician did not agree with the psychosis rating of the lay-interviewer, the psychosis rating was changed to the rating of the clinician and so the CIDI generated DSM-III-R diagnoses were based on the corrected CIDI psychosis ratings. At the NEMESIS baseline measurement, lifetime experiences of psychosis were assessed. A broad combined grouping of affective and non-affective psychosis was used as the outcome variable. In order to avoid the tautology that clinician-assessed experiences were used as a test for clinician-assessed psychosis, we used the original, *uncorrected* lay interviewer assessed CIDI self-report ratings as a screening tool (i.e. diagnostic test) for clinician-assessed DSM-III-R psychotic disorder.

Results

The prevalence of at least one self-reported, uncorrected "NCR experience" was 13.0%, of "secondary symptom" 0.5%, of "possible symptom" 4.2% and of "clinical symptom" 5.6%. The total prevalence of any type of self-reported psychotic experience was 18.1%. The total prevalence of DSM-III-R non-affective and affective psychosis (any psychosis) was 1.5%. The prevalence of psychotic disorder in the group with the additional selection criterion "lifetime contact with mental health services" (any psychosis MHS) was much higher at 6.4% (Fig. 2).

The likelihood ratio for a positive test result (a psychotic experience) for psychotic disorder was high for the category "clinical symptom" (23.4) (Table 1). The false positive rate in this category was low (4.2%), and the true positive rate (sensitivity) was high at 97.2%. After selection of subjects who had a history of contact with mental health services, the likelihood ratios of all categories decreased (Table 1), but was still higher than 10 for the category "clinical symptom". The post-test probability of the "clinical symptom" was highest (26.5%) (Table 2). The other psychotic experience ratings had low post-test probabilities in the range of 5.1–21.6. After applying the selection criterion of lifetime contact with mental health services, the post-test probabilities of all experience categories increased (Table 2, third column).

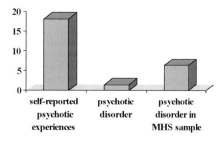

Fig. 2. Prevalence of any psychotic experience and psychotic disorder in a general population sample (n = 7076) and prevalence of psychotic disorder in sample with selection criterion "lifetime professional mental health contact" (MHS sample, n = 1352)

Table 1. Prevalence (%), true positives (true rate, %), false positives (false rate, %) and likelihood ratio positive test result (LR+) of CIDI items for affective and non-affective psychosis (any psychosis) and LR+ for any psychosis with selection criterion "lifetime professional mental health contact" (any psychosis MHS)

Type of psychotic experience	Any psychosis			Any psychosis MHS
	True rate	False rate	LR+ (95% CI)	LR+ (95% CI)
▌ Any psychotic experience	100.0	16.8	6.0 (5.7, 6.3)	3.7 (3.4, 4.0)
▌ Not clinically relevant experience	43.9	12.5	3.5 (2.8, 4.4)	2.3 (1.7, 3.0)
▌ Secondary symptom	7.5	0.4	18.0 (8.4, 38.4)	7.9 (3.3, 19.4)
▌ Possible symptom	57.0	3.4	16.8 (13.7, 20.7)	6.7 (5.2, 8.7)
▌ Clinical symptom	97.2	4.2	23.4 (20.8, 26.4)	11.1 (9.3, 13.4)

Any psychosis and psychotic experiences: n = 7076
Any psychosis MHS (lifetime) and psychotic experiences: n = 1352

Table 2. Post-test probability of CIDI items (PP, %) for affective and non-affective psychosis (any psychosis) and for any psychosis with selection criterion lifetime professional mental health contact (any psychosis MHS)

Type of psychotic experience [a]	Post-test Probability	
	Any psychosis	Any psychosis MHS
▌ Any psychotic experience	8.4 (7.7, 9.0)	20.0 (17.8, 22.1)
▌ Not clinically relevant experience	5.1 (4.6, 5.7)	13.3 (11.5, 15.1)
▌ Secondary symptom	21.6 (20.7, 22.6)	35.0 (32.5, 37.5)
▌ Possible symptom	20.5 (19.6, 21.5)	31.4 (28.9, 33.9)
▌ Clinical symptom	26.5 (25.4, 27.5)	43.1 (40.4, 45.7)

[a] Entered in the equation as dichotomous variable indicating presence or absence of the experience
Any psychosis and psychotic experiences: n = 7076
Any psychosis MHS and psychotic experiences: n = 1352

Conclusion

Some psychotic experiences have post-test probabilities on the order of 20% or higher with similarly high likelihood ratios. The presence of at least one clinical symptom had a post-test probability higher than 25% (26.5%). This indicates that out of 100 subjects with at least one clinical symptom, one quarter has a psychotic disorder and three-quarters does not have a psychotic disorder. In addition, the likelihood ratio of this category was higher than 10, i.e. satisfactory (Sackett et al. 1997), and the number of false positives was small. The diagnostic value was better in individuals who had had previous mental health care (although likelihood ratios may decrease because of diagnostic "admixture").

▮ Study 2

Background

This report describes a follow-up of individuals with recent onset of self-reported psychotic and/or psychosis-like experiences in the general population, examining their outcome in terms of stability of the psychotic experience, as well as functional impairment and need for care (Hanssen et al. 2002 a).

Method

This analysis is based on the three measurement points of the Dutch NEMESIS Study (see above), hereafter baseline, T1 (assessing the period between baseline and one year later) and T2 (assessing the period between T1 and 2 years later). A total of 7076 subjects between 18–64 years were enlisted at baseline. At T1, 5618 subjects participated for the second time; at T2 4848 subjects participated. In order to define a sample with incident psychotic experiences, individuals who had a diagnosis of any affective or non-affective psychotic disorder according to the DSM-III-R at baseline and at T1 were excluded from the analyses, as well as individuals who had had any rating of CIDI psychotic experiences in the 12 months before baseline. At T2, clinical re-interviews were conducted by telephone by a psychiatrist using the two positive psychosis items from the Brief Psychiatric Rating Scale (BPRS) (Overall and Gorham 1962) for all individuals who had a rating of NCR, possible or clinical symptom on any CIDI psychosis item. Two T2 psychosis outcomes were defined. The first was evidence of any psychotic experience at any level on either of the two BPRS items (score > 1). This outcome was used to examine the degree of stability from T1 to T2 (hereafter: stability outcome). The second outcome was defined in terms of severity and functional impairment and clinical judgement of need for care (hereafter: clinical outcome). This outcome was based on presence of two criteria: i) a BPRS score on either of the two psychosis items that was greater than pathology level in terms of severity and functional impairment (i.e. BPRS score > 3, see Lukoff et al. 1986) and ii) presence of clinical judgement of need for care according to the Camberwell Assessment of Need (Slade et al. 1996).

Results

A total of 4067 individuals were available for analysis. Of these, the number of subjects with incident psychotic experiences at T1 was 83 and at T2, the number of individuals with clinical outcome was 11 and with the stability outcome 47. In terms of relative risk, effect sizes of psychotic experiences at T1 for the clinical outcome at T2 was very high with odds ratio's varying from 46.5 to 94.2 (Table 3). The odds ratios for the stability outcome were more moderate, albeit still rather high (OR 14.8–24.9). In terms of post-test probabilities, the effect sizes for the clinical outcome were modest, with post-test probabilities ranging from 0.00 to 15.8 % (Table 3). Similar results were apparent for the

Table 3. 2-year clinical and stability outcome of different incident psychotic experiences at T1, expressed as odds ratios (OR) and post-test probabilities in % (PP)

CIDI psychotic experience rating [b]	OR (95% CI[a])		PP (95% CI)	
	Clinical outcome	Stability outcome	Clinical outcome	Stability outcome
▎ Any psychotic experience	65.1 (19.4–218.1)	22.8 (11.5–45.1)	7.6 (6.8, 8.4)	16.5 (15.3–17.6)
▎ NCR experience	46.5 (13.2–163.9)	24.9 (11.6–53.2)	7.6 (6.7, 8.4)	18.9 (17.7–20.1)
▎ Secondary experience	–	–	0.0	0.0
▎ Possible experience	94.2 (22.9–387.5)	24.7 (7.9–77.5)	15.8 (14.7, 16.9)	21.1 (19.8–22.3)
▎ Clinical experience	74.5 (14.5–381.4)	14.8 (3.2–67.9)	14.3 (13.2, 15.4)	14.3 (13.2–15.4)

[a] Confidence interval of OR not including unity denotes statistical significance
[b] CIDI symptom ratings entered in the equation as dichotomous variable indicating presence or absence of the symptom

stability outcome. For the clinical outcome, possible and clinical psychotic experiences had significantly higher post-test probabilities than NCR experiences, as indicated by non-overlapping confidence intervals (Table 3). For the stability outcome, differences between the different CIDI psychosis ratings were less marked.

Conclusion

Around 5–15% of individuals with incident self-reported psychotic experiences had developed an outcome defined in terms of functional impairment and need for care 2 years later. Psychotic experiences with distress/help-seeking behaviour, even if the interviewer doubted that they might have a basis in fact, had better predictive value for future functional impairment and clinical need than psychotic experiences without distress and help-seeking behaviour. This distinction in predictive value was specific for prediction of clinical need and was not apparent for prediction of presence of psychotic experiences at any level per se. In other words, the results show that psychotic experiences without distress have a better outcome whereas experiences accompanied by distress are associated with a more malignant course.

▮ Discussion part 1

Do these figures mean that psychotic experiences can be used as a screening tool for psychotic disorders? Arguably not. Although it would be relatively easy to collect self-reports on psychotic experiences in the general population, the cross-sectional analyses suggest that around 75% of those who test positive would be wrongly labelled with psychotic disorder. This might be acceptable in the case of a disease with a 100% mortality rate that strikes young people and for which an acceptable and successful cure is available, but it may not constitute good screening practice in the case of schizophrenia. Furthermore, if we assume that a treatment existed that could prevent a psychotic disorder from developing in a person with incident psychotic experiences, and that this treatment was effective 50% of the time, the numbers needed to treat given a 15% prediction rate would be 14 ([100/15]*2). The numbers needed to inconvenience (with a treatment that they do not need) would therefore be 13 (14-1). These figures do not look very appealing and are furthermore based on the rather optimistic assumption that an intervention in the pre-psychotic phase can be 50% effective. Therefore, prediction on the basis of psychotic and psychosis-like symptoms may not be very rewarding at the level of the general population.

One solution for the problems inherent to screening for rare psychotic disorders is to apply a series of selection filters that result in a very high baseline prevalence of psychotic disorders in the screening population. This is because the post-test probability is prevalence-dependent and increases as the prevalence of the disease in question rises (Hennekens and Buring 1987). Recent work in selected samples reports post-test probabilities of 40–70% on the basis of a variety of prodromal, developmental or symptomatic measures (Davidson et al. 1999; Klosterkotter et al. 2001; Phillips et al. 2000). In the current analyses, the diagnostic value of having a psychotic experience was better in individuals who had had previous mental health care. Screening in this group has the additional advantage that there is much less danger of stigmatisation in the case of a false positive test result, or of violating the right "not to know" in the case of a true positive test result, since these individuals have already developed help-seeking behaviour for a mental health problem.

▮ Psychological mechanisms mediating the transition to clinical states

Only a fraction of the individuals who report psychotic experiences, such as hallucinatory experiences and delusional ideation, will meet criteria for a clinical disorder (Peters et al. 1999; Tien, 1991; Van Os et al. 2000). Little is known about the mechanisms that mediate the relationship between non-clinical psychotic experience and subsequent clinical disorder. The study of these mechanisms would be particularly important in view of the interest in preventing individuals from making transitions from non-clinical to clinical psychotic states. It then becomes crucially important to understand what actually causes someone having psychotic experiences to develop illness behaviour.

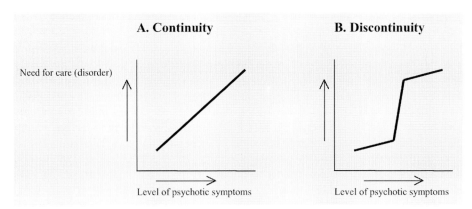

Fig. 3. Relationship between psychotic symptoms and psychotic disorder. In **A**, there is a continuous relationship between level of psychotic symptoms and need for care. In **B**, the initial increase is weak, but after a certain threshold the risk increases disproportionatel

It is important to distinguish between a truly continuous and quasi-continuous relationship between symptoms and disorder (Johns and van Os 2001). The relationship between symptoms and disorder may be truly linear, with an increasing number of symptoms increasing the risk for disorder (Fig. 3a). It may also be that psychotic symptoms behave like hypertension, which is on a direct continuum with continuous normal variation in blood pressure and in itself is not symptomatic, but beyond a certain threshold, the risk of somatic complications involving other organs increases exponentially (Fig. 3b). This possibility, the most likely one according to some (Hafner 1988, 1989), corresponds to a continuum-threshold relationship between symptoms of psychosis and clinical disorder. It would mean that an individual becomes much more likely to develop need for care caused by the psychotic symptoms themselves above a "critical" value of psychosis. Alternatively, someone with a certain level of psychosis may develop an abrupt, non-linear increase in need for care after exposure to additional interacting risk factors. In this case, the relationship between symptoms and disorder would be discontinuous.

If there is a discontinuous relationship, what are the factors that are additionally important in bringing about a marked change resulting in need for care? This chapter will be limited to a discussion of possible psychological factors. Symptoms vary in terms of frequency, degree of conviction, preoccupation, influence on behaviour, distress, and secondary attribution. Evidence suggests that the implausibility of the experience and degree of conviction may not be related to illness status (Garety and Hemsley 1994), whereas degree of preoccupation and distress do seem to be important. For example, Peters and colleagues (Peters et al. 1999) measured delusional ideation in the general population as well as in deluded patients using the Peters et al. Delusions Inventory (PDI). The PDI scores of the general population and the deluded patients showed a large degree of overlap and nearly 10 percent of the general population scored above the mean of the group with delusions. However, compared to patients, non-patients displayed significantly less distress, preoccupation and conviction regarding their unusual perceptual experiences and ideas. This would mean that in order to understand the transition from non-clinical to clinical states two interacting risks should be considered (Johns and van Os 2001). One determines the level of psychosis, or the position someone is going to occupy along the psychosis continuum, and one determines whether someone at a certain position is going to develop need for care. Thus, two persons at different positions along the continuum may differ with regard to number, frequency or severity of symptoms and because of this the person at the highest position may have a higher risk of developing overt disorder. Conversely, at each point of the continuum, two persons with the same level of psychosis may differ in that one copes well and does not develop illness behaviour, whereas the other may develop functional impairments and need for care.

Study 3

Background

Current hypotheses on psychological mechanisms of psychosis have emphasised that response to abnormal experiences is cognitively mediated by beliefs or appraisals (Bentall et al. 1994; Garety et al. 2001). Thus, the mere experience of voices itself may not lead to full-blown psychotic symptoms, but attributing the voice to an external malevolent source and giving it personal significance does. It is this interpretation that causes the associated distress and disability (Chadwick and Birchwood 1994; Morrison and Baker 2000) and thereby increases the risk of developing need for treatment. A prospective study design is best suited to validate these psychological mechanisms. Data from a follow-up study of a general population sample were analysed to investigate the hypothesis that a delusional interpretation and/or a depressed response to hallucinatory experiences predicts the later onset of clinical psychotic disorder (Krabbendam et al. 2002 a, b).

Methods

The analyses were based on the three measurement points of the Dutch NEM-ESIS study (see above), hereafter baseline, T1 (assessing the period between baseline and one year later) and T2 (assessing the period between T1 and 2 years later). The risk set consisted of individuals who i) had undergone both the baseline and the T1 interviews and had received no lifetime diagnosis of any DSM-III-R affective or non-affective psychotic disorder at either interview, ii) had had a CIDI interview at T2, and iii) at T2 had not missed re-interview by clinicians about the presence of psychotic symptoms if they had been eligible for this clinical re-interview. Baseline Hallucinatory Experience (HE) was broadly defined as any CIDI rating of NCR, secondary, possible or clinical symptom on any of the 4 CIDI hallucination items, and Delusional Ideation

(DE) at baseline and T1 was broadly defined as any CIDI rating of NCR, secondary, possible or clinical symptom on any of the 13 CIDI delusion items. Baseline presence of Depressed Mood (DM) was assessed by item E2 of the CIDI depression section ("Have you ever felt depressed most of the time for a period of two years or longer?"). At T1, the period between baseline and T1 was assessed and this rating thus reflects onset of DM one year before baseline. Three T2 psychosis outcomes were defined, based on the BPRS interview at T2 and clinical judgement of need for care: i) any psychotic experience at any level on either of the two BPRS items "unusual thought content" and "hallucinations" (score > 1, hereafter: BPRS psychotic-like experiences), ii) a BPRS score on either of the two psychosis items that was greater than pathology level in terms of severity and functional impairment (i.e. BPRS score > 3, hereafter: BPRS pathology-level psychosis) and iii) BPRS pathology-level psychosis and in addition presence of clinical judgement of need for care (hereafter: needs-based diagnosis of psychosis).

Results

The risk set consisted of 4672 individuals. The number of individuals with T2 BPRS psychotic-like experiences was 85 (1.8%), the number of individuals with BPRS pathology-level psychosis was 39 (0.8%) and 24 individuals (0.5%) had a need for care in relation to psychotic symptoms. At baseline interview, 287 individuals (6.1%) reported HE. Given the presence of HE at baseline, the increase in risk on the additive scale of having the psychosis outcome at T2 was much higher in the group with DE at T1 (n=30) than in those without DE at T1 (n=257) (see Table 4 and Fig. 4). The difference in risks between the groups with and without DE at T1 was statistically significant for each of the three psychosis outcomes (see Table 4). After adjustment for the effect of DE at baseline, the interactions between DE at T1 and HE at baseline remained significant for all three psychosis outcomes, indicating that the risk increasing effect of DE at T1 reflected the emergence of DE between baseline and T1. Similarly, given the presence of HE at baseline, the increase in risk on the additive scale of having the psychosis outcome at T2 was higher in the group with DM at T1 (n=24) than in those without DM at T1 (n=263) (see Table 4 and Fig. 4) and this effect remained after adjustment for baseline presence of DM.

In order to investigate whether the risk increasing effects of DE at T1 and DM at T1 overlapped, separate analyses were performed in which the interaction between DE and HE was adjusted for DM and the interaction between DM and HE was adjusted for DE. Adjustment for DM at T1 did not change the interaction between DE at T1 and HE at baseline (for all analyses, changes in risk difference coefficients were between 0.01% and 0.5%). In contrast, adjustment for the presence of DE at T1 reduced but not nullified the risk increasing effect of DM at T1 in those who reported hallucinatory experiences at baseline. After adjustment for DE, the risk difference between DM at T1 and no DM at T1 was 13.54% (95%CI –4.34, 31.42; $\chi^2=2.20$, df=1, p=0.138) for the outcome of BPRS psychotic-like experiences, 19.95% (95%CI 1.87, 38.02;

Table 4. Interactions between baseline hallucinatory experiences and delusion formation at T1 on the additive scale (risk difference)

	BPRS psychotic-like experiences (n=85)	BPRS pathology-level psychosis (n=39)	Needs-based diagnosis (n=24)
Increase in risk[a] associated with baseline hallucinatory experiences No delusion formation at T1 (n=257)	9.69% (5.93, 13.44)	6.04% (3.08, 8.99)	3.04% (0.92, 5.17)
Delusion formation at T1 (n=30)	29.22% (10.68, 47.75)	28.43% (11.05, 45.81)	21.76% (5.39, 38.13)
Risk difference	19.53% (0.61, 38.44)	22.39% (4.76, 40.02)	18.72% (2.22, 35.23)
Additive interaction[b]	$\chi^2=4.10$, $df=1$, $p=0.043$	$\chi^2=6.20$, $df=1$, $p=0.013$	$\chi^2=4.94$, $df=1$, $p=0.026$
Increase in risk associated with baseline hallucinatory experiences No depressed mood at T1 (n=263)	11.12% (7.15, 15.08)	6.94% (3.80, 10.07)	3.99% (1.57, 6.41)
Depressed mood at T1 (n=24)	28.13% (9.88, 46.37)	28.65% (10.43, 46.86)	20.83% (4.59, 37.08)
Risk difference	17.01% (−1.66, 35.67)	21.71% (3.22, 40.19)	16.84% (0.41, 33.27)
Additive interaction[b]	$\chi^2=3.19$, $df=1$, $p=0.074$	$\chi^2=5.30$, $df=1$, $p=0.021$	$\chi^2=4.04$, $df=1$, $p=0.045$

[a] Risk of having the psychosis outcome at T2
[b] Tests whether increase in risk in group with delusion formation or depressed mood at T1 is significantly greater than increase in risk in group without delusion formation or depressed mood at T1

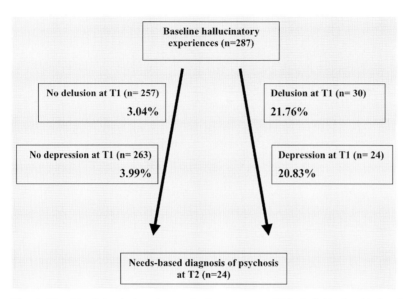

Fig. 4. The risk of developing the psychosis outcome at T2 in individuals with baseline hallucinatory experiences who developed delusion or depression at T1 compared to those who did not develop delusion or depression at T1

$\chi^2 = 4.68$, df $= 1$, p $= 0.031$) for BPRS pathology-level psychosis, and 14.18% (95% CI -1.34, 29.71; $\chi^2 = 3.21$, df $= 1$, p $= 0.073$) for the needs-based diagnosis of psychosis.

Conclusion

In the general population, the risk of developing clinical psychotic disorder in individuals with baseline self-reported hallucinatory experiences was much higher in those who developed delusional ideation than in those who did not. Similarly, the development of depressed mood in those with baseline self-reported hallucinatory experiences increased the risk for onset of clinical disorder, but this effect was partly mediated by the development of delusional ideation. Adjustment for lifetime presence of delusional ideation or depressed mood did not change the pattern of results, suggesting that the risk increasing effect reflects the effect of the emergence of delusional ideation or depressed mood between baseline and T1. In sum, delusional ideation and depressed mood may arise as a secondary response to hallucinatory experiences in the development of clinical psychotic disorder.

Study 4

Background

It follows from the previous results that the experience of hallucinations may give rise to secondary delusional interpretation. Analogous to the mediating role of cognitive beliefs and appraisals in the transition to clinical states, it can be hypothesised that similar mechanisms operate in the development of delusional thinking. This was investigated in the same general population sample but this time restricted to those individuals without previous evidence of any delusional ideation. It was hypothesised that subjects experiencing hallucinations with distress at baseline, compared to those without, would show a greater risk of developing delusions over the 3-year follow-up period (Hanssen et al. 2002 c).

Methods

This report is based on the three measurement points of the NEMESIS Study (see above). The study sample at T2 was restricted to subjects who did not report delusions at baseline and again at T1 in order to skew the sample towards individuals with truly incident delusions at T2. For the current analysis, ratings of NCR experiences and clinical symptoms on the four hallucination items at baseline were included in the analyses, as these are both indicative of presence of psychotic experience in the absence of doubt or secondary cause but crucially different in terms of subjective distress and help-seeking behaviour. Delusional ideation at T2 was measured with BPRS item "unusual thought content" (score > 1). In order to exclude misclassification at the lower end of the BPRS scoring range of the unusual thought content item, analyses were repeated with a more stringent definition of the BPRS "unusual thought content" item (score > 2) and with the clinical definition of delusions (score > 3).

Results

At baseline and limited to the risk set (n = 4236), 161 subjects reported lifetime occurrence of hallucinations without distress, and 32 subjects reported hallucinations with distress. The risk for delusion formation (BPRS score > 1) at T2 was 5 times greater in the individuals who at baseline were distressed by their hallucinations (OR = 25.0, 95% CI 9.3–67.8) than in the individuals who reported hallucinations without distress (OR = 4.9, 95% CI 2.0–11.9) (Table 5). This difference was statistically significant ($\chi^2 = 5.2$, df = 1, p = 0.02). After adjustment for a priori chosen covariates age, gender, urbanicity, ethnic group, neuroticism, experience of discrimination, experience of abuse before the age of 16 years, educational level, unemployment and single marital status, the difference remained robust $\chi^2 = 3.8$, df = 1, p = 0.05). Results were similar using the more stringent definition of delusions (score > 2), with again a highly significant difference in effect size ($\chi^2 = 8.7$, df = 1, p = 0.003) and for the clinical

Table 5. Comparison between hallucinations accompanied with and without distress regarding the formation of delusions three years later

	BASELINE: Hallucination with distress, OR (95% CI)	BASELINE: Hallucination without distress, OR (95% CI)	χ^2	df	p
T2: BPRS delusion >1	25.0 (9.3–67.8)	4.9 (2.0–11.9)	5.2	1	0.02
T2: BPRS delusion >1+ covariates	13.7 (4.4–42.4)	3.2 (1.2–8.4)	3.8	1	0.05
T2: BPRS delusion >2	50.4 (14.9–169.9)	0.9 (0.1–7.8)	8.7	1	0.003
T2: BPRS delusion >2+ covariates	25.1 (4.8–131.3)	0.5 (0.04–4.9)	8.5	1	0.004
T2: BPRS delusion >3	126.4 (26.8–595.3)	–[a]	–	–	–
T2: BPRS delusion >3+ covariates	136.2 (13.1–1414.3)	–[a]	–	–	–

[a] Predicts failure perfectly

definition of delusions (score >3): no individuals with hallucinations without distress developed clinically relevant delusional ideation, whereas the risk was very high in those whose hallucinatory experiences were accompanied by distress (Table 5).

Conclusion

Subjects who experienced negative emotional states associated with anomalous perceptual intrusions had a much greater risk of developing delusional ideation, including experiences of clinical relevance, than individuals who reported similar experiences without distress.

Study 5

Background

Another important determinant of the transition to clinical states may be the level of functional coping that the person mobilises in the face of stressful (psychotic) experiences (Claridge 1997; Lukoff et al. 1984; Nuechterlein and Dawson 1984; Romme et al. 1992). Active coping strategies, like problem solving, seeking help and distraction are reported to generate control and improve general functioning in people with a diagnosis of schizophrenia (Bak et al. 2001 b; Boschi et al. 2000). In contrast, symptomatic coping, characterised by going along with and indulging in the content of psychotic symptoms, diminishes the feeling of control. Passive coping strategies such as isolating oneself or getting involved in non-specific activities, are reported to be unrelated to control experience (Bak et al. 2001 a; Carr 1988). Previous studies suggested that individuals with psychiatric disorders tend to use more passive coping strategies than healthy controls (van den Bosch and Rombouts 1997; Vollrath et al. 1994). People with schizophrenia display the least efficient coping strategies such as withdrawal and avoidance in dealing with stressors, which results in poor control experiences (Hultman et al. 1997; Nicholson and Neufeld 1992; van den Bosch and Rombouts 1997). The present study investigated coping behaviour in individuals from the general population who had at least one experience of a psychotic symptom and no previous diagnosis of any psychotic disorder (Bak et al. 2002). It was hypothesised that presence of need for care would be associated with symptomatic coping strategies and less experience of control, whereas active coping strategies would reduce development of need for care status and increase the experience of control.

Methods

The study is based on the three measurement points of the NEMESIS study. The current analysis focused on subjects who had at least one experience of a psychotic symptom (NCR experience, possible or clinical symptom) and no previous diagnosis of any psychotic disorder at T2 (n = 191). To validate the T2 CIDI ratings, clinical re-interviews were conducted over the telephone by an experienced clinician using questions from the Structured Clinical Interview for DSM-III-R (SCID) (Spitzer et al. 1992). If the CIDI rating of the clinician did not coincide with the rating of the lay interviewer, the rating of the lay interviewer was replaced with the rating of the clinician. Telephone re-interviews were completed on 142 (74.4%) of the 191 subjects. In addition, 57 subjects were excluded from the analyses, because they had no NCR experience or clinical symptom rating left after re-interview, resulting in a sample of 85 subjects.

Coping, subjective distress with and perceived control over the psychotic experience were assessed using the Maastricht Assessment of Coping Strategies (MACS), a semi-structured interview administered by a clinician (Bak et al. 2001 a, b). The MACS focuses on 7 positive symptoms, suspiciousness, thought reading/broadcasting, passivity phenomena, thought insertion/interference, delusions of reference, hearing voices, and other hallucinations. The strategies mentioned by the patient can be scored in one of five domains of coping: 1) behavioural, 2) social, 3) cognitive, 4) care and 5) symptomatic, based on a previous factor analysis of 14 different coping strategies. Subjective distress and perceived control were assessed on a 7-point Likert scale. All 85 individuals were interviewed with the MACS. Since coping only has meaning in the presence of a symptom generating at least minimal distress, only the individuals with symptom observations that were associated with at least minimal presence of symptom distress were included in the analysis. A total of 47 individuals had at least one symptom observation associated with minimum distress. Of these, 19 had received a needs-based diagnosis of psychosis (defined as described above in the previous studies) and 28 did not have such a diagnosis.

Results

In the combined group of need for care and no need for care subjects, significant associations were apparent between the presence of coping and coping type, indicating differences in the frequency with which coping types were used (test statistic for the 5 coping factors – $\chi^2 = 74.54$, df = 4, p < 0.001). In both the need for care and the no need for care group, symptomatic coping was the most common strategy, followed by active problem solving and passive problem avoiding (Table 6). There was, however, a significant interaction between need for care status and coping type ($\chi^2 = 11.15$, df = 4, $P = 0.025$), also after correction for the two BPRS psychosis items as a measure of severity of psychotic symptoms ($\chi^2 = 10.88$, df = 4, $P = 0.028$). This interaction indicated that the two groups used one or more coping types with different frequencies. Examination of the relative distributions of coping type in both groups revealed that those with a need for care were much more likely to display symptomatic coping (OR = 6.07, 95% CI: 1.94–18.95), whereas the presence of the other four coping types was not different across the two groups (Table 6).

The presence of coping was not associated with perceived control (OR = 1.05, 95% CI: 0.97–1.13) and this remained so after adjustment for distress (OR = 1.05, 95% CI: 0.98–1.12). However, the association between the presence of coping and experience of control differed as a function of coping type (coping type κ control interaction term: $\chi^2 = 19.24$, df = 4, $P < 0.001$). Stratified analyses per coping type revealed that symptomatic coping was negatively associated with control (OR = 0.79; 95% CI: 0.63–0.98), whereas active problem solving was positively associated with experience of control (OR = 1.28; 95% CI: 1.10–1.49).

Conclusion

Symptomatic coping was used more frequently in the need for care group. This was not simply the result of the patient group having more severe psychotic experiences, since the interaction between need for care status and coping type was not reduced and remained significant after adjustment for both BPRS psychosis ratings. The use of coping strategies therefore differed between those with and without need for care independent of their differences in severity of symptoms. In addition, symptomatic coping was associated with less, and active problem solving with more perceived control over the psychotic experience.

Table 6. Presence of coping related to coping type and need for care status. For example, the fifth row relates to "symptomatic coping". In those with no need for care, out of 36 possible symptomatic coping observations, coping was present in 13 observations (36.11%). In subjects with need for care, out of 31 possible symptomatic coping observations, coping was present 77.24% of the observations (n = 24). The odds ratio of these two probabilities is 6.07, indicating that those with need for care were 6.07 times more likely to use symptomatic coping, where possible, compared to the other group

Coping type	No need for care (n = 28)		Need for care (n = 19)		χ^2 (1)	p	OR (95% CI)
	Coping absent	Coping present	Coping absent	Coping present			
Active problem solving	91 (84.26%)	17 (15.74%)	69 (74.19%)	24 (25.81%)	2.15	0.14	1.86 (0.81, 4.27)
Passive illness behaviour	107 (99.07%)	1 (0.93%)	90 (96.77%)	3 (3.23%)	1.02	0.31	3.57 (0.30, 42.03)
Active problem avoiding	134 (93.06%)	10 (6.94%)	117 (94.35%)	7 (5.65%)	0.23	0.64	0.80 (0.32, 2.00)
Passive problem avoiding	93 (86.11%)	15 (13.89%)	85 (91.40%)	8 (8.60%)	1.44	0.23	0.58 (0.24, 1.41)
Symptomatic	23 (63.89%)	13 (36.11%)	7 (22.58%)	24 (77.42%)	9,62	0.002	6.07 (1.94, 18.95)
Total	448 (88.89%)	56 (11.11%)	368 (84.79%)	66 (15.21%)	3.46	0.06	1.44 (0.98, 2.10)

▮ Discussion part 2

It is attractive to interpret the findings discussed in this section within the cognitive approach to psychotic symptoms, as outlined by previous authors (Bentall et al. 1994; Birchwood and Chadwick 1997; Garety et al. 2001; Morrison 2001). Central to the cognitive approach is the notion that the response to psychosis-like experiences is cognitively mediated by beliefs or appraisals. Thus, as stated earlier, the experience of voices itself may not necessarily lead to full-blown psychotic symptoms. Only when an individual appraises these experiences as externally caused and personally significant, is this identified as psychosis (Garety et al. 2001; Morrison 2001). Our findings suggest that transitions over the psychosis continuum are, at least in part, driven by the emotional and cognitive responses to anomalous perceptual intrusions. Subjects who experience negative emotional states associated with their hallucinations had a much greater risk of developing delusional ideation than individuals who reported similar experiences without distress. The development of delusional ideation in turn increased the risk for onset of clinical disorder.

Mechanisms of delusion formation

The hypothesis that delusions may arise as a secondary response to hallucinations in the development of clinical disorder is not new. According to Maher, delusions reflect perceptual abnormalities, that through normal reasoning leads to a mistaken conclusion (Maher 1974; Maher 1988). However, the fact that hallucinatory experiences not necessarily evoke delusional interpretation suggests involvement of other factors as well. Distress associated with the experiences is one important factor, as suggested by our findings and by previous authors (Escher et al. 2002; Freeman and Garety 1999; Morrison 2001; Morrison and Baker 2000). Negative emotions may make hallucinatory experiences personally significant or more intrusive, and so trigger the individual to search for explanations of the experiences. In addition, emotions may make the individual more prone to selective attentional processes and safety behaviours diminishing the opportunity to test the accuracy of the anomalous experience (Freeman et al. 2001; Garety et al. 2001).

Other mechanisms of delusion formation most likely involve cognitive processing. Empirical studies have yielded evidence for cognitive abnormalities in deluded patients (Garety and Freeman 1999), particularly, a probabilistic reasoning bias or a "jumping to conclusions" data gathering style (Dudley et al. 1997; Garety et al. 1991), a selective information processing bias focused at threat-related information (Bentall and Kaney 1989; Fear et al. 1996), an abnormal attributional style, i.e. strong externalising and personalising bias (Fear et al. 1996; Kinderman and Bentall 1997), and poor ability to understand and conceptualise the mental processes of other people (theory of mind) (Corcoran et al. 1995; Frith and Corcoran 1996; Janssen et al. 2003a). Even the experience of hallucinations itself may result from biases in cognitive processing in addition to sensory or perceptual abnormalities (Baker and Morrison 1998; Bentall et al. 1991).

The tendency to interpret anomalous perceptual experiences in a delusional way may be reinforced by the experience of social adversities. Evidence has linked traumatic experiences and adverse circumstances in childhood to later development of psychotic symptoms (Ellason and Ross 1997). Results of a comparison between patients with schizophrenia who were hearing voices and non-patients who were hearing voices, indicated that the disability incurred by hearing voices is associated with the reactivation of previous trauma and abuse (Honig et al. 1998). In the NEMESIS sample, experience of abuse before the age of 16 has been found to increase the risk of development of psychotic symptoms and disorder (Janssen et al. 2003 b). In the same sample, it was found that the experience of discrimination was associated with onset of delusional ideation (Janssen et al. 2003 c).

▪ Delusions and depression

Delusional ideation may in turn give rise to depressed feelings. In the study by Birchwood and Chadwick (1997), the depressive pathology in the patients with auditory hallucinations could be accounted for by the beliefs held by the individual about the power and intent of their voices, and not by voice topography or voice content. According to these authors, the sense of entrapment in the context of a threatening and powerful entity leads to feelings of powerlessness and depression. These beliefs and the negative emotional states they provoke may then contribute to the maintenance of psychotic symptoms and to the development of illness behaviour (Freeman and Garety 1999; Morrison 2001). Our finding that the risk increasing effect of depressed mood was partly mediated by the presence of delusional ideation may be explained along these lines.

The findings on the role of coping behaviour lend further support to this interpretation of our data. A coping strategy characterised by going along with and indulging in symptoms, yielding less experience of control, discriminates between those with and those without need for care in the context of psychotic symptoms. If distress, anxiety and depression in relation to psychotic illness are associated with perceived controllability, and feelings of subordination to omnipotent voices (Birchwood and Chadwick 1997; Morrison and Baker 2000), a symptomatic coping strategy of going along with the content of psychotic experiences may give rise to low perceived controllability and thus contribute to the development of need for care.

▪ Treatment issues

The proposed role for secondary beliefs and appraisals in the onset and maintenance of psychotic disorder has implications for treatment. Cognitive therapy focuses at the modification of cognitive processes (Alford and Beck 1994;

Beck 1976). Cognitive behavioural re-appraisal techniques could be instrumental in reducing the depression and fear generated by the voices and enhancing the perceived control over the experience. This may in some individuals prevent the formation of delusions and/or reduce the need for care (Chadwick and Birchwood 1994). Several studies have now evaluated the cognitive approach and have found that modification of beliefs can be successful in reducing the amount of time spent hallucinating as well as in the disruption caused by them (Gould et al. 2001; Haddock et al. 1998). Further elucidation of the cognitive processes involved in the onset and maintenance of clinical psychosis may contribute to the development of targeted psychological interventions.

References

Alford BA, Beck AT (1994) Cognitive therapy of delusional beliefs. Behav Res Ther 32:369–380
Bak M, Hanssen M, Bijl RV, Vollebergh W, Delespaul P, Van Os J (2003) When does experience of psychosis result in need for care? A prospective general population study. Schizophr Bull 429:349–358
Bak M, van der Spil F, Gunther N, Radstake S, Delespaul P, van Os J (2001a) Maastricht Assessment of Coping Strategies (MACS-I): a brief instrument to assess coping with psychotic symptoms. Acta Psychiatr Scand 103:453–459
Bak M, van der Spil F, Gunther N, Radstake S, Delespaul P, van Os J (2001b) MACS-II: does coping enhance subjective control over psychotic symptoms? Acta Psychiatr Scand 103:460–464
Baker CA, Morrison AP (1998) Cognitive processes in auditory hallucinations: attributional biases and metacognition. Psychol Med 28:1199–1208
Beck AT (1976) Cognitive therapy and the emotional disorders. International Universities Press. New York
Bentall RP, Baker GA, Havers S (1991) Reality monitoring and psychotic hallucinations. Br J Clin Psychol 30:213–222
Bentall RP, Kaney S (1989) Content specific information processing and persecutory delusions: an investigation using the emotional Stroop test. Br J Med Psychol 62:355–364
Bentall RP, Kinderman P, Kaney S (1994) The self, attributional processes and abnormal beliefs: towards a model of persecutory delusions. Behav Res Ther 32:331–341
Bijl RV, Ravelli A, van Zessen G (1998a) Prevalence of psychiatric disorder in the general population: results of The Netherlands Mental Health Survey and Incidence Study (NEMESIS). Soc Psychiatry Psychiatr Epidemiol 33:587–595
Bijl RV, van Zessen G, Ravelli A, de Rijk C, Langendoen Y (1998b) The Netherlands Mental Health Survey and Incidence Study (NEMESIS): objectives and design. Soc Psychiatry Psychiatr Epidemiol 33:581–586
Birchwood M, Chadwick P (1997) The omnipotence of voices: testing the validity of a cognitive model. Psychol Med 27:1345–1353
Boschi S, Adams RE, Bromet EJ, Lavelle JE, Everett E, Galambos N (2000) Coping with psychotic symptoms in the early phases of schizophrenia. Am J Orthopsychiatry 70:242–252
Carr V (1988) Patients' techniques for coping with schizophrenia: an exploratory study. Br J Med Psychol 61(Pt 4):339–352

Chadwick P, Birchwood M (1994) The omnipotence of voices. A cognitive approach to auditory hallucinations. Br J Psychiatry 164:190–201

Chapman LJ, Chapman JP, Kwapil TR, Eckblad M, Zinser MC (1994) Putatively psychosis-prone subjects 10 years later. J Abnorm Psychol 103:171–183

Chapman LJ, Edell WS, Chapman JP (1980) Physical anhedonia, perceptual aberration, and psychosis proneness. Schizophr Bull 6:639–653

Claridge G (1997) Schizotypy; implications for illness and health. Oxford University Press, Oxford

Claridge G, McCreery C, Mason O, Bentall R, Boyle G, Slade P, Popplewell D (1996) The factor structure of "schizotypal" traits: a large replication study. Br J Clin Psychol 35:103–115

Corcoran R, Mercer G, Frith CD (1995) Schizophrenia, symptomatology and social inference: investigating "theory of mind" in people with schizophrenia. Schizophr Res 17:5–13

Davidson M, Reichenberg A, Rabinowitz J, Weiser M, Kaplan Z, Mark M (1999) Behavioral and intellectual markers for schizophrenia in apparently healthy male adolescents. Am J Psychiatry 156:1328–1335

Dudley RE, John CH, Young AW, Over DE (1997) Normal and abnormal reasoning in people with delusions. Br J Clin Psychol 36:243–258

Eaton WW, Romanoski A, Anthony JC, Nestadt G (1991) Screening for psychosis in the general population with a self-report interview. J Nerv Ment Dis 179:689–693

Ellason JW, Ross CA (1997) Childhood trauma and psychiatric symptoms. Psychol Rep 80:447–450

Escher S, Romme M, Buiks A, Delespaul P, Van Os J (2002) Formation of delusional ideation in adolescents hearing voices: a prospective study. Am J Med Genet 114: 913–920

Falloon IR (1992) Early intervention for first episodes of schizophrenia: a preliminary exploration. Psychiatry 55:4–15

Fear C, Sharp H, Healy D (1996) Cognitive processes in delusional disorders. Br J Psychiatry 168:61–67

Freeman D, Garety PA (1999) Worry, worry processes and dimensions of delusions: an exploratory investigation of a role for anxiety processes in the maintenance of delusional distress. Behavioural and Cognitive Psychotherapy 27:47–62

Freeman D, Garety PA, Kuipers E (2001) Persecutory delusions: developing the understanding of belief maintenance and emotional distress. Psychol Med 31:1293–1306

Frith CD, Corcoran R (1996) Exploring 'theory of mind' in people with schizophrenia. Psychol Med 26:521–530

Garety P, Hemsley D (1994) Delusions: investigations into the psychology of delusional reasoning. Oxford University Press, Oxford

Garety PA, Freeman D (1999) Cognitive approaches to delusions: a critical review of theories and evidence. Br J Clin Psychol 38:113–154

Garety PA, Hemsley DR, Wessely S (1991) Reasoning in deluded schizophrenic and paranoid patients. Biases in performance on a probabilistic inference task. J Nerv Ment Dis 179:194–201

Garety PA, Kuipers E, Fowler D, Freeman D, Bebbington PE (2001) A cognitive model of the positive symptoms of psychosis. Psychol Med 31:189–195

Goldberg D, Huxley P (1980) Mental illness in the community: the pathway to psychiatric care. Tavistock Publications, London New York

Gould RA, Mueser KT, Bolton E, Mays V, Goff D (2001) Cognitive therapy for psychosis in schizophrenia: an effect size analysis. Schizophr Res 48:335–342

Haddock G, Morrison AP, Hopkins R, Lewis S, Tarrier N (1998) Individual cognitive-behavioural interventions in early psychosis. Br J Psychiatry (Suppl)172:101–106

Häfner H (1988) What is schizophrenia? Changing perspectives in epidemiology. Eur Arch Psychiatry Neurol Sci 238:63–72

Häfner H (1989) Application of epidemiological research toward a model for the etiology of schizophrenia. Schizophr Res 2:375–383

Häfner H, Loffler W, Maurer K, Hambrecht M, an der Heiden W (1999) Depression, negative symptoms, social stagnation and social decline in the early course of schizophrenia. Acta Psychiatr Scand 100:105–118

Hanssen M, Bak M, Bijl RV, Vollebergh W, van Os J (2002) Outcome of self-reported psychotic experiences in the general population: a prospective study. (Submitted manuscript)

Hanssen M, Bijl RV, Vollebergh W, Van Os J (2003) Self-reported psychotic experiences in the general population: a valid screening tool for DSM-III-R psychotic disorders? Acta Psychiatr Scand 107:369–377

Hanssen M, Krabbendam L, de Graaf R, Vollebergh W, van Os J (2003) The role of distress in delusion formation. Br J Psychiatry (in press)

Hennekens CH, Buring JE (1987) Epidemiology in medicine. Little, Brown and Company. Boston Toronto

Honi A, Romme MA, Ensink BJ, Escher SD, Pennings MH, deVries MW (1998) Auditory hallucinations: a comparison between patients and nonpatients. J Nerv Ment Dis 186:646–651

Hultman CM, Wieselgren IM, Ohman A (1997) Relationships between social support, social coping and life events in the relapse of schizophrenic patients. Scand J Psychol 38:3–13

Janssen I, Hanssen M, Bak M, Bijl RV, de Graaf R, Vollebergh W, McKenzie K, van Os J (2003c) Discrimination and delusional ideation. Br J Psychiatry 182:71–76

Janssen I, Krabbendam L, Bak M, Hanssen M, Vollebergh W, de Graaf R, van Os J (2003b) Childhood abuse as a risk factor for schizophrenia. Acta Psychiatr Scand (in press)

Janssen I, Krabbendam L, Jolles J, van Os J (2003a). Alterations in theory of mind in patients with schizophrenia and non-psychotic relatives. Acta Psychiatr Scand 108:110–117

Johns LC, van Os J (2001) The continuity of psychotic experiences in the general population. Clin Psychol Rev 21:1125–1141

Kinderman P, Bentall RP (1997) Causal attributions in paranoia and depression: internal, personal, and situational attributions for negative events. J Abnorm Psychol 106:341–345

Klosterkotter J, Hellmich M, Steinmeyer EM, Schultze-Lutter F (2001) Diagnosing schizophrenia in the initial prodromal phase. Arch Gen Psychiatry 58:158–164

Krabbendam L, Myin-Germeys I, Hanssen M, Bijl RV, de Graaf R, Vollebergh W, Bak M, van Os J (2002a) Hallucinatory experiences and onset of psychotic disorder: evidence that the risk is mediated by delusion formation. (Submitted manuscript)

Krabbendam L, Myin-Germeys I, Hanssen M, de Graaf R, Vollebergh W, van Os J (2002b) Depressed mood predicts onset of psychotic disorder in individuals who report hallucinatory experiences. (Submitted manuscript)

Kwapil TR, Miller MB, Zinser MC, Chapman J, Chapman LJ (1997) Magical ideation and social anhedonia as predictors of psychosis proneness: a partial replication. J Abnorm Psychol 106:491–495

Larsen TK, Friis S, Haahr U, Joa I, Johannessen JO, Melle I, Opjordsmoen S, Simonsen E, Vaglum P (2001) Early detection and intervention in first-episode schizophrenia: a critical review. Acta Psychiatr Scand 103:323–334

Lukoff D, Nuechterlein KH, Ventura J (1986) Manual for the expanded brief psychiatric rating scale. Schizophr Bull 12:594–602

Lukoff D, Snyder K, Ventura J, Nuechterlein KH (1984) Life events, familial stress, and coping in the developmental course of schizophrenia. Schizophr Bull 10:258–292

Maher BA (1974) Delusional thinking and perceptual disorder. J Individ Psychol 30:98–113

Maher BA (1988) Anomalous experience and delusional thinking: the logic of explanations. In: Oltmanns TF, Maher BA (eds) Delusional Beliefs. Wiley, New York, pp 77–114

McGorry PD, McFarlane C, Patton GC, Bell R, Hibbert ME, Jackson HJ, Bowes G (1995) The prevalence of prodromal features of schizophrenia in adolescence: a preliminary survey. Acta Psychiatr Scand 92:241–249

McGorry PD, Yung A, Phillips L (2001) Ethics and early intervention in psychosis: keeping up the pace and staying in step. Schizophr Res 51:17–29

Morrison AP (2001) The interpretation of intrusions in psychosis: an integrative cognitive approach to hallucinations and delusions. Behavioural and Cognitive Psychotherapy 29:257–276

Morrison AP, Baker CA (2000) Intrusive thoughts and auditory hallucinations: a comparative study of intrusions in psychosis. Behav Res Ther 38:1097–1106

Nicholson IR, Neufeld RW (1992) A dynamic vulnerability perspective on stress and schizophrenia. Am J Orthopsychiatry 62:117–130

Nuechterlein KH, Dawson ME (1984) A heuristic vulnerability/stress model of schizophrenic episodes. Schizophr Bull 10:300–312

Overall JE, Gorham DE (1962) The brief psychiatric rating scale. Psychol Rep 10:799–812

Peters ER, Joseph SA, Garety PA (1999) Measurement of delusional ideation in the normal population: introducing the PDI (Peters et al, Delusions Inventory). Schizophr-Bull 25:553–576

Phillips LJ, Yung AR, McGorry PD (2000) Identification of young people at risk of psychosis: validation of personal assessment and crisis evaluation clinic intake criteria. Aust N Z J Psychiatry 34(Suppl):S164–169

Poulton R, Caspi A, Moffitt TE, Cannon M, Murray R, Harrington H (2000) Children's self-reported psychotic symptoms and adult schizophreniform disorder: a 15-year longitudinal study. Arch Gen Psychiatry 57:1053–1058

Romme MA, Honig A, Noorthoorn EO, Escher AD (1992) Coping with hearing voices: an emancipatory approach. Br J Psychiatry 161:99–103

Rose G, Barker DJ (1978) Epidemiology for the uninitiated. What is a case? Dichotomy or continuum? Br Med J 2:873–874

Sackett DL, Richardson WS, Rosenberg W, Haynes RB (1997) Evidence-based medicine. Churchill Livingstone, New York

Slade M, Phelan M, Thornicroft G, Parkman S (1996) The Camberwell Assessment of Need (CAN): comparison of assessments by staff and patients of the needs of the severely mentally ill. Soc Psychiatry Psychiatr Epidemiol 31:109–113

Spitzer RL, Williams JB, Gibbon M, First MB (1992) The Structured Clinical Interview for DSM-III-R (SCID), I: history, rationale, and description. Arch Gen Psychiatry 49:624–629

Susser ES, Struening EL (1990) Diagnosis and screening for psychotic disorders in a study of the homeless. Schizophr Bull 16:133–145

Tien AY (1991) Distributions of hallucinations in the population. Soc Psychiatry Psychiatr Epidemiol 26:287–292

van den Bosch RJ, Rombouts RP (1997) Coping and cognition in schizophrenia and depression. Compr Psychiatry 38:341–344

Van Os J, Hanssen M, Bijl RV, Ravelli A (2000) Strauss (1969) revisited: a psychosis continuum in the general population? Schizophr Res 45:11–20

Van Os J, Verdoux H, Maurice Tison S, Gay B, Liraud F, Salamon R, Bourgeois M (1999) Self-reported psychosis-like symptoms and the continuum of psychosis. Soc Psychiatry Psychiatr Epidemiol 34:459–463

Verdoux H (2001) Have the times come for early intervention in psychosis? Acta Psychiatr Scand 103:321–322

Verdoux H, Maurice-Tison S, Gay B, Van Os J, Salomon R, Bourgeois ML (1998) A survey of delusional ideation in primary-care patients. Psychol Med 28:127–134

Vollrath M, Alnaes R, Torgersen S (1994) Coping and MCMI-II symptom scales. J Clin Psychol 50:727–736

World Health Organization (1990) Composite International Diagnostic Interview (CIDI); Version 1.0. World Health Organization, Geneva

▌ Discussion: Epidemiology and environment

WILLIAM W. EATON

Department of Mental Health, Bloomberg School of Public Health, Johns Hopkins University

The four papers represent widely varying perspectives and data. They are all informative, but it is difficult to draw a general summary message that applies to all. Therefore I comment on each one individually, making comparisons and drawing common conclusions where possible.

The paper "Schizophrenia and migration," by Jean-Paul Selten and Elizabeth Cantor-Graae, combines a thorough review of the literature on epidemiological studies of migration and schizophrenia, with a conceptual synthesis which includes a plausible neurological process explaining the effects of migration for the individual.

With respect to the review, it is nice to see the three-decade-long career of Benjamin Malzberg recognized. Malzberg was publishing his early monographs when Mort Kramer was still a doctoral student in biostatistics.

The literature includes many puzzles: the higher risk among internal migrants (mostly rural African Americans) in the United States, the higher risk among Black immigrants, but not south Asians, in the UK, and the higher risk among Surinamese, but not Turks, to the Netherlands; and other anomalies. These are not explained by country of origin (genetic or cultural effects), since the rates in the countries of origin are often or usually lower than the migrants. They are not explained by the stress of immigration since the effects endure, even to the second generation. They are not explained by diagnostic bias.

The authors state that biological hypotheses are not parsimonious because there are effects in the second generation. Second generation effects are well-explained by the hypothesis of *Cephalo-Pelvic Disproportion* (CPD) (Warner 1995); but this hypothesis has more trouble explaining the first generation effects. The CPD hypothesis has been challenged by a single, case control, self report study (Hutchinson et al. 1997). Half of the genetic material for the second generation (i.e., the mother's eggs) are formed in the country of origin, so that if there were an environmental factor that affected both the health of the mother and the formation of gametes, this would explain a two-generational effect, but not a third generation. It has been suggested that schizophrenia is a balanced polymorphism, similar to, but much more complex than, sickle cell anemia (Huxley et al. 1964). It has been further proposed that the advantageous side of the polymorphism is a tendency to separate from others under conditions of crowding (Stevens and Price 1996), possibly the "innate restlessness" from Ødegaard, but this tendency would not seem to be strong enough to produce the size of the differences often observed, and the situations of countries with highly deleted populations do not show a diminution in rate, in general. Another biological explanation might be that there is a rise in the level of assortative mating by personality with immigration. If "like married like" in terms of personality, instead of ethnic background or social class, the result would be an expansion in variation of a variety of personality traits, including those associated with the genetics of schizophrenia. (Elsewhere I have called this *Sociogenetic Lag* (2001).) But this would not explain the increased risk in the first generation. These hypotheses are not parsimonious, as the authors state.

Social hypotheses include the usual lower status of immigrants – but many immigrants are not of lower status; and many immigrant groups with lower status do not have higher rates. For more than a hundred years, it has been the common wisdom that lower socioeconomic status individuals are at higher risk for schizophrenia – this is actually the logic that sent me into sociology for a career. However, the most recent studies, all from Scandinavia, suggest higher risk among those born into upper, not lower, classes. So it is not social adversity per se, or lower socioeconomic status.

The authors propose uncertainty about social rank or status as the crucial variable. This is a good hypothesis, similar to one proposed earlier by Kleiner and Parker on "goal-striving stress" (1966). Table 1 shows results reorganized from that study – the psychotics have much greater discrepancies between their ideal and the actual selves. But, as the several categories of "self" in Table 1 imply, the central variable, "social rank or status," is not precisely defined. Ranking of individuals can occur with respect to wealth, income, prestige, power, and so forth. The group or population in which the rank is conceptualized is not stated: for example, is it the nation as a whole, or a city population – a macro level concept? Or, is it the primary group of individuals in the immediate social network? Animal studies imply that the primary group would be the most important: but since socioeconomic status varies by ethnic group, it may be relative rank within the ethnic or migrant group which is important – in effect deleting the power of the concept of rank. Use of the more general word "status" leaves open the possibility that uncertainty as to position itself, not rank, is important. Group membership, such as in a family, club, or ethnic group, is an example. This slight imprecision suggests a concept not dissimilar from Stonequist's *Marginal Man*, "the individual who through migration, education, marriage, or some other influence leaves one

Table 1. Goal striving stress scores from Parker and Kleiner (Eaton and Harrison 2001)

	General population	Treated psychotics
▌ Occupation	5.3	9.3
▌ Income	16.1	23.2
▌ Self	14.5	19.7
▌ Sample size	1464	1053

social group or culture without making a satisfactory adjustment to another and finds himself on the margin of each but a member of neither" (1937). For the marginal man, it is mobility itself that is the problem. The idea is generalized to membership in many groups, and, then, in effect, it becomes an aspect of the social identity, about which there is a strong literature in psychology, social psychology, and sociology (Baumeister 1986; Burke 1991; Giddens 1991; Scheibe 1995; Thoits 1991). Those with diffuse or uncertain social identities would be at high risk. The social identity is actually a process which occurs via frontal lobe cognitive systems which have been implicated in vulnerability to schizophrenia. Thus, the model could benefit by including a distribution of cognitive vulnerabilities, possibly inherited, which might interact with social position to produce uncertainty about social rank.

In spite of these criticisms, this new hypothesis builds carefully on prior work and unifies a wide range of research results. It is at least precise enough to evaluate empirically. One way to test it, for example, would be to look into the literature on subjective social class – a crucial variable for sociologists, especially those interested in class solidarity. According to this hypothesis, the discrepancy between objective measures of social class, and subjective measures, should be greater, and with more variation, among migrants than among non-migrants, and among persons with schizophrenia than those who do not have schizophrenia.

The paper "Course and outcome of schizophrenia: toward a new social biology of psychosis" by Glynn Harrison proposes the importance of social space in the etiology of schizophrenia. The proposal is somewhat similar in its orientation to the model of Selten and Cantor-Graae. Harrison notes, as I did above, the possibility that different components of social space, based on social networks or neighborhood, for example, may be important. The difference is that Harrison focuses on the social space itself – something I would call the social identity, as mentioned above – and Selten and Cantor-Graae focus on uncertainty as regards one specific aspect of the social space, that is, social rank. But we know from Dr. Harrison's other work that he is also interested in the cognitive problem-solving which is involved in sorting oneself through social space.

Harrison evaluates ideas about social space using data on the chronicity of schizophrenia in different cultures. An important focus is on the effects of the centers in the IPSS, DOSMeD, and ISoS studies, which were coordinated by the World Health Organisation. In my opinion these effects represent cultural differences, for the most part.

What is culture and how could it effect schizophrenia? Culture is knowledge, roles, and values shared by a group. Knowledge includes symbols and symbol systems; roles are shared expectations for behavior; values includes goals, attitudes and morals. Acquisition of culture varies by individual in any group, and each individual acquires many cultures. Culture is distinct from cultural products and expressions because, by this definition, it is mental. How can culture influence psychosis? It can affect the form of expression of a universal disease or problem – for example, the content of delusions as Carlos Leon showed many years ago. It can create certain tensions or possibilities for

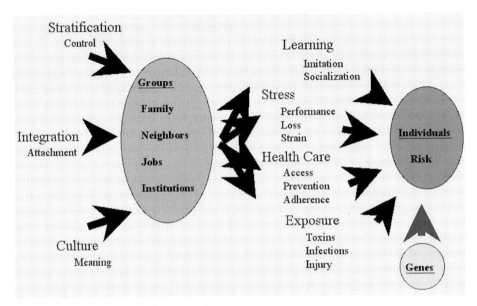

Fig. 1. Social processes in the human environment

local expressions which are not universal, such as the culture-bound syndromes like boufee delirante (Pichot 1986) or brief remitting psychosis (Susser 1994). The effects in the cross cultural studies of schizophrenia suggest that culture creates or expands on tensions which in turn change the risk for universal disorders, of which schizophrenia might possibly be one. Uncertainty about social rank, in the prior paper, and social space, in this paper, are mental concepts that affect risk for schizophrenia. Fig. 1 is a conceptual framework similar to that of Berkman and Glass (Berkman and Glass 2000), included in the paper by Harrison: it is slightly more detailed as regards "biological" environmental risk factors. Over the years I improved Fig. 1, with the help of Glynn Harrison and others, to Fig. 2. One difference is the section in the upper right, entitled "individual," which has to do with the psychological level of analysis. Uncertainty about social rank, and thoughts about social space, both pass through a mental synthesizing process which generates and maintains aspects of the social identity. As Fig. 1 shows, culture, associated with the innate drive for meaning, is associated with the tendency to achieve this mental synthesis. Thus, culture, a mental concept, gives us the opportunity to learn about this causal pathway. Focusing on India for future research, where results diverge, is recommended by Harrison for this reason, and I agree.

The paper "Childhood meningitis and adult schizophrenia" by Wagner Gattaz, André Abrahão, and Roberto Foccacia shows that meningitis increases risk for schizophrenia. In a way, this study reaffirms the need for a complete biosocial model, including exposure to infections (Fig. 2). An important aspect of the design is the use of the sibling control – a decision I agree with, be-

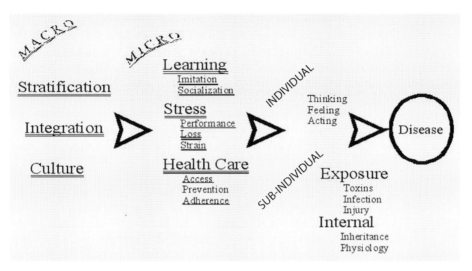

Fig. 2. Biosocial framework for the etiology of disease

cause it allows appropriate focus on the agent in question. The five-fold increase in prevalence (which is actually a relative risk, I believe) is convincing. The new and important aspect of this work, it seems to me, is to extend the period during which infections raise risk for schizophrenia beyond the fetal period, into and through the period of synaptogenesis. But there may be new insights from further information about the epidemic itself. Was it limited to São Paulo or was it part of a general epidemic throughout Brazil (from which we might learn other aspects of the infectious process) (Bryan et al. 1990)? Was the agent a virus or bacteria associated with schizophrenia in other studies? What was the case fatality rate (which would help characterize the survivors who are later at high risk for schizophrenia)? Is there a hypothesized mechanism which may, or may not, distinguish this cause from other early infections (or is it a more general cause such as fever)? A result of the matched design is the difficulty understanding how meningitis fits into the biosocial framework in general. For example, the prevalence of mental disorders was unusually high in the study groups – about 60%. Possibly this prevalence was high because living conditions that promoted the spread of meningitis also were associated with the prevalence of mental disorders. The most likely candidate might be socioeconomic status, poverty, or crowding, which are associated with transmission of enteroviruses, often the agents in meningitis. So, in order to fill out the biosocial model, it would be good to know more about the general characteristics of this epidemic.

The paper "Psychotic features in the general population: risk factors for what?" by Lydia Krabbendam, Manon Hanssen, Maarten Bak, and Jim van Os uses a multiwave survey to determine whether phenomena usually considered as signs and symptoms of psychosis, occurring individually, or without other necessary criteria for presence of disorder, can predict onset of the full disorder. An analysis similar to this was performed with longitudinal data from the Epidemiologic Catchment Area (ECA) Program data, but without the advantage of the clinical rating as an outcome (Tien and Eaton 1992). These studies raise the conceptual issue of the continuity of psychosis, as well as the methodologic topic of whether one can measure these putative signs and symptoms in the context of a survey – that is, without a psychiatrist, from a single highly structured interview in which most of the data are unedited and unquestioned reports from the subject. This is an important topic since the putative signs and symptoms are widespread in the general population and there is the tantalizing possibility of screening to locate and prevent new onsets.

It is helpful to define terms more precisely. Since symptoms and signs are indicators of disease, it may be helpful to avoid using terms which do not pre-judge the issue of the presence of disease. So I prefer to use the more in-clusive terms "complaints and behaviors" instead of "symptoms and signs," until I have judged that the disease is present. It is also awkward to use the term "risk factors" for aspects of thinking, feeling, and acting, that in another context are presenting features of the disorder. So I use the terms "precursor" for these features when it is not clear whether the disorder is present, and "prodrome" when they indicate ineluctable progress to full criteria for disorder (Eaton et al. 1995). The presence of prodrome can only be judged retrospectively.

The notion of this paper which is somewhat new is to screen via a *trajectory* towards disorder. Study 1 uses cross-sectional data to show that survey-style data on complaints and behaviors, obtained via the structured interview with the respondent in effect rating the responses, but without features of in-terrogation, cross-examination, and clinical rating probably often represents signs and symptoms, and serves as a screen for psychosis. Studies 2–4 focus on trajectories.

For the epidemiologist, incidence is a measure of the force of morbidity in the population. If we can measure that force after it is present, but before the disorder becomes fully apparent, we might be able to prevent the occurrence of the full-blown disorder. However, the usual way that epidemiologists think about incidence (Fig. 3, top) is constraining because it limits the information to dichotomies, albeit dichotomies observed over time (1994). In the context of development, it is useful to think about the force of incidence in terms of *intensification* and *acquisition* (Eaton et al. 1989). The bottom half of Fig. 3 shows a revised diagram, set up with three waves as in the paper by Krabben-dam et al. In the figure, each horizontal line or rectangle represents an indi-vidual case. The vertical width of the rectangle represents the intensity of the sign or symptom, and there is a criterion width which indicates sufficient in-tensity to regard the disorder itself as present, connecting the quantitative variation to the dichotomy of the epidemiologist. Case #3 from the top is re-presented in the bottom half as the ideal type in epidemiology: more or less instantaneous passage from no pathology at all, to the presence of disease. Case #5 is the slowly developing disorder, in which the sign or symptom is present to a lesser degree, but progresses over the time period of observation,

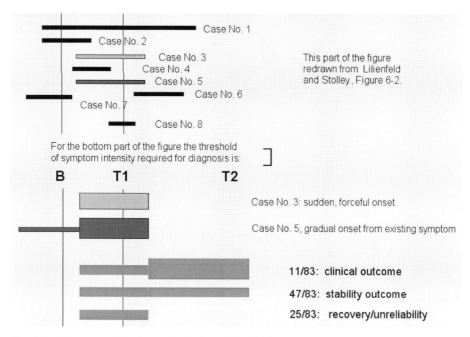

Fig. 3. Incidence, intensification, and the force of morbidity

to full a fledged disorder. This is the logic of study 2, with the minor exception that those with signs or symptoms during the year prior to the baseline are eliminated from the risk set. The difference in widths of the two sections of the case-5-rectangle amount to a trajectory, and if there were more waves of the survey, this trajectory could be estimated with more precision, and would have a quantitative aspect equivalent to a slope – the higher the slope, presumably, the more likely the onset. The slope could be used to estimate the force of morbidity in that individual, and a common or average slope would estimate the force in the population. The bottom three rectangles represent the three aspects of study 2: at T1 there is a new onset of signs or symptoms, which at T2 is divided into:

1) clinical cases;
2) the continuing presence of the signs or symptoms below the threshold of case definition; or
3) a recovery (which also might be thought of as measurement error).

Another way to think of the force of morbidity is the acquisition of symptoms and signs. Here the syndromal qualities of the signs and symptoms is important, as, under this formulation, it is impossible to judge the presence of the disease without observing the covariation of more than one sign and symptom. So the trajectory here becomes the rate at which signs and symptoms are added (Fig. 4) (Eaton 2001). Somewhere along the way to building a syndrome, the disease process becomes complete, and a set of not-too-closely-

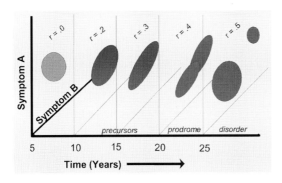

Fig. 4. Symptom acquisition and the force of morbidity

covaried signs and symptoms becomes so tightly covaried that it is certain that the disease will appear. Studies 3 and 4 of the paper by Krabbendam et al. approach the issue of screening in this fashion, addressing the issue of whether the presence of depression or delusion, together with a hallucination, predicts to psychosis (study 3); or whether hallucinations in the presence of distress predict to delusions (study 4).

These are wonderful concepts applied thoughtfully with unusual data. As the authors note, the predictive value is too low to actually be useful for screening and prevention. It is still not clear to me that the concept of hallucination or delusion, absent psychosis, is useful, because hallucinations and delusions, if we call them that, are so different among the five or ten percent who respond positively to survey questions, as compared to hallucinations and delusions among the less than one percent who are psychotic. I believe the majority of the positive responses are metaphors for private experiences, even if the linguistic designations for the metaphor are absent, whereas true hallucinations and delusions represent more or less accurate portrayals of private experiences.

This is the third symposium on the search for the causes of schizophrenia that I have participated in. We have not yet found "the" cause. But the amount of knowledge we now have about schizophrenia, compared to what existed 30 years ago, is truly phenomenal, and due in part to efforts such as this.

References

1. Baumeister RF (1986) Identity: Cultural Change and the Struggle for Self. Oxford University Press, New York
2. Berkman LF, Glass T (2000) Social integration, social networks, social support, and health. In: Berkman L, Kawachi I (eds) Social Epidemiology. Oxford University Press, Oxford
3. Bryan JP, de Silva HR, Tavares A, Rocha H, Scheld WM (1990) Etiology and mortality of bacterial meningitis in northeastern Brazil. Rev Infect Dis 12(1): 128–135
4. Burke PJ (1991) Identity process and social stress. Am Soc Rev 56:836–849
5. Eaton W (2001) The Sociology of Mental Disorders. Praeger, Westport, CT

6. Eaton WW, Badawi M, Melton B (1995) Prodromes and precursors: epidemiologic data for primary prevention of disorders with slow onset. Am J Psychiatry 152(7):967–972
7. Eaton WW, Kramer M, Anthony JC, Chee EML, Shapiro S (1989) Conceptual and methodological problems in estimation of the incidence of mental disorders from field survey data. In: Cooper B, Helgason T (eds) Epidemiology and the Prevention of Mental Disorders. Routledge, London, pp 108–127
8. Giddens A (1991) Modernity and Self-Identity: Self and Society in the Late Modern Age. Stanford University Press, Stanford, CA.
9. Hutchinson G, Takei N, Bhugra D, Fahy TA, Gilvarry C, Mallett R, Moran P, Leff J, Murray RM (1997) Increased rate of psychosis among African-Caribbeans in Britain is not due to an excess of pregnancy and birth complications. Br J Psychiatry 171:145–147
10. Huxley J, Mayr E, Osmond H, Hoffner A (1964) Schizophrenia as a genetic morphism. Nature 204:220–221
11. Lilienfeld DE, Stolley PD (1994) Foundations of Epidemiology. Oxford University Press, New York
12. Parker S, Kleiner RJ (1966) Mental Illness in the Urban Negro Community. Free Press, New York
13. Pichot P (1986) The concept of 'Bouffee delirante' with special reference to the Scandinavian concept of reactive psychosis. Psychopathology 19:35–43
14. Scheibe KE (1995) Self-Studies: The Psychology of Self and Identity. Praeger, Westport, CT
15. Stevens A, Price J (1996) Evolutionary Psychiatry: A New Beginning. Routledge, London
16. Stonequist EV (1937) The Marginal Man: A Study in Personality and Culture Conflict. Charles Scribner's Sons, New York
17. Susser EM (1994) Epidemiology of nonaffective acute remitting psychosis vs schizophrenia: sex and sociocultural setting. Arch Gen Psychiatry 51:294–301
18. Thoits PA (1991) On merging identity theory and stress research. Social Psychology Quarterly 54:101–112
19. Tien AY, Eaton WW (1992) Psychopathologic precursors and sociodemographic risk factors for the schizophrenia syndrome. Archives of General Psychiatry 49:37–46
20. Warner R (1995) Time trends in schizophrenia: changes in obstetric risk factors with industrialization. Schizophrenia Bulletin 21(3):483–500

Section 2
Precursors of schizophrenia

Early developmental abnormalities – risk for what?

D. John Done

Dept. Psychology, University of Hertfordshire, Hatfield, U.K. AL10 9AB

Introduction

The pathological process that leads to adult onset schizophrenia can be traced back to childhood in a substantial number of cases and this appears not to be restricted to cases with early onset. Brodaty (1999) reported a similar finding for schizophrenia with onset after the age of 50. This position emerges from quite different disciplines included epidemiological, neuropathological, structural brain imaging and neuropsychological studies of schizophrenia. In addition, the phenomenology and epidemiology of child onset schizophrenia strongly indicate that it is the same illness as adult-onset schizophrenia albeit with a much earlier age of onset (Asarnow and Tompson 1999; Nicolson et al. 2003; Asarnow et al. 2001). Thus theories about the aetiology and pathology of schizophrenia have started to embrace the discipline of developmental psychopathology, in which most theories about causality are complex, and dynamic rather than simple and deterministic (e.g. Sroufe 1997; Cicchetti and Cannon 1999; Kagan 1992; Harrington 2001). Initiating aetiological factors (e.g. genetic predisposition, obstetric complications etc.) might then offer a low risk for specific adult psychopathology, but high risk for a range of psychopathologies, since other causal factors tilt the developmental trajectory toward (i.e. increase risk), or away from (i.e. protective factors) a particular endpoint. I will argue here that evidence from cohort studies suggest that adult schizophrenia may well be an endpoint of one trajectory but other trajectories can occur given the same childhood risk factors. A starting point then is to outline the evidence base for early developmental factors in schizophrenia. Although 'early' legitimately covers the period from neonate through to adolescence, this paper will be concerned with the pattern of cognitive and behavioural features that characterise school-aged children at increased risk for schizophrenia. One reason for this restriction is that it makes discussion about risk more manageable. Developmental delay (e.g. age at first utterance, started to walk) are valid measures of abnormality in infancy, whereas their validity becomes limited in childhood, except for a small number of severely retarded individuals. Instead these become replaced by measures of vocabulary and motor skill. In addition, assessments in childhood and adolescence, when cohort members are at school, are typically more common. Thus trying to test hypotheses will stand a greater chance if these are pitched at developmental abnormalities at this age rather than an earlier age. With this evidence we can begin to sketch out a characteristic pattern of childhood risk factors for adult schizophrenia. Here we try to sketch out a set of risk factors in a manner akin to a set of symptoms that define DSM-IV Axis 1 disorders. Risk factors (A through G below) are organised into a hierarchy of signs based on the magnitude of effect size (e.g. odds ratios, relative risk, attribual risk, positive predictive value etc.), as well as their robustness (i.e. how well replicated) reported in published research.

(A) Early psychotic-like experiences. Limited to the Dunedin study (Poulton et al. 2000), although the odds ratio was high (5 or 16 depending on criterion) and providing a positive predictive value or PPV = 9% (assuming a 1% lifetime risk), which is the highest PPV reported to date.

(B) Having few friends, unpopularity, shunned by peers, schizoid. Reported in nearly every study (e.g. Malmberg et al. 1998; Davidson et al. 1999; Cannon et al. 2001; Brodaty et al. 1999; Johns et al. 1982; Watt et al. 1972; Ambelas 1992; Foerster et al. 1991), and in some studies provide the largest effect size. Earlier studies reported large effects of gender, with unpopularity being found for boys, but not girls (Watt et al. 1972; Foerster et al. 1991).

(C) Abnormal patterns of social and interpersonal behaviour. Various measures including general measures of social functioning (Davidson et al. 1999) or more specific ones, e.g. externalising, internalising or problem behaviours (e.g. Done et al. 1994). Reported in most studies, and sometimes providing the largest effect size (Done et al. 1994; Malmberg et al. 1998; Davidson et al. 1999; Cannon et al. 2001, 2002; Brodaty et al. 1999), although a few studies report small or no such effects (e.g. Jones et al. 1994; Cannon 1999). Some studies (e.g. Done et al. 1994; Watt et al. 1972) have reported a characteristic pattern in children who develop adult schizophrenia (hereon referred to as Pre-S children), but Davidson et al. (1999) with a larger sample report heterogeneity, some being withdrawn and others showing excessive externalising or antisocial tendencies.

(D) Language impairments. Typically these provide high odds ratios, but low attribual risk, i.e. only a small percent of the population fulfil criteria, but these are good predictors (Bearden et al. 2000). These are not disorders of expression/comprehension (Cannon et al. 2002), which would be the traditional criteria for rating a child as having a language impairment. The relatively small number of cases may therefore be cases with clear thought disorder (Ott et al. 2002), or a marked disorder of communication.

(E) Poor achievement in school. Most studies report below average academic grades in childhood (Jones et al. 1994; Cannon et al. 2002; David et al. 1997; Reichenberg et al. 2002) whereas others report effect sizes putting Pre-S children within the normal range of academic abilities (Cannon et al. 1999; Fuller et al. 2002).

(F) Neurological soft signs (primarily motor). Frequently reported in young Pre-S children (Leask et al. 2002; Jones et al. 1994; Walker et al. 1994; Isohanni et al. 2001; Niemi et al. 2003). These have included clumsiness (Leask et al. 2002), developmental delay (Jones et al. 1994), and choreoathetotic/other neuromotor abnormalities (Walker et al. 1994).

(G) Neurotic/anxious. There is considerable overlap between the concepts of neurosis, anxiety and internalising behaviour. Reported in some studies (Done et al. 1994; Jones 1994; Malmberg et al. 1998).

Why try to specify a childhood endophenotype for schizophrenia?

One reason for trying to move toward a specific characterisation of Pre-S children is that it can then be adopted as an endophenotype. That is to say it could provide greater specificity in the identification of gene carriers than relying on standardised diagnostic criteria such as DSM or ICD (Skuse 2001). A second reason, and the one focused on here, is that it provides greater efficiency in the identification of cases who might then benefit from appropriate preventive measures. This latter reason has been given added weight from the major developments in early intervention research and the belief that early interventions can limit the effects of a pathological process (McGlashan et al. 2001; McGlashan and Johanessen 1996). Perhaps the earlier the intervention then the greater its effectiveness. On this basis we might start to consider identification of cases in childhood and implement preventive measures. Such an ambition depends on the predictive validity and reliability of a specified endophenotype. Here is where there is a need for caution. Firstly the potential for error in quantitative estimates of risk coming out of case-control studies and secondly the measurement error inherent in birth or conscript cohorts which are opportunistic.

Clarke and Clarke (2000) note that outcomes of cohort studies (i.e. prospective) tend to reveal different results from case-control studies (i.e. follow-back or retrospective designs). In a prospective cohort study, cases deemed to be high risk (e.g. meeting criteria for the endophenotype) are identified and followed up. The high risk paradigm has of course been adopted in some 16 prospective cohort studies (Niemi et al. 2003). The criteria for selecting cases was principally genetic risk although other biological markers such as eye-movements have been used. No prospective study has been carried out to date in which a cognitive-behavioural endophenotype for schizophrenia has been defined according to risk factors A–G mentioned earlier. Empirical evidence for childhood risk factors has come from variations of the retrospective case-control study nested within a cohort. In case-control studies, one starts with the identification of cases (e.g. DSM-IV schizophrenia) and a matched group of controls and then examine available evidence for antecedent risk factors. Such nested case-control designs have typically utilised either birth cohorts e.g. NCDS (Done et al. 1991, 1994), NSHD (Jones et al. 1994; van Os et al. 1997), Dunedin cohort (Poulton et al. 2000; Cannon et al. 2002), and the North Finland 1966 cohort, or conscript cohorts such as the Swedish (Malmberg et al. 1998) and Israeli (Davidson et al. 1999) conscript cohorts. Case registers of patients and matched controls are identified and linked with records collected premorbidly during childhood/adolescence by teachers, parents, etc. A less robust case-control design has been used in which childhood information is obtained through structured interviews of parents or patients post onset of adult psychopathology typically using the Premorbid Social Adjustment scale (Cannon-Spoor et al. 1982).

Clarke and Clarke (2000) note some critical differences between case-control and true cohort studies (either retrospective or prospective). The former tend to start with homogeneous populations (e.g. DSM-IV criteria), and they also tend to reveal similar life paths for cases. To end up as a case there are only a few developmental trajectories that could have been taken. Cohort studies tend to yield more diverse and heterogeneous life paths, especially if the baseline is assessed when development is rapid and fluctuating, as it is in early childhood. Perhaps because of these differences, and a Western philosophy in which "... the present is continuous with the past." (Kagan and Zentner 1996), there has been a tendency for case-control studies to lend support to deterministic models in which causes early in development are seen as producing a linear sequence of psychological outcomes that ultimately lead to psychiatric disorder. The classic neurodevelopmental hypothesis of schizophrenia is a good example of a deterministic model. A disease process, affecting critical circuits in the brain, is initiated by a pre-/perinatal insult. The resulting lesion is expressed in adulthood, when developmental changes 'enable' the lesion to be expressed as a psychopathological disorder (Weinberger 1987; Marenco and Weinberger 2000). Here single events in childhood are seen as the cause of a later emergence of schizophrenia in adulthood, albeit with cognitive and behavioural abnormalities along the way. Prospective studies, on the other hand, tend to give more weight to a 'self righting tendency', where a substantial minority, or even majority of 'at risk' cases have a different outcome to that predicted (Clarke and Clarke 2000). The degree to which risk estimates differ in retrospective and prospective studies led Parker et al. (1995) to suggest that case-control studies '... are useful for suggesting connections between adult symptoms and childhood behaviour, but cannot provide data interpretable in terms of predictive risk' (p. 124).

There is another caution that we need to consider when evaluating the predictive validity and reliability of the proposed childhood endophenotype of schizophrenia. This is based on the opportunistic nature of the studies. Birth and conscript cohorts were not designed with schizophrenia in mind. Hence neurodevelopmental models of schizophrenia did not inform the choice of assessments. Cohorts such as these tend to use screening tools which assess characteristics which are distributed throughout the whole population rather than confined to a small subgroup with a life-time risk of only 1%. For example behaviour is typically assessed with scales measuring externalising or internalising subtypes of behaviour, which are known as good epidemiological tools to estimate mental health in study populations (Elander and Rutter 1996). However, these are manifest behaviours which can result from quite different underlying psychological causes. Siegal and Scovill (2000) identify 8 reasons for the emergence of childhood problem behaviour, including need for belonging, avoidance of boredom, personally seeking competence, seeking control of disruptive environments. As such, we might expect quite distinct forms of child psychopathology to produce excess externalising. Conduct problems in children with Asperger's syndrome can result from poor empathy or impaired social cognition (Klin and Volkmar 1995). Sensation seeking can lead to adolescent problem behaviour (Zuckerman 1979) and seeking control can be caused by rearing in adverse environments. Thus the reports of peer rejection, and deviant social behaviour in Pre-S children may well be proxy measures, i.e. they are surface manifestations of an underlying psychological state. So they may result from the psychotic-like experiences reported by Poulton et al. (2000), or perhaps impaired social reciprocity or even conduct disorder. In a retrospective case-control study of children seen in a psychiatric clinic (Cannon et al. 2001), hysterical symptoms and overactivity were noted in those who later developed adult onset affective psychosis whereas abnormal suspiciousness or sensitivity were elevated in the children who developed schizophrenia. Both sets of symptoms would be risk factors for peer rejection and excess externalising behaviour, yet the underlying psychological causes are different. As yet we have no evidence to indicate the reasons for peer rejection, or problem behaviour in Pre-S children. But such evidence could well provide a more specific characterisation of children at risk for schizophrenia, and may well explain the diversity of problem behaviours reported in Pre-S adolescents (Reichenberg et al. 2002). Excesses of both externalising and internalising behaviours have been reported as behavioural coping strategies in children with pervasive developmental disorders or children who have suffered adversity (Clarke and Clarke 2000). It seems a possibility that some of the antecedents noted above are proxy measures, and as such would be expected to show low specificity for schizophrenia.

▌ Specificity of childhood antecedents to schizophrenia

Individually childhood antecedents are risk factors for a variety of psychopathologies in adult life. Parker et al. (1995) report that 30–70% of children referred to clinics for psychological problems are reported by parents or teachers to have 'poor peer relationships'. Children rejected by their peers are at risk from a variety of psychopathological disorders, or serious adjustment problems, in adult life (Fergusson et al. 2003; Canon et al. 2002; Offord 1992). One explanation for multifinality could be that having few friends or being rejected by peers can occur for different reasons. Children with either conduct disorder or ADHD are both at high risk for being friendless and rejected by their peers. ADHD children are perceived as irritating, intrusive or disruptive by peers, whereas conduct disorder children are seen as bullies, intimidating or aggressive to their peers (Parker et al. 1995). Rubin et al. (1990) report that rejection by peers can result from either extreme social unassertiveness or alternatively low social interaction. In research on popularity and friendship in school-age children an important distinction is drawn between 'rejected' (i.e. shunned by peers) and 'neglected' (i.e. not seen as a close friend in sociometric studies) children. Risk of psychopathology in neglected children is much lower than that in rejected children (Asher and Dodge 1986). One would assume then that Pre-S children have few friends because they are the 'rejected' type, but as yet no sociometric data on Pre-S children has become available that could shed some light on this issue.

Less marked, but nevertheless significantly elevated, levels of externalising and internalising behaviour have been reported in children who develop bipolar/affective psychotic disorder, (Done et al. 1994; Van Os et al. 1997; Cannon et al. 2002; Jaffee et al. 2002). Robins and Ratcliffe (1978) and Moffitt (1993a) report that frequency and severity of externalising behaviours (most notably antisocial behaviour) in childhood is the most significant risk factor for adult antisocial personality. Internalising problems in children have been noted for those who develop an affective psychosis as well as non-psychotic anxiety/depressive disorder in adult life (Done et al. 1994; Cannon et al. 2002). However, other cohort studies have reported a normal pattern in non-psychotic affective disorder, especially with adult onset (Reichenberg et al. 2002; Jaffee et al. 2002; Sigurdsson 1999). In summary it would seem that excess of externalising and internalising can lead to widely differing pathological outcomes. Pre-S children though produce consistently elevated levels of problem behaviour relative to children who develop affective psychosis or bipolar disorder. Children who developed adult onset unipolar depression or anxiety disorders appear to show much reduced levels of either externalising or internalising behaviours.

It was reported earlier that externalising and internalising can be behavioural expressions of a more fundamental underlying psychological problem. As such the more moderate levels of externalising behaviour noted in children who develop affective disorders might arise for reasons quite different to the greater excesses noted in Pre-S children.

Reduced levels of academic ability, or even lower IQ scores, have been reported as a risk factor for a variety of outcomes in teenage/adult life. These include failing to escape from adversity (Kolvin et al. 1990), antisocial personality disorder (Moffitt 1993b), adult onset affective disorder (Done et al. 1994; van Os et al. 1997), and early onset affective disorder (Jaffee et al. 2002). However, a number of studies have failed to find any association between adult onset affective disorder and low academic ability in childhood (Reichenberg et al. 2002; Jaffee et al. 2002; Sigurdsson 1999). Typically the average lowering of IQ in children who develop a severe affective disorder is less than that for schizophrenia. Jones and Done (1997) reported IQ deficits in Pre-S children of 5 points, or 0.3 z-scores at age 8 in the NSHD cohort and 10 points, or 0.6 z-scores at age 11 in the NCDS cohort. In the Dunedin birth cohort, children who developed juvenile onset depression scored 3–6 IQ points below average (Jaffee et al. 2002), whereas those who developed schizophrenia scored consistently 0.5 z-scores, or 7–8 IQ points below the mean (Cannon et al. 2002). In this cohort though the children who developed adult onset depression showed no lowering of IQ compared to the control group without a psychiatric history.

Reduced neuromotor skills or neurological soft signs have been reported in children who develop affective psychosis (Leask et al. 2002), or juvenile, but not adult onset MDD (Jaffee et al. 2002).

Early language disorders have been reported as contributory causes for a diverse range of psychiatric disturbance in children (Howlin and Rutter 1987). Children with language disorder coupled with reduced IQ are at greater risk not only for psychiatric disturbance but persistence of the language disorder.

Premorbid psychotic-like experience and schizophrenia

This childhood risk factor deserves special consideration since recent indications would suggest continuity on the trajectory between childhood experience and adult onset schizophrenia (Poulton et al. 2000). This picture looks particularly promising since recent studies have reported that children who develop schizophrenia appear to suffer from the same illness as adults, the difference being age of onset (Asarnow and Tompson 1999; Nicolson et al. 2003; Asarnow et al. 2001). If childhood and adult onset schizophrenia differ only in terms of age of onset then a substantial proportion of adult onset cases might demonstrate subclinical levels of psychotic-like experience in childhood.

A number of studies have reported that psychotic-like phenomena are experienced by patients, without psychotic symptoms, who later develop schizophrenia. In one study identification of these experiences occurred eight years before onset of schizophrenia (Klosterkotter et al. 1997). Psychotic-like experiences have been reported in some 70% of nonpsychotic patients who develop schizophrenia one year later, compared to 4% who did not report any such experiences (Klosterkotter 2002). The risk for developing schizophrenia is then high in studies which examine outcomes of non-psychotic patients who report psychotic-like experiences. But these high estimates of risk are noted in a) adults, b) clinic-based populations of patients. As such this risk factor is recorded not long before the onset of illness, during a period that could be identified as the prodrome (Häfner et al. 1998). What then is the estimate of risk in children with psychotic-like experiences? There is only one study to date that can provide estimates of risk. In the Dunedin birth cohort study, Poulton et al. (2000) reported that early psychotic experiences provided a significantly increased risk of later schizophreniform disorder at age 26. Interestingly risk increased substantially when a strong criterion was used (odds ratios moved from 5 to 16 for low and high levels of reported psychotic-like experience, respectively). This conforms to the dose-response principle, i.e. the greater the degree of abnormality the greater the risk of schizophrenia. None of the cases in the Poulton et al. (2000) study who developed mania reported psychotic experiences in childhood suggesting specificity for a schizophreniform outcome. Increased risk was noted though in cases meeting criteria for anxiety disorder (20% compared to 10% in the normal controls). With a positive predictive value (PPV) for schizophrenia of 9 (assuming a lifetime morbid risk = 1%) and an attributable risk estimated of 42%, this measure provides much greater prediction than other childhood risk factors whose PPV = 3–5%

(Jones et al. 2000). This finding is well supported by evidence from the New York High Risk Study (Ott et al. 2002). Children who later developed schizophrenia scored high on both positive and negative thought disorder at age 9. However, since these are children living with a parent who suffers from schizophrenia their early thought disorder might be a consequence of disordered communication in the family (Tienari et al. 2002; Doane et al. 1981). The Dunedin cohort study is though unique as a population-based study, and given the size of effect and its relative specificity there is a real need for replication. A weakness of the study is the criterion of 'schizophreniform' disorder for caseness. Lifetime morbid risk of schizophreniform disorder in this cohort can be estimated at 6.6%, which is six times the estimate normally used when DSM-IV criteria for schizophrenia are used. As such their cases might have included schizotypal PD, who would only progress to full schizophrenia in a minority of cases (Johnson et al. 1999; Bernstein et al. 1993). Another reason for a degree of scepticism about the specificity of the outcome is that specificity was not found in a prospective study of schizotypy in students (Kwapil et al. 1999). In this study, students in their early 20's were followed up prospectively over 10 years. Those who reported subclinical, moderate psychotic-like experiences in their 20's demonstrated a 7.5-fold increase in risk for a spectrum of psychotic disorders, in their 30's (Kwapil et al. 1999). More cases met criteria for psychosis-NOS or bipolar disorder than schizophrenia; risk of schizotypal personality disorder was twice that of the control group and the 'at risk' group as a whole had poor follow-up scores on the Global Adjustment Scale. Thus whereas the study of Poulton et al. (2000) reported specificity for schizophreniform outcome, Kwapil et al. (1999) reported increased risk for a range of adverse outcomes. Extrapolating from findings obtained in a study of 20-year old students to estimate risk in children is a potentially error prone line of argument. For example, Kwapil et al. (1999) noted that the proportion reporting psychotic-like experiences dropped from 43% (aged 20ish) to 26% (aged 30ish) over the 10 year period. This might reflect the reduction of risk of schizophrenia that can be expected at this stage of the life cycle. In line with these findings though, Resch (2002) reported low reliability (r = 0.2–0.4) for BSABS psychotic-like experiences in a 6-month follow-up of children attending a psychiatric clinic, and suggested that these experiences did not resemble traits but transitory states in children.

▎ Summary

A childhood endophenotype has been proposed, based on a set of behavioural and cognitive risk factors. Each risk factor by itself appears to show an elevated risk for other forms of adult psychopathology. It is proposed that greater risk of schizophrenia is attributed to some factors given their reported effect size, and reliability in terms of replication across studies. Attributed risk is improved if the number of risk factors are summed in each case (Malmberg et al. 1998) and weighted on the basis of severity or deviation from the population mean. On the other hand current risk estimates are compromised by reliance on data from case-control studies nested within retrospective cohorts, rather than prospective population-based studies. This design will have a tendency to nurture deterministic neurodevelopmental models. Little can be discovered from such nested case-control studies on the matter of different developmental trajectories leading from an endophenotype. No one as yet has specified an 'at risk' group, based on a set of childhood risk factors, in a cohort and looked at their outcomes. To date all published studies in this field are case-control studies nested within a cohort. However the possibility for diverse trajectories is a plausible explanation for the low PPVs that have been reported for individual risk factors for schizophrenia. If the error of measurement is not responsible for the low PPV then multifinality could provide a better explanation. However the lack of construct validity for the assessments used in these case-control studies cannot be ruled out as the main reason for the low specificity of childhood risk factors. If reasons for peer rejection, excessive problem behaviours etc. could be identified, then estimates of risk might be greatly improved. It is critically important then that the evidence base from prospective studies be established so that we can obtain reliable risk estimates.

Strategies for a prospective study of a putative endophenotype

Setting up a truly prospective study specifically chosen to identify the positive predictive value of the endophenotype of schizophrenia will never happen, without the aid of an idiosyncratic benefactor. We would need to identify some 70 cases to provide adequate statistical power. The incidence rate for schizophrenia is very low and so we shall have to wait until the cohort reaches its late 20's, say 27, at which point some 50% of lifetime morbid risk is used up. So the time restriction of some 15–20 years means that we can only examine a cohort of children, rather than infants. A cohort of 14 000 twelve-year-olds would then be needed to identify 70 cases at age 27. However it is estimated that to screen such a cohort the cost would be $400K for 10 minutes of individual assessment. Assuming that our current understanding of the endophenotype would require a clinical interview, a neuropsychological assessment, as well as teacher and parent interview, then each child would require a minimum of 2 hours of assessment costing $5 million. A possible alternative though would be to use the current knowledge about the childhood endophenotype to identify plausible high risk candidates of childhood psychopathology and then follow these prospectively. This of course is fundamentally different to the traditional high risk strategy (e.g. Olin and Mednick 1999), in which cases are defined by family history rather than endophenotype. Good candidates would be childhood psychiatric disorders with diagnostic criteria that fit the endophenotype outlined earlier. Firstly, a follow-up of such a cohort would be a truly prospective design. Secondly, the comprehensive clinical interview, neuropsychological assessments and teacher/parental interviews would provide primary signs and symptoms, rather than the proxy measures we have at present. For example, children reported to have poor peer relations would be assessed to see whether the primary cause was poor social reciprocity (as in pervasive developmental disorders), aggressive behaviour (as in conduct disorder), social withdrawal (as in Cluster A personality disorders), or disorganised and interfering behaviour (as in ADHD). Thirdly, such cases would tend to be extreme cases on particular continua. So autistic children would be on the extreme end of the continuum for impaired social reciprocity and comprehension of social interaction, whereas conduct disordered children would be on the extreme end of the continuum for antisocial, intimidatory behaviour and aggression. We noted above that those children who developed schizophrenia rather than affective disorder seemed to deviate further from the population mean on risk factors A through G. The more marked a child's unpopularity, externalising and internalising (Bearden et al. 2000), early psychotic experience (Poulton et al. 2000), language impairment, lowering of IQ (David et al. 1997; Jones et al. 1994), then the greater the risk of schizophrenia for that child. Indeed this has led some to suggest a dose-response relationship (Jones 2002) between degree of deviance from the norm (the dose) and risk of schizophrenia (the response). In addition, risk for schizophrenia increases exponentially as the combination of risk factors increase (Malmberg et al. 1998).

▌ Candidates for prospective studies and the current evidence base

Personality disorders

PD's affect a sizeable percentage of the adolescent population. Community-based surveys have estimated the prevalence at 14–17% who meet DSM-III-R criteria for PD (Johnson et al. 1999; Bernstein et al. 1993). The argument for Cluster A (paranoid, schizoid or schizotypal) PD being a high risk candidate for adult onset schizophrenia is clearly a strong one. Klosterkotter et al. (1997) in a 8-year follow-up of adult patients seen in a psychiatric clinic reported that cases originally diagnosed with schizotypal personality disorder had a high risk of developing DSM-III-R schizophrenia at follow-up. Also in the Copenhagen 1962 High Risk Project, genetically high risk children had a substantially increased risk (relative risk = 14) for Cluster A PD compared to genetically low risk children (Olin and Mednick 1996). But Cluster B (borderline, antisocial and histrionic) would also appear to meet criteria as high risk candidates due to their lack of close friends, rejection by peers, and associated behaviour disorders (especially increased externalising), and poorer than average school performance (Bernstein et al. 1993).

Current evidence from prospective studies of childhood/adolescent personality disorders (PD)

Lofgren et al. (1991) reported continuity of personality disorder but no axis 1 disorders in a group of 6–10 year old borderline PD children followed up 10–20 years later. Johnson et al. (1999) followed up a community sample (n = 717) of adolescents (aged 14 years) through to age 22. Risk of Axis 1 mood disorders were increased in both Cluster A and B PD (OR = 5 and 4, respectively), and so were anxiety disorders (OR = 2 and 1.5, respectively). No mention is made of Axis 1 psychotic disorders and so it is likely that these were few in number. Nevertheless the data do suggest that outcomes are heterogeneous for adolescent Cluster A and B PDs. An alternative explanation could be that those with anxiety and depression could be going through the prodrome (Häfner et al. 1995) and might progress to schizophrenia at a later date. Bernstein and coworkers' (1993) community-based sample (n = 733) was much younger being followed up at age 16 and hence not much can be inferred given the low expected rates for schizophrenia at this age. However, two interesting issues emerge from the study. Firstly, stability is low over a 2 year period. Persistence of axis II disorders was as low as 6% for schizoid and reached a maximum of 43% for passive-aggressive PD. Secondly, the authors note a significant linear decline of 14% per year in risk of receiving a diagnosis of PD between the ages of 11 and 21 years. Thus there appears to be sizeable fluctuation over time, rather than stability of PD symptoms, in community-based populations.

Longitudinal research of community-based PD (as opposed to those attending a clinic) starting in adolescence is noted for its paucity. But interim conclusions from these studies would suggest that children, or adolescents, noted for poor peer relations, problem behaviour, poor academic performance, and also psychotic-like experiences (i.e. schizotypals) might a) develop a range of different forms of adult psychopathology, b) may show substantial change in developmental trajectory, with a possible decline in risk post-adolescence. In addition the estimated risk of schizophrenia in adulthood appears to be substantially lower for adolescent cases of PD when compared with the non-psychotic adult patients with schizotypal signs (Klosterkotter et al. 1997). The reduction in risk over time is frequently a sign of heterogeneous developmental trajectories. The narrower the time interval, the more likely it is that risk factor and outcome are on the same trajectory, whereas a wider time interval gives greater opportunity for the child to move onto a different developmental trajectory.

Pervasive developmental disorders

There is considerable conceptual overlap between diagnostic criteria for personality disorders and pervasive developmental disorders or PDD (Towbin 1997). Asperger's syndrome and PDD-NOS can be frequently misdiagnosed as schizoid or avoidant PD. Cases of PDD-NOS who are particularly prone to be misdiagnosed as a PD are those who avoid social contact, but have good language skills, or who express a wish for social contact, yet are aware of their disability. Ambelas (2003) noted the similarity between the clinical picture for Asperger's syndrome and the behavioural and neuromotor pattern reported by Leask et al. (2002) for Pre-S children in the National Child Development Study birth cohort. If there is similarity then it is more likely to be a similarity with the 'autistic spectrum' of disorders in PDD, rather than a particular diagnostic

Table 1. Comparison between the signs and symptoms in PDD children and those in Pre-S children

Sign/symptoms noted in PDD	Related patterns reported in Pre-S children
▮ Impaired social interaction	Peer acceptance anxiety (Done et al. 1994)
▮ Impaired gaze/facial expression	Poor eye contact (Walker et al. 1990) Negative facial expression (Grimes and Walker 1994)
▮ Lack of spontaneous sharing	?
▮ Lack of social reciprocity	?
▮ Restricted interest/stereotyped behaviour	Walker et al. (1990)
▮ Motor clumsiness/delayed motor milestones	Clumsiness (Leask et al. 2002), Delayed milestones (e.g. Jones et al. 1994)
▮ Poor peer relations	Various (e.g. Ambelas 1992; Foerster et al. 1991)
▮ Incoherent speech/loose associations	Thought disorder (Ott et al. 2002)
▮ Marked verbosity	Talking excess with teacher (Done et al. 1994)
▮ Poor prosody/volume adjustment	Bearden et al. (2000)

category (Allen et al. 2001). This spectrum can be considered as bounded by autism at the end marked 'most severe'. PDD-NOS manifest similar but typically milder symptoms and so these can be visualised toward the other end of the spectrum (Towbin 1997; Volkmar et al. 1995).

Comparing the two columns in Table 1 suggests that there might be considerable overlap between the pre-morbid characteristics of Pre-S children and those that characterise PDD. However, most of the risk factors for schizophrenia are underspecified, and so the matching is speculative. More detailed protocols of Pre-S children's psychosocial, linguistic and communicative abilities are necessary before one can assert whether there is a good pattern match.

Current evidence: are PDD children at increased risk for schizophrenia?

The evidence base provides a mixed picture. In a large cohort of 163 autistic adolescents and adults (mean age = 24) who had been repeatedly assessed over a number of years, only one case of DSM-III-R schizophrenia was ever recorded (Volkmar and Cohen 1991). Interestingly in some 41 cases either the teachers or the parents had reported at least two or more positive psychotic-like symptoms. Follow-ups of Asperger's syndrome are limited, partly due to the relatively recent inclusion of the diagnostic category into ICD-10 and DSM-IV. In the case of Asperger's syndrome, increased risk of schizophrenia has been reported (Tantam 1991; Klin and Volkmar 1995). Also Clarke et al. reported a high risk of adult psychosis in a select group of children with a DSM-III-R diagnosis of PDD. The descriptions of these children suggest that their childhoods were marked by PDD type symptoms without any reported psychotic-like symptoms.

This limited evidence base presents a rather unusual pattern. According to the dose-response principle, one would expect that the risk for schizophrenia is greater as the dose increases. Thus as one moves toward the autistic end of the spectrum, then the risk of schizophrenia should also increase. This though does not appear to be the case, and highlights the different results that can emerge from true cohort studies (i.e. where the 'at risk' cases are identified first and then followed up rather than case-control studies nested within a cohort (i.e. where the cases are selected according to their outcomes and risk for various factors is then estimated from data collected in childhood). Risk for schizophrenia may be greater in the less severe forms of PDD than it is for the more severe form, i.e. autism. However it is also noteworthy that the developmental trajectories of both autism and Asperger's syndrome can lead to a variety of psychiatric outcomes including conduct disorder and depression (Mesibov and Handlan 1995).

▌ Summary

A strategy is proposed in which cohorts of DSM/ICD categories of childhood onset psychopathology are followed up prospectively. This choice of strategy is based on the need a) to obtain risk estimates from prospectively collected data and b) to use assessments with better construct validity. Choice of diagnostic categories should be based on their similarity with the putative childhood endophenotype for schizophrenia. This endophenotype cannot only be described by a set of risk factors, but by a hierarchy of risk factors. On this basis, category A and B personality disorders and PDD are deemed more likely candidates than conduct disorder or ADHD, if poor peer relations/difficulty in forming friendships is primary. In both conduct disorder and ADHD, problems in forming friendships and low academic achievement appear secondary to the behavioural disturbance.

The evidence base from prospective cohorts of adolescent PD or PDD is very limited and as such one cannot be confident about any conclusions. Community-based studies of PD report increased risk of axis 1 disorders. These are predominantly mood or anxiety disorders, although there is the possibility that for some this may represent a prodromal phase of schizophrenia.

Autistic children appear to be at low risk for developing schizophrenia, although psychotic-like experiences are noted in a substantial minority of cases. Risk for schizophrenia may well be elevated in Asperger's type PDD or PDD-NOS.

▌ Deterministic models vs lifepath trajectories

Neurodevelopmental formulations of schizophrenia have typically been more deterministic than dynamic (Parker et al. 1995 provide a review of these different models). In deterministic models, adverse events early in childhood cause adult onset schizophrenia in some linear fashion (e.g. Marenco and Weinberger 2000). Animal models lend support to this formulation but typically the lesions are severe. Saunders et al. (2002) removed the medial-temporal cortex in neonate monkeys, and found a delayed effect. As adults there was substantial dysregulation of dopamine in the dorsolateral prefrontal cortex. The authors refer to this as a potential model for schizophrenia, suggesting that early focal injury to the temporal cortex had a delayed effect on DLPFC functioning. In this formulation, the trajectory is held to be linear with effect being delayed by many years. Perhaps then we might find a well-specified childhood endophenotype which leads to adult schizophrenia in such a linear fashion. However, alternative models are preferred in developmental psychopathology where a) estimates of risk are small, b) risk increases as the time interval between risk event and illness onset becomes narrower, and c) where there is multifinality suggesting different possible trajectories. Evidence outlined above would suggest that all of these features are found when one examines the relationship between childhood risk factors and adult onset schizophrenia. Alternative models might be either interactional models, i.e. risk factors interact to produce outcome, or transactional models, i.e. effects feedback to cause. Examples of these more complex aetiological models have been used to explain the transition from childhood to adulthood in both children with ADHD and extremely shy children. Like schizophrenia both have high heritability coefficients, and continuity is high over a short period (e.g. one year). Thapar et al. (1999) reported a heritability estimate for ADHD in the order of 70%, yet trajectories from childhood to adulthood are diverse, with only one third of all cases meeting criteria for ADHD as adults (Klein and Mannuzza 1991). Shyness also has a high estimate of heritability. In a prospective study extremely shy children were identified at age 9 and followed up at age 35 (Kerr et al. 1996). Childhood shyness ratings for extremely shy children correlated poorly with adult-rated shyness at age 35 ($r = +0.24$ for females and $+0.01$ for males). Kerr et al. note that although there is a statistically significant correlation indicating continuity, it is a very small effect, such that the life course of very shy children can be varied. Cicchetti and Cannon (1999) note that in various forms of developmental psychopathology 'epigenesis is probabilistic rather than predetermined'. If this principle can be applied to schizophrenia then critical causal factors, be they genetic or environmental factors, may well provide small relative risks for later schizophrenia. Likewise the evidence reported above would suggest that these early risk factors are risk factors for diverse outcomes. The most optimistic PPV to date is 9% (Poulton et al. 2000) but there is a need to replicate this. Most other PPVs are below 5 (Jones and Croudace 2000). It is generally assumed that these low PPVs result from poor specification of the exact childhood endophenotype for schizophrenia. With improved specification positive predictive power will improve. However, as noted by Clarke and Clarke (2000) we may well expect that the PPVs will reduce further when we conduct truly prospective studies.

A dynamic or transactional model appears to fit the available data better than a deterministic model. A number of aetiological factors having their effects at different stages of development would produce varied developmental trajectories leading to different endpoints. Low relative risks or PPVs for adult schizophrenia would then be expected for childhood antecedents. A child meeting the criteria for a high-risk endophenotype may well avoid ever developing schizophrenia because other factors will need to make their contribution between childhood and adulthood. However the more criteria that are met then the greater the constraints on alternative trajectories and hence the greater the risk for schizophrenia. It is also possible that there might be protective factors which mitigate the effects of early risk factors. In the quest for identifying early preventive measures it is important to have a better understanding of these possible developmental trajectories. These could provide valuable clues as to whether children with similar high-risk endophenotypes for schizophrenia can progress to adult outcomes other than schizophrenia.

▌ References

Allen DA, Steinberg M, Dunn M, Fein D, Feinstein C; Waterhouse L, Rapin I (2001) Autistic disorder versus other pervasive developmental disorders in young children: same or different? Euro Child and Adol Psychiat 10:67–78

Ambelas A (2003) Children, neurological soft signs and schizophrenia. British Journal of Psychiatry 182:362

Ambelas A (1992) Preschizophrenics: adding to the evidence, sharpening the focus. Brit J Psychiat 160:401–404

Asarnow JR, Tompson MC (1999) Childhood-onset schizophrenia: a follow-up study. Euro Child and Adol Psychiatry 8(suppl 1):9–12

Asarnow RF, Nuechterlein KH, Fogelson D, Subotnik KL, Payne DA, Russell AT, Asame J, Kuppinger H, Kendler KS (2001) Schizophrenia and schizophrenia-spectrum personality disorders in the first-degree relatives of children with schizophrenia: the UCLA family study. Archives of General Psychiatry 58:581–588

Bearden CE, Rosso IM, Hollister JM, Sanchez LE et al. (2000) A prospective cohort study of childhood behavioral deviance and language abnormalities as predictors of adult schizophrenia. Schizophrenia Bulletin 26:395–410

Bernstein DP, Cohen P, Velez N, Schwab-stone M, Siever LJ, Shinsato L (1993) Prevalence and stability of the DSM-III-R personality disorders in a community-based survey of adolescents. Am J Psychiatry 150:1237–1243

Brodaty H, Sachdev P, Rose N, Rylands K, Prender L (1999) Schizophrenia with onset after 50 years. Brit J Psychiat 175:410–415

Cannon M, Jones P, Gilvarry C, Rifkin L, McKenzie K, Foerster A, Murray RM (1997) Premorbid social functioning in schizophrenia and bipolar disorder: similarities and differences. American Journal Psychiatry 154:1544–1550

Cannon M, Jones P, Huttunen MO et al. (1999) School performance in Finnish children and later development of schizophrenia – a population based longitudinal study. Archives of General Psychiatry 56:457–463

Cannon M, Walsh E, Hollis C, Kargin M, Taylor E, Murray RM, Jones PB (2001) Predictors of later schizophrenia and affective psychosis among attendees at a child psychiatry department. British Journal of Psychiatry 178:420–426

Cannon M, Caspi A, Moffitt T et al. (2002) Evidence for early-childhood, pan-developmental impairment specific for schizophreniform disorder. Archives of General Psychiatry 59:449–455

Cannon-Spoor E, Potkin SG, Wyatt RJ (1982) Measurement of premorbid adjustment in chronic schizophrenia. Schizophrenia Bulletin 8:471–484

Cicchetti D, Cannon TD (1999) Neurodevelopmental process in the ontogeny and epigenesis of psychopathology. Developmental Psychopathology 11:375–393

Clarke A, Clarke A (2000) Early experience and the life path. Jessica Kingslet, London

David AS, Malmberg A, Brandt L, Allebeck P, Lewis G (1997) IQ and risk for schizophrenia: a population based cohort study. Psych Med 27:1311–1323

Davidson M, Reichenberg A, Rabinowitz J et al. (1999) Behavioural and intellectual markers for schizophrenia in apparently healthy male adolescents. Am J Psychiat 156:1328–1335

Doane JA, West KL, Goldstein MJ, Rodnick EH, Jones JE (1981) Parental communication deviance and affective style. Arch Gen Psychiat 38:679–685

Done DJ, Johnstone EC, Frith CD, Golding J, Shepherd PM, Crow TJ (1991) Complications of pregnancy and delivery in relation to psychosis in adult life: date from the British perinatal mortality survey sample. BMJ 302:1576–1580

Done DJ, Crow TJ, Johnstone EC, Sacker A (1994) Childhood antecedents of schizophrenia and affective illness: social adjustment at ages 7 and 11. BMJ 309:699–703

Elander J, Rutter M (1996) An update on the status of the Rutter parents' and Teachers' Scales. Child Psychol Psychiat Rev 1:31–35

Fergusson DM, Beautrais AL, Horwood LJ (2003) Vulnerability and resiliency in suicidal behaviours in young people. Psychol Med 33:61–73

Foerster A, Lewis S, Owen M, Murray R (1991) Pre-morbid adjustment in psychosis: effects of sex and diagnosis. Brit J Psychiat 158:171–176

Fuller R, Nopoulos P, Arndt S et al. (2002) Longitudinal assessment of premorbid cognitive functioning in patients with schizophrenia through examination of standardized scholastic test performance. Am J Psychiatry 159(7):1183–1189

Grimes K, Walker EF (1994) Childhood emotional expressions, educational attainment, and age of onset of illness in schizophrenia. J Abn Psychol 103:784–790

Häfner H, Mauer K, Löffler W et al (1995) Onset and early course of schizophrenia. In: Häfner H, Gattaz WF (eds) Search for the Causes of Schizophrenia, Vol III. Springer, Berlin, pp 43–65

Häfner H, Mauer K, Löffler W, an der Heiden W, Stein A, Konnecke R, Hambrecht M (1999) Onset and prodromal phase as determinants of the course. In: Gattaz WF, Häfner H (eds) Search for the Causes of Schizophrenia, Vol IV. Springer, Berlin, pp 35–59

Harrington R (2001) Causal processes in development and psychopathology. Brit J Psychiatry 179:93–94

Howlin P, Rutter M (1987) The consequences of language delay for other aspects of development. In: Yule W, Rutter M (eds) Language Development and Disorders. Clinics in Developmental Medicine No 1001/102, Blackwell, Oxford, pp 271–295

Isohanni M, Jones PB, Moilanen K et al (2001) Early developmental milestones in adult schizophrenia and other psychoses. A 31-year follow-up of Northern Finland 1966 Birth Cohort. Schizophrenia Research 52:1–19

Jaffee SR (2002) Differences in early childhood risk factors for juvenile-onset and adult-onset depression. Arch Gen Psychiat 59:215–222

John RS, Mednick SA, Schulsinger F (1982) Teacher reports as a predictor of schizophrenia and borderline schizophrenia: a bayesian decision analysis. J Abn Psychol 91:399–413

Johnson JG, Cohen P, Skodol AE, Oldham JM, Kaseen S, Brook JS (1999) Personality disorders in adolescence and risk of major mental disorders and suicidality during adulthood. Arch Gen Psychiat 56:805–811

Jones PB, Rodgers B, Murray R, Marmot M (1994) Child development risk factors for adult schizophrenia in the British 1946 birth cohort. Lancet 344:1398–1401

Jones PB, Croudace TJ (2000) Predicting schizophrenia in adults from teachers' reports in adolescence: perspectives on population-based intervention and indicated prevention. Schiz Res 41:177–178

Jones PB (2002) Risk factors for schizophrenia in childhood and youth. In: Häfner H (ed) Risk and Protective Factors in Schizophrenia: Towards a Conceptual Model of the Disease Process. Steinkopff, Darmstadt, pp 141–163

Kagan J (1992) Yesterday's premises, tomorrow's promises. Developmental Psychology 28:990–997

Kagan J, Zentner M (1996) Early childhood predictors of adult psychopathology. Harvard Review of Psychiatry 3:341–350

Kerr M, Lambert WW, Bem DJ (1996) Life course sequelae of childhood shyness in Sweden: comparison with the United States. Developmental Psychology 32:1100–1105

Klin A, Volkmar FR (1995) Asperger's syndrome. In: Cohen DJ, Volkmar FR (eds) Handbook of Autism and Pervasive Developmental Disorders. John Wiley & Sons, New York, pp 94–123

Klein RG, Mannuzza S (1991) Long-term outcome of hyperactive-children: a review. J Amer Acad Child and Adol Psychiat, 30:383–387

Klosterkotter J, Schultze-Lutter F, Gross G, Huber G, Steinmeyer EM (1997) Early experienced neuropsychological deficits and subsequent schizophrenic diseases: an 8-year average follow-up. Acta Psychiatr Scand 95:396–404

Klosterkotter J (2002) Predicting the inset of schizophrenia. In: Hafner H (ed) Risk and Protective Factors in Schizophrenia: Towards a conceptual model of the Disease Process. Steinkopff, Darmstadt, pp 193–207

Kolvin I, Miller FJW, Scott D McI, Gatzanis SRM, Fleeting M (1990) Continuities of deprivation? The Newcastle 1000 Family Study. Gower House, Aldershot

Kwapil TR, Chapman LJ, Chapman J (1999) Validity and usefulness of the Wisconsin Manual for assessing psychotic-like experiences. Schizophrenia Bulletin 25:363–375

Leask SJ, Done DJ, Crow TJ (2002) Adult psychosis, common childhood infections and neurological soft signs in a national birth cohort. British Journal of Psychiatry 181:387–392

Malmberg A, Lewis G, David A et al (1998) Premorbid adjustment and personality in people with schizophrenia. British Journal of Psychiatry 172:308–313

Marenco S, Weinberger DR (2000) The neurodevelopmental hypothesis of schizophrenia: following a trail of evidence from cradle to grave. Development and Psychopathology 12:501–527

McGlashan TH, Miller TJ, Woods SW (2001) Pre-onset detection and intervention research in schizophrenia psychoses: current estimates of benefit and risk. Schizophrenia Bulletin 27:563–570

McGlashan TH, Johannessen JO (1996) Early detection and intervention with schizophrenia: rationale. Schizophrenia Bulletin 22:201–221

Mesibov GB, Handlan S (1995) Adolescents and adults with autism. In: Cohen DJ, Volkmar FR (eds) Handbook of Autism and Pervasive Developmental Disorders. John Wiley & Sons, New York, pp 309–322

Moffitt TE (1993a) Adolescence-limited and life-course-persistent antisocial behaviour: a developmental taxonomy. Psychological Review 100:674–701

Moffitt TE (1993b) The neuropsychology of conduct disorder. Development and Psychopathology 5:135–151

Nicolson R, Brookner FB, Lenane M, Gochman P, Ingraham LJ, Egan MF, Kendler KS, Pickar D, Weinberger DR, Rapoport JL (2003) Parental schizophrenia spectrum disorders in childhood-onset and adult-onset schizophrenia. American Journal of Psychiatry 160:490–495

Niemi LT, Suvusaari JM, Tuulio-Henriksson A, Lonnqvist JK (2003) Childhood developmental abnormalities in schizophrenia: evidence from high-risk studies. Schizophrenia Research 60:239–258

Offord DR, Boyle MH, Racine YA, Fleming JE, Cadman DT, Blum HM, Byrne C, Links PS, Lipman EL, Macmillan HL et al (1992) Outcome, prognosis, and risk in a longitudinal follow-up study. Journal of American Academy of Child and Adolescent Psychiatry 31:916–923

Olin SS, Mednick SA (1999) Risk factors of psychosis: identifying vulnerable populations premorbidly. Schizophrenia Bulletin 22:224–240

Ott SL, Roberts S et al (2002) Positive and negative thought disorder and psychopathology in childhood among subjects with adulthood schizophrenia. Schizophrenia Research 58:231–239

Parker JG, Rubin KH, Price JM, DeRosier ME (1995) Peer relationships, child development, and adjustment: a developmental psychopathology perspective. In: Cicchetti D, Cohen DJ (eds) Developmental Psychopathology, Vol 2: Risk, Disorder and Adaptation. Wiley J, New York, pp 96–161

Poulton R, Caspi A, Moffitt TE, Cannon M, Murray R, Harrington H (2000) Children's self-reported psychotic symptoms and adult schizophreniform disorder. Arch Gen Psychiatry 57:1053–1058

Reichenberg A, Weiser M, Rabinowitz J et al (2002) A population-based cohort study of premorbid intellectual language, and behavioural functioning in patients with schizophrenia, schizoaffective disorder and nonpsychotic bipolar disorder. American J Psychiatry 159:2027–2035

Resch F, Parzer P, Poiutska L, Koch E, Meng H, Burgin D (2002) Specificity of basic symptoms in early onset schizophrenia. In: Häfner H (ed) Risk and Protective Factors in Schizophrenia: Towards a Conceptual Model of the Disease Process. Steinkopff, Darmstadt, pp 177–185

Robins LN, Ratcliff KS (1978) Risk factors in the continuation of childhood antisocial behavior into adulthood. Int J Ment Health 7:96–116

Rubin KH, LeMare LJ, Lollis S (1990) Social withdrawal in childhood: developmental pathways to peer rejection. In: Asher SJ, Coie JD (eds) Peer Rejection in Childhood. Cambridge Univ Press, New York, pp 217–249

Saunders RC, Kolachana BS, Bachevalier J, Weinberger DR (1998) Neonatal lesions of the medial temporal lobe disrupt prefrontal cortical regulation of striatal dopamine. Nature 393:169–171

Siegel AW, Scovill LC (2000) Problem behavior: The double symptom in adolescence. Development and Psychopathology 12:763–793

Sigurdsson E, Fombonne E et al (1999) Neurodevelopmental antecedents of early-onset bipolar affective disorder. Brit J Psychiat 174:121–127

Skuse DH (2001) Editorial: Endophenotypes and child psychiatry. Brit J Psychiat 178:395–396

Sroufe LA (1997) Psychopathology as an outcome of development. Development and Psychopathology 9:251–268

Tantum D (1991) Asperger's syndrome in adulthood. In: Frith U (ed) Autism and Asperger Syndrom. Cambs Univ Press, UK, pp 147–183

Thapar A, Holmes J, Poulton K, Harrington R (1999) Genetic basis of attention deficit and hyperactivity. Brit J Psychiat 174:105–111

Tienari P, Wynne LC, Sorri A, Lahti I et al. (2002) Genotype-environment interaction in the Finnish adoptive family study – interplay between genes and environment? In: Häfner H (ed) Risk and Protective Factors in Schizophrenia: Towards a Conceptual Model of the Disease Process. Steinkopff, Darmstadt, pp 29–39

Towbin KE (1997) Pervasive developmental disorder not otherwise specified. In: Cohen DJ, Volkmar FR (eds) Handbook of Autism and Pervasive Developmental Disorders. John Wiley & Sons, New York, pp 94–123

Van Os J, Jones P, Lewis G et al (1997) Developmental precursors of affective illness in a general population birth cohort. Arch Gen Psychiat 54:625–631

Volkmar FR, Klin A, Cohen DJ (1995) Diagnosis and classification of autism and related conditions; consensus and issues. In: Cohen DJ, Volkmar FR (eds) Handbook of Autismand Pervasive Developmental Disorders. John Wiley & Sons, New York, pp 94–123

Walker EF, Lewine RJ (1990) Prediction of adult-onset schizophrenia from childhood home movies of patients. Am J Psychiatry 147:1052–1056

Walker EF, Savole T et al. (1994) Neuromotor precursors of schizophrenia. Schizophrenia Bulletin 20:441–451

Walker EF, Walder DJ, Reynolds F (2001) Developmental changes in cortisol secretion in normal and at-risk youth. Development and Psychopathology 13:721–732

Watt NF, Stolorow RD, Lubensky AW et al (1972) Longitudinal changes in the social behaviour of children hospitalised for schizophrenia as adults. J Nerv Ment Dis 155:42–54

Weinberger DR (1987) Implications of normal brain development for the pathogenesis of schizophrenia. Arch Gen Psychiatry 44:660–669

Zuckerman M (1979) Sensation Seeking: Beyond the Optimal Level of Arousal. Erlbaum, Hillsdale, NJ

Are there specific risk factors for schizophrenia?

PREBEN BO MORTENSEN

National Centre for Register-based Research, University of Aarhus, Denmark

Introduction

The purpose of this paper is to review the evidence as to whether we can identify specific risk factors for schizophrenia or if, alternatively, these risk factors are shared between schizophrenia and other disorders. The main focus will be a comparison between schizophrenia, on the hand, and bipolar affective disorder, on the other, since this has represented the accepted dichotomy of psychoses for more than a century. However, this dichotomy has also repeatedly been challenged, and therefore, it seems worthwhile to review similarities and discontinuities as far as risk factors are concerned. Recent genetic studies have rekindled this debate. For example, the paper by Cardno and colleagues [14] concluded that there is a degree of overlap in the genes contributing to schizophrenic, schizoaffective and manic syndromes, and they also concluded that their results support an overlap in environmental risk factors for the schizophrenic and manic syndromes. Their conclusion is, to some extent, supported by results from molecular genetic studies, although their conclusions were not left unchallenged [30].

First, some of the basic descriptive epidemiology: in Fig. 1, the age- and gender-specific incidence of first admission with schizophrenia is shown (reproduced from [53]). When we compare this with the data for bipolar affective disorder (Fig. 2) (from Mortensen et al. [46]), we see conspicuous differences. For one, the overall incidence of schizophrenia is almost double that of bipolar affective disorder. Second, bipolar affective disorder has a considerably later peak age of onset, and third, the gender ratio is quite different between the two disorders with a male predominance especially among the young schizophrenic patients, and a less marked, but still significant, preponderance of women among bipolar affective disorder patients.

It should be noted that these curves should be interpreted with much caution; one definite limitation is the limited age span they cover, and also it should be noted that these curves only cover first treatment episodes in a hospital in- or outpatient setting which, of course, does not necessarily correspond to the real epidemiology of the disorders. Still, as some of these biases may be common for schizophrenia and bipolar disorder at least, these curves to me would suggest that the two disorders by far are not identical, even as far as basic age- and gender-specific rates are considered. In the following review, I would like to acknowledge the work by Dr. Tsuchiya from our group, as I follow some of the structure of his literature review [62].

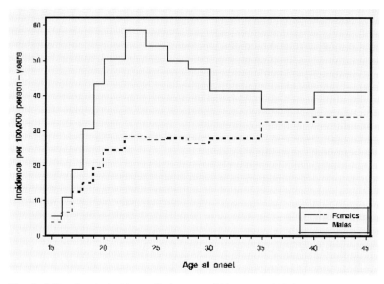

Fig. 1. Schizophrenia incidence (Pedersen and Mortensen 2001)

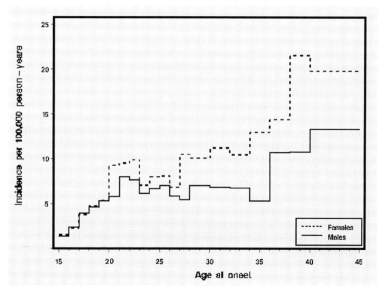

Fig. 2. Bipolar affective disorder incidence (Mortensen et al. 2003)

Ethnicity and migration

Repeated studies both in, for example, England [67], Holland [55], and Denmark [15, 43] have shown increased rates of schizophrenia in groups of immigrants. Studies of bipolar disorder have been fewer, and although some studies, e.g. among African-Caribbeans in London, have found differences between migrants and indigenous groups [63], some studies do not find such differences [23]. We have no Danish data that have currently addressed this specifically for bipolar disorder, but in a previous study [44], we found lower rates of admissions with manic-depressive psychosis in groups of immigrants. In conclusion, this is a factor that is associated with schizophrenia risk but currently there is less evidence regarding bipolar disorder.

∎ Obstetric complications

Numerous studies have found a relationship between schizophrenia and various pregnancy and birth complications both in terms of summary scores of complications and in terms of individual factors such as low birth weight (for reviews see [12, 13, 22, 65]). The studies in bipolar disorder are much fewer and generally smaller, and results are conflicting. Studies using general population controls did not find any differences [7, 56, 64], whereas other studies suggest a trend towards more complications in children who later develop bipolar disorder [31, 32, 34]. A recent Danish study based upon 196 cases and 4900 general population controls suggests no relationship to obstetric factors [49] and in summary there is much less evidence that obstetric complications may contribute to the etiology of bipolar affective disorder than what is the case for schizophrenia.

Prenatal exposure to infections has been linked to schizophrenia risk [8, 39, 69], and although studies of schizophrenia have also been conflicting [68] there is less epidemiological data to suggest any relationship between prenatal infections and bipolar affective disorder [7, 17, 20]. In the Dutch famine study, an association was found between intrauterine exposure to famine and schizophrenia [57]. This was replicated for affective disorders including bipolar disorder [5, 6] although the trend was weaker.

In summary, pre- and perinatal factors are less well studied for bipolar disorder than for schizophrenia but the current data would suggest that they are of less importance in bipolar disorder suggesting etiological differences between the disorders.

∎ Season of birth

A large body of literature reviewed by Torrey et al. [59] has demonstrated an excess risk of schizophrenia in individuals born during winter or spring months. Fewer studies have addressed this for bipolar disorder, and some have a positive association. However, in Danish data we have found no effect of seasonality for bipolar disorder and varying effect in schizophrenia [46].

Urbanicity of place of birth

This has been the topic of a number of studies from our group as well as other research centres. In most studies, some excess of schizophrenia associated with higher degrees of urbanicity of place of birth or upbringing has been found [33, 47, 52, 53]. Marcelis et al. [38] found a weaker but still significant association with urbanicity in manic-depressive psychosis in general including unipolar depression. In strong contrast to our schizophrenia findings [53], however, we found no association in a study of bipolar disorder with the exception of higher rates in those born in one of the three provincial cities with more than 100 000 inhabitants [46]. That is, no dose-response relationship whatsoever, and definitely a different pattern from that found in schizophrenia. We do not know the reason for the excess in those born in provincial cities, but suspect this pattern may be associated with different diagnostic traditions as the largest of the large provincial cities Aarhus has had a long-standing interest for bipolar disorder and lithium treatment. However, this explanation is, of course, speculative.

Socioeconomic status

Parental social class has been the subject of many studies in schizophrenia. The majority of these by and large find no associations [4] although a few recent studies [19, 37] find higher parental social class to be associated with schizophrenia. A similar pattern was found in bipolar disorder in some studies [21, 26, 51]. Recent Danish studies have found somewhat similar patterns in schizophrenia [9] and bipolar affective disorder [24], respectively, with a trend towards higher levels of education in parents to patients from both groups.

In summary, there is little evidence for a strong association between parental social variables and psychoses but no evidence of any specific evidence for either schizophrenia or bipolar disorder.

Premorbid adjustment

If we look at the premorbid adjustment in the patients themselves, measured variables in the socioeconomic domain as marital status or occupational status, patients hospitalized with schizophrenia deviate negatively from the controls for many years prior to the first admission [1, 24]. A similar but much less marked pattern is seen for patients with bipolar disorder.

Recent stressful life events

In a number of studies, this has been found to be associated with the onset of bipolar disorder [29, 54]. In contrast, there is much less evidence that this should be the case for schizophrenia [27].

▌ Early parental loss

A few studies [2] including our own recent data [61] suggest that early parental loss and especially loss of the mother may be associated with increased risk of being hospitalized with bipolar disorder later in life. In addition, it has been suggested that early parental loss may also be associated with schizophrenia (e.g. [2]).

▌ Head injury

Traumatic brain injuries have been studied relatively little as precursors for psychosis in larger scale epidemiological studies. In our own studies [45, 48], the strongest association was found for bipolar disorder, whereas the association with schizophrenia was much less clear and less marked.

▌ Relationship to childbirth

A highly increased rate of first onset of bipolar disorder has been noted within the first month after giving birth (e.g., Terp et al. [58]. The strong temporal relationship could suggest that there may be some direct biological or psychological association between the onset of bipolar disorder and childbirth whereas, based on the same study, this is much less likely to be the case for schizophrenia.

▌ Seizure disorders

Several studies have suggested an association between epilepsy and the risk of schizophrenia, in particular in connection with temporal lobe epilepsy [3]. Similar associations have been suggested for bipolar disorder and affective psychosis [36]. Unpublished Danish data by Bredkjaer et al. has suggested the same.

▌ Multiple sclerosis

Two studies have suggested that there may be an elevated risk for bipolar disorder in patients with multiple sclerosis. There is little certain knowledge as regards schizophrenia due to the difficulties in conducting this type of epidemiological study, and in general, of course, also it may be difficult to separate onset of mania symptoms due to steroid treatment of the underlying neurological disease.

▌ Rheumatoid arthritis

Reduced rates of rheumatoid arthritis have repeatedly been reported in patients with schizophrenia [41]. Very few studies of bipolar patients exist, but one study finding reduced rates in patients with schizophrenia found no association, positive or negative, in bipolar patients [40].

▌ Cancer

A number of studies have reported reduced incidences of various forms of cancer in patients with schizophrenia in particular in male patients [16, 41]. Some studies, however, have found the opposite trend for cancer in general [35] or for breast cancer, and it has been suggested that this could be linked to neuroleptic treatment [25, 66]. This may, however, be premature as methodological problems may explain the findings [42, 50]. Few studies have addressed this for patients with affective psychosis in general or specifically bipolar disorder [18]. However, generally no association with cancer risk has been found in large-scale epidemiological studies, meaning that the differing pattern in schizophrenia has not been found in bipolar disorder.

▌ Developmental precursors

A number of population-based cohort studies have reported on developmental precursors and biological markers for schizophrenia and affective disorders [11]. This has been summarized in a paper by Jones and Tarrant [28]. They conclude that many developmental precursors are shared between schizophrenia and affective disorder, although data generally do not allow specific conclusions regarding bipolar affective disorder. However, Cannon and coworkers in their study of the cohort in New Zealand found evidence for a specific set of impairments during early childhood in individuals who later developed schizophreniform disorder compared to other disorders [10]. The evidence regarding differences as regards developmental precursors for schizophrenia and bipolar disorders is as yet conflicting.

▌ Family history

There is probably no doubt that a family history of schizophrenia or bipolar disorder is the strongest risk factor for the two disorders, respectively. Most of the literature has suggested that there is limited overlap. However, an analysis of twin data by Cardno et al. [14] suggested that there may indeed be such an overlap. They also suggested that adopting a non-hierarchical approach when analyzing family history data might be relevant, which created some debate [30]. In our data, however, we indeed did find such overlap even when adopting a hierarchical approach to the analyses [46, 53]. The largest risk is

Table 1. Summary of various factors studied in schizophrenia and bipolar disorder

	Schizophrenia	Bipolar disorder
▌ Ethnicity and migration	+	?
▌ OCs	+	–
▌ Infections	+	–
▌ Season of birth	+	?
▌ Urbanicity of place of birth	+	–
▌ Socioeconomic status	+	+
▌ Premorbid adjustment	+	(+)
▌ Recent stress	–	+
▌ Early parental loss	(+)	+
▌ Head injury	?	(+)
▌ Childbirth	–	+
▌ Seizure disorders	+	(+)
▌ Multiple sclerosis	?	(+)
▌ Rheumatoid arthritis	+	(–)
▌ Cancer	+	–
▌ Developmental precursors	+	(+)
▌ Family history	+	+

+ Some evidence for association (positive or negative); (+) limited evidence suggesting association (positive or negative); ? no evidence for or against association; (–) limited evidence excluding association (positive or negative); – some evidence excluding association (positive or negative)

still associated with having a relative with the same disorder, but a history of other disorders also contributes to an increased risk.

If we try to summarize all this in Table 1, we see that many factors have maybe been studied relatively little in bipolar disorder compared to schizophrenia. However, given the evidence currently available, I think there would be much to suggest that there are substantial differences in the patterns of known risk factors for the two disorders.

▌ Conclusion

The conclusion of this comparative tour through risk factors for schizophrenia and bipolar affective disorder, for me, is that the differences by and large outweigh the similarities. Part of this discrepancy may be due to the fact that fewer studies have been performed in bipolar affective disorder, but where comparable evidence exists, both regarding simple demographic variables such as age and gender, and risk factors as pregnancy and birth complications, relatively distinct differences exist. However, this does not mean that there may not be a considerable overlap as regards familial risk of mental disorders. I believe it is undisputed that schizophrenia in the first-degree relatives is a stronger risk factor for schizophrenia than a family history of bipolar affective disorder, and the opposite would also be the case. However, a number of studies suggest that there is certainly an excess of affective disorders among first-degree relatives to schizophrenia patients, and this is also supported by our own data which I have shown. Therefore, although this overlap exists it would still be self-evident to me that the maintenance of the distinction between affective and non-affective psychoses is valuable, not only from a clinical point of view but also for the purpose of etiologic studies. However, it should be borne in mind also that this is not the same as saying that specific risk factors for schizophrenia exist. A number of the risk factors existing for schizophrenia may be shared with many other disorders, both mental disorders and possibly other disorders as neurological disorders, etc.

Finally, it is evident that very few studies have been conducted that allow us directly to compare the effect of individual risk factors across a broad range of mental disorders. Such studies might be very informative, both from an etiologic and a nosological point of view.

▌ References

1. Agerbo E (2003) Schizophrenia, marital and labour market status in the long run. Arch Gen Psychiatry (in press)
2. Agid O, Shapira B, Zislin J, Ritsner M, Hanin B, Murad H et al (1999) Environment and vulnerability to major psychiatric illness: a case control study of early parental loss in major depression, bipolar disorder and schizophrenia. Mol Psychiatry 4(2):163–172
3. Bredkjaer SR, Mortensen PB, Parnas J (1998) Epilepsy and non-organic non-affective psychosis. National epidemiologic study. Br J Psychiatry 172:235–238
4. Bresnahan M, Susser E (2003) Investigating socioenvironmental influences in schizophrenia: conceptual and design issues. In: Murray RM, Jones PB, Susser E, Van Os J, Cannon M (eds) The Epidemiology of Schizophrenia. Cambridge University Press, Cambridge, pp 5–17
5. Brown AS, Susser ES, Lin SP, Neugebauer R, Gorman JM (1995) Increased risk of affective disorders in males after second trimester prenatal exposure to the Dutch hunger winter of 1944–45. Br J Psychiatry 166(5):601–606
6. Brown AS, Van Os J, Driessens C, Hoek HW, Susser ES (2000) Further evidence of relation between prenatal famine and major affective disorder. Am J Psychiatry 157(2):190–195
7. Browne R, Byrne M, Mulryan N, Scully A, Morris M, Kinsella A et al (2000) Labour and delivery complications at birth and later mania. An Irish case register study. Br J Psychiatry 176:369–372
8. Buka SL, Tsuang MT, Torrey EF, Klebanoff MA, Bernstein D, Yolken RH (2001) Maternal infections and subsequent psychosis among offspring. Arch Gen Psychiatry 58(11):1032–1037
9. Byrne M, Mortensen PB (2003) Parental age and risk for schizophrenia. A case-control study. Arch Gen Psychiatry (in press)

10. Cannon M, Caspi A, Moffitt TE, Harrington H, Taylor A, Murray RM et al (2002) Evidence for early-childhood, pan-developmental impairment specific to schizophreniform disorder: results from a longitudinal birth cohort. Arch Gen Psychiatry 59(5):449–456

11. Cannon M, Jones P, Gilvarry C, Rifkin L, McKenzie K, Foerster A et al (1997) Premorbid social functioning in schizophrenia and bipolar disorder: similarities and differences. Am J Psychiatry 154(11):1544–1550

12. Cannon M, Jones PB, Murray RM (2002) Obstetric complications and schizophrenia: historical and meta-analytic review. Am J Psychiatry 159(7):1080–1092

13. Cannon M, Kendell R, Susser E, Jones P (2003) Prenatal and perinatal risk factors for schizophreni. In: Murray RM, Jones PB, Susser E, Van Os J, Cannon M, (eds) The Epidemiology of Schizophrenia. Cambridge University Press, Cambridge, pp 74–99

14. Cardno AG, Rijsdijk FV, Sham PC, Murray RM, McGuffin P (2002) A twin study of genetic relationships between psychotic symptoms. Am J Psychiatry 159(4): 539–545

15. Cantor-Graae E, Pedersen CB, McNeil TF, Mortensen PB (2003) Migration as a risk factor for schizophrenia: a Danish population-based cohort study. Br J Psychiatry 182:117–122

16. Cohen M, Dembling B, Schorling J (2002) The association between schizophrenia and cancer: a population-based mortality study. Schizophr Res 57(2/3):139–146

17. Crow TJ, Done DJ (1992) Prenatal exposure to influenza does not cause schizophrenia. Br J Psychiatry 161:390–393

18. Dalton SO, Mellemkjaer L, Olsen JH, Mortensen PB, Johansen C (2002) Depression and cancer risk: a register-based study of patients hospitalized with affective disorders, Denmark, 1969–1993. Am J Epidemiol 155(12):1088–1095

19. Done DJ, Crow TJ, Johnstone EC, Sacker A (1994) Childhood antecedents of schizophrenia and affective illness: social adjustment at ages 7 and 11. BMJ 309(6956):699–703

20. Done DJ, Johnstone EC, Frith CD, Golding J, Shepherd PM, Crow TJ (1991) Complications of pregnancy and delivery in relation to psychosis in adult life: data from the British perinatal mortality survey sample. BMJ 302(6792):1576–1580

21. Eisemann M (1986) Social class and social mobility in depressed patients. Acta Psychiatr Scand 73(4):399–402

22. Geddes JR, Verdoux H, Takei N, Lawrie SM, Bovet P, Eagles JM et al (1999) Schizophrenia and complications of pregnancy and labor: an individual patient data meta-analysis. Schizophr Bull 25(3):413–423

23. Grove W, Clayton PJ, Endicott J, Hirschfeld RM, Andreasen NC, Klerman GL (1986) Immigration and major affective disorder. Acta Psychiatr Scand 74(6): 548–552

24. Häfner H, Maurer K, Löffler W, an der Heiden W, Konnecke R, Hambrecht M (2002) The early course of schizophrenia. In: Häfner H, an der Heiden W, Resch F, Schröder J (eds) Risk and Protective Factors in Schizophrenia. Steinkopff, Darmstadt, pp 207–228

25. Halbreich U, Shen J, Panaro V (1996) Are chronic psychiatric patients at increased risk for developing breast cancer? Am J Psychiatry 153(4):559–560

26. Hare EH, Price JS, Slater E (1972) Parental social class in psychiatric patients. Br J Psychiatry 121(564):515–534

27. Hirsch S, Cramer P, Bowen J (1992) The triggering hypothesis of the role of life events in schizophrenia. Br J Psychiatry 18(suppl):84–87

28. Jones PB, Tarrant CJ (2000) Developmental precursors and biological markers for schizophrenia and affective disorders: specificity and public health implications. Eur Arch Psychiatry Clin Neurosci 250(6):286–291
29. Johnson SL, Roberts JE (1995) Life events and bipolar disorder: implications from biological theories. Psychol Bull 117(3):434–449
30. Kendler KS (2002) Hierarchy and heritability: the role of diagnosis and modeling in psychiatric genetics. Am J Psychiatry 159(4):515–518
31. Kinney DK, Yurgelun-Todd DA, Levy DL, Medoff D, Lajonchere CM, Radford-Paregol M (1993) Obstetrical complications in patients with bipolar disorder and their siblings. Psychiatry Res 48(1):47–56
32. Kinney DK, Yurgelun-Todd DA, Tohen M, Tramer S (1998) Pre- and perinatal complications and risk for bipolar disorder: a retrospective study. J Affect Disord 50(2/3):117–124
33. Lewis G, David A, Andreasson S, Allebeck P (1992) Schizophrenia and city life. Lancet 340(8812):137–140
34. Lewis SW, Murray RM (1987) Obstetric complications, neurodevelopmental deviance, and risk of schizophrenia. J Psychiatr Res 21(4):413–421
35. Lichtermann D, Ekelund J, Pukkala E, Tanskanen A, Lonnqvist J (2001) Incidence of cancer among persons with schizophrenia and their relatives. Arch Gen Psychiatry 58(6):573–578
36. Lyketsos CG, Stoline AM, Longstreet P, Ranen NG, Lesser R, Fisher R et al (1993) Mania in temporal lobe epilepsy. Neuropsychiatry Neuropsychol Behav Neurol 6(19):25
37. Makikyro T, Isohanni M, Moring J, Oja H, Hakko H, Jones P et al (1997) Is a child's risk of early onset schizophrenia increased in the highest social class? Schizophr Res 23(3):245–252
38. Marcelis M, Navarro-Mateu F, Murray R, Selten JP, Van Os J (1998) Urbanization and psychosis: a study of 1942–1978 birth cohorts in The Netherlands. Psychol Med 28(4):871–879
39. Mednick SA, Machon RA, Huttunen MD, Bonnett D (1988) Adult schizophrenia following prenatal exposure to an influenza epidemic. Arch Gen Psychiatry 45:189–192
40. Mors O, Mortensen PB, Ewald H (1999) A population-based register study of the association between schizophrenia and rheumatoid arthritis. Schizophr Res 40:67–74
41. Mortensen PB (2003) Mortality and physical illness in schizophrenia. In: Murray RM, Jones PB, Susser E, Cannon M (eds) The epidemiology of schizophrenia. Cambridge: Cambridge University Press, pp 275–287
42. Mortensen PB (1997) Breast cancer risk in psychiatric patients [letter]. Am J Psychiatry 154(4):589; discussion 589–590
43. Mortensen PB (1994) The occurrence of cancer in first admitted schizophrenic patients. Schizophr Res 12:185–194
44. Mortensen PB, Cantor-Graae E, McNeil TF (1997) Increased rates of schizophrenia among immigrants: some methodological concerns raised by Danish findings. Psychol Med 27(4):813–820
45. Mortensen PB, Mors O, Frydenberg M, Ewald H (2003) Head injury as a risk factor for bipolar affective disorder. J Affect Disord (in press)
46. Mortensen PB, Pedersen CB, Melbye M, Mors O, Ewald H (2003) Individual and familial risk factors for bipolar affective disorders in Denmark. Arch Gen Psychiatry (in press)

47. Mortensen PB, Pedersen CB, Westergaard T, Wohlfahrt J, Ewald H, Mors O et al (1999) Effects of family history and place and season of birth on the risk of schizophrenia. N Engl J Med 340(8):603–608
48. Nielsen AS, Mortensen PB, O'Callaghan E, Mors O, Ewald H (2002) Is head injury a risk factor for schizophrenia? Schizophr Res 55(1/2):93–98
49. Øgendahl BK (2002) Obstetric complications as risk factors for bipolar disorder. A Danish national register based study. National Centre for Register-based Research
50. Oksbjerg DS, Munk LT, Mellemkjaer L, Johansen C, Mortensen PB (2003) Schizophrenia and the risk for breast cancer. Schizophr Res 62(1/2):89–92
51. Petterson U (1977) Manic-depressive illness. A clinical, social and genetic study. Acta Psychiatr Scand 269(suppl):1–93
52. Pedersen CB, Mortensen PB (2001) Evidence of a dose-response relationship between urbanicity during upbringing and schizophrenia risk. Arch Gen Psychiatry 58:1039–1046
53. Pedersen CB, Mortensen PB (2001) Family history, place and season of birth as risk factors for schizophrenia in Denmark: a replication and reanalysis. Br J Psychiatry 179:46–52
54. Ramana R, Bebbington P (1995) Social influences on bipolar affective disorders. Soc Psychiatry Psychiatr Epidemiol 30(4):152–160
55. Selten JP, Slaets JP, Kahn RS (1997) Schizophrenia in Surinamese and Dutch Antillean immigrants to The Netherlands: evidence of an increased incidence. Psychol Med 27(4):807–811
56. Stober G, Kocher I, Franzek E, Beckmann H (1997) First-trimester maternal gestational infection and cycloid psychosis. Acta Psychiatr Scand 96(5):319–324
57. Susser E, Lin S (1992) Schizophrenia after prenatal exposure to the Dutch Hunger Winter of 1944–1945. Arch Gen Psychiatry 49:983–988
58. Terp IM, Engholm G, Moller H, Mortensen PB (1999) A follow-up study of postpartum psychoses: prognosis and risk factors for readmission. Acta Psychiatr Scand 100(1):40–46
59. Torrey EF, Rawlings RR, Ennis JM, Merrill DD, Flores DS (1996) Birth seasonality in bipolar disorder, schizophrenia, schizoaffective disorder and stillbirths. Schizophr Res 21(3):141–149
60. Tsuchiya K, Agerbo E, Byrne M, Mortensen PB (2003) Higher socioeconomic status of parents may increase risk for bipolar disorder in the offspring. Submitted 2003)
61. Tsuchiya K, Agerbo E, Mortensen PB (2003) Parental death and bipolar disorder: a robust association was found in early maternal suicide (submitted 2003)
62. Tsuchiya K, Mortensen PB, Byrne M (2003) Risk factors for bipolar disorder. Bipolar Disorders (in press)
63. Van Os J, Takei N, Castle DJ, Wessely S, Der G, MacDonald AM et al (1996) The incidence of mania: time trends in relation to gender and ethnicity. Soc Psychiatry Psychiatr Epidemiol 31(3/4):129–136
64. Verdoux H, Bourgeois M (1993) A comparative study of obstetric history in schizophrenics, bipolar patients and normal subjects. Schizophr Res 9(1):67–69
65. Verdoux H, Geddes JR, Takei N, Lawrie SM, Bovet P, Eagles JM et al (1997) Obstetric complications and age at onset in schizophrenia: an international collaborative meta-analysis of individual patient data. Am J Psychiatry 154(9):1220–1227

66. Wang PS, Walker AM, Tsuang MT, Orav EJ, Glynn RJ, Levin R et al (2002) Dopamine antagonists and the development of breast cancer. Arch Gen Psychiatry 59(12):1147–1154
67. Wessely S, Castle D (1991) Schizophrenia and Afro-Caribbeans. A case-control study. Br J Psychiatry 159:795–801
68. Westergaard T, Mortensen PB, Pedersen CB, Wohlfahrt J, Melbye M (1999) Exposure to prenatal and childhood infections and the risk of schizophrenia. Suggestions from a study of sibship characteristics and influenza prevalence. Arch Gen Psychiatry 56:993–998
69. Yolken RH, Torrey EF (1995) Viruses, schizophrenia, and bipolar disorder. Clin Microbiol Rev 8(1):131–145

Risk factors for schizophrenia in adolescents

M. Weiser, A. Reichenberg, J. Rabinowitz, H. Knobler, I. Grotto,
D. Nahon, K. Soares-Weiser, and M. Davidson

Chaim Sheba Medical Center, Tel-Hashomer, Israel

▌**Background.** Intellectual and behavioral abnormalities, non-psychotic psychiatric disorders, and drug abuse are sometimes present in adolescents who later develop schizophrenia. We followed a population-based cohort of adolescents with baseline assessments of intellectual and behavioral functioning, non-psychotic psychiatric disorders and drug abuse, and ascertained future hospitalization for schizophrenia.

▌**Methods.** Results of the medical and mental health assessments on 16- to 17 year-old male adolescents screened by the Israeli Draft Board were cross-linked with the National Psychiatric Hospitalization Case Registry, which contains data on all psychiatric hospitalizations in the country.

▌**Results.** Male adolescents who were later hospitalized for schizophrenia had significantly poorer test scores on all measures in comparison with adolescents not reported to the Psychiatric Registry, the magnitude of the differences was 0.3–0.5 standard deviations. Of the adolescents assigned a non-psychotic psychiatric diagnosis, 1.03% compared to only 0.23% of the adolescents without any psychiatric diagnosis were later hospitalized for schizophrenia. Of the patients with schizophrenia, 26.8% compared with only 7.4% in the general population of adolescents had been assigned a non-psychotic psychiatric diagnosis in adolescence (overall OR = 4.5, 95% CI = 3.6–5.6), ranging from OR = 21.5 (<2>95% CI = 12.6–36.6) for schizophrenia-spectrum personality disorders to OR = 3.6 (<2>95% CI = 2.1–6.2) for neurosis. The prevalence of self-reported drug abuse was higher in adolescents later hospitalized for schizophrenia (12.4%), compared with the prevalence of drug abuse in adolescents not later hospitalized (5.9%); adjusted RR = 2.033, 95% CI = 1.322–3.126.

▌**Conclusions.** These results reflect both the relatively common finding of impaired intellectual and behavioral functioning, the presence of non-psychotic psychiatric disorders, and drug abuse, in adolescents later hospitalized for schizophrenia, together with the relatively low power of these disorders in predicting schizophrenia.

▮ Introduction

Recent research suggests that the manifestation of schizophrenia is influenced by complex interactions between the known genetic, perinatal, familial, social and other environmental risk factors, with each factor contributing a relatively small part of the risk for the illness. An example may be a common functional polymorphism [Val 108/158 Met] in the catechol-o-methyltransferase gene, which accounts for a four-fold variation in enzyme activity and dopamine prefrontal catabolism of COMT, and slightly increases the risk for schizophrenia ($OR = 1.5$) (Egan et al. 2001). Other risk factors may include perinatal complications (Zornberg et al. 2000), late paternal age at conception (Malaspina et al. 2001), and subtle intellectual impairments (Reichenberg et al. 2000). Each specific risk factor by itself appears to make a very small contribution towards the clinical manifestation of schizophrenia. Furthermore, depending on the interactions with other risk factors and protective factors, the presence of a given risk factor might result in other, non-schizophrenia clinical manifestations (schizotypal personality disorder, for example), or behavioral or intellectual variants of no clinical significance. Identifying populations at risk for schizophrenia and dissecting out discreet factors contributing to the risk might constitute a reasonable strategy to understand and treat this condition (Tsuang et al. 2001).

The purpose of this paper is to present a series of studies on clinical characteristics of adolescents later hospitalized for schizophrenia. The studies presented here are a follow back or historical prospective study. This has the advantage that is drawn from an epidemiological population, not from a sample, and that it captures a very large population of cases, hence it can examine markers predicting vulnerability to the illness with high statistical power. This was done by merging the Israeli National Psychiatric Hospitalization Case Registry with the Draft Board Registry, which contains the scores of intellectual functioning and behavioral assessments, psychiatric diagnoses obtained at age 16–17 for the entire population, and records self-reported drug abuse for 15–20% of the population of males identified as having behavioral problems.

The following is a summary of intellectual and behavioral functioning (Davidson et al. 1999), non-psychotic psychiatric diagnoses (Weiser et al. 2001), and drug abuse (Weiser et al., submitted) that were identified as risk factors for schizophrenia in adolescence identified using this study design. Because the in-depth Draft Board assessment is applied only to males, these risk factors are relevant for male adolescents only.

▮ Method

Draft Board assessment

Israeli law requires that all adolescents between the ages of 16–17 undergo pre-induction assessment to determine their intellectual, medical and psychiatric eligibility for military service. This assessment is compulsory and is administered to the entire, unselected, population of Israeli adolescents. It includes individuals who will be eligible for military service, as well as those who will be excused from service based on medical, psychiatric or social reasons. The initial Draft Board assessment consists of an intelligence test battery and an interview assessing personality and behavioral traits conducted by a psychometrician, which are administrated to all male adolescents. Adolescents identified as problematic are referred for an in-depth psychosocial assessment, including screening for drug abuse. If a psychiatric diagnosis is likely, the adolescent is referred to a psychiatrist who assigns a psychiatric diagnosis where deemed appropriate. The draft board assessment is described in detail elsewhere (Gal 1986; Rabinowitz et al. 2000; Weiser et al. 2001).

The *intelligence test battery* yields a total score which is a highly valid measure of general intelligence equivalent to a normally distributed IQ score. The intellectual assessment is comprised of four sub-tests which assess arithmetic ability (Arithmetic-R), verbal abstraction and concept formation (Similarities-R), visuo-spatial abilities (RPM-R), and the ability to understand written instructions (OTIS-R).

The *behavioral assessment* is done by a trained psychometrician who administers a structured interview evaluating:

∥ *social functioning* which assesses social potency (e.g., likes to take charge, likes to be noticed at social events), and social closeness (e.g., sociable, have close interpersonal ties),
∥ *individual autonomy* which assesses personal autonomy, maturity and self-directed behavior (e.g., ability to function and make decisions independently),
∥ *organizational ability* which assesses compliance to time tables, self-mastery and self-care (e.g., ability to adhere to a schedule and tidiness responsibility), and
∥ *physical activity* which assesses the involvement in extra curricular activities concentrating in health-related physical activities (e.g., interest in sports and hiking).

The behavior is rated on a 1 (worst) to 5 (best) scale based on predetermined reliable and validated instructions. Examples of questions in the interview are: how many good friends do you have?, do you tend to be the center of attention at parties?, how often are you late for school?, do you consider yourself organized?, and who cleans your room? After this initial screening interview, those adolescents (approximately 15–20% of all male adolescents screened) who are suspected of having significant behavioral problems are referred for an in-depth psychosocial assessment.

Screening for drug abuse. All adolescents who meet the criteria for referral for the in-depth psychosocial assessment are first asked a general screening question: "Have you ever used drugs?" Those who respond affirmatively are then questioned in detail regarding the kind of drugs used, the frequency of drug use, and the psychological and physical effects of the drug. The interviewer assesses if the subject is addicted to drugs, if the use of drugs is daily and/or is a significant part of his life style or social life, and if these criteria are met, he is reported as a drug user in a yes/no format. Sporadic users are classified as non-users. Although the types of drugs used are not specified, data from several door-to-door studies on drug use between ages 12–18, carried out by the Israeli health authorities in 1989, 1992 and again in 1995, the time period that the data reported here were collected, indicate that the majority of drug users in this age group principally used marijuana.

The *mental health assessment* is a comprehensive psychosocial examination performed by a clinical social worker or psychologist, who inquires about personal and family history, previous psychological and psychiatric treatments, interpersonal relationships, self-esteem, self-injurious and anti-social acts, and functioning within the family and in school. If the clinician suspects that the adolescent suffers from psychopathology, a provisional diagnosis is suggested, and the adolescent is then referred for evaluation to a board-certified psychiatrist experienced in evaluating adolescents. Adolescents who had previously been treated by mental health professionals, or who had been hospitalized, are required to present treatment summaries and/or discharge letters. Diagnoses during the time covered by this study were based on ICD-9 criteria. In cases of co-morbidity, the examining psychiatrist decides which diagnosis is most clinically significant, and only that diagnosis is recorded, without the co-morbid condition. For the sake of simplicity, personality disorders were divided into three groups: schizophrenia-spectrum personality disorders (schizotypal and paranoid personality disorders), anti-social personality disorder, and other personality disorders (avoidant, dependent, histrionic, obsessive-compulsive, narcissistic, borderline or schizoid personality disorders). Because the ICD-9 code for affective disorders includes affective disorder with or without psychotic features, and because we were interested in future schizophrenia in adolescents with *non-psychotic* psychiatric diagnoses, adolescents diagnosed with affective disorders in the draft board were not included in the analysis, as some of the adolescents with affective disorders had psychotic as well as affective symptoms.

The National Psychiatric Hospitalization Case Registry is a complete listing of all psychiatric hospitalizations in the country, including the diagnosis assigned and coded upon admission and discharge by a board-certified psychiatrist at the facility. During the time covered by this study, ICD 9 diagnoses were used by the registry. All inpatient psychiatric facilities in the country, including psychiatric hospitals, day hospitals and psychiatric units in general hospitals, are required by law to report all admissions and discharges to the registry.

Study populations

Due to periodic changes in Draft Board procedure, each of the three research questions addressed utilized the assessments of adolescents examined by the draft board during slightly different time periods and therefore examined slightly different, but overlapping populations assessed by the Draft Board during the 1980s and 1990s. Follow-up periods ranged from 4–15 years, and the risk for schizophrenia in this population was 0.46–0.52%, which is compatible with the age-adjusted incidence of schizophrenia in other studies carried out in Israel (Levav et al. 1993) and the United States (Bromet 1995). In order to lessen the chance of including patients in the prodrome or initial stages of their disease, individuals who had a psychiatric hospitalization prior to the Draft Board assessment or within one year from the date of Draft Board assessment were excluded. The analyses of the intelligence tests and behavioral assessment scores of the cases were compared to the mean scores of a control group made up of all individuals tested at the same age and attending the same high school who were found eligible for military service and did not appear in the Psychiatric Hospitalization Registry. Matching cases to non-cases by high school attended at the time of testing was an attempt to control for educational and social opportunities.

▌ Results

The analysis of behavioral and intelligence test scores focused on examining the extent to which test scores could be used to correctly classify draftees as cases or controls. Five hundred and nine cases were compared to their matched control schoolmates using a paired samples t-test. As a group, individuals destined to develop schizophrenia (n = 509) obtained statistically significant lower (worse) scores on all measures as compared to matched non-cases (n = 9,215) and to the entire population (all p values were lower than 0.0001). The differences between future cases and controls ranged from 0.3–0.5 standard deviations. To examine the extent to which the behavioral and intelligence measures discriminated between the cases and matched controls, the distribution of the scores in these two groups were compared. For this analysis the mean score of the non-case matched comparisons was used. The most pronounced differences were in social functioning, where 8.3% of cases had the lowest score and 35.1% had the second to lowest score, whereas only 0.8% and 6.2% of non-cases, respectively, had scores in these categories. Thus, although a high proportion of cases perform below the range of *their* comparisons, as a group, future schizophrenics perform over the entire range of possible normal performance (i.e. comparing the distribution of all cases to the distribution of all controls).

The follow-up of adolescents with non-psychotic psychiatric diagnoses found that having any non-psychotic psychiatric disorder in adolescence increased the risk of future hospitalization for schizophrenia, compared with the risk for schizophrenia in the entire cohort of adolescents. The prevalence of non-psychotic psychiatric disorders in future schizophrenia patients was 26.8%, as compared to 7.4% of non-psychotic, non-major affective psychiatric disorders in the general population of adolescents (OR = 4.5, 95% CI = 3.6–5.6).

The non-psychotic psychiatric diagnoses assigned by Draft Board psychiatrists, and the risk for later hospitalization for schizophrenia showed an association was found between the different disorders in adolescence, and schizophrenia. The magnitude of this association differed between the different diagnostic groups. For example, patients with a registry diagnosis of schizophrenia were about 21.5 times more likely to have had a pre-morbid diagnosis of schizophrenia-spectrum personality disorder in adolescence, compared with the prevalence of schizophrenia-spectrum personality disorder in the general population of adolescents. On the other hand, patients with a registry diagnosis of schizophrenia were only about 3.6 times more likely to have had a pre-morbid diagnosis of neurosis in adolescence, compared with the prevalence of neurosis in the general population of adolescents.

Among the adolescents who were identified by the Draft Board screening process as having behavioral disturbances and were systematically asked about drug abuse, subjects with baseline drug abuse were two times more likely (12.4% vs. 5.9%, adjusted RR = 2.033, 95% CI = 1.322–3.126) to be later hospitalized for schizophrenia, in comparison to adolescents who did not report drug use. This effect was specific for schizophrenia, as the rate of drug abuse in patients later hospitalized for affective disorders was not different than the rate of drug abuse in the entire cohort: 5.1% of the adolescents later hospitalized for affective disorder reported using drugs in the Draft Board, vs. the 5.9% rate of drug abuse in the cohort, RR = 0.9075, 95% CI = 0.2813–2.9272. The observed association between drug abuse and later hospitalization with schizophrenia was maintained after controlling for the presence of below-normal intellectual functioning, below-normal social functioning, and/or the presence of a non-psychotic psychiatric disorder in the Draft Board assessment (Wald Chi-square = 6.53, df = 1, p = 0.0106, RR = 1.70, 95% CI: 1.13–2.56).

The observed overall increase in drug use before the onset of illness might be explained by self-medication of the non-psychotic symptoms often preceding psychosis in schizophrenia patients. Consistent with this, it would be expected that the prevalence of drug abuse would increase as the first psychotic episode draws closer. To investigate this assumption, we evaluated the association between drug abuse and risk for future schizophrenia in the years preceding the first psychiatric admission. A Kaplan-Meier survival analysis found that those individuals who abused drugs were hospitalized farther from the Draft Board assessment, rather than closer to it (log rank = 8.54, df = 1, p = 0.0035). The finding that adolescents who abuse drugs were hospitalized farther from, rather than closer to hospitalization does not support the hypothesis that pre-morbid drug abuse reflects self-medication of non-psychotic symptoms preceding the onset of psychosis. This interpretation was also supported by finding that patients who abused drugs had a later mean age of first hospitalization, compared to those who did not report abusing drugs (23.48 ± 2.23 years vs. 21.98 ± 2.6 years, respectively; t = 2.79, df = 261, p = 0.006).

The comparison of social functioning in future schizophrenia patients with social functioning of those male adolescents in this cohort who were not later hospitalized found that future schizophrenia patients who abused drugs had non-significantly better social functioning compared with future schizophrenia patients who did not abuse drugs (2.65 ± 1.06 vs. 2.36 ± 0.80, t = 1.69, p = 0.092), a finding which does not support the hypothesis that drug abuse reflects self-medication of pre-morbid social withdrawal.

∎ Discussion

These data confirm and extend existing reports indicating that as a group, individuals destined to develop schizophrenia manifest subtle intellectual and behavioral abnormalities before the symptoms essential to diagnose schizophrenia manifest. In addition, 26.8% of the males hospitalized for schizophrenia suffered from non-psychotic psychiatric disorders in adolescence, in comparison to 7.4% prevalence of non-psychotic psychiatric disorders in the general population of adolescents. These findings are consistent with and extend previous studies (Jones et al. 1993; Done et al. 1994) which found that persons with schizophrenia often suffer from behavioral and emotional disturbances years before the manifestation of psychosis. More unique are the findings of the follow-up, which found that adolescents with non-psychotic psychiatric disorders had an increased risk for future schizophrenia (1.03%), as compared with the risk for schizophrenia in the entire population (0.46%). Taken together, these may indicate that although many patients with schizophrenia have behavioral deviations in adolescence, these behavioral deviations alone lack the specificity necessary to predict future schizophrenia, because the vast majority of adolescents who have low scores on assessments of intelligence or behavior, or have non-psychotic psychiatric disorders, do not later suffer from schizophrenia.

Another singular finding of this report is the gradient of association between the various psychiatric disorders and future schizophrenia. While the OR of persons with other personality disorders and neuroses were 3.6–3.9, adolescents with anti-social personality disorder, mental retardation or drug abuse had OR in the range of 7–9.

Moreover, adolescents with schizophrenia-spectrum personality disorders (SSPD's) had an OR of 21.5. It could be hypothesized that those non-psychotic psychiatric disorders with higher ORs share more genetic or environmental factors in common with schizophrenia. This makes sense particularly for the SSPDs, which are phenomenologically more similar to schizophrenia (Siever et al. 1993).

The data presented here are consistent with high-risk studies (Parnas et al. 1993; Erlenmeyer-Kimling 2000) of children and siblings of persons with schizophrenia that found increased prevalence of non-psychotic symptoms and diagnoses in these persons, and increased prevalence of schizophrenia at follow-up. Furthermore, the finding that adolescents with SSPDs have increased chances of future schizophrenia replicates and expands other studies, which found that magical thinking (Chapman et al. 1994; Kwapil et al. 1997) and schizotypal symptoms (Fenton and McGlashan 1989) increase the risk of future schizophrenia. The findings in this report replicate very closely a recently published paper with a similar design (Lewis et al. 2000), which followed conscripts screened by the Swedish Draft Board for Future Hospitalization for Schizophrenia. That study reported that 38% of the future patients had a diagnosis of non-psychotic psychiatric disorder at age 18, with OR of 4.6 for neurosis, 8.2 for personality disorder, 5.5 for alcohol abuse, and 14.0 for substance abuse. The great similarity of the findings in that paper with the present report support the reliability of the data reported here.

Drug abuse, mainly marijuana, was also found to be a risk factor for schizophrenia. In a cohort of 50 413 male adolescents who were suspected of having behavioral problems, those adolescents who self-reported abuse of drugs at age 16–17 were 2 times more likely to be later hospitalized for schizophrenia. These data are compatible with the one previous, longitudinal study on Swedish army conscripts which utilized a similar study design, and found that over a 15 year follow-up, the relative risk of hospitalization for schizophrenia in heavy cannabis users (more than fifty occasions) was 6.0, compared to non-users (Andreasson et al. 1987). Similarly, a retrospective study in which patients with schizophrenia were asked about the use of cannabis before the onset of the illness reported higher rates of cannabis use in patients compared with controls (Hambrecht and Häfner 2000). Taken together these findings indicate that use of drugs might interact with other risk factors contributing to the manifestations of schizophrenic symptoms in vulnerable individuals. Support to this idea is drawn from a report which found that the density of canabinoid receptors was increased in the dorsolateral prefrontal cortex in subjects with schizophrenia, compared with controls (Dean et al. 2001). This increased density of canabinoid receptors might be an example of an underlying brain pathology which increases vulnerability, and when the vulnerable brain is exposed to the trigger (illicit drugs), this may increase the risk of later symptom manifestation. Yet another view (Chambers et al. 2001) of the association between schizophrenia and drug abuse before the onset of overt psychosis is based on evidence that developmental neuropathology in hippocampal and pre-frontal cortical pathways contributes both to symptoms of schizophrenia and to vulnerability to addictive behavior, via dysfunctional interactions with the nucleus accumbens.

The finding that drug use is more prevalent among adolescents who develop schizophrenia farther from, rather than closer to the questioning about drug use is not consistent with the explanation that illicit drugs are used to ameliorate the anxiety, depression, and confusion that characterize prodromal schizophrenia. Another possibility is that drug use is actually an effective treatment of prodromal symptoms, and thus is associated with delay of first hospitalization.

▌ Limitations

The diagnoses assigned by Draft Board psychiatrists are not research but clinical diagnoses, raising concerns about their accuracy. However all the psychiatrists working for the Draft Board are board-certified, received their postgraduate education after the introduction of DSM III, and are instructed and supervised on a regular basis for quality and consistency. The three-stage screening procedure used by the Draft Board dictates that even before the adolescent is referred to the psychiatrist, both the interviewer assessing personality and behavioral traits, and the clinical social worker or clinical psychologist identify him as having significant behavioral problems. In addition, the clinical social worker or clinical psychologist assigns a tentative diagnosis, so that the psychiatric diagnosis assigned reflects the consensus diagnosis between them and the psychiatrist. Disagreements between the two are resolved by consensus with the help of another, senior psychiatrist.

A related concern is the fact that the case registry diagnoses are clinical, not research diagnoses. However, these diagnoses too are assigned by board-certified psychiatrists who have had the benefit of observing the patient throughout one or more hospitalizations, and had been trained and re-trained in the use of the diagnostic criteria of the ICD 9. Moreover, studies which have compared clinical diagnoses of schizophrenia assigned in hospitals in the US (Pulver et al. 1988) and in Israel (Knobler 2000) with research diagnoses have shown a high degree of concordance.

The results are limited to males since the Draft Board administers behavioral tests only to males (females undergo intelligence testing only). Since male patients are more likely than female patients to be hospitalized for schizophrenia (Munk-Jorgensen 1985), and since male patients may suffer from a more severe form of illness (Meltzer et al. 1997), the more severely ill schizophrenic patients might be overrepresented in this study.

The prevalence of non-psychotic psychiatric diagnoses made by the Draft Board in the population of adolescents, approximately 7.4%, is lower than the prevalence of psychiatric disorders found in some, but not all, other studies (Roberts et al. 1998). One reason for the relatively low prevalence rates observed may be that the Draft Board screening procedure sets a high threshold for diagnosis of minor psychiatric disturbances, compared with screening instruments used in epidemiological surveys. For example, diagnoses such as specific phobias (included here in the "anxiety" category), which are relatively common in epidemiological surveys, are less common in the present sample.

The Draft Board assessment is intended to screen adolescents before military service, and not specifically to detect recruits who will manifest schizophrenia, and the instruments used reflect this. It is clear that the optimal design of a study assessing the association between intellectual and behavioral functioning, non-psychotic psychiatric diagnoses, and drug abuse in adolescence with later hospitalization for schizophrenia would screen subjects using structured research instruments which specifically assess intellectual and behavioral functioning known to be impaired in patients with schizophrenia, and to ascertain diagnoses both of the non-psychotic psychiatric disorders at baseline and of schizophrenia using the SCID or similar instruments. However, the incidence of schizophrenia in the population is between 0.5–1%, and not all patients have abnormal intellectual and behavioral functioning, non-psychotic psychiatric disorders, or abuse drugs before manifesting psychosis. In order to yield significant results, this hypothetical protocol would therefore necessitate screening of hundreds of thousands of adolescents and then following them for years, a project which is probably not feasible in the near future.

Conclusions

The results of this study, based on the screening of an entire population of 16–17 year old males, indicate that years before the onset of illness, future schizophrenia patients have subtle impairments in intellectual and behavioral functioning, and that non-psychotic psychiatric disorders in adolescence are associated with future schizophrenia. Drug abuse is also associated with future schizophrenia, and is probably not due to self-medication of pre-morbid symptoms.

References

Andreasson S, Allebeck P et al (1987) Cannabis and schizophrenia. A longitudinal study of Swedish conscripts. Lancet 2(8574):1483–1486

Bromet EJ, Dew MA, Eaton W (1995) Epidemiology of psychosis with special reference to schizophrenia. In: Tsuang MT, Tohen M, Zahner GEP (eds) Psychiatric Epidemiology. John Wiley & Sons, New York, pp 283–300

Chambers RA, Krystal JH et al (2001) A neurobiological basis for substance abuse comorbidity in schizophrenia. Biol Psychiatry 50(2):71–83

Chapman LJ, Chapman JP et al (1994) Putatively psychosis-prone subjects 10 years later. J Abnorm Psychol 103(2):171–183

Davidson M, Reichenberg A et al (1999) Behavioral and intellectual markers for schizophrenia in apparently healthy male adolescents [in process citation]. Am J Psychiatry 156(9):1328–1335

Dean B, Sundram S et al (2001) Studies on [3H]CP-55940 binding in the human central nervous system: regional specific changes in density of cannabinoid-1 receptors associated with schizophrenia and cannabis use. Neuroscience 103(1):9–15

Done DJ, Crow TJ et al (1994) Childhood antecedents of schizophrenia and affective illness: social adjustment at ages 7 and 11 [see comments]. BMJ 309(6956):699–703

Egan MF, Goldberg TE et al (2001) Effect of COMT Val108/158 Met genotype on frontal lobe function and risk for schizophrenia. Proc Natl Acad Sci USA 98(12):6917–6922

Erlenmeyer-Kimling L (2000) Neurobehavioral deficits in offspring of schizophrenic parents: liability indicators and predictors of illness. Am J Med Genet 97(1):65–71

Fenton WS, McGlashan TH (1989) Risk of schizophrenia in character disordered patients. Am J Psychiatry 146(10):1280–1284

Gal R (1986) The selection, classification and placement process. In: Gal R (ed) A Portrait of the Israeli Soldier. Greenwood Press, Westport, CT, pp 77

Hambrecht M, Häfner H (2000) Cannabis, vulnerability, and the onset of schizophrenia: an epidemiological perspective. Aust N Z J Psychiatry 34(3):468–475

Jones PB, Bebbington P et al (1993) Premorbid social underachievement in schizophrenia. Results from the Camberwell Collaborative Psychosis Study. Br J Psychiatry 162:65–71

Knobler HY (2000) First psychotic episodes among Israeli youth during military service. Mil Med 165(3):169–172

Kwapil TR, Miller MB et al (1997) Magical ideation and social anhedonia as predictors of psychosis proneness: a partial replication. J Abnorm Psychol 106(3):491–495

Levav I, Kohn R et al (1993) An epidemiological study of mental disorders in a 10-year cohort of young adults in Israel. Psychol Med 23(3):691–707

Lewis G, David AS et al (2000) Non-psychotic psychiatric disorder and subsequent risk of schizophrenia: cohort study [in process citation]. Br J Psychiatry 177:416–420

Malaspina D, Harlap S et al (2001) Advancing paternal age and the risk of schizophrenia. Arch Gen Psychiatry 58(4):361–367

Meltzer HY, Rabinowitz J et al (1997) Age at onset and gender of schizophrenic patients in relation to neuroleptic resistance. Am J Psychiatry 154(4):475–482

Munk-Jorgensen P (1985) The schizophrenia diagnosis in Denmark. A register-based investigation. Acta Psychiatr Scand 72(3):266–273

Parnas J, Cannon TD et al (1993) Lifetime DSM-III-R diagnostic outcomes in the offspring of schizophrenic mothers. Results from the Copenhagen High-Risk Study. Arch Gen Psychiatry 50(9):707–714

Pulver AE, Carpenter WT et al (1988) Accuracy of the diagnoses of affective disorders and schizophrenia in public hospitals. Am J Psychiatry 145(2):218–220

Rabinowitz J, Reichenberg A et al (2000) Cognitive and behavioural functioning in men with schizophrenia both before and shortly after first admission to hospital. Cross-sectional analysis. Br J Psychiatry 177:26–32

Reichenberg A, Rabinowitz J et al (2000) Premorbid functioning in a national population of male twins discordant for psychoses. Am J Psychiatry 157(9):1514–1516

Roberts RE, Attkisson CC et al (1998) Prevalence of psychopathology among children and adolescents. Am J Psychiatry 155(6):715–725

Siever LJ, Kalus OF et al (1993) The boundaries of schizophrenia. Psychiatr Clin North Am 16(2):217–244

Tsuang MT, Stone WS et al (2001) Genes, environment and schizophrenia. Br J Psychiatry 40(suppl):18–24

Weiser M, Reichenberg A et al: Self-reported drug abuse in male adolescents with behavioural disturbances, and follow-up for future schizophrenia. Biol Psychiatry 54(6):655-660

Weiser M, Reichenberg A et al (2001) Association between nonpsychotic psychiatric diagnoses in adolescent males and subsequent onset of schizophrenia. Arch Gen Psychiatry 58(10):959–964

Zornberg GL, Buka SL et al (2000) Hypoxic-ischemia-related fetal/neonatal complications and risk of schizophrenia and other nonaffective psychoses: a 19-year longitudinal study. Am J Psychiatry 157(2):196–202

Cannabis as a causal factor for psychosis – a review of the evidence

John Witton[1], Louise Arseneault[2], Mary Cannon[3], and Robin Murray[3]

[1] National Addiction Centre, Institute of Psychiatry, King's College London, UK
[2] Social, Genetic, and Developmental Psychiatry Research Centre, Institute of Psychiatry, King's College London, UK
[3] Division of Psychological Medicine, Institute of Psychiatry, King's College London, UK

Abstract

Adults suffering from psychosis have high rates of cannabis use. However, there remains controversy as to whether this is a cause or consequence of the psychosis. This review tests the hypothesis that cannabis can cause psychosis by reviewing studies verifying three important criteria for causality in psychiatry: association, temporal priority, and direction, with the emphasis put on prospective longitudinal population-based studies that tested temporal priority. Evidence supports a causal role for cannabis in the development of psychosis but it appears that cannabis use is neither a sufficient nor a necessary cause for psychosis. Rather, it is a component cause – part of a complex constellation of factors leading to psychosis. On an individual level, cannabis use appears to confer only a two- to three-fold increase in the relative risk for later schizophrenia. On a population level, elimination of cannabis use could lead to a 7–13% reduction in incidence of schizophrenia. Thus, some cases of psychotic disorder could be prevented by discouraging cannabis use, particularly among vulnerable youths. More research is needed to better understand the mechanisms by which cannabis causes psychosis.

Introduction

There is little dispute that cannabis intoxication can trigger brief episodes of psychotic symptoms and that it can produce short-term exacerbation or recurrences of pre-existing psychotic symptoms (Mathers and Ghodse 1992; Negrete et al. 1986; Thornicroft 1990; Hall and Degenhardt in press). However, there remains controversy about whether cannabis use can actually cause schizophrenia (Johns 2001). More than 10 years ago, a review by Thornicroft (1990) examined the evidence supporting an association between cannabis and psychosis from clinical and epidemiological studies, but reached no firm conclusion regarding causality. The paper concluded by stressing the importance of prospective longitudinal population-based cohort studies to elucidating the potential causal influence of cannabis on psychosis.

Now, fifteen years after the publication of the first evidence that cannabis may be a causal risk factor for later schizophrenia (Andréasson et al. 1987), four prospective epidemiological studies have further examined the question (Van Os et al 2002; Zammit et al. 2002; Arseneault et al. 2002; Fergusson et al. 2003). We review this evidence within the framework of established criteria for determining causality.

▌ What is a cause?

Rothman and Greenland (1998) have defined a cause of a specific disease occurrence as "*an event, condition or characteristic that preceded that disease occurrence, and without which the disease would either not have occurred at all, or would not have occurred until some later time*". The same authors also used pictures of 'causal pies' as a device to explain the concept of *necessary* and *sufficient* causes (Fig. 1). Each pie can be thought of as a constellation of causes that inevitably leads to disease occurrence, each constellation being *sufficient* for causation. Each slice in the pie represents a *component* cause. Each component is necessary for the disease to occur from that particular causal constellation. A disease may have many different sufficient causes. A particular component cause may also be part of several different sufficient causal constellations and therefore lead to a disease in conjunction with different component causes. Any component cause that is an active agent in all the sufficient

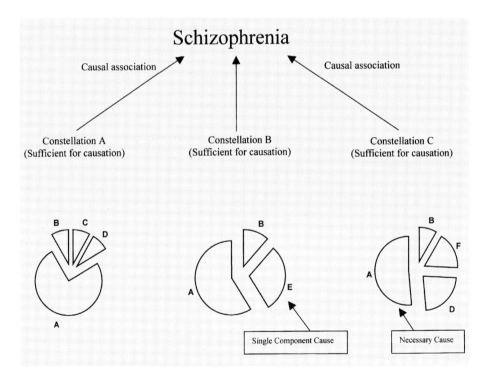

Fig. 1. Causal pie model

causes for a disease outcome is deemed a *necessary* cause. The disease will not occur without it. For the purposes of this review, the evidence that cannabis is a causal factor for schizophrenia will be assessed for association, temporal priority, and direction, the three defining criteria of a cause (Susser 1991).

∎ Cannabis and psychosis: evidence for association

Four major national surveys (from the USA, the UK, Australia, and the Netherlands) have compared rates of cannabis use among people with schizophrenia and among the general population (Johns 2001).

The US National Epidemiological Catchment Area study (Robins and Regier 1991) indicated that 50% of those identified with schizophrenia also had a diagnosis of substance use disorder (abuse or dependence), compared with 17% of the general population (Regier et al. 1990). People who used cannabis on a daily basis were 2.4 times more likely to report psychotic experiences than non-daily cannabis users, even after controlling for a variety of confounding variables such as sociodemographic factors, social role, and psychiatric conditions (Tien and Anthony 1990).

In contrast, the UK National Psychiatric Morbidity Survey reported that both 5% of patients with schizophrenia or delusional disorders and 5% of the general population reported using cannabis during the year prior to interview (Farrell et al. 1998). The low rates of cannabis use reported in this study might be explained by the exclusive use of self-reports to assess cannabis use among the two high-risk groups, potentially creating a problem of underreporting cannabis use.

The more representative Australian National Survey of Mental Health and Well-Being found that 12% of those diagnosed with schizophrenia also had met ICD-10 criteria for cannabis use disorder (Hall and Degenhardt 2000). After statistically adjusting for other disorders and socio-demographic factors, individuals who met the ICD-10 criteria for cannabis dependence were nearly three times as likely to report that they had been diagnosed with schizophrenia than those without cannabis dependence disorder. Finally, a population-based study conducted in the Netherlands reported that cannabis use was more prevalent among those subjects with psychotic symptoms at the initial assessment (15.3%) than those without (7.7%) (Van Os et al. 2002).

Local surveys in the United Kingdom have found high rates of cannabis use in psychiatric patients under treatment. A study of patients with psychotic illnesses in contact with mental health services in South London found that 40.4% reported trying cannabis at least once in their life (Menezes et al. 1996). Another study showed that 51% of a patient sample detained under the 1983 Mental Health Act reported lifetime use of cannabis (Wheatley 1998). A recent study in Scotland indicated that 7% of schizophrenia patients reported problematic use of drugs (4% related specifically to cannabis use) compared to 2% of controls (McCreadie, 2002). Also, nearly 20% of 352 people suffering from schizophrenia and other related psychoses in a central London area reported lifetime cannabis use (Duke et al. 2001). This group included individuals living in the community as well as hospitalised patients and took place in areas with notable deprivation; unfortunately, the absence of controls prevents us from comparing this rate with that for the general population. Finally, a study examining psychotic patients at a hospital in South London showed that 38.8% of patients and 21.9% of controls were using cannabis (Grech et al. 1998).

The elevated rates of cannabis use among people with schizophrenia raise the question of whether the cannabis use is a consequence or a cause of the condition? Studies examining temporal priority between the drug consumption and the diagnosis help answer this question.

∎ Cannabis and psychosis – evidence for temporal priority and direction

In order to establish temporal priority, we need to have prospective reports of cannabis use, collected before the onset of schizophrenia, and hence, unbiased by later outcome. Ideally these studies should use population-based samples.

Prospective studies

So far, there are four population-based samples in which use of cannabis was assessed in adolescence, before diagnosis of schizophrenia outcomes: three cohort studies and one longitudinal population-based survey. These samples are described below and summarised in Table 1. The results are summarised in Table 2.

∎ The Swedish Conscript Cohort.

For many years, the only evidence as to whether cannabis use might predispose to later psychosis came from a cohort study of 50 087 Swedish conscripts who were followed up using record-linkage techniques based on inpatient admissions for psychiatric care (Andréasson et al. 1987). A dose-response relationship was observed between cannabis use at conscription (age of 18) and schizophrenia diagnosis 15 years later. Self-reported 'heavy cannabis users' (i.e. who had used cannabis more than 50 times) were 6 times more likely than non-users to have been diagnosed with schizophrenia 15 years later. However, more than half of these heavy users had a psychiatric diagnosis other than psychosis at conscription and when this confound was controlled for, the relative risk decreased to 2.3 (but nonetheless remained statistically significant). Of note, very few heavy cannabis users (3%) went on to develop schizophrenia, indicating that cannabis use may serve to increase the risk for schizophrenia only among individuals already vulnerable to developing psychosis. The authors concluded that "*Cannabis should be viewed as an additional clue to the still elusive aetiology of schizophrenia*".

A follow-up study of the same Swedish Conscript Cohort has recently been carried out (Zammit et al. 2002). Consistent with the original findings, this report showed that 'heavy cannabis users' by the age of 18 years were 6.7 times more likely than non-users to be diagnosed with schizophrenia 27 years later.

Table 1. Epidemiological studies on cannabis use and schizophrenia

Authors	Study design, year of enrolment (N)	Sex	Number of participants	Follow-up (years)	Age of cannabis users	Outcome	N (%) of outcome	Diagnostic criteria
Swedish Conscript Cohort (Sweden)	Andréasson et al., 1987	Conscript cohort 69–70 (~ 50000)	Males	45570	15	18	1. Inpatient admission for schizophrenia	246 (0.5)	ICD 8
	Zammit et al., 2002	Conscript cohort 69–70 (~ 50 000)	Males	50053	27	18	1. Hospital admission for schizophrenia	362 (0.7)	ICD 8/9
NEMESIS (the Netherlands)	Van Os et al., 2002	Population based study 96 (7076)	Males and females	4104	3	Between 18 and 64	1. Any level of psychotic symptoms 2. Pathology level of psychotic symptoms 3. Need for care	38 (0.9) 10 (0.3) 7 (0.2)	BPRS (Brief Psychiatric Rating Scale)
Dunedin Study (New Zealand)	Arseneault et al., 2002	Birth cohort 72–73 (1037)	Males and females	759	11	15	Schizophreniform disorder 1. Symptoms 2. Diagnosis	25 (3.3)	DSM-IV

Table 2. Findings from epidemiological studies on cannabis use and schizophrenia

	Risk (OR, 95% CI)	Adjusted risk (OR, 95% CI)	Confounding variables controlled for	Dose-response relationship	Specificity of risk factor	Specificity of outcome
Swedish conscript cohort	1. 6.0 (4.0–8.9) for those who used cannabis >50 times at 18 2. 6.7 (4.5–10.0) for those who used cannabis >50 times at age 18	2.3 (1.0–5.3) 3.1 (1.7–5.5)	– psychiatric diagnosis at conscription – parents divorced – diagnosis at conscription – IQ score – Social integration – disturbed behaviour – cigarette smoking – place of upbringing	yes yes	no yes	N/A yes
NEMESIS	1. 3.25 (1.5–7.2) 2. 28.54 (7.3–110.9) 3. 16.15 (3.6–72.5) for cannabis use at baseline (age 16–17)	2.76 (1.2–6.5) 24.17 (5.44–107.5) 12.01 (2.4–64.3)	– age – sex – ethnic group – single marital status – education – urbanicity – discrimination	yes	yes	N/A
Dunedin Study	1. 6.91 (5.1–8.7) (B)* 2. 4.50 (1.1–18.2) Users by the age of 15 and continued at 18 * Beta of multiple linear regression	6.56 (4.78–8.34)* 3.12 (0.7–13.3) * Beta of multiple linear regression	– sex – social class – psychotic symptoms prior to cannabis use	N/A	yes	yes

This risk held when the analysis was repeated on a sub-sample of men who used cannabis only, as opposed to using other drugs as well. The risk was reduced but remained significant after controlling for other potential confounding factors such as disturbed behaviour, low IQ score, growing up in a city, cigarette smoking, and poor social integration. In order to control for the possibility that cannabis use might be a consequence of prodromal manifestations of psychosis, the analyses were repeated on a subsample of individuals who developed schizophrenia at least five years after conscription; the findings obtained were similar to those with the entire cohort. The authors concluded that the findings are *"consistent with a causal relationship between cannabis use and schizophrenia"*.

▌ **The Dutch NEMESIS sample.** An analysis of the Netherlands Mental Health Survey and Incidence Study (NEMESIS) (Van Os et al. 2002) goes beyond the reliance on hospital discharge register data for outcomes and examines the effect of cannabis use on psychotic symptoms among the general population. In this study, 4 045 psychosis-free and 59 subjects with self-reported symptoms of psychosis were assessed at baseline and then were assessed one year later, and again three years after the baseline assessment. For those subjects who reported psychotic symptoms, an additional clinical interview was conducted by an experienced psychiatrist or psychologist (at baseline and at three-year follow-up). Compared to non-users, individuals using cannabis at baseline were nearly three times more likely to manifest psychotic symptoms at follow-up. This risk remained significant after statistical adjustment for a range of factors including ethnic group, marital status, educational level, urbanicity, and discrimination. The authors also found a dose-response relationship with the highest risk (odds ratio = 6.8) being observed for the highest level of cannabis use. Further analysis revealed that lifetime history of cannabis use at baseline was a stronger predictor of psychosis three years later than the use of cannabis at follow-up. This suggests that the association between cannabis use and psychosis is not merely the result of short-term effects of cannabis use leading to an acute psychotic episode. Use of other drugs did not explain the risk associated with cannabis use for later psychosis: although use of other drugs was associated with psychosis outcomes, the effects were not significant after taking into account cannabis use. The authors concluded that this study confirms *"that cannabis use is an independent risk factor for the emergence of psychosis in psychosis-free persons and that those with an established vulnerability to psychotic disorders are particularly sensitive to its effects, resulting in a poor outcome."* However, the relatively short time-lag between baseline and follow-up assessments in this study tends to provide more support for an *association* between cannabis use and psychosis, rather than verifying *temporal priority*.

▌ **The Christchurch Health and Development Study.** The *association* between cannabis use and psychosis was also investigated in the Christchurch Study, a birth cohort of 1265 individuals from the South Island of New Zealand who have been studied for more than 20 years. Linkage between cannabis dependence disorder and levels of psychotic symptoms at ages 18 and 21 was examined taking into account several potential confounding factors including previous psychotic symptoms level (Fergusson et al. 2003). Statistical control for previous psychotic symptoms clarifies the temporal sequencing by attempting to rule out an alternative explanation, that is, psychotic symptoms cause cannabis dependence. The findings indicated concurrent associations between cannabis dependence disorder and rates of psychotic symptoms both at ages 18 and 21; individuals meeting diagnostic criteria for cannabis dependence disorder at age 18 had a rate of psychotic symptoms that was 3.7 times higher than those without cannabis dependence problems, and 2.3 times higher for those with cannabis dependence disorder at age 21. Moreover, after controlling for an exhaustive list of confounding factors including anxiety disorder, deviant peer affiliations, exposure to childhood sexual or physical abuse, educational achievement, and most importantly psychotic symptoms at the previous assessment, the association remained strong and significant at age 21. The authors concluded that *"the findings are clearly consistent with the view that heavy cannabis use may make a causal contribution to the development of psychotic symptoms since they show that independently of pre-existing psychotic symptoms and a wide range of social and contextual factors, young people who develop cannabis dependence show elevated rate of psychotic symptoms."*

▌ **Dunedin Multidisciplinary Health and Development Study.** The Dunedin Multidisciplinary Health and Development Study (Silva and Stanton 1996) is a study of a general-population birth cohort of 1037 individuals born in Dunedin, New Zealand, in 1972–1973 (96% follow-up rate at age 26). Although small, this study has unique advantages:

▌ it has information on self-reported psychotic symptoms at age 11, before the onset of cannabis use;

▌ it allows the examination of the age of onset of cannabis use in relation to later outcome, as self-reports of cannabis use were obtained at ages 15 and 18; and

▌ it does not rely on treatment data for outcomes as the entire cohort were assessed at age 26 using a standardised psychiatric interview schedule yielding *DSM-IV* (American Psychiatric Association 1994) diagnoses (Poulton et al. 2000).

This allowed the examination of schizophrenia outcome both as a continuum (by examination of symptoms) and as a disorder (DSM-IV schizophreniform disorder) in this population. Of note, in obtaining a schizophreniform diagnosis, the interview protocol ruled out psychotic symptoms occurring while under the influence of alcohol and drugs.

Those subjects using cannabis at ages 15 and 18 had higher rates of psychotic symptoms at age 26, compared to non-users (Arseneault et al. 2002). This remained significant after controlling for quasi-psychotic symptoms at age 11 years, i.e. predating the onset of cannabis use. The effect was stronger with earlier use (i.e. by 15 rather than 18 years). In addition, onset of cannabis use by age 15 was associated with an increased likelihood of meeting diag-

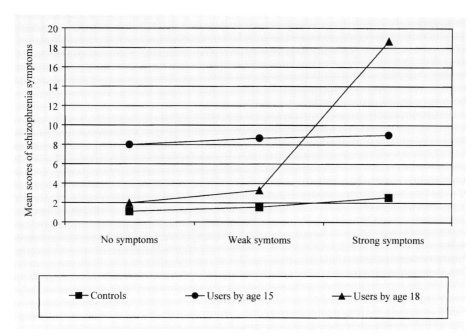

Fig. 2. Interaction between cannabis use at age 18 and psychotic symptoms at age 11 in predicting adult schizophrenia symptoms

nostic criteria for schizophreniform disorder at age 26. Indeed, 10.3% of the age-15 cannabis users in this cohort were diagnosed with schizophreniform disorder at age 26, as opposed to 3% of the controls. After controlling for age-11 psychotic symptoms, the risk for adult schizophreniform disorder remained elevated (odds ratio = 3.1) though was no longer statistically significant, possibly due to power limitation.

Cannabis use by age 15 did not predict depressive outcomes at age 26 (indicating specificity of the outcome) and the use of other illicit drugs in adolescence did not predict schizophrenia outcomes over and above the effect of cannabis use (indicating specificity of the exposure). A significant exacerbation or interaction effect was found between cannabis use by age 18 and age-11 psychotic symptoms (Fig. 2). This effect indicates that age-18 cannabis users had elevated scores on the schizophrenic symptom scale only if they had reported psychotic symptoms at age 11. The authors concluded that *"using cannabis in adolescence increases the likelihood of experiencing symptoms of schizophrenia in adulthood."*

▌ Methodological issues

Before coming to a conclusion about cannabis as a causal risk factor for schizophrenia, it is important to point out some methodological limitations in the four population-based longitudinal studies we have just discussed.

Firstly, a variety of measures of schizophrenia outcome were used in these studies: hospital discharge, pathology-level of psychosis, psychotic symptoms, and schizopheniform disorder. The heterogeneity of the outcome makes it difficult to draw a firm conclusion on schizophrenia from the findings reported by these studies. However, it is at least reassuring that all studies converge in showing an elevated risk for "psychosis" in later life amongst cannabis users.

Secondly, all measures of cannabis use were based on self-reports and were not supplemented by urine or hair analysis. In particular, the reliability of non-anonymous interviews with conscripts as a source of information about drug use may be questioned (under-reporting would not be surprising in this situation). However, Andréasson et al. (1987) argued that this problem would create an underestimation of the risk associated with cannabis use for later schizophrenia. This is true only if participants underreport their cannabis use, regardless of whether they have schizophrenia or not. The Dunedin Study and the Christchurch Study may be less open to this criticism as participants have learned after many years of involvement with the studies that all information they provide remains strictly confidential; their answers are likely to provide a reasonably good estimate of actual levels of drug use in those populations (Arseneault et al. 2002; Fergusson et al. 2003).

Thirdly, there is limited information on other illicit drug use. It would be informative to gather more precise information about other illicit drugs used by young people to more effectively control for possible confounding effects of, for example, stimulant drug use.

Fourthly, there is the question of whether prodromal manifestations of schizophrenia preceded cannabis use leaving the possibility that cannabis use may be a consequence of emerging schizophrenia rather than a cause of it. Schizophrenia is typically preceded by psychological and behavioural changes years before the onset of diagnosed disease (Cannon et al. 1997; Jones et al. 1994; Malmberg et al. 1998). It is, then, possible that cannabis use may be a consequence of early emerging schizophrenia or characteristics predisposing to schizophrenia rather than itself independently contributing to the development of the disorder. Thus, it is crucial to control for these early signs of psychosis to clearly establish temporal priority between cannabis use and adult psychosis. To date, the Dunedin Study is the only study to demonstrate clear temporal priority by showing that adolescent cannabis users are at increased risk of experiencing schizophrenic symptoms in adult life, even after taking into account childhood psychotic symptoms that preceded the onset of cannabis use.

Finally, there was limited statistical power in the smaller studies using self-reports of schizophrenia and symptom outcomes (in the Christchurch and Dunedin studies) for examining such a rare outcome disorder. It will be important for future studies to examine larger population samples in order to assess a greater number of individuals with psychotic disorders.

▌ Alternative explanations

One might speculate that cannabis is a "gateway drug" for the use of harder drugs (Kazuo and Kandel 1984) and that individuals who use cannabis heavily might also be using other substances such as amphetamines, phencyclidine and LSD which are thought to be psychotogenic (Murray et al. in press). Support for this explanation is provided by recent findings showing that use of other drugs among young adults is almost always preceded by cannabis use (Fergusson and Horwood 2000). This is especially true for heavy cannabis users (50 times of more per year) who were 140 times more likely to move on to other illicit drugs, than people who did not use cannabis previously. However, in the Dunedin, Christchurch, Dutch, and Swedish studies, the association between cannabis and schizophrenia held even when adjusting for the use of other drugs (Zammit et al. 2002; Van Os et al. 2002; Arseneault et al. 2002; Fergusson et al. 2003).

A second possibility is that individuals who use cannabis in adolescence continue to use this illicit substance in adulthood and because cannabis use intoxication can be associated with transient psychotic symptoms (Verdoux in press), this could account for the observed association. The Dunedin study is the only study for which psychiatric interview explicitly ruled out schizophrenia symptoms if these occurred only following substance use.

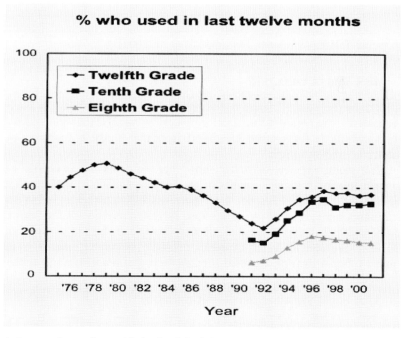

Fig. 3. Trends in annual use of cannabis in the United States in 2001. (From: Johnston, O'Malley, and Bachman 2002)

A third possibility is that early-onset cannabis use is a proxy measure for poor premorbid adjustment which is known to be associated with schizophrenia (Cannon et al. 1997, 2002). However, Arseneault et al. (2002) found that cannabis use was specifically related to schizophrenia outcomes, as opposed to depression, suggesting specificity in longitudinal association rather than general poor premorbid adjustment. Having said this, other evidence supports an association between cannabis use and depression (Degenhardt et al. in press; Patton et al. 2002).

▓ Is cannabis a causal risk factor for psychosis?

We have shown that all the available population-based studies have found that cannabis use is associated with later schizophrenia outcomes (see Table 1). All these studies support the concept of *temporal priority* by showing that cannabis use most probably preceded schizophrenia. These studies also provide evidence for *direction* by showing that the association between adolescent cannabis use and adult psychosis persists after controlling for many potential confounding variables such as disturbed behaviour, low IQ, place of upbringing, cigarette smoking, poor social integration, sex, age, ethnic groups, level of education, unemployment, single marital status, and previous psychotic symptoms. Further evidence for a causal relationship is provided by the presence of a dose-response relationship between cannabis use and schizophrenia (Andréasson et al. 1987; Van Os et al. 2002; Zammit et al. 2002); specificity of exposure, i.e. cannabis use (Arseneault et al. 2002; Van Os et al. 2002; Zammit et al. 2002; Fergusson et al. 2003) and specificity of the association to schizophrenia-related outcomes (Arseneault et al. 2002).

What kind of cause is it?

Thus, on the best evidence currently available, cannabis use is likely to play a causal role in regard to schizophrenia. However, further questions now arise. How strong is the causal effect and is cannabis use a *necessary* or *sufficient* cause of schizophrenia?

The studies reviewed earlier show that cannabis use is clearly not a *necessary* cause for the development of psychosis, since it is obvious that all adults with schizophrenia have not used cannabis in adolescence. It is also clear that cannabis use is not a *sufficient* cause for later psychosis since the majority of adolescent cannabis users did not develop schizophrenia in adulthood. Therefore we can conclude that cannabis use is a *component* cause, among possibly many others, forming a causal constellation that leads to adult schizophrenia.

What might the other component causes be?

Unfortunately we obtain little insight on component causes other than cannabis from the studies reviewed in this chapter. Cannabis use appeared to increase the risk of schizophrenia outcomes primarily among those individuals vulnerable by virtue of psychotic symptoms prior to diagnosable schizophrenia outcome (Arseneault et al. 2002; Van Os et al. 2002). Verdoux (in press) has shown that among cannabis users, adverse psychological effects were more common in those rated as 'psychosis prone'. However the interaction is not a simple one.

A case control study by McGuire et al. found an association between the development or recurrence of psychosis in the context of cannabis use and genetic predisposition, reporting that schizophrenic patients with a history of heavy cannabis use were 10 times more likely to have a family history of schizophrenia than those with psychosis who had not used cannabis (McGuire et al. 1995).

Three "high-risk studies" explored further the role of cannabis use in the development of psychotic symptoms in groups of young people considered to be at high risk of developing psychotic symptoms. An analysis of the Edinburgh High Risk Study found that both individuals at high genetic risk of schizophrenia (by virtue of two affected relatives) and individuals with no family history of schizophrenia were at increased risk of psychotic symptoms after cannabis use (Miller et al. 2001). A study of French undergraduate university students showed that the acute effects of cannabis were stronger among participants with high vulnerability for psychosis (by virtue of psychotic symptoms) (Verdoux et al. 2003). Those vulnerable participants reported increased level of perceived hostility and unusual perceptions, and also decreased level of pleasure associated with the experience of using cannabis. Also, an Australian study followed up a group of 100 individuals who presented to an early intervention service (Phillips et al. 2002). Cannabis use or dependence at entry to the study was not associated with the development of psychotic illness (transition to psychosis) over a 12-month period of follow-up after entry to the study. However, the low level of reported cannabis use amongst the group could indicate that the sample may not be representative of the population of "prodromal" individuals.

How strong is the causal effect?

Can we say anything about the strength of the causal effect of cannabis for schizophrenia? We are somewhat hampered in this endeavour, since the strength of any particular cause depends on the prevalence of the other component causes in the population (Rothman and Greenland 1998). As we have discussed above, we do not have a clear view of all the other component causes in the 'schizophrenia constellation'. We can make some broad suggestions. A component cause, even if it is very common, will rarely cause a disorder if the other component causes in the causal constellation are rare. That will hold regardless of the prevalence of the component cause of interest in the population or its role in the pathophysiology of the disorder. On the other hand, the rarer a component cause relative to its partners in any sufficient cause, the stronger that component cause will appear. Since cannabis use is relatively common in the population but appears to cause schizophrenia rarely, it would follow that at least one of the other component cause in the causal constellation is rare. Indeed, as Table 2 shows, cannabis use appears to confer only a two- or three-fold increase in relative risk for schizophrenia. Does this mean that we should not worry about cannabis as a causal factor?

There is another way of looking at this issue. Once causality is assumed, the strength of a particular association from a public health point of view can be assessed with the Population Attributable Fraction (PAF). This gives a measure of the number of cases of the disorder in the population that could be eliminated (i.e. would not occur) by removal of a harmful causal factor. The PAF for the Dunedin study is 8. In other words, removal of cannabis use from the New Zealand age-15 population would have led to an 8% reduction in the incidence of schizophrenia in that population. The NEMESIS group reported higher PAFs, possibly because of outcome measures they used did not exclusively include clinical psychosis cases (i.e. need for care). These are not insignificant figures from a public health point of view. However, the possibility of eliminating cannabis use totally from the population is rather remote and it may be advisable to concentrate on those for whom adverse outcome are more common.

A further factor is that the Dunedin study showed that cannabis use in early adolescence (first reported use at age 15) was associated with the strongest effects on schizophrenia outcomes. Trends of cannabis use among adolescents in Western countries indicate that cannabis users under the age of 16 is a fairly new phenomenon that has appeared only since the early 1990s (see Figure 3) (Johnston et al. 2002). One would therefore predict an increase in rates of schizophrenia over the next 10 years. Although the majority of young people are able to use cannabis in adolescence without harm, a vulnerable minority experiences adverse outcomes. Epidemiological evidences suggest that cannabis use among psychologically vulnerable young adolescents should be strongly discouraged by parents, teachers, and health practitioners alike. Findings also suggest that the youngest cannabis users are most at risk (Arseneault et al. 2002); this may be because their cannabis use becomes long-standing or because the still developing brain is more susceptible to the effects of cannabis.

▌ Conclusion

We have tried to determine whether cannabis is a cause of schizophrenia, and if so, whether it is a necessary or a sufficient cause. Recent empirical evidence suggests that cannabis is not a necessary cause for schizophrenia; nor is it a sufficient cause. Cannabis use is rather a component cause, part of a complex constellation including possibly some necessary causes such as genetic predisposition that leads to the development of schizophrenia. The other components of this causal constellation remain to be determined.

▌ References

American Psychiatric Association (1994) Diagnostic and Statistical Manual of Mental Disorders (4th edn) (DSM-IV). American Psychiatric Association, Washington, DC

Andréasson S, Allebeck P, Engström A, Rydberg U (1987) Cannabis and schizophrenia: a longitudinal study of Swedish conscripts. Lancet 11:1483–1485

Arseneault L, Cannon M, Poulton R, Murray R, Caspi A, Moffitt TE (2002) Cannabis use in adolescence and risk for adult psychosis: longitudinal prospective study. British Medical Journal 325:1212–1213

Cannon M, Caspi A, Moffitt TE, Harrington H, Taylor A, Murray RE, Poulton R (2002) Evidence for early, specific, pan-developmental impairment in schizophreniform disorder: results from a longitudinal birth cohort. Archives of General Psychiatry 59:449–457

Cannon M, Jones P, Gilvarry C, Rifkin L, McKenzie K, Foerster A, Murray RM (1997) Premorbid social functioning in schizophrenia and bipolar disorder: similarities and differences. American Journal of Psychiatry 154:1544–1550

Cantwell R, Brewin J, Glazebrook C, Dalkin T, Fox R, Medley I, Harrison G (1999) Prevalence of substance abuse in first-episode psychosis. British Journal of Psychiatry 174:150–153

Degenhardt L (2003) The link between cannabis use and psychosis: furthering the debate. Psychological Medicine 33:3–6

Degenhardt L, Hall W, Lynskey M et al (2004) The association between cannabis use and depression: a review of the evidence. In: Castle DJ, Murray R (eds) Marijuana and Madness. Cambridge University Press, Cambridge, UK (in press)

Duke PJ, Pantelis C, McPhillips MA, Barnes TRE (2001) Comorbid non-alcohol substance misuse among people with schizophrenia. British Journal of Psychiatry 179:509–513

Farrell M, Howes S, Taylor C, Lewis G, Jenkins R, Bebbington P, Jarvis M, Brugha T, Gill B, Meltzer H (1998) Substance misuse and psychiatric comorbidity: an overview of the OPCS National Psychiatric Comorbidity Survey. Addictive Behavior 23:909–918

Fergusson DM, Horwood LJ (2000) Does cannabis use encourage other forms of illicit drug use? Addiction 95:505–520

Fergusson DM, Horwood LJ, Swain-Campbell NR (2003) Cannabis dependence and psychotic symptoms in young people. Psychological Medicine 33:15–21

Grech A, Takei N, Murray R (1998) Comparison of cannabis use in psychotic patients and controls in London and Malta. Schizophrenia Research 29:22

Hall W, Degenhardt L (2002) Cannabis use and psychosis: a review of clinical and epidemiological evidence. Australian and New Zealand Journal of Psychiatry 34:26–34

Hall W, Degenhardt L (2004) Is there a specific "cannabis psychosis"? In: Castle DJ, Murray R (eds) Marijuana and Madness. Cambridge University Press, Cambridge, UK (in press)

Hambrecht M, Häfner H (1996) Substance abuse and the onset of schizophrenia. Biological Psychiatry 40:1155–1163

Hill AB (1965) The environment and disease: association or causation? Proceedings of the Royal Society of Medicine 58:295–300

Johns A (2001) Psychiatric effects of cannabis. British Journal of Psychiatry 178:116–122

Johnston LD, O'Malley PM, Bachman JG (2001) Monitoring the Future national results on adolescent drug use: overview of key findings (NIH Publication No. 02-5105). National Institute on Drug Abuse, Bethesda, MD

Jones P, Rodgers B, Murray R, Marmot M (1994) Child developmental risk factors for adult schizophrenia in the British 1946 birth cohort. Lancet 344:1398–1402

Kazuo Y, Kandel DB (1984) Patterns of drug use from adolescence to young adulthood: II. sequences of progression. American Journal of Public Health 74:668–672

Malmberg A, Lewis G, David A, Allebeck P (1998) Premorbid adjustment and personality in people with schizophrenia. British Journal of Psychiatry 172:308–313

Mathers DC, Ghodse AH (1992) Cannabis and psychotic illness. British Journal of Psychiatry 161:648–653

McCreadie RG (2002) Use of drugs, alcohol and tobacco by people with schizophrenia: case-control study. British Journal of Psychiatry 181:321–323

McGuire PK, Jones P, Harvey I, Williams M, MacGuffin P, Murray RM (1995) Morbid risk of schizophrenia for relatives of patients with cannabis-associated psychosis. Schizophrenia Research 15:277–281

Menezes PR, Johnson S, Thornicroft G, Marshall J, Prosser D, Bebbington P, Kuipers E (1996) Drug and alcohol problems among individuals with severe mental illnesses in South London. British Journal of Psychiatry 168:612–619

Miller P, Lawrie SM, Hodges A, Clafferty R, Cosway R, Johnstone CE (2001) Genetic liability, illicit drug use, life stress and psychotic symptoms: preliminary findings from the Edinburgh study of people at high risk for schizophrenia. Social Psychiatry and Psychiatric Epidemiology 36:338–342

Murray R, Grech A, Phillips P et al (2003) What is the relationship between substance abuse and schizophrenia? In: Murray R, Jones P, Susser E, Van Os J, Cannon M (eds) The Epidemiology of Schizophrenia. Cambridge University Press, Cambridge, UK (in press)

Negrete JC, Knapp WP, Douglas D, Bruce Smith W (1986) Cannabis affects the severity of schizophrenia symptoms: results of a clinical survey. Psychological Medicine 16:515–520

Patton GC, Coffrey C, Carlin JB, Degenhardt L, Lynskey M, Hall W (2002) Cannabis use and mental health in young people: cohort study. British Medical Journal 325:1195–1198

Phillips LJ, Curry C, Yung AR, Yuen HP, Adlard S, McGorry S (2002) Cannabis use is not associated with the development of psychosis in an 'ultra' high-risk group. Australian and New Zealand Journal of Psychiatry 36:800–806

Poulton R, Caspi A, Moffitt TE, Cannon M, Murray R, Harrington H (2000) Children's self-reported psychotic symptoms and adult schizophreniform disorder: a 15-year longitudinal study. Archives of General Psychiatry 57:1053–1058

Regier D, Farmer ME, Rae DS, Locke BZ, Keith SJ, Judd LL, Goodwin FK (1990) Comorbidity of mental disorders with alcohol and other drug abuse: results from the epidemiologic catchment area (ECA) study. Journal of the American Medical Association 264:2511–2518

Robins LN, Regier DA (1991) Psychiatric Disorders in America: The Epidemiologic Catchment Area Study. The Free Press, New York

Rothman KJ, Greenland S (eds) (1998) Modern epidemiology, second edition. Lippincott-Raven, Philadelphia

Silva PA, Stanton WR (eds) (1996) From Child to Adult: The Dunedin Multidisciplinary Health and Development Study. Oxford University Press, Auckland

Susser M (1991) What is a cause and how do we know one? A grammar for pragmatic epidemiology. American Journal of Epidemiology 133:635–648

Thornicroft G (1990) Cannabis and psychosis. British Journal of Psychiatry 157:25–33

Tien AY, Anthony JC (1990) Epidemiological analysis of alcohol and drug use as risk factors for psychotic experiences. Journal of Nervous and Mental Disease 178:473–480

Van Os J, Bak M, Hanssen M, Bijl RV, De Graaf R, Verdoux H (2002) Cannabis use and psychosis: a longitudinal population-based study. American Journal of Epidemiology 156:319–327

Verdoux H (2004) Cannabis and psychosis proneness. In: Castle DJ, Murray R (eds) Marijuana and Madness. Cambridge University Press, Cambridge, UK (in press)

Verdoux H, Gindre C, Sorbara F, Tournier M, Swendson JD (2003) Effects of cannabis and psychosis vulnerability in daily life: an experience sampling test study. Psychological Medicine 33:23–32

Wheatley M (1998) The prevalence and relevance of substance use in detained schizophrenic patients. Journal of Forensic Psychiatry 9:114–129

Zammit S, Allebeck P, Andréasson S, Lundberg I, Lewis G (2002) Self-reported cannabis use as a risk factor for schizophrenia: further analysis of the 1969 Swedish conscript cohort. British Medical Journal 325:1199–1201

Discussion:
Schizophrenia – diverse etiologies, common pathogenesis

T. H. McGlashan and R. E. Hoffman

Yale University School of Medicine, New Haven, USA

Introduction: the session papers

In this session on the Precursors of Schizophrenia our speakers have presented data about pathways to schizophrenia that are at first glance quite diverse. Indeed, the time-honored notion that schizophrenia is a heterogeneous group of disorders appears validated by the diversity of the accumulated findings.

Dr. Done provides a scholarly review of developmental psychopathology and associated childhood disorders. He identifies childhood signs, symptoms, and behaviors that may constitute a "childhood endophenotype for schizophrenia". These include having few friends, abnormal social/interpersonal behavior, early psychotic-like experiences, language impairments, poor school achievement, neurologic soft signs, and neurotic/anxious behavior. Such constellations of abnormalities are found frequently in childhood personality disorders, pervasive developmental disorders, and ADHD. Dr. Done questions the degree to which endophenotypic constellations within these childhood disorders predict the development of schizophrenia, and recommends tracking them longitudinally in order to determine this.

Dr. Soares-Weiser details data from the Israeli military and hospital registers showing that many males who later develop schizophrenia show social and cognitive deficits, drug abuse, and carry non-psychotic adolescent diagnoses at the time of conscription. The findings are consistent with a neurodevelopmental model of schizophrenia. While the positive predictive values of these phenomenologies for later schizophrenia are low, the associations are still significant, suggesting linkage of some kind(s) with schizophrenia.

Dr. Murray outlines evidence supporting the idea that cannabis is a causal factor in some cases of schizophrenia. The issue raises questions about pathophysiology, i.e., in what manner might cannabis be causal to schizophrenia?

Dr. Mortensen uses large data sets from the Danish Registers to test the associations of a remarkably heterogeneous set of risk factors with schizophrenia and bipolar disorder. His data suggest that the two disorders are (paradoxically) both dimensionally continuous and categorically specific.

Heterogeneity could not be better exemplified by this collection of papers. Schizophrenia is somehow related to childhood disorders, deficits in early social and cognitive functioning, drug abuse (especially cannabis), absence of rheumatoid arthritis, urban birth, obstetrical complications, immigrant status, family history of severe mental illness, and so on. How do we make sense of this panoply of associated "risk" factors? In keeping with the central theme of this conference on the causes of schizophrenia, my discussion will attempt to describe a model of schizophrenia that may encompass and explain this diversity.

▌ A connectivity model of schizophrenia

My colleague Ralph Hoffman and I consider the final common pathway to schizophrenia to be the reduction of cortical synaptic connections beyond a critical threshold [7, 9, 12]. We base this formulation on evidence from the postmortem and neuroimaging findings of the brains of schizophrenic patients, and from computerized neural network modeling that simulates the consequences of reduced connectivity.

As reviewed [12], postmortem evidence for reduced synaptic connectivity in schizophrenia is found in 1) increased neuronal density seen histologically as reduced neuropil without neuronal loss (the neuropil is made up of extra-neuronal microstructures including synapses), 2) reduced spine densities and small dendritic arbors on the pyramidal cells of the prefrontal cortex, and 3) decreased synaptic "products" in postmortem tissue such as synaptic protein mRNA expression or synaptophysin in the prefrontal cortex. Neuroimaging findings include reduced brain volume, especially reduced gray matter volume, and increased extra-cerebral (sulcal) spinal fluid.

Computerized neural network models provide a mathematical quasi-validation of the connectivity hypothesis, or of what happens as a result of this interstitial cortical tissue attenuation. These models simulate the working of many interconnected and communicating units, i.e., neurons [6]. The outputs of such systems are seldom linearly related to the input. In fact, output often feeds back to input in a self-organizing fashion, much like the human brain. The results can often be unpredictable phasic shifts in network function and organization. Sometimes the organization simulates normal cognitive mental function such as speech perception and memory; sometimes it simulates pathologic mental states such as delusions [8] or hallucinations [7].

The system alteration which changes such a network from simulating normal brain processes to one simulating pathological brain processes is a reduction of the connections between the network units, i.e., pruning connections. The process is highly nonlinear. Mild pruning of connections of a speech perception network, for example, will increase the accuracy and capacity of the network [7]. Once the pruning eliminates 40% or more of the connections, however, the network begins to function aberrantly. This is seen in an increase of network processing errors (simulating cognitive impairment) and the emergence of output in the absence of input [7].

Translating computer simulations back to biology, mild pruning of synaptic connections may be an important normal neurobiological brain process that supports learning, an example being the reduction (pruning) of brain song-center synapses in conjunction with bird-song imprinting [2, 3]. Pruning beyond a critical threshold, however, may lead to disruptions of normal cognitive processes, among them being the generation of mental content in the absence of afferent inputs, an ictal-like creation of perceptions, thoughts, or feelings that are autonomous and experienced as being generated independently of will, i.e., the cardinal first-rank symptoms of schizophrenia. Severe pruning also leads to a deterioration of cognitive functioning.

Integrating the postmortem and imaging findings with the computer simulations of pruning network connections, Dr. Hoffman and I hypothesize that the final common pathway to schizophrenia is the reduction of synaptic connectivity beyond a critical threshold. The key element is the functional loss of connectedness, not the anatomic loss of neurons. Neurotoxicity and neuronal loss are not part of this model. Active psychosis is the result of reduced connectivity, not vice versa. Active psychosis may be extraordinarily damaging to a person's reputation and ability to function, but we do not regard it as being neurobiologically toxic. As such we consider the term neurodegeneration to be misleading insofar as it implies loss of neuronal cell bodies. A "degeneration" is involved in schizophrenia, but it involves the loss of neuropil (synapses), not neurons. A better term, perhaps, is neuroregression, which suggests a loss and change without cell body dissolution.

The processes of synaptogenesis and synaptic elimination are the key neurobiological elements of the model. As initially delineated by Huttenlocher [9, 10], these processes fluctuate over normal development. Postnatal brain development includes cortical synaptogenetic over-elaboration followed by a gradual reduction in synaptic density that is close to 60% of the childhood maximum. The reduction is not uniform over development across the cortex. For example, it is complete by age 2 in the occipital cortex, but not complete until adolescence in the prefrontal and association areas (the latter fact led to the hypothesis that schizophrenia was a disorder of too much synaptic pruning, originally articulated by Feinberg [5]). In adulthood, synaptic elimination appears to be balanced by a similar rate of synaptogenesis to effect a plateau in synaptic density.

We hypothesize that the critical psychotic threshold of synaptic connectivity can be reached by one or a combination of three pathways. The first two involve the loss of connectivity through synaptic elimination that reaches the critical threshold (see Fig. 1). The first pathway is neurodevelopmental wherein synaptic density is reduced at birth or in childhood (because of genetics and/or negative perinatal events) and followed by a normal rate of pruning in adolescence that reduces the density below the critical threshold. The second is neuroregressive wherein the synaptic density is normal to start with but is followed by an accelerated rate of pruning in adolescence that reduces density below threshold.

The third pathway is neuromodulatory, not neuroanatomic. Synaptic connectivity is functionally reduced by shifting balances in brain synaptic neurochemicals such as dopamine, glutamate, GABA, etc., whereby interneuron communication is altered. Since neurons themselves are not lost, connectivity reductions are potentially reversible with antipsychotic drug treatment and/or attenuation of environmental stress. In contrast, the loss of connectivity via the anatomic pathways is less easily reversible.

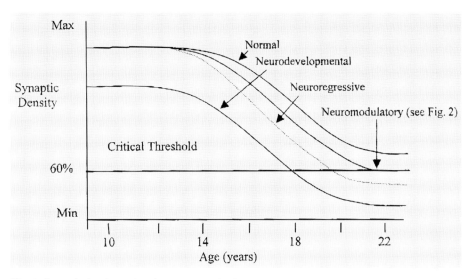

Fig. 1. Synaptic density and pathways to psychosis

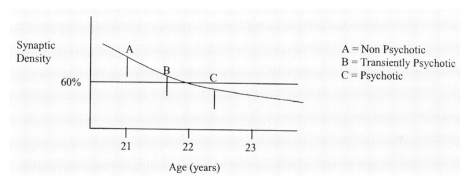

Fig. 2. Neuromodulatory "dips" in functional synaptic connectivity along a neuroanatomically determined level of synaptic density

Neuromodulatory changes in synaptic connectivity are illustrated in Fig. 2. Vertical lines A, B, and C represent reversible, functional "dips" in synaptic density associated, for example, with temporary hyperdopaminergia secondary to stressful experiences. We chose short vertical lines to illustrate that these changes are brief in time (days and weeks rather than years) and account for a limited percent of the overall synaptic density. According to the critically reduced connectivity theory, such neuromodulatorily induced fluctuations occur constantly in everyone. They are normal processes that can, as illustrated by A, B, and C in Fig. 2, become a sufficient cause of psychosis, but *only* in persons with levels of synaptic connectivity that are already close to the critical threshold as determined by developmental neuro*anatomic* processes.

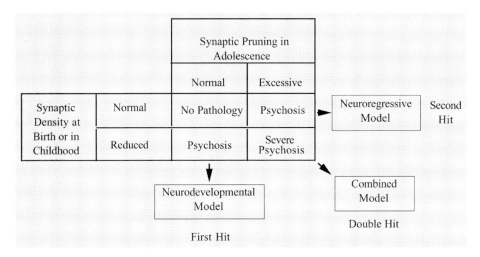

Fig. 3. Neuroanatomic pathways to critically reduced synaptic connectedness

The two anatomic pathways to critically reduced connectivity determine most of the heterogeneity in clinical presentation, lifetime course, and prognosis of schizophrenia. Fig. 3 illustrates this interaction. In the neurodevelopmental model early (baseline) synaptic density is reduced, a situation often referred to as the "first hit". In the neuroregressive model, the rate of synaptic pruning in adolescence is excessive, a situation referred to as the second hit. If synaptic density is reduced both neurodevelopmentally and neuroregressively, severe psychosis ensues as a result of a double hit to synaptic connectivity.

▌ The precursors of schizophrenia and the connectivity model: discussion

The final pathway in the reduced synaptic connectivity (RSC) model is clear and mechanistically uniform, i.e., it is a final "common" pathway of critically reduced cortical connectivity. The roads leading into the final pathway are also distinct and limited in number. All together, however, they may account for most, if not all, of the heterogeneity of schizophrenia. This includes the impressive mélange of risk factors carefully collected, studied, and presented by this session's speakers.

According to the RSC model, the endophenotypic behaviors linked to forms of childhood psychopathology detailed by Dr. Done can be sufficient (i.e., true or valid) risk factors for schizophrenia if, but only if, they are associated with attenuated levels of synaptic density in childhood, i.e., the period of life considered "premorbid" in those who do eventually develop psychosis. As their psychopathologies usually emerge prior to adolescence, any loss of connectivity would be neurodevelopmentally determined, i.e., a first hit. The findings presented by Dr. Soares-Weiser fit here as well. Some of the non-psychotic disorders and social and cognitive deficits displayed by the Israeli military conscripts may also be true risk factors via the same neurodevelopmental pathway. However, since the conscripts are clearly adolescents, neuroregressive or second hit processes may also be contributing. The presence of second hit attenuation of synaptic density would be particularly suspect if the disorders and deficits noted at evaluation were of recent, i.e., adolescent, onset.

Dr. Murray marshals impressive data about the place of cannabis as a causal factor in schizophrenia. By the RSC model we would hypothesize that cannabis does this by a dose-dependent functional (neuromodulatory) attenuation of synaptic connectivity to a point below the critical threshold. How cannabis does this neurochemically is still largely speculative. Perhaps, like the dissociative agent ketamine [1, 11], it blocks NMDA-receptor glutamate neurotransmission (C. D'Sousa, personal communication, 2003). The effect of this reduction of functional connectivity is probably not large insofar as only a small minority of cannabis users actually develop psychosis. Furthermore, the RSC model would maintain that the small minority who do go "over the edge" are already highly vulnerable because of prior first and/or second hit neuroanatomic reductions in synaptic density that are sufficient to bring the person close to the critical threshold. It has been reported, for example, that the development and/or recurrence of acute psychosis in those who use cannabis may be associated with the presence of schizophrenia in a first-degree relative [13]. A similar example can be seen with amphetamine abuse where heavy use is unlikely to lead to paranoid psychosis in the absence of a genetic [15] or schizotypal proneness [14] for psychosis.

In this model, cannabis is a sufficient causal factor if, and only if, other necessary causal factors are present. If neuroanatomically determined levels of synaptic connectivity are just above the critical threshold as in B of Fig. 2, cannabis use may result in psychosis that coincides with use but that is reversible with abstinence. If second hit processes continue to attenuate connectivity in the same person, however, cannabis use may ultimately precipitate a psychosis that does not remit with abstinence.

Dr. Mortensen's epidemiological comparison of risk factors for schizophrenia and bipolar disorder, here reproduced in Table 1, suggests to me that the two disorders share reduced synaptic connectivity as the primary pathophysiologic mechanism, i.e., that a continuum of psychosis does exist. The differences between the disorders, furthermore, are likely to be determined by the location in the brain of such reductions and the degree of first versus second hit contributions to the reductions.

Dr. Mortensen's comparison of risk factors does little to suggest where in the cortex we might find differences in regions of reduced connectivity between schizophrenia and bipolar disorder. Data relevant to this question should become available soon via comparative neuroimaging studies. Dr. Mortensen's data, however, do suggest that schizophrenia is more severe than bipolar disorder neurodevelopmentally. The onset is earlier. Evidence of brain deficits prior to onset is stronger in the form of more frequent obstetrical complications, early infections, developmental precursors, and poor premorbid adjustment. Bipolar disorder, in contrast, is more intact neurodevelopmentally

Table 1. Epidemiologic risk factors for schizophrenia and bipolar disorder (from Mortensen)

	Schizophrenia	Bipolar disorder
‖ Ethnicity (migration)	+	?
‖ OCS	+	–
‖ Infections	+	–
‖ Season of birth	+	?
‖ Urbanicity of place of birth	+	–
‖ Socioeconomic status	(–)	(–)
‖ Premorbid adjustment	+	(+)
‖ Recent stress	–	+
‖ Early parental loss	?	+
‖ Head injury	?	(+)
‖ Childbirth	–	+
‖ Seizure disorders	+	(+)
‖ Multiple sclerosis	?	(+)
‖ Rheumatoid arthritis	+	–
‖ Cancer	+	–
‖ Developmental precursors	+	(+)
‖ Family history	+	+

and, perhaps as a consequence, more environmentally attuned and stress-reactive. On Dr. Mortensen's list, for example, bipolar disorder is more associated with recent stress, early parental loss, and the postpartum challenges of childbirth.

The stress-diathesis hypothesis of schizophrenia postulates that the clinical manifestations of disorder are related to the degree of environmental stress and the interaction of this stress with the individual's degree of genetic-constitutional vulnerability for schizophrenia. A similar interaction may be active in determining the clinical vicissitudes of bipolar disorder. If, however, bipolar disorder is more neurodevelopmentally intact than schizophrenia, we would expect a different kind of diathesis or response to stress. In fact, we do see rather striking differences in established forms of each disorder. Bipolar patients appear capable of an intact but exaggerated response to environmental stress and stimuli. Schizophrenia patients, on the other hand, either have a blunted response to environmental stress and stimuli in the form of negative symptoms, or their very capacity to respond disorganizes under pressure in the form of active psychosis. These differences may be determined in the early neurodevelopmental stages of persons at risk for each disorder, with those evolving to schizophrenia receiving less brain "hardware" in the form of premorbid synaptic density from those evolving to bipolar disorder.

Dr. Mortensen's risk factor comparisons confirm the importance of genetics in both disorders. Furthermore, closer scrutiny suggests that the genetic influences are both distinctive within disorders and continuous across disorders. Distinctive means the disorders mostly breed true across generations within affected families, i.e., schizophrenia begats schizophrenia and bipolar begats bipolar. Occasionally, however, they do not "breed true" and there is genetic continuity across disorders [4]. How this relates to the RSC model of schizophrenia is unclear. Genetic continuity between schizophrenia and bipolar disorder supports reduced synaptic connectivity in the pathogenesis of the latter. It may be that reduced connectivity is pathogenic for both disorders, with the location and severity of the connectivity deficit being distributed differently across the cerebral cortex in ways that are determined by diagnosis-specific forces, genetic or otherwise.

The effects of migration (ethnicity) and urban birth on the incidence of disorders appear specific to schizophrenia. This is hard to understand in light of the commonly held belief that these phenomena are stress induced, because bipolar disorder, as discussed, is clearly stress-responsive. To me these comparisons suggest that there is much about the immigration and urbanization effects that we do not understand, and that we should not be satisfied with stress-response as the sole explanation.

▌ Conclusion

Our speakers have provided us with a rich selection of phenomenologies that are risk or antecedent factors associated with schizophrenia. In a sense these phenomenologies are etiologic, or provide clues to several etiologies. They are also remarkably numerous and diverse in nature, and one can see why many of the thinkers about schizophrenia consider it to be a group of disorders with separate etiologies.

I both agree and disagree. I agree that schizophrenia has multiple etiologies, but I disagree that each etiology generates a different disorder. Schizophrenia, as presented here, is actually quite uniform in its pathophysiology. The final path is one of critically reduced synaptic connectivity, and all etiologies, diverse as they are, lead into this final path via three processes, neurodevelopmental, neuroregressive, and neurohumoral. The combination of different etiologies and processes gives us the heterogeneity or diversity of expression of schizophrenia, but the confluence of these etiologies and processes into a final common path also gives us the homogeneity of schizophrenia as a uniform, and uniformly disabling, presence in all cultures in all parts of the world.

▌ References

1. Adler CM, Malhotra AK, Elman I, Goldberg T, Egan M, Pickar D, Breier A (1999) Comparison of ketamine-induced thought disorder in healthy volunteers and thought disorder in schizophrenia. American Journal of Psychiatry 156:1646–1649

2. Bock J, Braun K (1999) Filial imprinting in domestic chicks is associated with spine pruning in the associative area, dorsocaudal neostriatum. European Journal of Neuroscience 11:2566–2570
3. Bock J, Wolf A, Braun K (1996) Influence of the N-Methyl-D-aspartate receptor antagonist DL-2-amino-5-phosphonovaleric acid on auditory filial imprinting in the domestic chick. Neurobiology of Learning and Memory 65:177–188
4. Cardno AG, Rijsdijk FV, Murray RM, McGuffin P (2002) A twin study of genetic relationships between psychotic symptoms. American Journal of Psychiatry 159: 539–545
5. Feinberg I (1983) Schizophrenia: caused by a fault in programmed synaptic elimination during adolescence? Journal of Psychiatric Research 17:319–334
6. Hoffman RE (1987) Computer simulation of neural information processing and the schizophrenia-mania dichotomy. Archives of General Psychiatry 44:178–188
7. Hoffman RE, McGlashan TH (1997) Synaptic elimination, neurodevelopment, and the mechanism of hallucinated "voices" in schizophrenia. American Journal of Psychiatry 154:1683–1689
8. Hoffman RE, McGlashan TH (1993) Parallel distributed processing and the emergence of schizophrenic symptoms. Schizophrenia Bulletin 19:119–140
9. Huttenlocher PR (1979) Synaptic density in the human frontal cortex: developmental changes and effects of aging. Brain Research 163:195–205
10. Huttenlocher PR, Dabholkar AS (1997) Regional differences in synaptogenesis in human cerebral cortex. Journal of Comparative Neurology 387:167–178
11. Krystal JH, Karper LP, Seibyl JP, Freeman GK, Delaney R, Bremner JD, Heninger GR, Bowers MB, Charney DS (1994) Subanesthetic effects of the noncompetitive NMDA antagonist, ketamine, in humans. Archives of General Psychiatry 51:199–214
12. McGlashan TH, Hoffman RE (2000) Schizophrenia as a disorder of developmentally reduced synaptic connectivity. Archives of General Psychiatry 57:637–648
13. McGuire PK, Jones P, Harvey I, Williams M, McGuffin P, Murray RM (1995) Morbid risk of schizophrenia for relatives of patients with cannabis-associated psychosis. Schizophrenia Research 15:277–281
14. Satel SL, Edell WS (1991) Cocaine-induced paranoia and psychosis proneness. American Journal of Psychiatry 148:1708–1711
15. Tatetsu S (1972) Methamphetamine psychosis. In: Ellinwood EH, Cohen S (eds) Current Concept on Amphetamine Abuse. DHEW Publication No. (HSM) 72-9085. US Government Printing Office, Washington, DC

Section 3
Pathophysiological mechanisms

Genetic liability, brain structure and symptoms of schizophrenia

ANDREW MCINTOSH, HEATHER WHALLEY, DOMINIC JOB, EVE JOHNSTONE, and STEPHEN LAWRIE

Division of Psychiatry, Royal Edinburgh Hospital, Edinburgh, UK

Introduction

Over 100 structural MRI (sMRI) studies of schizophrenia have demonstrated that the structure of the brain in vivo is different from that of healthy controls. When the brain abnormalities arise and how they relate to the clinical symptoms are less certain. Such questions are not only of interest for theoretical reasons, but are also relevant to clinicians who may seek to detect schizophrenia at an earlier stage or perhaps to prevent it altogether. A better understanding of regional brain anomalies and their relationship to clinical symptoms may also inform us of the presence of subsyndromes (endophenotypes) and the boundaries of schizophrenia with other illnesses such as affective disorder.

The timing of structural brain changes in schizophrenia and their relationship to symptoms and genetic liability to the disorder have been addressed using a number of experimental paradigms. Using imaging, structural and functional abnormalities have been described in affected individuals once the diagnosis has become clear. Often these patients have been unwell for many years and have had considerable exposure to antipsychotic medication. Some studies have compared the brains of patients with schizophrenia occurring in the context of a multiply affected family ('familial schizophrenia') with the brains of patients with no family history ('sporadic schizophrenia') with an aim to separate the effects of genes for schizophrenia with the effects contingent upon diagnosis. However, the assumption that a given patient has a sporadic or familial form of illness is not without difficulty and studies using this design generally do not effectively address the question of timing. Other studies have examined monozygotic twins discordant for schizophrenia and, although the circumstances of twin birth limit the degree to which these results may be generalised, these studies provide useful information about the relative strength of genetic and environmental influences. Studies of the wider family have also provided useful information in this regard.

The problem remains however that, without prospective study, structural and functional brain changes occurring premorbidly in those destined to develop schizophrenia may be difficult to separate from the effects of genes which lead to structural brain changes but which do not lead to psychosis. For this reason, high risk studies have prospectively studied individuals at increased risk of schizophrenia with a view to clarifying these issues. Because high risk studies have tended to select subjects on the basis of a family history of schizophrenia, these studies have also further informed the study of relationships between brain abnormalities and genetic risk.

▌ Structural MRI of schizophrenia

Early sMRI studies were generally small in size and used area measures such as the ventricle to brain ratio (VBR). sMRI methodology has greatly improved and, in particular, thin contiguous slicing through the brain has facilitated accurately measuring of regional brain volumes. Studies consistently show differences between controls and people with schizophrenia and two meta-analytic reviews of more than 50 individual studies have summarised our knowledge of the location and extent of these regional differences (Wright et al. 2000; Lawrie and Abukmeil 1998).

Lawrie and Abukmeil (1998) located articles using a search of Medline and a hand search of seven psychiatric journals. Studies were included in the review if they included patients with DSM-III-R schizophrenia and if volumes of one or more cerebral structures were reported. No statistical analysis was performed but median differences were reported for several structures. Whole brain volume was reduced by approximately 3% and CSF volume increased by around 18%. Lateral ventricular volume was increased by approximately 22%, although a larger difference was found for the body of the lateral ventricles (47–50%) and occipital horns (28–31%). Prefrontal lobes were reduced by approximately 1.5% (right) to 3% (left). Temporal lobes (–6% left and –9.5% right) were also smaller in schizophrenic subjects as were the amygdala-hippocampal complexes (6.5%-L, 5.5%-R). Wright et al. (2000) used similar searching techniques but combined studies that compared the same region of interest using random effects meta-analysis. Whole brain volume was reduced by approximately 2% in schizophrenic patients. Whole brain grey matter was reduced by approximately 4%, although no significant difference was found for whole brain white matter. Lateral ventricles were approximately 20 to 30% larger in schizophrenic patients compared to controls and this difference was greater still for the body of the lateral ventricles which were approximately 47–48% larger in schizophrenic subjects. Left and right hemispheres, frontal and temporal lobes were all reduced significantly on the order of 3 to 5%. Some temporal lobe structures were, however, reduced to a greater extent. Although superior temporal gyri volumes did not differ between patients and controls, the difference was significant when the anterior or posterior portions were considered separately. The right and left amygdala-hippocampal complex, amygdala, hippocampus and parahippocampus were significantly reduced on the order of between 5% (left amygdala-hippocampal complex) and 11% (left parahippocampus). The only subcortical grey matter to be increased in size was the globus pallidus which was increased in volume by between 18% (left) and 21% (right).

More recent studies have examined smaller structures by separating them from surrounding structures using parcellation or by voxel-based analysis. Limbic structures have been the source of most interest with differences in

Table 1. Summary of findings from sMRI in schizophrenia

Region	Findings
▌ Whole brain volume	50+ studies. Reduced by approximately 3%. Grey matter decreased by around 4%. White matter volume differences are unclear and may not be different from healthy controls
▌ Frontal lobes	50+ studies. Reductions of approximately 3% compared to controls
▌ Temporal lobes	100+ studies. Whole temporal lobe reduced by approximately 5–6%. Reductions also found in planum temporale and anterior/posterior superior temporal gyrus
▌ Basal ganglia	25+ studies. Increased globus pallidus size by around 18% left to 21% right. Association found between enlargement and antipsychotic exposure (Chakos et al. 1994). Caudate and putamen do not consistently show enlargement
▌ Thalamus	6+ studies. Early studies (Andreasen et al. 1994) showed decreases in volume although several negative studies also exist. Meta-analysis shows significant differences between patients and controls overall
▌ Hippocampus	10+ studies. Consistent reductions shown in most studies of around 4%
▌ Parahippocampus	8+ studies. Parahippocampus reduced by between 8% right and 11% left
▌ Amygdala	7+ studies. Early findings were −ve although several recent studies have shown reductions compared to controls. Overall reduced by around 9% compared to controls
▌ Insula	2+ Studies, most showing reductions
▌ Lateral ventricles	20+ studies. Increased by approximately 22%, although a larger difference is found for the body of the lateral ventricles (47–50%) and the occipital horns (28–31%). Enlargement of lateral ventricles may be greater in men
▌ Third ventricle	33+ studies. Consistently show enlargement averaging 26% overall

the hippocampus, insula and amygdala being repeatedly found (Wright et al. 1999; Levitt et al. 2001; O'Driscoll et al. 2001; Job et al. 2002).

▌ Imaging genetic risk and schizophrenia

A family history of schizophrenia has long been established as one of the strongest risk factors for the development of the disorder in unaffected probands (Cannon and Jones 1996). In comparison, other risk factors have generally weaker effects that are less consistently replicated. However, the positive relationship between family history and risk of schizophrenia need not necessarily be explained by genes for schizophrenia. The finding could be explained by abnormal early environmental factors (e.g. discordant parenting, infection), or an increased liability to obstetric complications or gene-environment interactions. Adoption studies of unaffected relatives has shown that the risk to schizophrenia is not ameliorated by being raised by a family with no background of genetic risk and obstetric studies suggest that OCs are unlikely to provide a plausible explanation for the familiality of the illness (van Erp et al. 2002; McIntosh et al. 2002). Therefore, the likely explanation for increased familial risk is the presence of genes which raise the liability to schizophrenia more directly. Some twin and family studies have additionally performed CT or MRI scans and provide additional information about brain structure in affected and unaffected relatives. The rationale for such studies is relatively strong. Firstly, schizophrenia is associated with cerebral abnormalities and is a highly heritable disorder. Secondly, brain volumes themselves are highly heritable (Baare et al. 2001a; Carmelli et al. 1998) and make good candidates for both linkage and association analyses (Faraone et al. 2003).

▌ Twin studies

Studies of monozygotic twins discordant for schizophrenia have the potential to distinguish environmental from genetic effects. In the context of these studies, greater neuroanatomical similarity would be presumed to reflect common genetic effects and greater difference to reflect environmental effects. Studies of discordant monozygotic twins are however limited by the unusual circumstances of twin birth and differences between twins may be a reflection of different gene expression or gene-environment interaction. Notwithstanding these potential limitations, studies of discordant MZ twins have enhanced our understanding of genetic and environmental influences in schizophrenia.

Generally, the results from CT and MRI have been consistent: unaffected relatives have a degree of quantitative brain anomaly which is intermediate between that of their affected relatives and healthy controls. Such findings suggest that a degree of brain anomaly is inherited at least by a proportion of those who never develop schizophrenia. Studies of discordant monozygotic (MZ) twins have the added ability to quantify the effect of environmental factors on subsequent illness. In a study of 15 pairs of MZ twins discordant for schizophrenia (Suddath et al. 1990), it was the affected twin which had larger ventricles, reduced temporal lobe grey matter and reduced hippocampal volumes. These findings are difficult to explain without the effect of environmental factors or gene-environment interactions. However, no differences were found in either frontal lobe volume or white matter. Since frontal lobe volume has been shown to be consistently reduced in schizophrenia (Lawrie and Abukmeil 1998; Wright et al. 2000) compared to non-related healthy controls, it is possible that a reduced frontal lobe volume may predispose to psychosis while a reduction in temporal lobe grey matter and hippocampal volumes might be associated more closely with the onset of illness itself.

A further study of monozygotic twin pairs discordant for schizophrenia used 15 pairs of discordant monozygotic twins, 14 pairs of discordant dizygotic twins and 29 healthy twin pairs matched on a number of important confounders (Baare et al. 2001 b). Frontal brain volumes were smaller in affected versus unaffected monozygotic twins but were not apparent for the same sibwise comparison within the discordant dizygotic twin group. Irrespective of zygosity however, affected twins had smaller whole brain, hippocampal and parahippocampal volumes than their healthy co-twin. Unaffected co-twins had smaller whole brain volumes than twins from unaffected sibships. These findings suggest that frontal brain volumes are associated with the development of illness itself and that small whole brain, hippocampal and parahippocampal volumes may also be associated with the development of illness. The relationship of these brain regions to genetic vulnerability could however not be excluded due to the relatively small sample sizes. Whole brain volume however, appeared to be both a marker of illness and genetic vulnerability. A further study specifically examining differences in thalamic and caudate volumes in discordant MZ twins (Bridle et al. 2001) found larger caudate nuclei in affected twins but found no differences in thalamic volumes between twin pairs.

In an attempt to further characterise the significance and extent of grey matter deficits in affected and unaffected co-twins, Cannon (2002) conducted an MRI study of discordant MZ and DZ twins along with a sample of demographically matched control twins. The study used a relatively novel technique of constructing three-dimensional probabilistic maps of the cortex. Cortical maps were used to compute 3D vector deformation fields which allowed researchers to compute a measure to reflect grey matter density at each cortical point. Differences between well twins and their schizophrenic co-twin were found in the region of the dorsolateral prefrontal cortex, superior temporal gyrus and superior parietal lobule and were associated with measures of disease severity and cognitive function. No relationship was found with duration of illness or antipsychotic drug treatment. A cortical map of grey matter density associated with genetic proximity to affected patients found deficits in the polar and dorsolateral prefrontal cortex. These findings suggest that different cortical areas may be associated with genetic and disease-specific influences. Medial prefrontal and medial temporal lobe structures could not be assessed in this approach as they could not be extracted using the surface extraction method employed in the study.

The functional significance of structural abnormalities in twins discordant for schizophrenia has been investigated in few studies, probably because of the practical limitations of this kind of research. Berman (1992) measured cortical blood flow in monozygotic twins discordant and concordant for schizophrenia and a group of healthy co-twins. Three conditions were studied: a resting task, the Wisconsin Card Sorting Test and a number matching task designed to act as a non-specific active control task. During the task, all affected subjects from MZ twin pairs showed hypofrontality compared to their well sibling. However, well siblings of schizophrenic MZ twins showed no significant differences compared to healthy twins from unaffected pairs suggesting that hypofrontality is related to non-genetic factors. Hypofrontality in the schizophrenic co-twins was also associated with a higher life time exposure to antipsychotic medication. A further publication by the same group (Weinberger et al. 1992) examined the relationship between functional deficits and regional brain volumes measured by MRI in both healthy MZ and twins discordant for schizophrenia. Differences between discordant MZ twin pairs in prefrontal dysfunction measured during the Wisconsin Card Sort Test were found to be related to differences in left hippocampal volume. Within the affected twin group alone, prefrontal activation was strongly related to both right and left hippocampal volumes. A third publication (Goldberg et al. 1994) from the group examined intra-pair differences in anatomic structures, prefrontal rCBF and cognitive function. The study found left hippocampal volume to be related to a parameter of verbal memory and prefrontal rCBF to be related to psychotic symptom scores and preservation on the Wisconsin Card Sort Test. These findings suggest that prefrontal and medial temporal lobe regions are important in the aetiology of psychotic symptoms and cognitive dysfunction.

▌ sMRI studies of the 'extended' family

The underlying rationale of examining the first degree relatives of patients with schizophrenia is that they share approximately 50% of their genome and that common differences versus controls probably reflect genetic factors, while differences between unaffected and affected relatives presumably represent disease-specific effects. A similar degree of abnormality in relatives and patients implies that the volume alterations are not related to the disease itself but are probably related to genetic factors. In some cases, however, studies may be small and of low statistical power rendering a conclusion of no difference between two groups insecure. It is clear that these studies cannot distinguish genetic and environmental causation, but as schizophrenia is usually found to reflect mainly genetic factors, with a relatively small unique environmental effect, and almost no familial environment involvement (McGuffin et al. 1994), the commonalities between patients and their relatives are probably genetic in origin.

Most of these relatives' studies have examined the volumes of the lateral ventricles (LVs) and/or the AHCs. Only one study has reported significantly enlarged LVs in relatives as compared to controls (Sharma et al. 1998), although most of the studies in siblings (Cannon et al. 1998; Seidman et al. 1999; Staal et al. 2000) or offspring (Keshavan et al. 1997, 2002; Lawrie et al. 2001; Schreiber et al. 1999) give results in that direction. The few comparisons of patients and sibs are, on the other hand, universally significant (Cannon et al. 1998; Sharma et al. 1998; Staal et al. 2000; McDonald et al. 2002), as are the twin studies, suggesting stronger environmental and phenotypic effects. Indeed, in older 'obligate gene carriers' lateral ventriculomegaly (Sharma et al. 1998; McDonald et al. 2002) has yet to be externally replicated (Steel et al. 2002). An increased VBR in relatives may therefore primarily reflect a reduction in brain volume, although the results on sMRI are equivocal. While some studies find the brain is smaller in relatives than controls (Keshavan et al.

1997, 2002; Cannon et al. 1998), and/or no patient-relative differences (Cannon et al. 1998; McDonald et al. 2002; Seidman et al. 1999), many of the former type of study find no differences (Seidman et al. 1999; Sharma et al. 1998; McDonald et al. 2002), and one of the latter did (Steel et al. 2002).

The evidence from relatives' studies is similarly inconclusive for most other brain regions, in some cases because of insufficient studies and in others due to low power. There are, for example, isolated reports of abnormal cerebral torque (Sharma et al. 1999), but the most consistent abnormalities in patients (Table 2) have not been found in relatives (Bartley et al. 1993; Frangou et al. 1997); and findings of abnormal sylvian fissure (Honer et al. 1995) and AHC asymmetry (Schreiber et al. 1999) have yet to be replicated (Bartley et al. 1993). There is however a degree of agreement with the twin and automated studies reviewed above for fronto-temporal differences with the changes greatest in schizophrenic subjects, intermediate in relatives and smallest in con-

Table 2. Summary of sMRI findings relating to psychosis and genetic risk

Study design	Principal findings
▮ Schizophrenia vs. controls	Numerous volume reductions, particularly in temporal lobe, hippocampus, parahippocampus and amygdala
▮ Familial versus non-familial schizophrenia	Difficulties with design and replication make interpretation difficult
▮ Twin studies	*Differences between affected and non-affected MZ twins (non-genetic effects)* Ventricular enlargement, reduced whole brain, frontal & temporal lobe and hippocampal volumes. *Differences between non-affected MZ twin and unaffected controls (genetic effects)* Whole brain & frontal lobe volume reductions. Left hippocampus also shows genetically mediated volume reductions
▮ Extended family studies	Lateral ventricles, amygdala and hippocampus appear to be disease related. Genetic effects also include 3V, thalamus and amygdala and hippocampal reductions
▮ Obligates	Amygdala-hippocampal complex volume reductions appear related to symptoms. Frontal and temporal lobe reductions appear to be more closely associated with genetic carrier status. Very few studies so far
▮ High risk studies	*Symptom effects* Reductions in amygdala-hippocampal complexes, parahippocampus, thalamus, anterior cingulate, medical prefrontal lobe appear to be related to genetic liability to schizophrenia at baseline. Right temporal lobe volume reductions were also found over time associated with symptoms *Genetic effects* Smaller left and right prefrontal lobes, thalami and hippocampus

trols. The main support for this is from ROI studies in relatives with trends from a large study using sophisticated segmentation algorithms (Cannon et al. 1998), and from studies contrasting patients with their unaffected relatives (Staal et al. 2000; McDonald et al. 2002; Steel et al. 2002). Preliminary voxel-based morphometry (VBM) analyses of the latter study suggest both frontal and temporal reductions, with common genetic and disease effects. Small (Keshavan et al. 1997, 2002; Schreiber et al. 1999) and large studies (Lawrie et al. 2001) of high risk offspring have not found such differences, and neither have medium-sized studies which do not control for family membership (Sharma et al. 1998). It appears that the relatively small effects require automated approaches and should control for within family clustering.

The importance of statistical power is again illustrated in studies of the third ventricle (3V) and the thalamus (the increase in the former probably reflecting reductions in the latter and other surrounding structures). The only negative studies of the third ventricle in relatives (n = 15, Schreiber et al. 1999) and the thalamus (n = 11, Keshavan et al. 1997) are the two smallest offspring studies and Keshavan et al. (2002) found thalamus reductions when they increased the sample size to 19 (although differences have been found with samples as small as six). While most of the available literature suggests 3V increases and/or thalamus reductions in relatives more than controls, the only significant patient-relative difference reported is for the thalamus (Staal et al. 1998). Thalamus reductions, which were related to genetic liability but not psychotic symptoms in the Edinburgh High Risk Study (Lawrie et al. 2001 and see below), may therefore be genetically mediated risk markers not related to the disease itself. Ventricular enlargement may be related to disease-specific or other environmental effects rather than genetic liability.

What the relatives' studies are clear about, however, is that amygdala-hippocampal complex (AHC) reductions are both genetic and disease related. Relatives have smaller AHCs than controls (Keshavan et al. 1997, 2002; Schreiber et al. 1999; Seidman et al. 1999; Lawrie et al. 2001), and schizophrenics have smaller AHCs than relatives (Lawrie et al. 2001; O'Driscoll et al. 2001; Steel et al. 2002), although there are some negative studies (Staal et al. 2000). There are suggestions that the reductions may be more marked anteriorly (Keshavan et al. 2002; O'Driscoll et al. 2001), and on the left side (Keshavan et al. 2002; Lawrie et al. 2001). There is, however, good evidence for hippocampal differences as well (Waldo et al. 1994; Harris et al. 2002; Seidman et al. 2002; van Erp et al. 2002).

Functional studies of unaffected family members and their close relatives have been conducted and are also relevant to the understanding of structural findings. A SPECT study of 19 schizophrenic patients, 36 first degree relatives and 34 unrelated healthy controls found decreased left inferior prefrontal cortex and anterior cingulate perfusion in both relatives and schizophrenic patients compared to controls (Blackwood et al. 1999). Increases in perfusion were also found in schizophrenics and relatives compared to controls in the periventricular white matter, occipital-frontal fasciculus and internal capsule. A further study by O'Driscoll et al. (1999) used positron emission tomography (PET). The first degree relatives of schizophrenic patients with eye tracking dysfunction (ETD) showed decreased perfusion in the frontal eye fields compared to those without ETD and healthy controls. The authors suggest that hypoperfusion of the frontal eye fields may be caused by genes which predispose to schizophrenia.

▮ Studies of obligate carriers

Studies of the healthy relatives of schizophrenic subjects have provided a useful design in which to study the effects of genes which raise the liability to schizophrenia. Such studies are generally unconfounded by the effects of medication and are not associated with the expression of the illness itself. However, the proportion of genes shared with the affected relative may be much less than 50% and the relative importance of shared genetic factors is likely to be less the more distant the relationship. A potentially stronger design is to consider the unaffected relatives of schizophrenic probands who have both a parent and a child with schizophrenia (Fig. 1). Unaffected 'obligate carriers' can therefore be assumed to have transmitted the genotype from one generation to the next without succumbing to the illness themselves. They also share approximately 50% of their genes with both relatives, and since both are affected, the shared genes are more likely to contain alleles which increase the genetic liability to schizophrenia.

Sharma et al (Sharma et al. 1998, 1999) were one of the first to use the 'obligate carrier' approach to studying the effects of genes for schizophrenia. Thirty one people with schizophrenia were compared to 39 unrelated controls and 57 relatives, of whom 11 were presumed 'obligate carriers'. Obligate carriers had larger left and right lateral ventricles volumes than any other group. A subsequent study by Steel et al. (2002) compared 6 affected sibships of three individuals in which one sibling was an affected subject with schizophrenia, one was a presumed obligate carrier with a child with schizophrenia and one

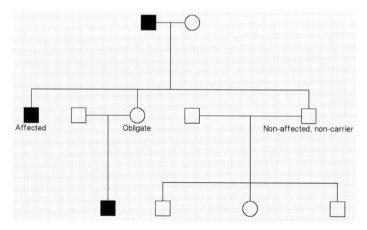

Fig. 1. Schematic showing affected patients and obligate carriers of schizophrenia

sibling had no children with schizophrenia ('non-obligate'). In terms of cortical structures (WB, FL, TL), obligates resembled their non-obligate unaffected siblings, both having significantly larger volumes than their affected siblings. However, the amygdala-hippocampal complex was significantly smaller in schizophrenic siblings and their obligate siblings than it was in the non-affected non-obligate sibling. Premorbid IQ, measured by the NART, was also unexpectedly higher in the sample of obligate carriers.

Positron emission tomography (PET) has been used to compare obligate carriers with stable schizophrenic patients and healthy controls in one study which used $H_2^{15}O$ to examine the functional correlates of verbal fluency (Spence et al. 2000). The 'normal' functional response is said to be characterised by left dorsolateral prefrontal cortex (DLPFC) activation and deactivation of the left superior temporal gyrus (STG) and was found in both normal controls, obligate carriers and affected patients. The same research group found similar results in asymptomatic patients with schizophrenia in an earlier study (Dye et al. 1999) who showed similar responses to both normal controls and a further group of six patients with schizophrenia. Previously replicated findings of reduced fronto-temporal connectivity (Frith et al. 1995; Fletcher et al. 1999; Lawrie et al. 2002a) in schizophrenia were not replicated in either study suggesting that at least some patterns of dysconnectivity may be related to psychotic symptoms rather than be markers of genetic liability.

▮ Studies of familial and sporadic schizophrenia

Studies of the ventricle to brain ratio (VBR) in 'sporadic versus familial' schizophrenia provide less consensus, as one of the originators of the distinction noted in a review of the early studies (Lewis 1990). Patients without a family history of schizophrenia may have repeatedly been shown to have higher VBRs and more marked ventriculomegaly than family history-positive patients (Vita et al. 1994; DeQuardo et al. 1996), and some notable large studies (n > 100) may have failed to find an association between family history and the VBR (Johnstone et al. 1989; Jones et al. 1994); but several studies do report such an association (Owens et al. 1985) , including those which go some way to supporting the distinction (Vita et al. 1994; Silverman et al. 1998a). It may be that schizophrenics without an obvious genetic loading are more likely to have had environmental triggers which may increase the VBR, but determining sporadic status is not easy when many healthy relatives are likely to be carrying the gene(s) and, especially in families where there is a poor knowledge of family psychiatric history an affected subject may be misclassified as 'sporadic' (Johnstone et al. 1995). The limited resolution of CT studies increases measurement error and the use of VBR may have further compounded these difficulties. Indeed, the few sMRI studies to have adopted similar approaches have all reported similar or greater abnormalities in familial cases (Schwarzkopf et al. 1991; Roy and Crowe 1994; Falkai et al. 2002; Harris et al. 2002), with the exception of McDonald et al. (2002), and some suggest specific genetic effects in frontal and temporal lobes, the ventricles and the basal ganglia.

▌ Individual gene effects in schizophrenia

Individual gene effects might best be quantified by relating their presence or expression to clinical features and/or regional brain volumes in both affected subjects and their well relatives. To date, however, very few studies have attempted to use this method. Difficulties with this approach are almost certainly contingent on the fact that few specific gene effects have been consistently replicated in schizophrenia. Kunugi et al (1999) looked at the relationship between the neurotrophin-3 A3 allele and regional brain volumes in schizophrenia and bipolar disorder. The results showed A3 allelic status to be associated with reduced volumes in schizophrenic but not bipolar subjects. This unconfirmed finding suggests that bipolar subjects may be subject to genetic or environmental factors which ameliorate the effects of this gene. Without further information about the clinical associations of A3 allelic status, it is difficult to draw any firm conclusions from this study. ApoE status has also been related to hippocampal volume in schizophrenia (Fernandez et al. 1999; Hata et al. 2002), although the results are inconsistent.

The catechol-O-methyl transferase (COMT) is a potential candidate gene for schizophrenia, having a role in dopamine metabolism and also a relationship between its expression and prefrontally medicated cognition. A study of 175 patients with schizophrenia, 219 unaffected siblings and 55 controls (Egan et al. 2001) demonstrated a dose-like effect of COMT genotype expression and performance on the Wisconsin Card Sorting Test. COMT allelic expression was further related to brain physiology during a working memory task in three subgroups (n=11–16) of the original sample. Met allele load predicted a stronger prefrontal response and in a subsequent analysis of 104 trios it was shown that the Val allele was preferentially transmitted to schizophrenic offspring. These findings suggest that the COMT Val allele may raise the liability to schizophrenia possibly by an impairment of dopamine function and consequent impairment of executive function. At the time of going to press, there had been no independent replication of this finding to the knowledge of any of the authors.

▌ Studies of the schizophrenia spectrum

Schizotypy and schizoid personality disorder have been postulated to be genetic variants of schizophrenia which lie along a spectrum of illness. Schizotypal disorder is presumed to be more closely associated with schizophrenia and the diagnosis increases the risk of developing schizophrenia several-fold. The results of structural MRI studies of schizotypal disorder might therefore reflect the expression of genes for schizophrenia or brain abnormality preceding the onset of psychosis.

CT studies have compared schizotypal subjects with controls and also with schizophrenic subjects. CT studies found larger VBRs than in unaffected siblings and healthy non-related controls (Dickey et al. 2002; Silverman et al. 1998b; Siever et al. 1995). This finding might reflect a decrease in total brain substance generally or a more specific loss or absence of tissue around the boundaries of the ventricles themselves. MRI studies have also compared schizotypal subjects with healthy controls and suggest that schizotypal subjects have lower brain volumes (Cannon et al. 1994; Dickey et al. 2000) and that ventricle size is intermediate between that of schizophrenia and healthy controls (Buchsbaum et al. 1997). A further finding in schizotypal disorder is of reduced STG volumes (Dickey et al. 1999; Downhill, Jr. et al. 2001), perhaps a reflection of abnormal language in those subjects. A further study (Dickey et al. 2003), currently in press, reports no difference in fusiform gyrus volume in schizotypal subjects compared to controls although volumes were negatively correlated with measures of illusions and magical thinking. A relative paucity of studies in this area makes it difficult to draw any firm conclusions.

High risk studies

High risk studies follow a cohort of unaffected individuals at increased risk of schizophrenia prospectively through the period of high risk (circa 23 in males, 26 in women) in the knowledge that some subjects will become affected. This design overcomes several of the difficulties of case-control studies. Subjects can be scanned and interviewed repeatedly over the period of risk allowing any effects to be unconfounded by the effects of medication or positive symptoms. Imaging findings may be associated to symptoms or neuropsychological performance and subjects who develop schizophrenia may be scanned before medication has been prescribed. In addition, because the matter of who will develop schizophrenia is not known, investigators are less liable to observer bias.

In spite of the considerable advantages of 'high risk' studies, they have many practical limitations. Patient attrition, cost and the tendency for both staff and technology to change over time has meant that few centres have undertaken this study design. The first high risk imaging study to be completed was the Copenhagen high risk project (CHRP), although the scans (CT) were not repeated over time (Cannon 1993). Two further studies are ongoing, both using sMRI, the Edinburgh High Risk Study (EHRS) and the Australian High Risk Study (AHRS). The Australian High Risk Study will be covered in detail in the chapter by McGuire.

The Copenhagen High Risk Study

The Copenhagen High Risk Study (Mednick 1966) concerned the children of mothers with schizophrenia. Subjects received a CT scan of the brain and neuropsychological assessments. High risk subjects were compared to healthy controls with no family history of mental illness that were matched to high risk subjects on age, sex social class and IQ. CT scans were not repeated over time and the main results compare the scans from high risk subjects with healthy controls. Their results suggest that widened fissures and sulci are positively associated to genetic risk but that only schizophrenic subjects have enlarged ventricles (Cannon et al. 1989). A subsequent study of 16 twin pairs discordant for schizophrenia (Zorrilla et al. 1997) found that the sulci to brain ratio and VBR differed between the twin pairs suggesting an environmental effect or gene-environment interaction.

Edinburgh High Risk Study

The Edinburgh High Risk Study concerns the families of known patients throughout Scotland whose consultant thought might have a family history of schizophrenia. Healthy family members were included if they had at least two close relatives with a confirmed diagnosis of schizophrenia using the OPCRIT computer program (McGuffin et al. 1991). 162 high risk subjects provided some data and 150 had at least one sMRI scan in the first phase of the study between 1994 and 1999. Two control groups were also recruited. The first consisted of healthy non-related controls matched as closely as possible for age and sex. The second consisted of patients with first schizophrenic episodes but without a known family history of psychosis. High risk subjects were further classified at each of up to 3 interviews, according to the Present State Examination, into the following categories:

0 Symptom free;
1 Any fully rated non-psychotic PSE item (e.g., tension, depression, anxiety);
2 Any partially rated psychotic symptom;
3 Any fully rated psychotic symptom;
4 Catego S+ schizophrenia.

The increased liability to schizophrenia, presumably of genetic origin, was also quantified. Genetic liability to schizophrenia was measured in two ways. The first is an ordinal measure of genetic liability rated from lowest to highest: two or more first degree relatives with schizophrenia, one family member with schizophrenia and one or more second degree relatives with schizophrenia and finally, two or more first degree relatives with schizophrenia. The other method employs simple matrix algebra to provide a continuous measure of genetic liability which should, in theory, provide more information about risk (Lawrie et al. 2001). High risk subjects and controls were reassessed every eighteen months. Assessments performed included neuropsychological testing and clinical examinations and an MRI scan of the brain. Obstetric complications were also assessed from maternal recall and health service records (McIntosh et al. 2002) and the mothers of subjects and controls were interviewed with a view to obtaining information about childhood behaviour (Miller et al. 2002).

Numerous differences in neuropsychological measures were shown (Byrne et al. 2003). In general, controls performed best followed by high risk subjects followed by first episode patients. After controlling for IQ high risk subjects performed worse on the Hayling sentence completion test and the Rivermead

Behavioural Memory Test (RBMT) of delayed memory. Both measures were negatively correlated with both measures of genetic liability used in the study.

Early region of interest analysis of the first 100 MRI scans found the amygdala-hippocampal complex to be approximately 4% smaller than controls and about 4% larger than subjects with schizophrenia (Lawrie et al. 1999). Thalamic size was also smaller in high risks compared to controls. An increase in third ventricular volume was found in high risk subjects compared to controls, although this was not significant after the correlation in volumes between subjects from the same family had been taken into account (Lawrie et al. 1999). Voxel-based morphometry confirms these early results and also shows medial prefrontal and temporal lobe reductions in grey matter density with a gradient which is greatest in first episodes, intermediate in high risks and lowest in controls (Job et al. 2002). Within high risk subjects, higher genetic liability was associated with smaller left and right prefrontal lobes and smaller left and right thalami (Lawrie et al. 2001).

Changes in brain size were also measured using repeat scans in the 66 high risk subjects and 20 healthy controls (Lawrie et al. 2002 c). Changes within the high risk group were also compared for subgroups according to whether or not they had fully rated psychotic symptoms in the first phase of the study. No differences were found between controls and high risk subjects. When high risks with symptoms were compared to those without symptoms however, several other differences emerged. Those with psychotic symptoms showed a greater reduction in right temporal lobe volume compared to those without symptoms and similar, though non-significant differences were also reported in respect of the left temporal lobe and the prefrontal cortex bilaterally. Over the same time period, neuropsychological measures also continued to favour controls over high risk subjects and those with psychotic symptoms performed less well than those without particularly in the area of memory (Cosway et al. 2002). Decline in memory performance also appeared greatest in those with symptoms though the change was not statistically significant.

Early fMRI findings from the Edinburgh High Risk Study

Functional Magnetic Resonance Imaging (fMRI) has been used to examine the functional correlates of performance on the Hayling sentence completion test (Whalley et al. 2003). All participants were initially presented with a series of sentences with the last word missing and asked to think of an appropriate word to complete the sentence and press a button when they had done so. The sentences differed in their degree of constraint (4 levels) and were presented in randomised blocks, along with rest periods. High constraint consisted of sentences in which a single last word was strongly suggested by the form of the sentence (e.g. 'Bob proposed but she turned him..'). Low constraint sentences allowed for more than one possible completion (e.g., 'His ability to work was…'). Behavioural data was also obtained for word appropriateness and reaction time.

In a previous study using a similar paradigm, 8 patients with DSM IV schizophrenia were compared to 10 healthy controls matched for age and IQ

(Lawrie et al. 2002b). Correlation coefficients between the BOLD response in the left temporal cortex (x = –54, y = –42, z = 3) and left dorsolateral prefrontal cortex (x = –39, y = 12, z = 24) were significantly lower in the schizophrenic group and were negatively correlated with the severity of auditory hallucinations suggesting a relative disconnection in the schizophrenic group.

The study paradigm was then applied to all participants in the second phase of the Edinburgh High Risk Study. High risk subjects with and without psychotic symptoms were compared with a group of healthy controls. Differences in activation between all high risk subjects and controls were assumed to represent 'genetic' effects and differences between high risks without psychotic symptoms and those with psychotic symptoms were assumed to represent 'state' or disease-related effects.

Preliminary results have been obtained from the first 100 subjects to be assessed. This sample consists of 21 normal controls and 69 high risk subjects. Of the 69 high risk subjects, 27 had one or more partially or fully rated psychotic symptoms from the PSE and 42 did not. None of the controls had psychotic symptoms. There were no significant differences on several demographic variables or on reaction time or 'word appropriateness' scores.

For the sentence completion versus rest comparison, high risk subjects with psychotic symptoms versus all those without symptoms showed greater activation in the left parietal lobe. No other group differences were found. Control subjects showed greater activation ('genetic effect') than high risk subjects as a whole in the right medial frontal gyrus, the left posterior lobe of the cerebellum and also the thalamic nuclei in relation to increasing task difficulty.

▍ Conclusions

sMRI studies of patients with schizophrenia have established that multiple cortical and subcortical regions are affected. Because the patients in these studies have often been ill for many years it has been difficult to tease out the brain changes associated with genetic or environmental liability from those which occur premorbidly and those which may be contingent upon psychotic symptoms or their treatment.

The results of twin and relative studies have shed light on many of these issues. Discordant monozygotic twin studies in particular can control for sources of genetic and between family environmental variations in cerebral structure that occurs between unrelated individuals. There is some evidence that prefrontal and medial lobe deficits appear to be associated both with disease specific and genetic effects. It is however possible that the disease specific effects are complex gene-environmental interactions, although this hypothesis is difficult to test without further knowledge of specific environmental risks (van Erp et al. 2002). Unfortunately, information regarding genetic risk factors has generally been more equivocal and poorly replicated. Twin and relative studies are however still confounded by treatment and disease processes and as a result there findings are often inconclusive. This problem is made worse by issues of low statistical power and the practical difficulties underlying the execution of such studies.

The realisation over the last ten years of high risk studies in which demographic, clinical, neuropsychological and imaging data is collected on subjects at increased risk of schizophrenia before the matter of who will be affected has become clear has been a significant advance. Such studies have the potential ability to clarify the brain changes which are associated with genetic loading, those which are present premorbidly and those which are associated with the development and continuation or illness or its treatment. To date, three studies have now published both imaging and neuropsychological data though many more have been published on the basis of more restricted data sets.

Many cerebral regions appear to be associated with both genetic risk and psychotic symptoms. Explanations for this include the possibility that disease processes are already underway in those destined to develop schizophrenia before the first symptom becomes apparent. Unfortunately practical considerations limit the age at which an unaffected cohort may be ascertained, although recruitment of an unaffected cohort of children remains an interesting possibility. A further explanation for the failure to more clearly separate genetic and symptom related effects is the relative crudeness of region of interest methods. Many studies consider the 'prefrontal cortex' as a whole, when the region shows considerable functional specialisation. It is possible that voxel-based morphometry (VBM) and parcellation will overcome some of these difficulties. However, there is no consensus about the optimal way in which to measure changes over time using VBM. Advances in high risk research may therefore be as likely to come from technological advances as they are from new paradigms or larger studies.

References

Andreasen NC, Arndt S, Swayze V, Cizadlo T, Flaum M, O'Leary D, Ehrhardt JC, Yuh WT (1994) Thalamic abnormalities in schizophrenia visualized through magnetic resonance image averaging [comment]. Science 266:294–298

Baare WF, Hulshoff Pol HE, Boomsma DI, Posthuma D, de Geus EJ, Schnack HG, van Haren NE, van Oel CJ, Kahn RS (2001a) Quantitative genetic modeling of variation in human brain morphology. Cerebral Cortex 11:816–824

Baare WF, van Oel CJ, Hulshoff Pol HE, Schnack HG, Durston S, Sitskoorn MM, Kahn RS (2001b) Volumes of brain structures in twins discordant for schizophrenia. Archives of General Psychiatry 58:33–40

Bartley AJ, Jones DW, Torrey EF, Zigun JR, Weinberger DR (1993) Sylvian fissure asymmetries in monozygotic twins: a test of laterality in schizophrenia. Biological Psychiatry 34:853–863

Berman KF, Torrey EF, Daniel DG, Weinberger DR (1992) Regional cerebral blood flow in monozygotic twins discordant and concordant for schizophrenia. Archives of General Psychiatry 49:927–934

Blackwood DHR, Glabus MF, Dunan J, O'Carroll RE, Muir WJ, Ebmeier KP (1999) Altered cerebral perfusion measured by SPECT in relatives of patients with schizophrenia: correlations with memory and P300. British Journal of Psychiatry 175: 357–366

Bridle N, Pantelis C, Wood SJ, Coppola R, Velakoulis D, McStephen M, Tierney P, Le TL, Torrey EF, Weinberger DR (2001) Thalamic and caudate volumes in monozygotic twins discordant for schizophrenia. Australian and New Zealand Journal of Psychiatry 36:347–354

Buchsbaum MS, Yang S, Hazlett E, Siegel BV Jr, Germans M, Haznedar M, O'Flaithbheartaigh S, Wei T, Silverman J, Siever LJ (1997) Ventricular volume and asymmetry in schizotypal personality disorder and schizophrenia assessed with magnetic resonance imaging. Schizophrenia Research 27:45–53

Byrne M, Clafferty BA, Cosway R, Grant E, Hodges A, Whalley HC, Lawrie SM, Cunningham-Owens DG, Johnstone EC (2003) Neuropsychology, genetic liability and psychotic symptoms in those at high risk of schizophrenia. Journal of Abnormal Psychology 112:38–48

Cannon M, Jones P (1996) Schizophrenia [review]. Journal of Neurology, Neurosurgery & Psychiatry 60:604–613

Cannon TD, Mednick SA, Parnas J (1989) Genetic and perinatal determinants of structural brain deficits in schizophrenia. Archives of General Psychiatry 46:883–889

Cannon TD, Mednick SA, Parnas J, Schulsinger F, Praestholm J, Vestergaard A (1994) Developmental brain abnormalities in the offspring of schizophrenic mothers. II. Structural brain characteristics of schizophrenia and schizotypal personality disorder. Archives of General Psychiatry 51:955–962

Cannon TD, Thompson PM, van Erp TG, Toga AW, Poutanen VP, Huttunen M, Lönnqvist J, Standerskjold-Nordenstam CG, Narr KL, Khaledy M, Zoumalan CI, Dail R, Kaprio J (2002) Cortex mapping reveals regionally specific patterns of genetic and disease-specific gray-matter deficits in twins discordant for schizophrenia. Proceedings of the National Academy of Sciences of the United States of America 99:3228–3233

Cannon TD, van Erp TG, Huttunen M, Lönnqvist J, Salonen O, Valanne L, Poutanen VP, Standerskjold-Nordenstam CG, Gur RE, Yan M (1998) Regional gray matter, white matter and cerebrospinal fluid distributions in schizophrenic patients, their siblings and controls. Archives of General Psychiatry 59:35–41

Carmelli D, DeCarli C, Swan GE, Jack LM, Reed T, Wolf PA, Miller BL (1998) Evidence for genetic variance in white matter hyperintensity volume in normal elderly male twins. Stroke 29:1177–1181

Chakos MH, Lieberman JA, Bilder RM, Borenstein M, Lerner G, Bogerts B, Wu H, Kinon B, Ashtari M (1994) Increase in caudate nuclei volumes of first-episode schizophrenic patients taking antipsychotic drugs. American Journal of Psychiatry 151:1430–1436

Cosway R, Byrne M, Clafferty R, Hodges A, Grant E, Morris J, Abukmeil SS, Lawrie SM, Miller P, Owens DG, Johnstone EC (2002) Sustained attention in young people at high risk for schizophrenia. Psychological Medicine 32:277–286

DeQuardo JR, Goldman M, Tandon R (1996) VBR in schizophrenia: relationship to family history of psychosis and season of birth. Schizophrenia Research 20:275–285

Dickey CC, McCarley RW, Shenton ME (2002) The brain in schizotypal personality disorder: a review of structural MRI and CT findings [review]. Harvard Review of Psychiatry 10:1–15

Dickey CC, McCarley RW, Voglmaier MM, Niznikiewicz MA, Seidman LJ, Frumin M, Toner S, Demeo S, Shenton ME (2003) A MRI study of fusiform gyrus in schizotypal personality disorder. Schizophrenia Research 64(1):35–39

Dickey CC, McCarley RW, Voglmaier MM, Niznikiewicz MA, Seidman LJ, Hirayasu Y, Fischer I, Teh EK, Van Rhoads R, Jakab M, Kikinis R, Jolesz FA, Shenton ME (1999) Schizotypal personality disorder and MRI abnormalities of temporal lobe gray matter. Biological Psychiatry 45:1393–1402

Dickey CC, Shenton ME, Hirayasu Y, Fischer I, Voglmaier MM, Niznikiewicz MA, Seidman LJ, Fraone S, McCarley RW (2000) Large CSF volume not attributable to ventricular volume in schizotypal personality disorder. American Journal of Psychiatry 157:48–54

Downhill JE Jr, Buchsbaum MS, Hazlett EA, Barth S, Lees RS, Nunn M, Lekarev O, Wei T, Shihabuddin L, Mitropoulou V, Silverman J, Siever LJ (2001) Temporal lobe volume determined by magnetic resonance imaging in schizotypal personality disorder and schizophrenia. Schizophrenia Research 48:187–199

Dye SM, Spence SA, Bench CJ, Hirsch SR, Stefan MD, Sharma T, Grasby PM (1999) No evidence for left superior temporal dysfunction in asymptomatic schizophrenia and bipolar disorder. British Journal of Psychiatry 175:367–374

Egan MF, Goldberg TE, Kolachana BS, Callicott JH, Mazzanti CM, Straub RE, Goldman D, Weinberger DR (2001) Effect of COMT Val108/158 Met genotype on frontal lobe function and risk for schizophrenia. Proceedings of the National Academy of Sciences of the United States of America 98:6917–6922

Falkai P, Honer WG, Alfter D, Schneider-Axmann T, Bussfeld P, Cordes J, Blank B, Schonell H, Steinmetz H, Maier W, Tepest R (2002) The temporal lobe in schizophrenia from uni- and multiply affected families. Neuroscience Letters 325:25–28

Faraone SV, Seidman LJ, Kremen WS, Kennedy D, Makris N, Caviness VS, Goldstein J, Tsuang MT (2003) Structural brain abnormalities among relatives of patients with schizophrenia: implications for linkage studies. Schizophrenia Research 60:125–140

Fernandez T, Yan WL, Hamburger S, Rapoport JL, Saunders AM, Schapiro M, Ginns EI, Sidransky E (1999) Apolipoprotein E alleles in childhood-onset schizophrenia. American Journal of Medical Genetics 88:211–213

Fletcher P, McKenna PJ, Friston KJ, Frith CD, Dolan RJ (1999) Abnormal cingulate modulation of fronto-temporal connectivity in schizophrenia. Neuroimage 9:337–342

Frangou S, Sharma T, Sigmundson T, Barta P, Pearlson G, Murray RM (1997) The Maudsley Family Study 4. Normal planum temporale asymmetry in familial schizophrenia. British Journal of Psychiatry 170:328–333

Frith CD, Friston KJ, Herold S, Silbersweig D, Fletcher P, Cahill C, Dolan RJ, Frackowiak RS, Liddle PF (1995) Regional brain activity in chronic schizophrenic patients during the performance of a verbal fluency task. British Journal of Psychiatry 167:343–349

Goldberg TE, Torrey EF, Berman KF, Weinberger DR (1994) Relations between neuropsychological performance and brain morphological and physiological measures in monozygotic twins discordant for schizophrenia. Psychiatry Research: Neuroimaging 55:51–61

Harris JG, Young DA, Rojas DC, Cajade-Law A, Scherzinger A, Nawroz S, Adler LE, Cullum CM, Simon J, Freedman R (2002) Increased hippocampal volume in schizophrenics' parents with ancestral history of schizophrenia. Schizophrenia Research 55:11–17

Hata T, Kunugi H, Nanko S, Fukuda R, Kaminaga T (2002) Possible effect of the APOE epsilon 4 allele on the hippocampal volume and asymmetry in schizophrenia. American Journal of Medical Genetics 114:641–642

Honer WG, Bassett AS, Squires-Wheeler E, Falkai P, Smith GN, Lapointe JS, Canero C, Lang DJ (1995) The temporal lobes, reversed asymmetry and the genetics of schizophrenia. NeuroReport 7:221–224

Job DE, Whalley HC, McConnell S, Glabus M, Johnstone EC, Lawrie SM (2002) Structural gray matter differences between first-episode schizophrenics and normal controls using voxel-based morphometry. Neuroimage 17:880–889

Johnstone EC, Lang FH, Owens DGC, Frith CD (1995) Determinants of the extremes of outcome in schizophrenia. British Journal of Psychiatry 167:604–609

Johnstone EC, Owens DGC, Bydder GM, Colter N, Crow TJ, Frith CD (1989) The spectrum of structural brain changes in schizophrenia: age of onset as a predictor of cognitive and clinical impairments and their cerebral correlates. Psychological Medicine 19:-91

Jones PB, Harvey I, Lewis SW, Toone BK, van Os J, Williams M, Murray RM (1994) Cerebral ventricle dimensions as risk factors for schizophrenia and affective psychosis: an epidemiological approach to analysis. Psychological Medicine 24:995–1011

Keshavan MS, Dick E, Mankowski I, Harenski K, Montrose DM, Diwadkar V, DeBellis M (2002) Decreased left amygdala and hippocampal volumes in young offspring at risk for schizophrenia. Schizophrenia Research 58:173–183

Keshavan MS, Montrose DM, Pierri JN, Dick EL, Rosenberg D, Talagala L, Sweeney JA (1997) Magnetic resonance imaging and spectroscopy in offspring at risk for schizophrenia: preliminary studies. Progress in Neuropsychopharmacology and Biological Psychiatry 21:1285–1295

Kunugi H, Hattori M, Nanko S, Fujii K, Kato T, Nanko S (1999) Dinucleotide repeat polymorphism in the neurotrophin-3 gene and hippocampal volume in psychoses. Schizophrenia Research 37:271–273

Lawrie SM, Abukmeil SS (1998) Brain abnormality in schizophrenia. A systematic and quantitative review of volumetric magnetic resonance imaging studies. British Journal of Psychiatry 172:110–120

Lawrie SM, Buechel C, Whalley HC, Frith CD, Friston KJ, Johnstone EC (2002a) Reduced frontotemporal functional connectivity in schizophrenia associated with auditory hallucinations. Biological Psychiatry 51:1008–1011

Lawrie SM, Buechel C, Whalley HC, Frith CD, Friston KJ, Johnstone EC (2002b) Reduced frontotemporal functional connectivity in schizophrenia associated with auditory hallucinations. Biological Psychiatry 51:1008–1011

Lawrie SM, Whalley HC, Abukmeil SS, Kestelman JN, Miller P, Best JJ, Owens DG, Johnstone EC (2002c) Temporal lobe volume changes in people at high risk of schizophrenia with psychotic symptoms. British Journal of Psychiatry 181:138–143

Lawrie SM, Whalley HC, Abukmeil SS, Kestelman JN, Miller P, Best JJK, Owens DGC, Johnstone EC (2001) Brain structure, genetic liability and psychotic symptoms in subjects at high risk of developing schizophrenia. Biological Psychiatry 49:811–823

Lawrie SM, Whalley HC, Kestelman JN, Abukmeil SS, Byrne M, Hodges A, Rimmington JE, Best JJK, Owens DGC, Johnstone EC (1999) Magnetic resonance imaging of the brain in people at high risk of developing schizophrenia. Lancet 353:30–33

Levitt JG, Blanton RE, Caplan R, Asarnow R, Guthrie D, Toga AW, Capetillo-Cunliffe L, McCracken JT (2001) Medial temporal lobe in childhood-onset schizophrenia. Psychiatry Research 108:17–27

Lewis SW (1990) Computerised tomography in schizophrenia 15 years on. British Journal of Psychiatry 157:16–24

McDonald C, Grech A, Toulopoulou T, Schulze K, Chapple B, Sham P, Walshe M, Sharma T, Sigmundson T, Chitnis X, Murray RM (2002) Brain volumes in familial and non-familial schizophrenic probands and their unaffected relatives. American Journal of Medical Genetics 114:616–625

McGuffin P, Asherson P, Owen M, Farmer A (1994) The strength of the genetic effect. Is there room for an environmental influence in the aetiology of schizophrenia? [comment] [review]. British Journal of Psychiatry 164:593–599

McGuffin P, Farmer A, Harvey I (1991) A polydiagnostic application of operational criteria in studies of psychotic illness. Development and reliability of the OPCRIT system. Archives of General Psychiatry 48:764–770

McIntosh AM, Holmes S, Gleeson S, Burns JK, Hodges AK, Byrne MM, Dobbie R, Miller P, Lawrie SM, Johnstone EC (2002) Maternal recall bias, obstetric history and schizophrenia. British Journal of Psychiatry 181:520–525

Mednick SA (1966) A longitudinal study of children with a high risk for schizophrenia. Mental Hygiene 50:522–535

Miller PM, Byrne M, Hodges A, Lawrie SM, Johnstone EC (2002) Childhood behaviour, psychotic symptoms and psychosis onset in young people at high risk of schizophrenia: early findings from the Edinburgh high risk study. Psychological Medicine 32:173–179

O'Driscoll GA, Benkelfat C, Florencio PS, Wolff AL, Joober R, Lal S, Evans AC (1999) Neural correlates of eye tracking deficits in first-degree relatives of schizophrenic patients: a positron emission tomography study. Archives of General Psychiatry 56:1127–1134

O'Driscoll GA, Florencio PS, Gagnon D, Wolff AV, Benkelfat C, Mikula L, Lal S, Evans AC (2001) Amygdala-hippocampal volume and verbal memory in first-degree relatives of schizophrenic patients. Psychiatry Research 107:75–85

Owens DGC, Johnstone EC, Crow TJ, Frith CD, Jagoe JR, Kreel L (1985) Lateral ventricular size in schizophrenia: relationship to the disease process and its clinical manifestations. Psychological Medicine 15:27–41

Roy MA, Crowe RR (1994) Validity of the familial and sporadic subtypes of schizophrenia [review]. American Journal of Psychiatry 151:805–814

Schreiber H, Baur-Seack K, Kornhuber HH, Wallner B, Friedrich JM, De Winter IM, Born J (1999) Brain morphology in adolescents at genetic risk for schizophrenia assessed by qualitative and quantitative magnetic resonance imaging. Schizophrenia Research 40:81–84

Schwarzkopf SB, Nasrallah HA, Olson SC, Bogerts B, McLaughlin JA, Mitra T (1991) Family history and brain morphology in schizophrenia: an MRI study. Psychiatry Research 40:49–60

Seidman LJ, Faraone SV, Goldstein JM, Kremen WS, Horton NJ, Makris N, Caviness VS, Tsuang MT (1999) Thalamic and amygdala-hippocampal volume reductions in first degree relatives of patients with schizophrenia: an MRI-based morphometric analysis. Biological Psychiatry 46:941–954

Seidman LJ, Faraone SV, Goldstein JM, Kremen WS, Horton NJ, Makris N, Toomey N, Kennedy D, Caviness VS, Tsuang MT (2002) Left hippocampal volume as a vulnerability indicator for schizophrenia. Archives of General Psychiatry 59(9):839–849

Sharma T, Lancaster E, Lee D, Lewis S, Sigmundson T, Takei N, Gurling H, Barta P, Pearlson G, Murray R (1998) Brain changes in schizophrenia. Volumetric MRI study of families multiply affected by schizophrenia – the Maudsley Family Study 5. British Journal of Psychiatry 173:132–138

Sharma T, Lancaster E, Sigmundson T, Lewis S, Takei N, Gurling H, Barta P, Pearlson G, Murray R (1999) Lack of normal pattern of cerebral asymmetry in familial schizophrenic patients and their relatives – The Maudsley Family Study. Schizophrenia Research 40:111–120

Siever LJ, Rotter M, Losonczy M, Guo SL, Mitropoulou V, Trestman R, Apter S, Zemishlany Z, Silverman J, Horvath TB (1995) Lateral ventricular enlargement in schizotypal personality disorder. Psychiatry Research 57:109–118

Silverman JM, Smith CJ, Guo SL, Mohs RC, Siever LJ, Davis KL (1998a) Lateral ventricular enlargement in schizophrenic probands and their siblings with schizophrenia related disorders. Biological Psychiatry 43:97–106

Silverman JM, Smith CJ, Guo SL, Mohs RC, Siever LJ, Davis KL (1998b) Lateral ventricular enlargement in schizophrenic probands and their siblings with schizophrenia-related disorders. Biological Psychiatry 43:97–106

Spence SA, Liddle PF, Stefan MD, Hellewell JSE, Sharma T, Friston KJ, Hirsch SR, Frith CD, Murray RM, Deakin JFW, Grasby PM (2000) Functional anatomy of verbal fluency in people with schizophrenia and those at genetic risk. British Journal of Psychiatry 176:52–60

Staal WG, Hulshoff Pol HE, Schnack H, Hoogendoorn MLC, Jellema K, Kahn RS (2000) Structural brain abnormalities in patients with schizophrenia and their healthy siblings. American Journal of Psychiatry 157:416–421

Staal WG, Hulshoff Pol HE, Schnack H, van der Schot AC, Kahn RS (1998) Partial volume decrease of the thalamus in relatives of patients with schizophrenia. American Journal of Psychiatry 155:1784–1786

Steel R, Whalley HC, Miller P, Best JJK, Johnstone EC, Lawrie SM (2002) Structural MRI of the brain in presumed carriers of genes for schizophrenia, their affected and unaffected siblings. Journal of Neurology, Neurosurgery and Psychiatry 72:455–458

Suddath RL, Christison GW, Torrey EF, Casanova MF, Weinberger DR (1990) Anatomical abnormalities in the brains of monozygotic twins discordant for schizophrenia [comment] [erratum appears in N Engl J Med 1990 May 31; 322(22): 1616]. New England Journal of Medicine 322:789–794

van Erp TG, Saleh PA, Rosso IM, Huttunen M, Lönnqvist J, Pirkola T, Salonen O, Valanne L, Poutanen VP, Standerskjold-Nordenstam CG, Cannon TD (2002) Contributions of genetic risk and fetal hypoxia to hippocampal volume in patients with schizophrenia or schizoaffective disorder, their unaffected siblings and healthy unrelated volunteers. American Journal of Psychiatry 159:1514–1520

Vita A, Dieci M, Giobbio GM, Garbarini M, Morganti C, Braga M, Invernizzi G (1994) A reconsideration of the relationship between structural abnormalities and family history of schizophrenia. Psychiatry Research 53:41–55

Waldo MC, Cawthra E, Adler LE, Dubester S, Staunton M, Nagamoto H, Baker N, Madison A, Simon J, Scherzinger A, Drebing C, Gerhardt G, Freedman R (1994) Auditory sensory gating, hippocampal volume and catecholamine metabolism in schizophrenics and their siblings. Schizophrenia Research 12:93–105

Weinberger DR, Berman KF, Suddath R, Torrey EF (1992) Evidence of dysfunction of a prefrontal-limbic network in schizophrenia: a magnetic resonance imaging and regional cerebral blood flow study of discordant monozygotic twins. American Journal of Psychiatry 149:890–897

Wright IC, Ellison ZR, Sharma T, Friston KJ, Murray RM, McGuire PK (1999) Mapping of grey matter changes in schizophrenia. Schizophrenia Research 35:1–14

Wright IC, Rabe-Hesketh S, Woodruff PW, David AS, Murray RM, Bullmore ET (2000) Metaanalysis of regional brain volumes in schizophrenia. American Journal of Psychiatry 157:16–25

Zorrilla LT, Cannon TD, Kronenberg S, Mednick SA, Schulsinger F, Parnas J, Praestholm J, Vestergaard A (1997) Structural brain abnormalities in schizophrenia: a family study. Biological Psychiatry 42:1080–1086

The hippocampus and schizophrenia

STEPHAN HECKERS

Department of Psychiatry, Massachusetts General Hospital – East, Charlestown, MA, USA

Introduction

It is now widely accepted that schizophrenia is associated with abnormalities of the brain. The details, however, are unclear: Which neural circuits are affected and which remain intact? When do structural and functional abnormalities develop in the brain? How can brain abnormalities explain the clinical features?

There has never been a shortage of observations and speculations to provide answers to these three questions. When Emil Kraepelin introduced the concept of dementia praecox, in the 5th edition of his textbook of psychiatry (Kraepelin 1896), he was convinced that a single disease mechanism could explain dementia paranoides, hebephrenia, and catatonia. He suggested that the patients suffer from an autointoxication and, accordingly, he classified dementia praecox as an endocrine disorder. Only one year later, the first postmortem study of dementia praecox was published by Alois Alzheimer, then a young psychiatrist in Frankfurt (Alzheimer 1897). Alzheimer studied 5 brains of dementia praecox patients and concluded that the illness affected primarily the cerebral cortex. Kraepelin incorporated these new findings into his system of psychiatric diseases and redefined dementia praecox as a disorder of the prefrontal cortex (Kraepelin 1913).

The strong link between schizophrenia and the prefrontal cortex continues to dominate the field of schizophrenia research (Goldman-Rakic 1999; Lewis and Lieberman 2000). It was only in the early 1970s that the limbic system hypothesis of schizophrenia was proposed (Stevens 1973; Torrey and Peterson 1974). The term "limbic system" refers to a set of brain regions with prominent connections to the hypothalamus, including the septum, cingulate gyrus, amygdala, and hippocampus (Gloor 1997). James Papez (Papez 1937) and Paul McLean (MacLean 1952) had proposed that the limbic system is the neural circuitry governing emotions. The limbic system appeared to be a reasonable candidate to explain the positive symptoms (i.e., hallucinations and delusions) and the marked abnormalities of affect seen in schizophrenia. Therefore, the first report of smaller hippocampal volume in schizophrenia (Bogerts et al. 1985) was seen as a confirmation of the limbic system hypothesis of schizophrenia (Bogerts 1997; Csernansky and Bardgett 1998). A substantial body of literature now supports the notion that the structure and function of the hippocampus are abnormal in schizophrenia (Dwork 1997; Harrison and Eastwood 2001; Heckers 2001; Heckers and Konradi 2002; Weinberger 1999). The majority of studies have provided further evidence for the original finding of a smaller hippocampus in schizophrenia. Here I will review some of this evidence with a focus on the time course of hippocampal volume change, the underlying mechanisms, and the functional implications.

▪ When does hippocampal volume change in schizophrenia?

The hippocampus is located in the ventromedial temporal lobe, next to the amygdala and the parahippocampal gyrus (Van Hoesen 1997). The hippocampus is small, occupying only 3–4 cm^3 in each hemisphere (i.e., less than 1% of the total brain volume). The first study of hippocampal volume in schizophrenia reported a 31% reduction in patients with schizophrenia (Bogerts et al. 1985). Recent meta-analyses (Nelson et al. 1998; Wright et al. 2000) and reviews (Heckers 2001; McCarley et al. 1999) have concluded that smaller hippocampal volume is one of the most replicated brain abnormalities in schizophrenia. However, hippocampal volume change is much more subtle than originally reported (i.e., typically in range of 5–10% decrease compared to control samples) and is not diagnostic for schizophrenia.

Several conditions associated with smaller hippocampal volume (e.g., temporal lobe epilepsy, amnesia, and dementia) are linked to a traumatic brain injury or a progressive loss of hippocampal neurons, but that is not the case for schizophrenia. How can we then explain the subtle hippocampal volume decrease in schizophrenia?

Neuroimaging studies have provided some interesting clues. Whereas the initial neuroimaging studies confirmed the postmortem finding of smaller hippocampal volume in chronic patients with schizophrenia, more recent studies have now established this finding also in schizophrenic patients at the time of their first hospitalization or their first presentation with psychotic symptoms (Barr et al. 1997; Bogerts et al. 1990; DeLisi et al. 1991; Hirayasu et al. 1998; Hoff et al. 1992; Lawrie et al. 2001; Niemann et al. 2000; Ohnuma et al. 1997; Phillips et al. 2002; Razi et al. 1999; Sumich et al. 2002; Velakoulis et al. 1999; Wood et al. 2001). This finding makes it unlikely that smaller hippocampal volume in schizophrenia is due to chronic effects of suffering from a psychiatric illness or being treated with psychotropic medication. This notion has gained even further support by the finding of smaller hippocampal volume in subjects who are at risk to develop schizophrenia. For example, Pantelis et al. studied 75 subjects who were genetically at risk to develop schizophrenia (Pantelis et al. 2003). Twenty-three of the study subjects developed a psychotic illness (including schizophrenia, schizoaffective disorder, bipolar disorder, and major depression with psychotic features) within the course of one year after structural brain images were acquired. When the brain images of those at-risk subjects who did and those who did not develop a psychotic illness were compared, the right hippocampus was found to be smaller in the psychotic subjects. Furthermore, cortico-limbic regions such as the cingulate gyrus and parahippocampal gyrus continued to show further progression of volume change, but not the hippocampus. These and other data (Lawrie et al. 1999) provide compelling evidence that hippocampal pathology is present before the onset of clinical symptoms. These data also raise the important question whether hippocampal volume change is more closely linked to psychosis, rather than schizophrenia, since more than half of the at-risk subjects developed a psychotic illness other than schizophrenia (Pantelis et al. 2003).

The hypothesis that hippocampal volume reduction in schizophrenia indicates the presence of risk genes (Tsuang 2000; Weinberger 1999) is substantially strengthened by the finding that hippocampal volumes of first-degree relatives of schizophrenic probands are larger than those of schizophrenic patients but significantly smaller compared with a healthy control sample (Seidman et al. 2002). If smaller hippocampal volume confers a risk to develop schizophrenia, it is crucial to understand the additional factor that makes the genetic risk clinically apparent. In addition, smaller hippocampal volume could confer a more general risk for the development of psychiatric illnesses, with different additional factors leading to distinct psychopathologies (e.g., schizophrenia, bipolar disorder, PTSD) (Gilbertson et al. 2002; Sapolsky 2002). The combination of genetic and neuroimaging techniques in the study of complex gene-gene and gene-environment interactions holds the promise to uncover the genetic risk factors and their interactions with non-genetic stressors.

▌ Are regions of the hippocampus differentially affected?

The neuroimaging studies that report, on average, a 6% smaller hippocampal volume in schizophrenia have provided widely disparate estimates of normal hippocampal volume. In fact, the estimates range between 0.4 cm^3 (Pearlson et al. 1997) and 6.39 cm^3 (Bryant et al. 1999). It appears that the seemingly trivial task of estimating hippocampal volume from serial sections could benefit from more attention to the anatomical details of this complex brain structure. More importantly, the acquisition of high-resolution images and subsequent analysis using standardized, anatomically informed protocols (Pruessner et al. 2000) allows us to test the hypothesis that not all but specific regions of the hippocampus are affected in schizophrenia.

The human hippocampus is an elongated structure along the inferior horn of the lateral ventricle. On coronal sections through the body of the hippocampus it is easy to appreciate the classic seahorse-shaped configuration of the hippocampus and adjacent parahippocampal gyrus (Duvernoy 1998; Gloor 1997) (Fig. 1). Stained postmortem specimens reveal a three-layered organization of this primitive cortical structure: Most neuronal cell bodies are localized in the densely packed pyramidal cell layer, whereas the rich dendritic arborization as well as the intrinsic and extrinsic fiber pathways are located in the two cell-poor layers, the stratum oriens and the stratum radiatum/lacunosum/moleculare (Gloor 1997). This three-layered cortex can be subdivided into the dentate gyrus (DG), the cornu Ammonis sectors CA1–4, and the subiculum.

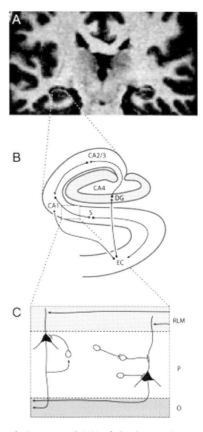

Fig. 1. Anatomy of the human hippocampus. **A** High resolution coronal MRI of the human hippocampus. **B** Schematic diagram of the regions of the human hippocampal formation and their major connections. The entorhinal cortex (EC) sends direct projections and indirect projections via the dentate gyrus (DG) and cornu Ammonis sector CA2/3 to CA1, from which output is relayed via the subiculum (S) back to EC. **C** The laminar organization of the human hippocampus. Input arrives at dendrites of pyramidal cells in the stratum radiatum/lacunosum/moleculare (RLM), output leaves via fibers in the stratum oriens (O). The two neuronal types in the pyramidal cell layer are the pyramidal shaped principal cells and the nonpyramidal shaped interneuron

The hippocampus is closely connected with the neighboring parahippocampal gyrus, especially its anterior region, the entorhinal cortex. Highly processed and integrated multimodal sensory information arrives in the entorhinal cortex and is then relayed into the hippocampus (Van Hoesen 1982). It is generally believed that the intricate architecture of this entorhinal-hippocampal system provides the anatomical basis for the encoding of information into and retrieval from long-term memory (Amaral and Insausti 1990; Eichenbaum and Cohen 2001; Witter et al. 2000). Two major inputs arise from layer 2 of the entorhinal cortex and reach sector CA1 (direct pathway) and the DG (indirect pathway). The input into DG is relayed via the mossy fiber pathway to

CA2/3 and via Schaffer collaterals to CA1. Output from CA1 reaches the subiculum and the entorhinal cortex. Multimodal sensory information, converging on the entorhinal cortex, is processed via the direct and indirect pathway, which enables the hippocampus to compare previously stored information with novel sensory data (Witter et al. 2000). This appears to be the essential operation of the hippocampus: to detect novelty through a mismatch of stored and current input, to associate various sensory features of the same object, and to recognize a match between current and previously stored input.

How does the subtle hippocampal volume reduction seen in schizophrenia affect this intricate network underlying memory formation? Deficits in each node of the hippocampal circuitry may produce quite different patterns of neural dysfunction. A recent study (Wang et al. 2001) reported a selective reduction of hippocampal volume in the subiculum, but this inference was not based on an identification of hippocampal subdivisions but rather on mapping the hippocampal volume maps onto the expected map of the normal human hippocampus. It is now possible to visualize hippocampal sectors in vivo (Zeineh et al. 2002) and it will be exciting to see this improved technology being used in the study of schizophrenia.

In addition to the hippocampal architecture seen in coronal sections, several authors have proposed a further distinction of hippocampal anatomy and function along an anterior-posterior axis. This began when retrograde tracer injections in regions of the prefrontal cortex were followed along the anterior-posterior extent of the hippocampus in the nonhuman primate (Barbas and Blatt 1995; Goldman-Rakic et al. 1984). The implication of such an anterior-posterior gradient of prefrontal-hippocampal projections did not become fully appreciated until structural and functional neuroimaging studies provided evidence for regionally specific functions of the hippocampus. The most relevant debate in this context is the HIPER (*Hip*pocampal *E*ncoding/*R*etrieval) model by Lepage and colleagues (Lepage et al. 1998) and the rebuttal of this model by Schacter and Wagner (Schacter and Wagner 1999). Although the details of this model, which proposes an anterior-posterior gradient of hippocampal activation during the performance of memory tasks, have to be tested more thoroughly, it is generally accepted that one function of the human hippocampus, memory retrieval, is linked to posterior but not anterior aspects of the hippocampus (Schacter and Wagner 1999). This is of interest, since the lateral aspects of the prefrontal cortex are connected primarily with the posterior parahippocampal/hippocampus complex, whereas medial aspects of the prefrontal project are connected primarily with the anterior hippocampus (Barbas and Blatt 1995; Goldman-Rakic et al. 1984). Taken together, there is now emerging evidence that anterior-posterior segments of the human hippocampus might be part of distinct neural circuits, subserving different functions.

Several studies have provided volume estimates for anterior and posterior segments of the hippocampus in schizophrenia (Becker et al. 1996; Bogerts et al. 1990, 1993; Hirayasu et al. 1998; Hoff et al. 1992; Kasai et al. 2003; McCarley et al. 1993; Narr et al. 2001; Rajarethinam et al. 2001; Razi et al. 1999; Rossi et al. 1994; Shenton et al. 1992; Staal et al. 2000; Whitworth et al. 1998; Yeo et al. 1997). So far, the results are equivocal and more work needs to be done.

However, in contrast to the parcellation of the hippocampus in coronal sections, the anterior-posterior axis of the hippocampus does not provide readily identifiable criteria for a cytoarchitectural map. The most reliable landmark is the uncus, which is formed by two sheets of hippocampal tissue in the anterior part of the hippocampus (Duvernoy 1998) and which occupies more than 50% of the total hippocampal volume. It is of interest to know that the shape and volume of the uncus are much more variable than the posterior part of the human hippocampus (Gertz et al. 1972). This could indicate that the anterior aspects of the human hippocampus are more responsive to evolutionary pressure, resulting in unique functional implications of the normal hippocampus and greater vulnerability for the development of neuropsychiatric deficits.

Although smaller hippocampal volume is now established as a reliable brain abnormality in schizophrenia, it is not found in all patients. In fact, hippocampal volume of most schizophrenic patients is well within the normal range and accurate classification into schizophrenia and/or control groups purely based on hippocampal volume estimates is poor. It appears that adding additional information about hippocampal shape improves the classification into schizophrenia/control groups (Csernansky et al. 1998, 2002; Shenton et al. 2002; Wang et al. 2001). It remains to be seen, whether adding information about hippocampal function would increase the diagnostic yield even further.

Ultimately it will be important to study the detailed anatomical architecture of the hippocampus at the level of functionally defined subregions and individual cell populations. For some of these questions we need the superior resolution of postmortem preparations of the human hippocampus.

▌ What is the mechanism of smaller hippocampal volume in schizophrenia?

Most pathological conditions that lead to hippocampal volume reduction are associated with a decreased number of hippocampal neurons, often in conjunction with an increased number of glial cells (Graham 2002). It is intriguing that this is not the case in schizophrenia: Hippocampal volume is reduced, but overall hippocampal neuron number is normal (Heckers et al. 1991b; Walker et al. 2002). How can we explain subtle volume differences in the context of overall normal neuron number?

One possible scenario is the selective reduction of neuronal subpopulations, which could remain undetected if the number of all neurons is studied. This resembles current theories of pathology in the dorsolateral prefrontal cortex and anterior cingulate cortex, where the overall density of neurons is not significantly decreased (Heckers 1997) (and maybe even increased (Selemon and Goldman-Rakic 1999), but where subpopulations of interneurons appear to be decreased. For example, chandelier interneurons, located in layer 3 and inhibiting the axon initial segment of pyramidal cells, appear to be selectively decreased in schizophrenia (Lewis and Lieberman 2000; Lewis et al. 1999). Similarly, the density of interneurons but not pyramidal cells is decreased in the anterior cingulate cortex in schizophrenia (Benes 1998).

Several recent studies have provided preliminary evidence that subpopulations of interneurons are also affected in the hippocampus in schizophrenia. Approximately 10–20% of all neurons in the human hippocampus can be classified as nonpyramidal cells (Jones and Yakel 1999). Benes et al. provided the initial evidence for neuron-specific changes in the hippocampus in schizophrenia by showing that nonpyramidal cell density is decreased but that pyramidal cell density remains unaltered (Benes et al. 1998). The class of nonpyramidal cells that uses GABA as their major neurotransmitter has been designated *hippocampal interneuron* (Freund and Buzsaki 1996; Parra et al. 1998). Subpopulations of hippocampal interneurons can be defined by their protein expression. For example, the calcium-binding proteins parvalbumin (PV), calbindin (CB), and calretinin (CR) are expressed in largely nonoverlapping subsets of hippocampal interneurons. All three types of interneurons express the hallmark enzyme glutamic acid decarboxylase (GAD) and all establish short-ranging connections to neighboring cells, but each has distinct functional characteristics and they are affected differentially in neurological and psychiatric disorders (Brady and Mufson 1997; DeFelipe et al. 1993). For example, patients with temporal lobe epilepsy show selective deficits of chandelier cells, resulting in decreased inhibition at the axon initial segment and serious consequences for the inhibitory control of the pyramidal cell (DeFelipe 1999). Several studies have now also provided evidence for specific changes in the expression of calcium-binding proteins in SZ (Reynolds et al. 2001). For example, Zhang et al. reported that the density of parvalbumin-positive but not calbindin-positive interneurons is decreased in the hippocampus in schizophrenia (Zhang and Reynolds 2002). This is in line with a recent GAD in situ hybridization study that estimated the density of all interneurons in the hippocampus in schizophrenia and bipolar disorder (Heckers et al. 2002). In contrast to bipolar disorder, which was characterized by a significant decrease of GAD mRNA-positive neurons in the hippocampus, the schizophrenic subjects showed more subtle decreases. This is compatible with the notion that only some but not all hippocampal interneurons are affected in schizophrenia.

Studies of the hippocampus in schizophrenia have investigated only hippocampal neurons with cell bodies in the pyramidal cell layer. Since the vast majority of neurons in the human hippocampus are located in the pyramidal cell layer, this appears to be a reasonable first step. However, it is well known that the various subpopulations of interneurons are also populating the two cell-poor layers, the stratum oriens (SO) and the stratum radiatum/lacunosum/moleculare (SRLM) (Freund and Buzsaki 1996). It would be of great interest to study these neurons since they have considerable influence on the function of the pyramidal cells.

Furthermore, selective changes of neurons in SO and SRLM could elucidate a surprising finding of hippocampal pathology in schizophrenia. Two stereological studies of hippocampal volume and cell number (Heckers et al. 1991 a; Walker et al. 2002) have reported that the volume of the pyramidal cell layer is normal in schizophrenia, but that the overall volume of the hippocampus (encompassing all three layers) is decreased in schizophrenia. This is similar to the finding by Colter et al. who reported decreased white matter in the parahippocampal gyrus in schizophrenia (Colter et al. 1987). Another possible mechanism for a selective decrease of SO and SRLM volume in schizophrenia is abnormal hippocampal connectivity. The major intrinsic fiber pathways (mossy fibers, Schaffer collaterals) as well as the major afferent connection (perforant pathway) run within the SO and SRLM. These pathways myelinate much later than most other white matter tracts in the human brain, typically at the end of the second decade of life (Benes et al. 1994). Could abnormalities of hippocampal connectivity lead to the volume change seen in MRI studies? If so, do they have functional implications? Functional neuroimaging techniques are needed to study the functional implications of abnormal hippocampal structure in schizophrenia.

▌ What are the functional implications of a smaller hippocampus in schizophrenia?

The human hippocampus is crucial for the encoding of sensory data into long-term memory and the subsequent retrieval of previously stored information. The domains of memory most affected by damage to the hippocampus are the two forms of declarative memory, i.e., the memory for facts (semantic memory) and events (episodic memory). It is therefore not surprising that many patients with significant hippocampal volume reduction, as seen, e.g., in temporal lobe epilepsy and dementia, present with deficits of declarative memory. Is the subtle hippocampal volume loss in schizophrenia also associated with abnormal cognitive function (Weiss and Heckers 2001)?

Initial studies have addressed this question by correlating hippocampal volume with performance scores on neuropsychological tests (Bilder et al. 1995; Colombo et al. 1993; Szeszko et al. 2002; Weinberger et al. 1992). It is surprising that the evidence points to an association of hippocampal volume decrease with cognitive deficits outside of the domain of declarative memory. For example, Weinberger et al. reported an association of anterior hippocampal volume decrease with impaired frontal lobe function (Weinberger et al. 1992), whereas Szeszko et al. reported that decreased anterior hippocampal volume in schizophrenia was associated with impaired function on executive and motor tasks (Szeszko et al. 2002). A recent study of hippocampal volume and memory function in first-degree relatives of schizophrenic probands has now provided evidence that smaller hippocampal volume, especially in the left hemisphere, is associated with deficits of declarative memory in first-degree relatives (Seidman et al. 2002). It would be of great interest to know if similar relationships exist in schizophrenic patients.

To demonstrate convincingly that hippocampal function is impaired in schizophrenia we would need to have some indication of abnormal activity of hippocampal neurons. Earlier neuroimaging studies have reported abnormalities of hippocampal glucose metabolism and blood flow as indices of pathological hippocampal activity in schizophrenia (Buchsbaum et al. 1992; Gur et al. 1995; Nordahl et al. 1996; Tamminga et al. 1992). Of interest, some of these studies of schizophrenic patients have documented an increase of medial temporal lobe regional cerebral blood flow (Friston et al. 1992; Kawasaki et al. 1992, 1996; Liddle et al. 1992). When resting blood flow values were correlated with clinical symptoms, increased left medial temporal lobe blood flow in schizophrenia was associated with more severe psychopathology in general (Friston et al. 1992; Liddle et al. 1992) or with more prominent positive symptoms (delusions and hallucinations) (Liddle et al. 1992). These studies have been interpreted as evidence that hippocampal hyperactivity (or the lack of inhibition) is involved in the pathogenesis of delusions and hallucinations.

This hypothesis was confirmed and extended by more recent neuroimaging studies which measured regional cerebral blood flow in schizophrenic patients during the experience of auditory hallucinations (Weiss and Heckers 1999). The still limited number of studies has demonstrated activation of a network of brain regions involved in the processing of auditory information and language, and two studies have revealed increased activation of the hippocampal formation. Specifically, the studies by Silbersweig et al. (1995) and Dierks et al. (1999) have documented activation of the hippocampal formation during the experience of auditory hallucinations. It is unclear whether the hippocampal activation seen in these studies occurs early in the generation of the hallucinatory experience or whether it is involved in the top-down processing of representations generated in the primary and secondary auditory cortices, e.g., to monitor the source of an auditory representation.

▌ Impaired memory function of the hippocampus in schizophrenia

Functional neuroimaging now allows the detailed study of brain activation during task performance. This makes it possible to test directly the hypothesis that hippocampal function is impaired in schizophrenia, e.g., while learning or remembering test items. The first evidence for abnormal hippocampal recruitment during a memory task in schizophrenia came from a study of word-stem cued recall (Heckers et al. 1998). While normal subjects activated a right frontal-temporal network to retrieve previously studied words, schizophrenic patients failed to recruit the hippocampus. Instead, the schizophrenic patients showed robust and significantly increased activation of prefrontal cortex regions. Furthermore, schizophrenic patients with and without the deficit syndrome lacked the normal hippocampal recruitment but differed in prefrontal cortex activation during memory retrieval (Heckers et al. 1999). Compared to the control group, hippocampal activity was continuously increased in schizophrenia and was not modulated by environmental contingencies (Fig. 2). Increased hippocampal activity at baseline and impaired recruitment during episodic memory retrieval might represent the functional correlate of an abnormal cortico-hippocampal interaction in schizophrenia (Fletcher 1998). A recent study of tone recognition in schizophrenia has confirmed increased regional cerebral blood flow values in the hippocampus (Medoff et al. 2001). Furthermore, the increased hippocampal rCBF was more pronounced in patients off antipsychotic medication, which confirms previous evidence that

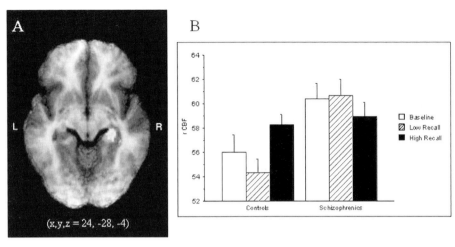

Fig. 2. Impaired hippocampal recruitment during memory retrieval in schizophrenia. **A** PET statistical map comparing blood flow between control subjects and schizophrenic patients during memory retrieval. The right hippocampal region (at coordinates 24, −28, and −4) was significantly less activated in the schizophrenia group. **B** Means (together with standard error bars) of relative rCBF during baseline, low recall, and high recall conditions in the right hippocampus

antipsychotic drugs normalize hippocampal dysfunction in schizophrenia (Todtenkopf and Benes 1998).

We have recently confirmed and extended our finding of decreased hippocampal recruitment during word-stem cued recall in schizophrenia (Weiss et al. 2003 b). Subjects counted either the number of meanings or T-junctions of words seen only once or repeated four times. This created four different levels of processing, ranging from shallow (T-junction, one time) to deep (meaning, 4 time). Subsequently, O^{15}-PET scans were acquired while subjects completed word-stems with previously studied items. Control subjects recalled more words overall, but both groups demonstrated similar performance benefits following deeper encoding. Both item repetition and the use of a semantic encoding task were associated with memory retrieval-related hippocampal recruitment in control, but not schizophrenic participants. Like in our original study, patients with schizophrenia again demonstrated greater activation of prefrontal cortex during word retrieval. This study provides evidence that, despite a lack of hippocampal recruitment, patients with schizophrenia show intact modulation of memory performance following deep and shallow encoding. Impaired hippocampal recruitment, in concert with greater prefrontal activation, may reflect a specific deficit in conscious recollection in schizophrenia.

Previous neuropsychological studies have reported that schizophrenic patients are impaired during retrieval tasks when the targets are not shown (i.e., free recall), but are less or not impaired when forced to make an Old/New decision in response to targets and lures. We have recently completed a functional magnetic resonance imaging (fMRI) study which revealed that schizophrenic patients show normal hippocampal activation patterns during forced choice recognition of previously seen words (Weiss et al. 2003 a). Of interest, the schizophrenic patients showed this normal pattern of hippocampal recruitment despite a significantly smaller hippocampal volume. This provides evidence that not all hippocampal functions are impaired and that smaller hippocampal volume is not necessarily associated with impaired hippocampal function in schizophrenia.

In addition to the evidence of impaired hippocampal function during cued recall, there is now also evidence of impaired hippocampal recruitment during memory encoding in schizophrenia. Eyler-Zorilla et al. compared brain activation between healthy and schizophrenic subjects during the viewing of novel or repeated pictures (Eyler Zorilla et al. 2002). Only the control subjects demonstrated hippocampal activation in response to novel pictures, whereas schizophrenic subjects showed a decrease of hippocampal activity, despite similar reaction time and accuracy during the experiment and normal recognition of the study objects after scanning. This study provides evidence for abnormal hippocampal responses during the detection of novelty in schizophrenia.

In summary, functional neuroimaging studies of the hippocampus in schizophrenia have linked increased activity to the expression of positive symptoms (delusions and hallucinations) and revealed decreased hippocampal recruitment during novelty detection and cued word recall, but not during forced choice recognition of previously studied words. This evidence of abnormal hippocampal function in schizophrenia needs to be replicated and extended. It is especially important to combine morphometric and functional approaches and to characterize the relationship of functional abnormalities of the hippocampus and clinical features.

▌ How can hippocampal pathology explain the features of schizophrenia?

Deficits of declarative memory are one of the most robust cognitive deficits in schizophrenia (Aleman et al. 1999; Heinrichs 2001). The recent neuroimaging studies reviewed above support the notion that hippocampal dysfunction contributes to some of these memory deficits seen in patients with schizophrenia. In addition, there is intriguing evidence that one form of memory associated with the hippocampus, i.e., episodic memory, is selectively impaired in schizophrenia (Danion et al. 1999; Huron et al. 1995; Tendolkar et al. 2002). Episodic memory is closely linked to self representation (autonoetic awareness) and makes it possible for us to "travel back in time" to recollect details of the original event (Tulving and Markowitsch 1998; Wheeler 2000). A selective impairment of episodic memory in schizophrenia could explain the disconnection of self and object representation seen in schizophrenia (Churchland 2002).

Several models of abnormal cortical-hippocampal function have been advanced to explain abnormal mental representations in schizophrenia. Roberts (1963) suggested in his paper "Schizophrenia and the brain" that a functional disturbance of the hippocampus could potentially explain "the production of psychosis" (Roberts 1963). Venables and Hemsley introduced a hippocampal model of impaired information processing in schizophrenia to explain their findings of abnormal auditory sensory gating and the inability to ignore irrelevant stimuli in schizophrenic patients (Hemsley 1993; Venables 1992). Neural network models of hippocampal function have expanded on such concepts and have provided evidence that abnormal hippocampal-cortical interactions can give rise to psychotic features and cognitive deficits in schizophrenia (Chen 1995; Meeter et al. 2002; Schmajuk 2001). I have previously suggested that delusions and hallucinations originate from an abnormal interaction between the hippocampal formation and the association cortex (Heckers 2001).

▪ Conclusion

The hippocampus is a recent addition to the list of candidates for the neural basis of schizophrenia. This is, at least in part, due to the fact that, for a long time, the hippocampus had been viewed merely as an extension of the olfactory system. The formulation of the limbic system as the neural circuit underlying affect regulation and the discovery of the critical role of the medial temporal lobe for long-term memory has put the hippocampus in the center of current neuroscience. After just 18 years of study, there is now compelling evidence that hippocampal structure is abnormal in schizophrenia. Further, we have emerging evidence that hippocampal function is abnormal and might be relevant for the explanation of memory deficits in schizophrenia. However, the etiology and pathogenesis of hippocampal abnormalities in schizophrenia remain unknown. Further studies are needed to explore the details of hippocampal pathology in schizophrenia.

▪ References

Aleman A, Hijman R, de Haan EHF, Kahn RS (1999) Memory impairment in schizophrenia: a meta-analysis. Am J Psychiatry 156:1358–1366

Alzheimer A (1897) Beiträge zur pathologischen Anatomie der Hirnrinde und zur anatomischen Grundlage einiger Psychosen. Monatsschrift für Psychiatrie und Neurologie 2:82–120

Amaral DG, Insausti R (1990) Hippocampal formation. In: Paxinos G (ed) The Human Nervous System. Academic Press, San Diego, CA

Barbas H, Blatt GJ (1995) Topographically specific hippocampal projections target functionally distinct prefrontal areas in the rhesus monkey. Hippocampus 5:511–533

Barr WB, Ashtari M, Bilder RM, Degreef G, Lieberman JA (1997) Brain morphometric comparison of first-episode schizophrenia and temporal lobe epilepsy. Br J Psychiatry 170:515–519

Becker T, Elmer K, Schneider F, Schneider M, Grodd W, Bartels M, Heckers S, Beckmann H (1996) Confirmation of reduced temporal limbic structure volume on magnetic resonance imaging in male patients with schizophrenia. Psychiatry Res 67:135–143

Benes FM (1998) Model generation and testing to probe neural circuitry in the cingulate cortex of postmortem schizophrenic brain. Schizophr Bull 24:219–230

Benes FM, Kwok EW, Vincent SL, Todtenkopf MS (1998) A reduction of nonpyramidal cells in sector CA2 of schizophrenics and manic depressives. Biol Psychiatry 44:88–97

Benes FM, Turtle M, Khan Y, Farol P (1994) Myelination of a key relay zone in the hippocampal formation occurs in the human brain during childhood, adolescence, and adulthood. Arch Gen Psychiatry 51:477–484

Bilder RM, Bogerts B, Ashtari M, Wu H, Alvir JM, Jody D, Reiter G, Bell L, Lieberman JA (1995) Anterior hippocampal volume reductions predict frontal lobe dysfunction in first episode schizophrenia. Schizophr Res 17:47–58

Bogerts B (1997) The temporolimbic system theory of positive schizophrenic symptoms. Schizophrenia Bull 23:423–435

Bogerts B, Ashtari M, Degreef G, Alvir JM, Bilder RM, Lieberman JA (1990) Reduced temporal limbic structure volumes on magnetic resonance images in first episode schizophrenia. Psychiatry Res 35:1–13

Bogerts B, Lieberman JA, Ashtari M, Bilder RM, Degreef G, Lerner G, Johns C, Masiar S (1993) Hippocampus-amygdala volumes and psychopathology in chronic schizophrenia. Biol Psychiatry 33:236–246

Bogerts B, Meertz E, Schönfeldt-Bausch R (1985) Basal ganglia and limbic system pathology in schizophrenia. A morphometric study of brain volume and shrinkage. Arch Gen Psychiatry 42:784–791

Brady DR, Mufson EJ (1997) Parvalbumin-immunoreactive neurons in the hippocampal formation of Alzheimer's diseased brain. Neuroscience 80:1113–1125

Bryant NL, Buchanan RW, Vladar K, Breier A, Rothman M (1999) Gender differences in temporal lobe structures of patients with schizophrenia: a volumetric MRI study. Am J Psychiatry 156:603–609

Buchsbaum MS, Haier RJ, Potkin SG, Nuechterlein K, Bracha HS, Katz M, Lohr J, Wu J, Lottenberg S, Jerabek PA et al (1992) Frontostriatal disorder of cerebral metabolism in never-medicated schizophrenics. Arch Gen Psychiatry 49:935–942

Chen EY (1995) A neural network model of cortical information processing in schizophrenia. II – Role of hippocampal-cortical interaction: a review and a model. Can J Psychiatry 40:21–26

Colombo C, Abbruzzese M, Livian S, Scotti G, Locatelli M, Bonfanti A, Scarone S (1993) Memory functions and temporal-limbic morphology in schizophrenia. Psychiatry Res 50:45–56

Csernansky JG, Bardgett ME (1998) Limbic-cortical neuronal damage and the pathophysiology of schizophrenia. Schizophrenia Bull 24:231–248

Csernansky JG, Joshi S, Wang L, Haller JW, Gado M, Miller JP, Grenander U, Miller MI (1998) Hippocampal morphometry in schizophrenia by high dimensional brain mapping. Proc Natl Acad Sci USA 95:11406–11411

Csernansky JG, Wang L, Jones D, Rastogi-Cruz D, Posener JA, Heydebrand G, Miller JP, Miller MI (2002) Hippocampal deformities in schizophrenia characterized by high dimensional brain mapping. American Journal of Psychiatry 159:2000–2006

Danion JM, Rizzo L, Bruant A (1999) Functional mechanisms underlying impaired recognition memory and conscious awareness in patients with schizophrenia. Arch Gen Psychiatry 56:639–644

DeFelipe J (1999) Chandelier cells and epilepsy. Brain 122:1807–1822

DeFelipe J, Garcia Sola R, Marco P, del Rio MR, Pulido P, Ramon y Cajal S (1993) Selective changes in the microorganization of the human epileptogenic neocortex revealed by parvalbumin immunoreactivity. Cerebral Cortex 3:39–48

DeLisi LE, Hoff AL, Schwartz JE, Shields GW, Halthore SN, Gupta SM, Henn FA, Anand AK (1991) Brain morphology in first-episode schizophrenic-like psychotic patients: a quantitative magnetic resonance imaging study. Biol Psychiatry 29:159–175

Dierks T, Linden DE, Jandl M, Formisano E, Goebel R, Lanfermann H, Singer W (1999) Activation of Heschl's gyrus during auditory hallucinations. Neuron 22: 615–621

Duvernoy HM (1998) The Human Hippocampus. Springer, Berlin

Dwork AJ (1997) Postmortem studies of the hippocampal formation in schizophrenia. Schizophrenia Bull 23:403–421

Eichenbaum H, Cohen NJ (2001) From Conditioning to Conscious Recollection. Memory Systems of the Brain. Oxford University Press, Oxford

Eyler Zorilla LT, Jeste DV, Paulus M, Brown GG (2002) Functional abnormalities of medial temporal cortex during novel picture learning among patients with chronic schizophrenia. Schizophrenia Res 59:187–198

Fletcher P (1998) The missing link: a failure of fronto-hippocampal integration in schizophrenia. Nature Neuroscience 1:266–267

Freund TF, Buzsaki G (1996) Interneurons of the hippocampus. Hippocampus 6:347–470

Friston KJ, Liddle PF, Frith CD, Hirsch SR, Frackowiak RS (1992) The left medial temporal region and schizophrenia. A PET study. Brain 115:367–382

Gertz SD, Lindenberg R, Piavis GW (1972) Structural variations in the rostral human hippocampus. Hopkins Medical Journal 130:367–376

Gilbertson MW, Shenton ME, Ciszewski A, Kasai K, Lasko NB, Orr SP, Pitman RK (2002) Smaller hippocampal volume predicts pathological vulnerability to psychological trauma. Nature Neuroscience 5:1242–1247

Gloor P (1997) The Temporal Lobe and Limbic System. Oxford University Press, New York

Goldman-Rakic PS (1999) The physiological approach: functional architecture of working memory and disordered cognition in schizophrenia. Biol Psychiatry 46:650–661

Goldman-Rakic PS, Selemon LD, Schwartz ML (1984) Dual patthways connecting the dorsolateral prefrontal cortex with the hippocampal formation and parahippocampal cortex in the rhesus monkey. Neuroscience 12:719–743

Graham DI (ed) (2002) Greenfield's Neuropathology, 7th edn. Edward Arnold, London

Gur RE, Mozley PD, Resnick SM, Mozley LH, Shtasel DL, Gallacher F, Arnold SE, Karp JS, Alavi A, Reivich M, Gur RC (1995) Resting cerebral glucose metabolism in first-episode and previously treated patients with schizophrenia relates to clinical features. Arch Gen Psychiatry 52:657–667

Harrison PJ, Eastwood SL (2001) Neuropathological studies of synaptic connectivity in the hippocampal formation in schizophrenia. Hippocampus 11:508–519

Heckers S (1997) Neuropathology of schizophrenia: cortex, thalamus, basal ganglia, and neurotransmitter-specific projection systems. Schizophrenia Bull 23:403–421

Heckers S (2001) Neuroimaging studies of the hippocampus in schizophrenia. Hippocampus 11:520–528

Heckers S, Goff D, Schacter DL, Savage CR, Fischman AJ, Alpert NM, Rauch SL (1999) Functional imaging of memory retrieval in deficit vs nondeficit schizophrenia. Arch Gen Psychiatry 56:1117–1123

Heckers S, Heinsen H, Beckmann H (1991a) The hippocampus and schizophrenia. Biol Psychiatry 29:223S

Heckers S, Heinsen H, Geiger B, Beckmann H (1991 b) Hippocampal neuron number in schizophrenia. A stereological study. Arch Gen Psychiatry 48:1002–1008

Heckers S, Konradi C (2002) Hippocampal neurons in schizophrenia. Journal of Neural Transmission 109:891–905

Heckers S, Rauch SL, Goff D, Savage CR, Schacter DL, Fischman AJ, Alpert NM (1998) Impaired recruitment of the hippocampus during conscious recollection in schizophrenia. Nature Neuroscience 1:318–323

Heckers S, Stone D, Walsh J, Shick J, Koul P, Benes FM (2002) Differential hippocampal expression of glutamic acid decarboxylase 65 and 67 messenger RNA in bipolar disorder and schizophrenia. Arch Gen Psychiatry 59:521–529

Heinrichs RW (2001) In Search of Madness: Schizophrenia and Neuroscience. Oxford University Press, Oxford

Hemsley DR (1993) A simple (or simplistic?) cognitive model for schizophrenia. Behav Res Ther 31:633–645

Hirayasu Y, Shenton ME, Salisbury DF, Dickey CC, Fischer IA, Mazzoni P, Kisler T, Arakaki H, Kwon JS, Anderson JE et al (1998) Lower left temporal lobe MRI volumes in patients with first-episode schizophrenia compared with psychotic patients with first-episode affective disorder and normal subjects. Am J Psychiatry 155:1384–1391

Hoff AL, Riordan H, O'Donnell D, Stritzke P, Neale C, Boccio A, Anand AK, DeLisi LE (1992) Anomalous lateral sulcus asymmetry and cognitive function in first-episode schizophrenia. Schizophrenia Bull 18:257–272

Huron C, Danion JM, Giacomoni F, Grange D, Robert P, Rizzo L (1995) Impairment of recognition memory with, but not without, conscious recollection in schizophrenia. Am J Psychiatry 152:1737–1742

Jones S, Yakel JL (1999) Inhibitory interneurons in hippocampus. Cell Biochemistry & Biophysics 31:207–218

Kasai K, Shenton ME, Salisbury DF, Hirayasu Y, Lee C-U, Ciszewski AA, Yurgelun-Todd D, Kikinis R, Jolesz FA, McCarley RW (2003) Progressive decrease of left superior temporal gyrus gray matter volume in patients with first-episode schizophrenia. Am J Psychiatry 160:156–164

Kawasaki Y, Maeda Y, Sakai N, Higashima M, Yamaguchi N, Koshino Y, Hisada K, Suzuki M, Matsuda H (1996) Regional cerebral blood flow in patients with schizophrenia: relevance to symptom structures. Psychiatry Res 67:49–58

Kawasaki Y, Suzuki M, Maeda Y, Urata K, Yamaguchi N, Matsuda H, Hisada K, Suzuki M, Takashima T (1992) Regional cerebral blood flow in patients with schizophrenia. A preliminary report. Eur Arch Psychiatry Clin Neurosci 241:195–200

Kraepelin E (1896) Psychiatrie. Ein Lehrbuch für Studirende und Aerzte. Fünfte, vollständig umgearbeitete Auflage. Johann Ambrosius Barth, Leipzig

Kraepelin E (1913) Psychiatrie. Ein Lehrbuch für Studierende und Ärzte. Achte, vollständig umgearbeitete Auflage. 3. Band. Klinische Psychiatrie, 2. Teil

Lawrie SM, Whalley H, Kestelman JN, Abukmeil SS, Byrne M, Hodges A, Rimmington JE, Best JJK, Owens DGC, Johnstone EC (1999) Magnetic resonance imaging of brain in people at high risk of developing schizophrenia. Lancet 353:30–33

Lawrie SM, Whalley HC, Abukmeil SS, Kestelman JN, Donnelly L, Miller P, Best JJ, Owens DG, Johnstone EC (2001) Brain structure, genetic liability, and psychotic symptoms in subjects at high risk of developing schizophrenia. Biological Psychiatry 49:811–823

Lepage M, Habib R, Tulving E (1998) Hippocampal PET activations of memory encoding and retrieval: the HIPER model. Hippocampus 8:313–322

Lewis DA, Lieberman JA (2000) Catching up on schizophrenia: natural history and neurobiology. Neuron 28:325–334

Lewis DA, Pierri JN, Volk DW, Melchitzky DS, Woo TU (1999) Altered GABA neurotransmission and prefrontal cortical dysfunction in schizophrenia. Biol Psychiatry 46:616–626

Liddle PF, Friston KJ, Frith CD, Jones T, Hirsch SR, Frackowiak RSJ (1992) Patterns of cerebral blood flow in schizophrenia. Br J Psychiatry 160:179–186

MacLean PD (1952) Some psychiatric implications of physiological studies of fronto-temporal portion of limbic system (visceral brain). Electroencephalogr Clin Neurophysiol 4:407–418

McCarley RW, Shenton ME, O'Donnell BF, Faux SF, Kikinis R, Nestor PG, Jolesz FA (1993) Auditory P300 abnormalities and left posterior superior temporal gyrus volume reduction in schizophrenia. Arch Gen Psychiatry 50:190–197

McCarley RW, Wible CG, Frumin M, Hirayasu Y, Levitt JJ, Fischer IA, Shenton ME (1999) MRI anatomy of schizophrenia. Biol Psychiatry 45:1099–1119

Medoff DR, Holcomb HH, Lahti AC, Tamminga CA (2001) Probing the human hippocampus using rCBF: Contrasts in schizophrenia. Hippocampus 11:543–550

Meeter M, Talamini LM, Murre JMJ (2002) A computational approach to memory deficits in schizophrenia. Neurocomputing 44:929–936

Narr KL, Thompson PM, Sharma T, Moussai J, Blanton R, Anvar B, Edris A, Krupp R, Rayman J, Khaledy M, Toga AW (2001) Three-dimensional mapping of temporo-limbic regions and the lateral ventricles in schizophrenia: gender effects. Biological Psychiatry 50:84–97

Nelson MD, Saykin AJ, Flashman LA, Riordan HJ (1998) Hippocampal volume reduction in schizophrenia as assessed by magnetic resonance imaging: a meta-analytic study. Arch Gen Psychiatry 55:433–440

Niemann K, Hammers A, Coenen VA, Thron A, Klosterkotter J (2000) Evidence of a smaller left hippocampus and left temporal horn in both patients with first episode schizophrenia and normal control subjects. Psychiatry Research 99:93–110

Nordahl TE, Kusubov N, Carter C, Salamat S, Cummings AM, O'Shora-Celaya L, Eberling J, Robertson L, Huesman RH, Jagust W, Budinger TF (1996) Temporal lobe metabolic differences in medication-free outpatients with schizophrenia via the PET-600. Neuropsychopharmacology 15:541–554

Ohnuma T, Kimura M, Takahashi T, Iwamoto N, Arai H (1997) A magnetic resonance imaging study in first-episode disorganized-type patients with schizophrenia. Psychiatry and Clinical Neurosciences 51:9–15

Pantelis C, Velakoulis D, McGorry PD, Wood SJ, Suckling J, Phillips LJ, Yung AR, Bullmore ET, Brewer W, Soulsby B et al (2003) Neuroanatomical abnormalities before and after onset of psychosis: a cross-sectional and longitudinal MRI comparison. Lancet 361:281–288

Papez JW (1937) A proposed mechanism of emotion. Archives of Neurology and Psychiatry 38:725–743

Parra P, Gulyas AI, Miles R (1998) How many subtypes of inhibitory cells in the hippocampus? Neuron 20:983–993

Pearlson GD, Barta PE, Powers RE, Menon RR, Richards SS, Aylward EH, Federman EB, Chase GA, Petty RG, Tien AY (1997) Medial and superior temporal gyral volumes and cerebral asymmetry in schizophrenia versus bipolar disorder. Biol Psychiatry 41:1–14

Phillips LJ, Velakoulis D, Pantelis C, Wood SJ, Yuen HP, Yung AR, Desmond P, Brewer W, McGorry PD (2002) Non-reduction in hippocampal volume is associated with higher risk of psychosis. Schizophrenia Res 58:145–158

Pruessner JC, Li LM, Serles W, Pruessner M, Collins DL, Kabani N, Lupien S, Evans AC (2000) Volumetry of hippocampus and amygdala with high-resolution MRI and three-dimensional analysis software: minimizing the discrepancies between laboratories. Cerebral Cortex 10:433–442

Rajarethinam R, DeQuardo JR, Miedler J, Arndt S, Kirbat R, Brunberg JA, Tandon R (2001) Hippocampus and amygdala in schizophrenia: assessment of the relationship of neuroanatomy to psychopathology. Psychiatry Research 108:79–87

Razi K, Greene KP, Sakuma M, Ge S, Kushner M, DeLisi LE (1999) Reduction of the parahippocampal gyrus and the hippocampus in patients with chronic schizophrenia. Br J Psychiatry 174:512–519

Reynolds GP, Zhang ZJ, Beasley CL (2001) Neurochemical correlates of cortical GABAergic deficits in schizophrenia: selective losses of calcium binding protein immunoreactivity. Brain Research Bulletin 55:579–584

Roberts DR (1963) Schizophrenia and the brain. Journal of Neuropsychiatry 5:71–79

Rossi A, Stratta P, Mancini F, Gallucci M, Mattei P, Core L, Di Michele V, Casacchia M (1994) Magnetic resonance imaging findings of amygdala-anterior hippocampus shrinkage in male patients with schizophrenia. Psychiatry Res 52:43–53

Sapolsky RM (2002) Chickens, eggs and hippocampal atrophy. Nature Neuroscience 5:1111–1113

Schacter DL, Wagner AD (1999) Medial temporal lobe activations in fMRI and PET studies of episodic encoding and retrieval. Hippocampus 9:7–24

Schmajuk NA (2001) Hippocampal dysfunction in schizophrenia. Hippocampus 11:599–613

Seidman LJ, Faraone SV, Goldstein JM, Kremen WS, Horton NJ, Makris N, Toomey R, Kennedy D, Caviness VS, Tsuang MT (2002) Left hippocampal volume as a vulnerability indicator for schizophrenia. Arch Gen Psychiatry 59:839–849

Selemon L, Goldman-Rakic P (1999) The reduced neuropil hypothesis: a circuit based model of schizophrenia. Biol Psychiatry 45:17–25

Shenton ME, Gerig G, McCarley RW, Szekely G, Kikinis R (2002) Amygdala-hippocampal shape differences in schizophrenia: the application of 3D shape models to volumetric MR data. Psychiatry Research Neuroimaging 115:15–35

Shenton ME, Kikinis R, Jolesz FA, Pollak SD, LeMay M, Wible CG, Hokama H, Martin J, Metcalf D, Coleman M et al (1992) Abnormalities of the left temporal lobe and thought disorder in schizophrenia. A quantitative magnetic resonance imaging study. N Engl J Med 327:604–612

Silbersweig DA, Stern E, Frith C, Cahill C, Holmes A, Grootoonk S, Seaward J, McKenna P, Chua SE, Schnorr L et al (1995) A functional neuroanatomy of hallucinations in schizophrenia. Nature 378:176–179

Staal WG, Hulshoff Pol HE, Schnack HG, Hoogendoorn ML, Jellema K, Kahn RS (2000) Structural brain abnormalities in patients with schizophrenia and their healthy siblings. Am J Psychiatry 157:416–421

Stevens JR (1973) An anatomy of schizophrenia? Arch Gen Psychiatry 29:177–189

Sumich A, Chitnis XA, Fannon DG, O'Ceallaigh S, Doku VC, Falrowicz A, Marshall N, Matthew VM, Potter M, Sharma T (2002) Temporal lobe abnormalities in first-episode psychosis. Am J Psychiatry 159:1232–1234

Szeszko PR, Strous RD, Goldman RS, Ashtari M, Knuth KH, Lieberman JA, Bilder RM (2002) Neuropsychological correlates of hippocampal volumes in patients experiencing a first episode of schizophrenia. Am J Psychiatry 159:217–226

Tamminga CA, Thaker GK, Buchanan R, Kirkpatrick B, Alphs LD, Chase TN, Carpenter WT (1992) Limbic system abnormalities identified in schizophrenia using positron emission tomography with fluorodeoxyglucose and neocortical alterations with deficit syndrome. Arch Gen Psychiatry 49:522–530

Tendolkar I, Ruhrmann S, Brockhaus A, Pukrop R, Klosterkötter J (2002) Remembering of knowing: electrophysiological evidence for an episodic memory deficit in schizophrenia. Psychological Medicine 32:1261–1271

Todtenkopf MS, Benes FM (1998) Distribution of glutamate decarboxylase 65 immunoreactive puncta on pyramidal and nonpyramidal neurons in hippocampus of schizophrenic brain. Synapse 29:323–332

Torrey EF, Peterson MR (1974) Schizophrenia and the limbic system. Lancet 2:942–946

Tsuang M (2000) Schizophrenia: genes and environment. Biol Psychiatry 47:210–220

Tulving E, Markowitsch HJ (1998) Episodic and declarative memory: role of the hippocampus. Hippocampus 8:198–204

Van Hoesen GW (1982) The parahippocampal gyrus: new observations regarding its cortical connections in the monkey. Trends Neurosci 5:345–350

Van Hoesen GW (1997) Ventromedial temporal lobe anatomy, with comments in Alzheimer's disease and temporal injury. J Neuropsychiatry Clin Neurosci 9:331–341

Velakoulis D, Pantelis C, McGorry PD, Dudgeon P, Brewer W, Cook M, Desmond P, Bridle N, Tierney P, Murrie V et al. (1999) Hippocampal volume in first-episode psychoses and chronic schizophrenia: a high-resolution magnetic resonance imaging study. Arch Gen Psychiatry 56:133–141

Venables PH (1992) Hippocampal function and schizophrenia. Experimental psychological evidence. Ann NY Acad Sci 658:111–127

Walker MA, Highley JR, Esiri MM, McDonald B, Roberts HC, Evans SP, Crow TJ (2002) Estimated neuronal populations and volumes of the hippocampus and its subfields in schizophrenia. Am J Psychiatry 159:821–828

Wang L, Joshi SC, Miller MI, Csernansky JG (2001) Statistical analysis of hippocampal asymmetry in schizophrenia. Neuroimage 14:531–545

Weinberger D, Berman K, Suddath R, Torrey E (1992) Evidence of dysfunction of a prefrontal-limbic network in schizophrenia: A magnetic resonance imaging and regional cerbral blood flow study of discordant monozygotic twins. Am J Psychiatry 149:890–897

Weinberger DR (1999) Cell biology of the hippocampal formation in schizophrenia. Biol Psychiatry 45:395–402

Weiss AP, Zalesak M, De Witt I, Goff D, Kunkel L, Heckers S (2004) Impaired hippocampal function during the detection of novel words in schizophrenia. Biological Psychiatry (in press)

Weiss AP, Heckers S (1999) Neuroimaging of hallucinations: a review of the literature. Psychiatry Research: Neuroimaging 92:61–74

Weiss AP, Heckers S (2001) Neuroimaging of declarative memory in schizophrenia. Scandinavian Journal of Psychology 42:239–250

Weiss AP, Schacter DL, Goff DC, Rauch SL, Alpert NM, Fischman AJ, Heckers S (2003b) Impaired hippocampal recruitment during normal modulation of memory performance in schizophrenia. Biol Psychiatry 53:48–55

Wheeler MA (2000) Episodic memory and autonoetic awareness. In: Tulving E, Craig FIM (eds) The Oxford handbook of memory. Oxford University Press, Oxford, pp 597–608

Whitworth AB, Honeder M, Kremser C, Kemmler G, Felber S, Hausmann A, Wanko C, Wechdorn H, Aichner F, Stuppaeck CH, Fleischhacker WW (1998) Hippocampal volume reduction in male schizophrenic patients. Schizophrenia Res 31:73–81

Witter MP, Wouterlood FG, Naber PA, Van Haeften T (2000) Anatomical organization of the parahippocampal-hippocampal network. In: Scharfman HE, Witter MP, Schwarcz R (eds) The Parahippocampal Region. Implications for Neurological and Psychiatric Diseases. Annals of the New York Academy of Sciences, New York, pp 1–24

Wood SJ, Velakoulis D, Smith DJ, Bond D, Stuart GW, McGorry PD, Brewer WJ, Bridle N, Eritaia J, Desmond P et al (2001) A longitudinal study of hippocampal volume in first episode psychosis and chronic schizophrenia. Schizophrenia Research 52:37–46

Wright IC, Rabe-Hesketh S, Woodruff PW, David AS, Murray RM, Bullmore ET (2000) Meta-analysis of regional brain volumes in schizophrenia. Am J Psychiatry 157:16–25

Yeo RA, Hodde-Vargas J, Hendren RL, Vargas LA, Brooks WM, Ford CC, Gangestad SW, Hart BL (1997) Brain abnormalities in schizophrenia-spectrum children: implications for a neurodevelopmental perspective. Psychiatry Research Neuroimaging 76:1–13

Zeineh MM, Engel SA, Thompson PM, Bookheimer SY (2002) Dynamics of the hippocampus during encoding and retrieval of face-name pairs. Science 299:577–580

Zhang ZJ, Reynolds GP (2002) A selective decrease in the relative density of parvalbumin-immunoreactive neurons in the hippocampus in schizophrenia. Schizophrenia Res 55:1–10

Neuroimaging studies of auditory verbal hallucinations

Philip McGuire

Institute of Psychiatry, London, SE5 8AF, UK

Introduction

Auditory hallucinations are a central feature of schizophrenia and a source of distress and disability for many patients. Although often responsive to treatment, in about a third of patients they are resistant to treatment or only partially improve (Shergill et al. 1999). In patients with schizophrenia auditory hallucinations of speech (auditory verbal hallucinations) are the most common type, and these usually involve derogatory phrases addressed to the patient in the second person (Junginger and Frame 1985).

Until recently little was known of the mechanisms underlying auditory hallucinations, but the development and application of neuroimaging has significantly advanced our understanding in this area. More generally, one can consider auditory hallucinations as a model for psychotic symptoms in general: understanding the mechanisms underlying hallucinations may reveal deficits that are fundamental to psychotic phenomena. For example, Frith and Done (1987) suggests that all positive symptoms may reflect an impairment in cognitive self-monitoring.

This chapter will review data from neuroimaging studies that have provided clues to the mechanisms underlying auditory hallucinations. The main focus will be on functional neuroimaging work, although structural imaging studies will also be discussed.

Functional neuroimaging

'Capturing' neural activity during hallucinations

Two broad methodological approaches have been used in functional imaging studies of auditory hallucinations. One has been to use functional neuroimaging to 'capture' the pattern of brain activity in patients while they are actually experiencing hallucinations inside the scanner. With this design images collected when a patient is experiencing hallucinations are compared with images collected when the same individual is not hallucinating, ideally in the same scanning session. The difference in activity between the two states may thus be related to the presence of hallucinations. In most of these studies, the subject signals the presence or absence of hallucinations by pressing a button or moving their finger.

This approach has been used with single photon emission tomography (SPET), positron emission tomography (PET) and most recently with functional magnetic resonance imaging (fMRI). Early studies generally identified one or two regions which were significantly more active in the hallucinating than the non-hallucinating state. However, while there was some overlap across studies, different investigations tended to identify activation in different brain areas. These included the left inferior frontal cortex (McGuire et al. 1993), the cingulate gyrus (Cleghorn et al. 1992), the thalamus and basal ganglia (Silbersweig et al. 1995), the parahippocampal cortex (Liddle et al. 1992) and the lateral temporal cortex (Dierks et al. 1999). One factor in this apparent inconsistency may have been the limited power of some of these early studies: because of the risks of radiation, those using SPET and PET involved a relatively small number of images in each subject. In contrast, as it does not involve radiation, larger numbers of images can be acquired using fMRI. In our most recent study using the 'capture' approach, we used fMRI and were able to collect multiple images corresponding to hallucinations in each patient. This revealed a distributed network of areas active during hallucinations that included all of the areas individually identified in previous studies (Shergill et al. 2000). These recent data suggest the experience of auditory verbal hallucinations seems to involve several different brain regions, including the inferior frontal, anterior cingulate and temporal cortex, the parahippocampal region and subcortical structures. The specificity of these findings to auditory hallucinations, as opposed to hallucinations in other modalities, has been demonstrated by comparing the correlates of auditory and somatic hallucinations in the same patient. These within-subject comparisons indicated the former were particularly associated with activation in the lateral temporal cortex while the latter involved the somatosensory cortex (Shergill et al. 2001).

Cognitive processes impaired in hallucinators

A complementary approach to that described above is to use imaging techniques to study normal cognitive processes that are thought to be impaired in patients with auditory verbal hallucinations. According to Frith's model (1992), the key deficit underlying verbal hallucinations is a failure to recognise that self-generated inner speech is endogenous in origin. This impairment in self-monitoring leads to the mid-identification of inner speech as 'alien' and its perception as external speech.

Verbal self-monitoring can be examined implicitly by asking subjects to imagine another person's speech. When patients who are prone to hallucinations do this they show attenuated activation in the temporal, parahippocampal and cerebellar cortex, areas that have been implicated in the monitoring of inner speech (McGuire et al. 1995; Shergill et al. 2001) and in cognitive self-monitoring more generally (Blakemore et al. 2002). Similar functional differences between patients who are prone to hallucinations and controls are evident when subjects are required to generate inner speech at increasing rates, another task that implicitly increases the demands on verbal self-monitoring (Shergill et al. 2003). While these paradigms may engage verbal self-monitoring, patients who suffer from hallucinations have no difficulty in performing them and they do not elicit any abnormalities at the behavioural level (Evans et al. 1999; Aleman et al. 2003 a). This is in contrast with another task which engages self-monitoring more directly. When patients with hallucinations speak and hear a distorted version of their own voice 'on-line' (i.e. as they are speaking, in real time), they tend to mis-identify their own speech as alien (Cahill et al. 1999; Johns and McGuire 1999). This misattribution of self-generated verbal material as being of external origin is thought to be one of the fundamental deficits underlying auditory verbal hallucinations (Frith 1992), suggesting that this paradigm may be particularly useful in investigating the basis of this symptom. Subjects are especially liable to mis-identify their own speech when its content is emotionally negative (Johns et al. 2001), consistent with the predominantly negative content of hallucinations in schizophrenia. When healthy volunteers perform this task they engage the inferior frontal, cingulate, temporal and cerebellar cortex (McGuire et al. 1996; Fu et al. 2001). Patients with schizophrenia with hallucinations and delusions differ from controls and from patients with no hallucinations in that they are more likely to misattribute their own speech as alien and this is associated with differential activation of the lateral temporal cortex (Fu et al. 2001).

While these neuroimaging data are consistent with an impairment in self-monitoring in patients with hallucinations, they could also reflect deficits in other processes. Patients' beliefs and expectations may influence how they appraise sensory stimuli, particularly when these are anomalous (Garety et al. 2001), and such 'top-down' processes may thus contribute to the experience of auditory hallucinations (Bentall and Slade 1985).

We have examined the role of top-down processes by modifying the verbal self-monitoring paradigm described above. In this modified version, subjects do not speak, but are required to decide whether distorted speech that they hear was self- or externally-generated. Even though the task does not involve self-monitoring, patients with hallucinations are more likely than controls or patients with no hallucinations to mis-recognise their own distorted speech as alien, particularly when the speech has an emotional content (Allen et al. 2003). In healthy volunteers, the correct identification of one's own voice under these conditions is associated with the engagement of inferior frontal, dorsolateral prefrontal and anterior cingulate cortex, suggesting that these regions might mediate top-down effects on the processing of auditory verbal material (Allen, Amaro et al., in press).

Another way of studying how such influences might affect brain function is by examining the effect of imagery on auditory processing. Imagining a tone of a given frequency significantly enhances the detection of tones at that frequency presented in white noise (Farah and Smith 1983). In patients with schizophrenia, this effect of imagery on perception seems to be correlated with the severity of auditory hallucinations (Aleman et al. 2003 b), suggesting that the mechanisms underlying this effect might be relevant to the perception of hallucinations. In controls, imagining a tone significantly increases activation in the auditory cortex and thalamus when subjects are subsequently presented with an auditory tone of the same frequency (Amaro et al. 2003). We are currently investigating the correlates of this paradigm in patients with and without hallucinations.

Structural MRI

Structural neuroimaging has mainly been used to study the disorder of schizophrenia, as opposed to auditory hallucinations, and there have been relatively few investigations that have sought to examine the correlates of hallucinations. Although Barta (1991) reported a striking inverse correlation between the volume of the left superior temporal cortex and the severity of hallucinations, this finding has not been consistently replicated (De Lisi et al. 1994), and other work using a region of interest approach has linked volumetric changes in this region to formal thought disorder, rather than hallucinations (Shenton et al. 1992; Vita et al. 1994). Studies that have used a voxel-based approach have also produced inconsistent findings. Wright et al. (1995) found a link between auditory hallucinations and reduced left temporal grey matter volume but another study did not (Chua et al. 1997), and the relationship between verbal hallucinations and the structure of the brain in schizophrenia thus remains unclear.

Functional imaging studies of schizophrenia (reviewed in McGuire and Frith 1996) and of patients with auditory hallucinations (McGuire et al. 1995; Shergill et al. 2003) suggest that the temporal relationship between activation in prefrontal and temporal cortex may be abnormal. These findings could reflect faulty communication between areas involved in the generation and perception of inner speech, and there is currently great interest in the use of diffusion tensor imaging (DTI) as a means of examining anatomical connectivity in patients with hallucinations. At present these studies are ongoing but should yield results in the near future.

Clinical applications

One striking way in which data from imaging studies of hallucinations has been used in clinical practice is with transcranial magnetic stimulation (TMS). Functional imaging data that indicates areas which are active during hallucinations can be used to select the region to target with TMS, and this approach has been used in recent TMS studies (Hoffman et al. 2003). Imaging data has also informed cognitive psychological models of hallucinations (Seal et al. 2004), which form a rational basis for the development of new psychological interventions for hallucinations.

▌ Conclusions

Neuroimaging has provided new information that has improved our understanding of the mechanisms underlying auditory hallucinations, mechanisms that may also be relevant to other psychotic phenomena.

▌ References

Aleman A, Bocker KB, Hijman R, de Haan EH, Kahn RS (2003a) Cognitive basis of hallucinations in schizophrenia: role of top-down information processing. Schizophrenia Research 1926:1–11

Aleman A, Koen A, Böcker B, Hijman R, de Haan E, Kahn R (2003) Cognitive basis of hallucinations in schizophrenia: role of top-down information processing. Schizophrenia Research 64:175–185

Allen P, Johns L, Fu C, Broome M, Brammer M, Vythelingum N, McGuire PK (2004) Misattribution of external speech in patients with delusions and hallucinations. Schizophrenia Research (in press)

Barta PE, Pearlson GD, Powers RE et al (1990) Auditory hallucinations and smaller superior temporal gyral volume in schizophrenia. American Journal of Psychiatry 39:784–788

Bentall RP, Slade PD (1985) Reality testing and auditory hallucinations: a signal detection analysis. British Journal of Clinical Psychology 24:159–169

Blakemore SJ, Wolpert DM, Frith CD (2002) Abnormalities in the awareness of action. Trends in Cognitive Sciences 6:237–242

Cahill C, Silbersweig D, Frith C (1996) Psychotic experiences induced in deluded patients using distorted auditory feedback. Cognitive Neuropsychiatry 1:201–211

Cleghorn JM, Franco S, Szechtman B et al (1992) Towards a brain map of auditory hallucinations. American Journal of Psychiatry 149:1062–1069

Chua S, Wright I, Murray RM, Friston KJ, Liddle PF, McGuire PK (1997) Grey matter correlates of syndromes in schizophrenia: a semi-automated analysis of structural magnetic resonance images. British Journal of Psychiatry 170:406–410

DeLisi L, Hoff AL, Neale C, Kushner M (1994) Asymmetries in the superior temporal lobe in male and female first-episode schizophrenic patients: measures of the planum temporale and superior temporal gyrus by MRI. Schizophrenia Research 12:19–28

Dierks T, Linden DEJ, Jandl M, Formisano E, Goebel R, Lanfermann H, Singer W (1999) Activation of Heschl's gyrus during auditory hallucinations. Neuron 22:615–621

Evans C, McGuire PK, David A (2000) Is auditory imagery defective in patients with auditory hallucinations? Psychological Medicine 30(1):137–148

Farah M J, Smith AF (1983) Perceptual interference and facilitation with auditory imagery. Perceptiion & Psychophysics 33(5):475–478

Frith CD, Done DJ (1987) Towards a neuropsychology of schizophrenia. British Journal of Psychiatry 153:437–443

Frith CD (1992) The Cognitive Neuropsychology of Schizophrenia. Erlbaum, Taylor & Francis, Hove, UK

Fu C, Vythelingum N, Andrew C, Brammer M, Amaro Jr E, Williams S, McGuire PK (2001) Alien voices ... who said that? Neural correlates of impaired verbal self-monitoring in schizophrenia. Neuroimage 13:1052

Garety PA, Kuipers E, Fowler D, Freeman D, Bebbington PE (2001) A cognitive model of the positive symptoms of psychosis. Psychological Medicine 31:189–195

Hoffman RE, Hawkins KA, Gueorguieva R, Boutros NN, Rachid F, Carroll K, Krystal JH (2003) Transcranial magnetic stimulation of left temporoparietal cortex and medication-resistant auditory hallucinations. Archives of General Psychiatry 60(1): 49–56

Johns L, McGuire PK (1999) Verbal self-monitoring and auditory hallucinations in schizophrenia. Lancet 353:469–470

Johns L, Rossell S, Ahmad F, Frith C, Hemsley D, Kuipers L, McGuire PK (2001) Auditory verbal hallucinations and defective verbal self-monitoring in schizophrenia. Psychological Medicine 31:705–715

Junginger J, Frame CL (1985) Self-report of the frequency and phenomenology of verbal hallucinations. The Journal of Nervous & Mental Disease 173:149–155

Liddle PF, Friston KJ, Frith CD, Hirsch SR, Jones T, Frackowiak RSJ (1992) Patterns of cerebral blood flow in schizophrenia. British Journal of Psychiatry 160:179–186

McGuire PK, Syed GMS, Murray RM (1993) Increased blood flow in Broca's area during auditory hallucinations in schizophrenia. Lancet 342:703–706

McGuire PK, Silbersweig DA, Wright I, Murray RM, David AS, Frackowiak R, Frith CD (1995) Abnormal perception of inner speech: a physiological basis for auditory hallucinations. Lancet 346:596–600

McGuire PK, Silbersweig DA, Frith CD (1996) Functional neuroanatomy of verbal self-monitoring. Brain 119:907–917

McGuire PK, Frith CD (1996) Disordered functional connectivity and schizophrenia. Psychological Medicine 26:663–667

Seal M, Aleman A, McGuire P (2004) Alluring imagery, unanticipated speech and deceptive memory: neurocognitive models of auditory verbal hallucinations in schizophrenia. Cognitive Neuropsychiatry 9:43–72

Shenton ME, Kikinis R, Jolesz FA, Pollack SD, LeMay M, Wible CG, Hokama H, Martin J, Metcalf D, Coleman M, McCarley RW (1992) Abnormalities of the left temporal lobe and thought disorder in schizophrenia. A quantitative magnetic resonance imaging study. New England Journal of Medicine 327:604–612

Shergill S, Murray RM, McGuire PK (1998) Auditory hallucinations: a review of psychological treatments. Schizophrenia Research 32:137–150

Shergill S, Bullmore E, Williams S, Brammer M, Murray RM, McGuire PK (2000) Functional anatomy of auditory verbal imagery in patients with auditory verbal hallucinations. American Journal of Psychiatry 157:1691–1693

Shergill S, Brammer M, Williams S, Murray RM, McGuire PK (2000) Mapping auditory hallucinations in schizophrenia using functional magnetic resonance imaging. Archives of General Psychiatry 57:1033–1038

Shergill S, Cameron L, Brammer M, Williams S, Murray RM, McGuire PK (2002) Modality-specif neural correlates of auditory and somatic hallucinations. Journal of Neurology, Neurosurgery & Psychiatry 71:688–690

Shergill S, Fukuda R, Brammer M, Murray RM, McGuire PK (2002) Modulation of temporal cortical activity during generation of inner speech. Human Brain Mapping 16:219–227

Shergill S, Fukuda R, Brammer M, Murray RM, McGuire PK (2003) Impaired monitoring of inner speech in schizophrenia. British Journal of Psychiatry 182:525–531

Vita A, Dieci M, Giobbio GM, Caputo A, Ghiringhelli M, Garbarini M, Medini AP, Morganti C, Tenconi F, Cesana B, Invernizzi G (1995) Language and thought disorder in schizophrenia: brain morphological correlates. Schizophrenia Research 15:243–251

Vita A, Dieci M, Giobbio GM, Caputo A, Ghiringhelli M, Garbarini M, Medini AP, Morganti C, Tenconi F, Cesana B, Invernizzi G (1995) Language and thought disorder in schizophrenia: brain morphological correlates. Schizophrenia Research 15:243–251

Wright IC, McGuire PK, Poline J-B, Travere JM, Murray RM, Frackowiak RSJ, Friston KJ (1995) A voxel-based method for the statistical analysis of grey and white matter density applied to schizophrenia. Neuroimage 2:244–252

Gender differences in schizophrenia

HEINZ HÄFNER

From Schizophrenia Research Unit, Central Institute of Mental Health, Mannheim/Germany

Introduction

Sex differences, whether in the premorbid stage, age at onset, symptomatology, brain morphology or illness course, are a long-pursued, but still fascinating topic of schizophrenia research.

Material and method

Our analyses will be based on relevant literature and a *population-based* sample of 232 first illness episodes of a broad diagnosis of schizophrenia (ICD-9: 295, 297, 298.3 and 298.4), the ABC sample (=84% of first admissions). The patients were 12 to 59 years old and came from a semi-urban, semi-rural German population of 1.5 million. A detailed description of the sample has been given elsewhere (Häfner et al. 1993a, 2003). The patients were assessed using the PSE (Wing et al. 1974), the SANS (Andreasen 1983), the PIRS (Biehl et al. 1989), the DAS (World Health Organization 1988; Jung et al. 1989), and other instruments immediately upon hospitalisation in order to be able to compare them at identical stages of illness. Premorbid social development, the onset and early course of the disorder were assessed retrospectively using the IRAOS interview (Häfner et al. 1992, 1999a, 2003). A subsample of 57 patients was compared with controls drawn from the population register, matched for age, sex and place of residence and interviewed using the IRAOS. Further illness course, from first admission on, was assessed prospectively in a subsample of 115 first-episode cases at five cross sections (six months, one, two, three and five years after first admission) over five years (Fig. 1).

Results

Gender differences in the type of onset and symptomatology of first-episode schizophrenia

The literature mostly reports a greater frequency of an insidious type of onset and of negative symptoms for men and a greater frequency of positive and affective symptoms for women (Castle 1999).

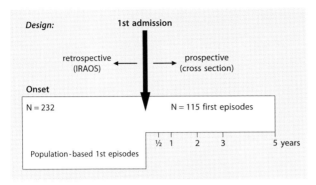

Fig. 1. ABC Schizophrenia Study: medium-term course (Source: Häfner and an der Heiden 1999)

We undertook to test these results by comparing diagnoses, subtypes, symptom clusters and symptoms between men and women. As shown in Table 1, significant differences were found in none of the cross-sectional data on the clinical or the operationalised diagnoses, scores or symptoms at first admission, i.e. in the psychotic episode.

The three categories of symptoms of illness onset: positive, negative, unspecific, showed no difference between men and women (Table 1). Nor did the 10 most frequent initial symptoms show significant gender differences, except one item, worrying, which is also significantly more frequent in women in general-population studies (Table 2).

Types of onset, defined as acute (≤1 month), subacute (1 months to 1 year) and chronic (>1 year), showed no significant gender difference (Table 3). Nor did the six *symptom clusters* – which represent empirical subtypes – that we derived from the psychotic prephase up to first admission differ in age of onset or frequency *when controlled for age* (Table 4).

Results from comparative neuropsychological studies are inconsistent (Goldstein and Lewine 2000; Fitzgerald and Seeman 2000). Goldberg et al. (1995) for example studied four independent samples of men and women with schizophrenia using a large test battery, but did not find any substantial neuropsychological gender differences.

To conclude, when identical early stages of illness are carefully compared by taking age into account, as Jablensky (1995) writes, "there is no unequivocal evidence of consistent sex differences" in the types of onset or symptom profiles.

Gender difference in the morbid risk

In the literature the male-female ratio of the annual incidence and lifetime risk of schizophrenia varies considerably from 0.70 to 3.47/10 000. But comparisons between the sexes are very difficult, because the male and female rates across the life-cycle are uneven and show great differences. We have shown that the highly uneven age-of-onset distributions of men and women consti-

Table 1. Comparison of clinical and operationalised diagnoses and CATEGO subclasses, scores and index of definition at first admission (=in the first psychotic episode) between men and women – ABC study sample of 232 first-episode cases (=84% of 276 first admissions) (Source: Häfner 2002)

Diagnosis (%)[*]	Females n = 124	Males n = 108	p
Schizophrenia broad definition (ICD-9: 295, 297, 298.3/4)	100%	100%	
Schizophrenia ICD 295	87.1%	88.0%	NS
Operationalised diagnosis			
CATEGO ICD 295	79.0%	73.1%	NS
CATEGO class S+	73.4%	67.6%	NS
CATEGO: affective psychosis	13.7%	13.0%	NS
Scores (mean values)[**]			
PSE: index of definition	7.47	7.49	NS
CATEGO: total score	40.67	41.44	NS
CATEGO subscores:			
DAH (delusions, hallucinations)	10.83	10.01	NS
BSO (behaviour, speech)	8.04	7.85	NS
SNR (specific neurotic syndrome)	7.11	7.68	NS
NSN (non-specific neurotic syndrome)	14.69	15.91	NS

[*] chi^2-tests
[**] t-tests

Table 2. Percentages of men and women presenting the ten most frequent earliest signs of schizophrenia reported by the patients[1] ABC first-episode sample n = 232. (Source: Häfner et al. 1995, modified)

	Total (n = 232) %	Men (n = 108) %	Women (n = 124) %	p
▮ Restlessness	19	15	22	
▮ Depression	19	15	22	
▮ Anxiety	18	17	19	
▮ Trouble with thinking and concentration	16	19	14	
▮ Worrying	15	9	20	*
▮ Lack of self-confidence	13	10	15	
▮ Lack of energy, slowness	12	8	15	
▮ Poor work performance	11	12	10	
▮ Social withdrawal, distrust	10	8	12	
▮ Social withdrawal, communication	10	8	12	

[1] Based on closed questions in the IRAOS interview, multiple counting possible.
All items tested for sex differences; *: p ≤ 0.05

Table 3. Age at first admission and frequency of symptom clusters in the psychotic prephase (from first positive symptom to first admission) of the first psychotic episode in men and women with schizophrenia (Source: Häfner 2000 b)

Cluster	Non-specific, negative, depressive	Delusional	Psychotic thought disorder	Auditory hallucina-tions, substance abuse	Disorganisa-tion/psychotic thought disorder	Low values on all dimensions
Sex:						
males (%)	49.2	45.2	40.6	48.4	50.0	42.3
females (%)	50.8	54.8	59.4	51.6	50.0	57.7
$Chi_2 = 1.1$, df: 5; p=0.95						
Age at first admission (years) (both sexes) F=0.293, df=5; p=0.91	31.1	29.8	29.9	29.3	30.3	31.4

Table 4. Type of onset and type of initial symptoms of schizophrenia – ABC first-episode sample n = 232. (Source: Häfner et al. 1995, modified)

	Total n = 232 (%)	Men n = 108 (%)	Women n = 124 (%)
Type of onset			
Acute (≤1 month)	18	19	17
Subacute (>1 month ≤1 year)	15	11	18
Insidious or chronic (>1 year)	68	70	65
Type of first symptoms*			
Negative or non-specific	73	70	76
Positive	7	7	6
Both	20	22	19

* The variables listed, except "worrying", showed no significant sex differences

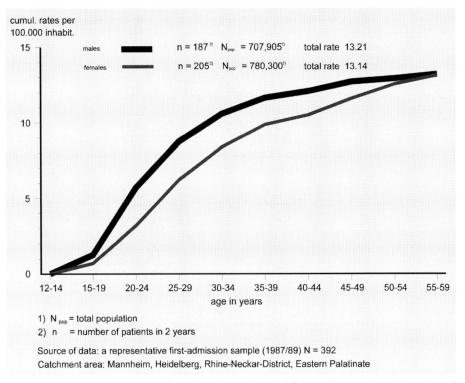

Fig. 2. Cumulative incidence rates for schizophrenia, broad definition (ICD-9: 295, 297, 298.3 and 298.4) Source: Häfner et al. 1991)

tute a methodological pitfall difficult to tackle (Hambrecht et al. 1994). Low upper age limits of the samples studied produce an overrepresentation of young males and an underrepresentation of female late-onset cases (e.g. Bland 1977) and, hence, explain a large part of the male predominance reported by the majority of studies on the topic (Hambrecht et al. 1992; Häfner and an der Heiden 1997; see also Seeman 1982; Lewine et al. 1984; Castle et al. 1993; Goldstein and Lewine 2000). The rare methodologically sophisticated studies show that until age 55 or 60 years there is a trend towards convergence in the male-female lifetime prevalence rates for schizophrenia of a broad, but precise diagnostic definition (e.g. Jablensky et al. 1992; Häfner and an der Heiden 1997). But it is unlikely that the rates would continue to converge if schizophrenia and schizophrenia-like delusional disorders of old age (late paraphrenia etc.) with their markedly higher incidence rates for women (Harris and Jeste 1988; Castle and Murray 1993; van Os et al. 1995; Häfner et al. 2001) were included.

We calculated cumulative incidence rates until age 60 years – a good indicator of the age-related lifetime risk – as based on five-year age bands of the population studied. As Fig. 2 shows, men consumed their lifetime risk until age-band 30 to 35 years more rapidly than women did. From that age on, however, women caught up with men, finally reaching almost the same lifetime rate at about 13/100 000.

This result provided further support for the hypothesis that the disorder as such is essentially the same in men and women at least until age 60 years.

Normal gender differences in development and behaviour

The developmental psychology of behaviour and gender, reviewed for example by Maccoby and Jacklin (1974), has shown that boys and young men exhibit a higher frequency of aggressive behaviour, antisocial aggression in particular, than girls and young women do, who display more prosocial or inhibited aggression and a greater acceptance of authority. From puberty on, the mental health risks of males and females, too, follow different lines, males showing a greater frequency of attention deficit disorder, dissocial behaviour, aggressiveness and antisocial personality and females a greater frequency of anxiety and affective disorders (Rutter et al. 1970; Shepherd et al. 1971; Achenbach et al. 1987; Esser et al. 1992).

Rosenfield (2000) distinguished between externalising disorders also including antisocial behaviour and substance abuse, more frequent in men, and internalising disorder including anxiety and depression, more frequent in women (see also Achenbach 1989). He attributed these disorders to "different socialisation processes in men and women – and different genetic and hormonal dispositions". In that respect these behavioural dispositions are very likely not accounted for by the disease process of schizophrenia.

Gender differences in the antecedents of schizophrenia and premorbid behaviour

As shown by studies based on population birth cohorts (Jones et al. 1995; Isohanni et al. 1998 a, b), from school age on behavioural anomalies as antecedents of schizophrenia manifest themselves several years later in girls than in boys (Crow et al. 1995).

Walker et al. (1995) compared childhood videos of siblings discordant for schizophrenia. Like normal children, boys later falling ill with schizophrenia exhibit primarily externalising behaviours (e.g. hyperactivity, physical and verbal aggression) somewhat earlier than girls do, who manifest mainly "internalising" behaviours, e.g. shyness, social withdrawal, depressive mood and social anxiety (Fig. 3).

Gender differences in premorbid functioning

Retrospective studies of patients and prospective studies of children of women suffering from schizophrenia have consistently found a greater frequency of premorbid social and occupational dysfunctioning for males than females (McGlashan and Bardenstein 1990; Mueser et al. 1990 a; Moldin 2000). This was also shown by the Israeli conscript study of 16- to 17-year-old adolescents with follow-ups of 4 to 10 years until first admission (Weiser et al. 2000).

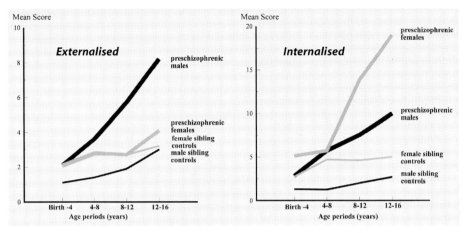

Fig. 3. Antecedents of schizophrenia in childhood and youth: comparison of preschizophrenic and control siblings, mean externalized/internalized behaviour problem scores by age period and sex (Source: Walker et al. 1995)

In studies that define illness onset by first contact, gender differences in premorbid functioning become contaminated not only with the "normal" behavioural differences, but also with the prodromal stage of the disorder. This initial stage, characterised by negative symptoms, functional impairment and social disability, has a 3 to 4 year earlier onset in men. In these cases, the gender differences can probably be explained partly by normal behavioural differences, partly by the difference in age of onset, involving age-related or developmental deficits.

Determinants and consequences of the gender difference in age at onset

Nearly one hundred years ago, Kraepelin (1909–15) reported women's several years higher age at first admission. Angermeyer and Kühn (1988) found only in three out of 53 studies a higher age for men. The pooled data of the World Health Organization ten-country study (Jablensky et al. 1992) revealed a 3.4 years higher mean age of onset for women versus men (Hambrecht et al. 1992, 1994).

In the ABC first-episode sample mean age at the emergence of the first sign of the disorder, first negative, first positive symptom and at the climax of the first episode showed a parallel and significant difference of three to four years between men and women.

Looking at the distribution of onsets over the entire age range, we found for men an early and steep increase with a maximum between 15 and 25 years (Fig. 4). After that peak the onset rates for men fell continually. Women's rates of onset rose slightly more slowly, reached a lower peak and after a decline a second, somewhat smaller peak around menopause. The same pattern also emerged in Castle et al. (1993) study, based on the Camberwell case register,

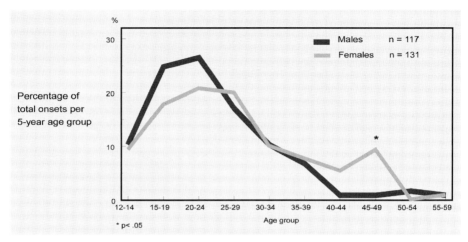

Fig. 4. Distribution of age at onset of schizophrenia (first ever sign of mental disorder) by sex (ICD-9: 295, 297, 298.3 and 298.4), ABC Schizophrenia Study (Source: Häfner et al. 1993 b)

and in our analysis of all first admissions for a diagnosis of schizophrenia in a one-year period from the Danish case register (Löffler et al. 1994).

Testing the oestrogen hypothesis at different levels

From the distribution of onsets across the female life-cycle we inferred that the protective effect was accounted for by oestrogen secretion. A protective effect of oestrogen had previously been suggested by Mendelson et al. 1977, Seeman 1981, Loranger 1984, Häfner 1987, Lewine 1988 and Seeman 1996. It had been shown very early that short-term oestrogen applications lead to a dose-dependent modulation of the dopaminergic (DiPaolo and Falardieu 1985; Fields and Gordon 1982; Hruska 1986) and the serotonergic systems (Sumner and Fink 1995).

Together with Wagner Gattaz we tested the oestrogen hypothesis by a four-week oestrogen treatment of ovariectomised rats and found a significant attenuation of apomorphine-stimulated dopaminergic behaviour compared with two control groups. We were able to demonstrate that oestrogen reduces the sensitivity of D2 receptors (Häfner et al. 1991; Gattaz et al. 1992).

A decade of experimental oestrogen studies has since then shown that the sex hormone has potent neuromodulatory and neuroprotective effects. Sumner and Fink (1995), Fink et al. (1998), Shughrue et al. (1997), Sumner et al. (1999), McEwen et al. (1981), Woolley and McEwen (1994) showed that oestrogen has similar, functional effects not only on D2-receptors, but also on 5-HT_{A2} glutamate (NMDA) and GABA receptors on both the neurochemical and the genomic level. The basic neuroprotective mechanisms include interactions with free radical detoxifying systems and the inhibition of the cellular liquid peroxidation (Behl 2002).

To test the applicability of the results of our animal experiments to human schizophrenia we compared 32 women with schizophrenic and 29 women with depressive episodes, both with normal menstrual cycles (Riecher-Rössler et al. 1994a, b). We found significant negative correlations between increasing oestrogen plasma levels and schizophrenia symptom scores in both groups of women, but no correlation with depressive symptom scores in either group. An analogous variation in symptom severity over the menstrual cycle has also been reported by Hallonquist et al. (1993), and similar clinical observations had previously been published by Dalton (1959) and Endo et al. (1978).

Noteworthy in this context is also the finding that twins or cases with a family history of schizophrenia show no or small gender differences in age of onset (DeLisi et al. 1994; Kendler and Walsh 1995; Albus and Maier 1995; Könnecke et al. 2000).

For this reason we tested the hypothesis that the protective effect of oestrogen in women wanes with increasing strength of genetic predisposition to illness, operationalised by one or more first-degree relatives diagnosed with schizophrenia. As Fig. 5 shows, in familial cases the gender difference in age of onset fell from 4.2 to a non-significant 1.6 years, and this reduction was almost entirely accounted for by women. In contrast, in sporadic cases the gender difference attained a highly significant 4.9 years. The other major aetiological risk factor, obstetric complications, had a similar, but weaker effect. Hence, it seems that the weaker a person's predisposition to illness, the stronger the protective effect of oestrogen.

The causal effect of this hormone on schizophrenia has recently been proven by Kulkarni et al. (2002) with adjunctive treatment of acute psychotic episodes in two successful intervention studies of women and men.

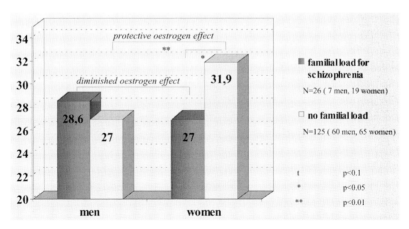

Fig. 5. Age at first psychotic symptom by gender and familial load (ABC first-episode sample n = 232) (Source: Könnecke et al. 2000)

Consequences of the gender difference in age at onset

Provided that an early onset is associated with a greater severity of illness, men, lacking the protective effect of oestrogen, would be expected to develop the most severe forms of the disorder fairly early. In women, as long as they produce enough oestrogen, the disease should be slightly milder until menopause. From premenopause on women should not only show higher incidence rates, as in fact depicted in Table 5, but also present more severe forms of the disorder.

A comparison of symptom scores in early- and late-onset schizophrenia (age at onset 20 years or younger versus 40 years or older) by gender yielded different age trends for men and women, which is in line with our hypothesis and several other studies, e.g. Harris and Jeste's (1988) (Table 6). Four out of eight symptom scores were significantly lower for late-onset men. In contrast, late-onset women showed not a single symptom score significantly lower and one, the SANS global score denoting negative symptomatology, significantly

Table 5. Onset of schizophrenia by age and sex – ABC first-episode sample n = 232 (Source: Häfner and Nowotny 1995)

Age at first psychotic symptom	n	Men (%)	Women (%)	m/f ratio
12–20 yrs.	49	57	43	1.33
21–35	136	48	52	0.92
36–59	47	32	68	0.47*

* Odds ratio = 2.16 (sex ratio in the age group against the sex ratio in the remaining age groups); p < 0.05
m/f = male/female

Table 6. Symptomatology at onset: young and old in comparison (age at first psychotic symptom < 21 years vs. ≥ 40 years) (Source: Häfner et al. 1998 a)

Symptomatology	Men			Women		
	Young n = 28	vs. Wilcoxon	Old n = 9	Young n = 21	vs. Wilcoxon	Old n = 24
DAS	12.1	0.02*	↓5.7	10.0	0.95	10.5
BSO	8.6	0.29	7.3	8.9	0.44	7.9
SNR	10.7	0.11	7.3	8.2	0.42	7.1
NSN	18.9	0.03*	↓11.4	13.0	0.58	13.8
Total score	50.3	0.02*	↓31.8	40.0	0.80	39.2
SANS	9.3	0.29	6.6	6.7	0.08t	↑9.5
PIRS	10.7	0.29	8.4	9.8	0.73	10.5
DAS-M	3.0	0.06t	↓1.8	1.9	0.61	1.8

higher compared with early-onset cases. These gender-different age trends in the severity of the first psychotic episode support our hypothesis of a clearly age-dependent protective effect emanating from the age-dependent oestrogen secretion.

In clear agreement with our results at the symptom level, Lewine et al. (1997), who studied the interaction of sex and age of onset in schizophrenia, found a poorer cognitive outcome for early-onset males (< 25 years) compared with late-onset males and a poorer outcome for late-onset females compared with their early-onset counterparts.

In line with our hypothesis are also the results of several long-term studies showing that postmenstrual women have a poorer symptom-related course and outcome (Opjordsmoen 1991).

Gender-specific illness behaviour and its effect on the course of the disorder

To analyse sex differences in the first illness episode in greater detail we compared all the 303 single items from the instruments we used for measuring symptoms, functional impairment and social disability (PSE, SANS, PIRS, DAS and IRAOS) in the first episode. Controlling for multiple testing we found no significant gender differences in the positive and negative core symptoms.

The most pronounced gender difference emerged with socially adverse behavioural items, such as self-neglect, reduced interest in a job, social withdrawal and deficits of communication, which were all significantly more frequent in men (Table 7). Only one – socially favourable – behavioural item was significantly more frequent in women: overadaptiveness/conformity. The cumulative prevalence of drug and alcohol abuse – assessed on IRAOS data – was also significantly more frequent in men, as was also shown by several

Table 7. Behavioural items with significant sex differences (from a total of 303 PSE, PIRS, SANS, DAS and IRAOS items)* – ABC first-episode sample, n = 232 (Source: Häfner 1998)

More frequent in women	More frequent in men
Cumulative until first admission	
– restlessness	– drug abuse
	– alcohol abuseb
Cross-sectional: at first admission	
– overadaptiveness/conformity	– self-neglect
	– reduced interest in a job
	– social inattentiveness
	– deficits of free time activities
	– deficits of communication
	– social disability (overall estimate)
	– loss of interests
	– deficits of personal hygiene

* Validated by split-half method for Â-correction

other studies (Mueser et al. 1990b, 1992; Soyka 1994; Kessler et al. 1994; Jenkins et al. 1997; Kandel 2000). In view of the aforementioned gender differences in normal development and behaviour and the consistent reports from population studies of a higher frequency of conduct disorders, disruptive, antisocial and violent behaviour and of substance abuse among young men in comparison with their female counterparts (Choquet and Ledoux 1994; Döpfner et al. 1997), we are here probably dealing with reflections of normal gender- and age-specific behaviour.

▌ Gender differences in course, outcome and quality of life

A wealth of studies have reported a poorer short- and medium-term course of schizophrenia for men compared with women. The difference has turned out to be accounted for by the social and not the symptom-related course (Biehl et al. 1986; Salokangas et al. 1987; Häfner et al. 1999b).

In our study mean symptom scores over 5 years after first admission – the CATEGO global score (Fig. 6) and the four subscores – indeed showed no significant gender difference. By contrast, the social course of schizophrenia (cf. Table 7) was significantly poorer for men throughout the 5-year follow-up period studied (Fig. 7). This result lends support to our hypothesis that men's socially unfavourable illness behaviour might contribute to their poorer social

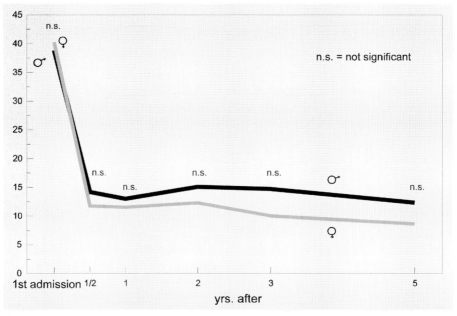

Fig. 6. Five-year course of schizophrenia (from first admission – 6 cross sections) for men and women by the CATEGO total score (ABC first-episode follow-up subsample n = 115) (Source: Häfner 1998)

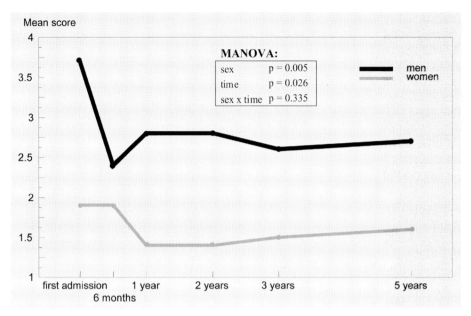

Fig. 7. Socially negative behaviour over five years after first admission for schizophrenia by sex (ABC first-episode follow-up subsample n = 115) (Source: Häfner et al. 1998 b)

course, whereas women's higher tendency to prosocial behaviour, cooperativeness and compliance might influence the social course favourably.

For a reliable assessment of the social course of a disorder it is necessary to proceed from a baseline: the level of social development at the onset of the disorder. We chose six key social roles, i.e. school education, occupational training, employment, own income, own accommodation, marriage or stable partnership. These roles indicate the level of social development at illness onset, which usually is the higher, the higher the patient's age.

A comparison of social-role performance at illness onset by gender revealed significant advantages for women in the domains of employment, own income and marriage or stable partnership in particular (Table 8). From these results we inferred that men's more poorer social course is explained not only by their socially adverse illness behaviour, but also – due to the disorder's three to four years earlier intrusion in men's social biographies – by their lower baseline of social development at illness onset.

Predicting five-year social outcome (after first admission)

We tested to what extent these two variables, along with the traditional prognostic variables of the disorder, predict social outcome. Fig. 8 illustrates two models: on the right a stepwise logistic regression including symptoms at first admission measured by the PSE, type of onset, age at first psychotic symptom and gender. Significant negative predictors of 5-year social outcome, operationalised by the ability to earn one's living, were the number of non-fulfilled so-

Table 8. Social "baseline" at illness onset: social-role performance of men and women at the emergence of the first sign of mental disorder – ABC first-episode sample n = 232 (Source: Häfner 1996, modified)

Age (in years)	Men n = 108 22.5 (%)		Women n = 124 25.4 (%)	Total n = 232 24.0 (%)
▌ School education	70		69	70
▌ Occupational training	41	NS	38	39
▌ Employment	37	*	52	45
▌ Own income	44	NS	55	50
▌ Own accommodation	39	*	54	47
▌ Marriage or stable partnership	28	**	52	41

t: $p \leq 0.1$, * $p \leq 0.05$, ** $p \leq 0.01$; NS = not significant

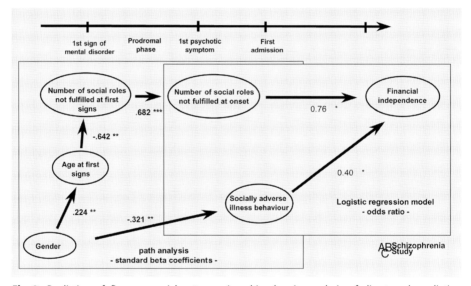

Fig. 8. Prediction of five-year social outcome in schizophrenia: analysis of direct and mediating causal factors (ABC first-episode follow-up subsample n = 115) (Source: Häfner 2000 b)

cial roles at psychosis onset and the number of items of socially adverse illness behaviour at first admission. Symptomatology and type of onset had no significant effect and age and gender merely that mediated by the first two variables. This is clearly shown in the pathanalytic model on the left, which revealed highly significant correlations of age at onset and gender with the two mediating variables: social development at illness onset and illness behaviour. This means that the poorer social course of schizophrenia in young men compared with premenopausal women, instead of reflecting a gender-different illness, is basically a result of

1) the protective effect of oestrogen in women, mediated by the higher stage of social development at illness onset, and

2) the socially adverse illness behaviour of men. The fact that these two predictors are associated with young age makes it understandable why women's advantageous social course is lost after menopause.

Sex differences in the long-term course of schizophrenia

The Mannheim first-admission cohort (an der Heiden et al. 1995, 1996) of the WHO Disability Study (n=70) was assessed at 10 cross sections over 15.6 years after first admission. The repeated measurements, based on the PSE total score, demonstrated a relatively high degree of stability in the mean symptom scores over the long-term course. But women, showing significantly lower symptom scores only in the first 1.5 years after first admission primarily because of their shorter first episodes, attained the level of male scores in the long-term. From two to 15.6 years after first admission, men and women showed almost equal symptom levels (Fig. 9).

Medium- and long-term studies on schizophrenia almost invariably show considerable differences in social status between men and women: An der Heiden et al. (1995) in the 14-year follow-up of their first-admission cohort found

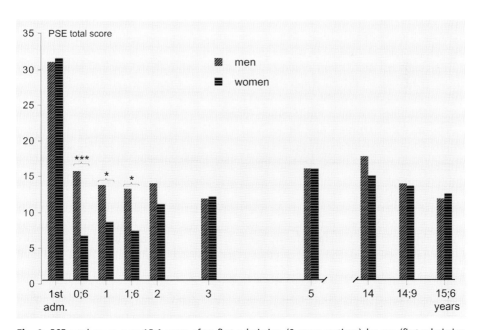

Fig. 9. PSE total score over 15.6 years after first admission (9 cross sections) by sex (first-admission sample of the WHO "Disability Study" Mannheim cohort n=70) (Source: Häfner 2000c)

Table 9. Living situation of schizophrenic men and women 15.5 years after first admission – WHO "Disability Study" Mannheim cohort n = 70 at inclusion in the study (Source: Häfner 2003)

	Women n = 22	Men n = 34	
Mean age[+]	44 years	41 years	NS
Outcome			
▌ symptoms or disability			
▌ present	59%	62%	NS
Living situation			
▌ never married	23%	71%	**
▌ married[+]	42%	19%	t
▌ lives with a spouse/partner[+]	53%	28%	*
▌ lives in a home[+]	5%	28%	t
▌ own children[+]	45%	26%	*
Employment status			
▌ has a regular job	26%	31%	NS

NS not significant; t: $p \leq 0.1$; * $p \leq 0.05$, ** $p \leq 0.001$
[+] n = 51 due to missing data
Based on data from an der Heiden et al. 1996

that 71% of the male patients, but only 23% of the female patients had never married. Consequently, only 28% of the men, but 53% of the women were living with a spouse and 28% of the men, but only 5% of the women were living in a supervised apartment or home. Naturally, more than twice as many women as men had children. Interestingly, however, there was no significant sex difference in employment status, which coincided with the equal measures of social disability for men and women (Table 9).

The fact that women fare better in real life than men is obviously also accounted for by women's more favourable social conditions at illness onset and socially less adverse behaviour in the course of the illness.

Coping with illness

I. Weber (1996) from our group looked into cognitive coping with the illness and subjective life satisfaction in the fairly homogeneous Mannheim cohort (an der Heiden et al. 1995) 15.5 years after first admission by using a life goal and satisfaction questionnaire (FNL: Fragebogen zu Lebenszielen und Lebenszufriedenheit; Kraak and Nord-Rüdiger 1989), based on Lehman's (1983 a, b) interaction model. She assessed subjective importance of life goals, goal achievement and life domain-specific satisfaction and found no correlation between symptom measures and social disability, on the one hand, and overall life satisfaction, on the other. But patients and controls showed significant dif-

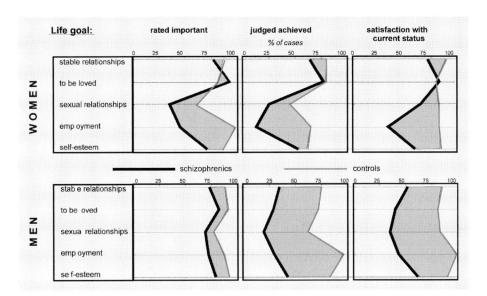

Fig. 10. Life-goal importance, achievement and satisfaction of men (n = 30) and women (n = 18) with schizophrenia 15.5 years after first admission compared with age- and sex-matched controls (first-admission sample of the WHO "Disability Study" Mannheim cohort n = 70). Based on data from Weber 1996 (Source: Häfner 2000 a)

ferences: 82% of the control men and 84% of the control women reported a high degree of overall life satisfaction, whereas only 43% of the male and 58% of the female patients with schizophrenia did so (Fig. 10).

Many life goals were considered less or slightly less important by patients with schizophrenia than by healthy controls. On the other hand, to be loved or to maintain stable relationships and self-esteem were almost equally important to both patients and healthy individuals. But only male patients considered sexual relationships and employment as important as did healthy controls. Women had significantly reduced their expectations in these life domains during the lengthy course of the illness obviously as a means of coping with their diminished capacities and chances. As a consequence, women with schizophrenia were generally more satisfied than their male counterparts, whose goal achievement and satisfaction with current status differed more markedly from their high expectations and from those of healthy controls. Nonetheless, women managed to achieve, to a greater extent than male patients, some of their highly valued aspirations in the domain of interpersonal relationships. Again, it was their illness behaviour that contributed to the more favourable social situation, to their better coping with illness-related deficits and, as a result, to their slightly higher life satisfaction compared with men suffering from schizophrenia.

▌ Summary and conclusions

Our studies showed that the nuclear process of schizophrenia until age 60 years does not essentially differ between the sexes. But, due to age-dependent developmental and neurohormonal gender differences in normal behaviour and in age of schizophrenia onset, the social course and severity of the disorder show considerable differences across the life-cycle: men fare poorly particularly at younger age, but significantly better at a later age, women fare considerably better until the age of menopause, but worse afterwards.

▌ References

Achenbach TM (1989) Internalizing disorders: subtyping based on parental questionnaires. In: Schmidt MH, Remschmidt H (eds) Needs and Prospects of Child and Adolescent Psychiatry. Hogrefe and Huber Publishers, Toronto, Lewiston, Bern, pp 83–92

Achenbach TM, Verhulst FC, Baron GD, Althaus M (1987) A comparison of syndromes derived from the Child Behavior Checklist for American and Dutch boys aged 6–11 and 12–16. J Child Psychology Psychiatry 28:437–453

Andreasen NC (1983) The scale for the assessment of negative symptoms (SANS). University of Iowa, Iowa City

Albus M, Maier W (1995) Lack of gender differences in age at onset in familial schizophrenia. Schizophrenia Res 18:51–57

an der Heiden W, Krumm B, Müller S, Weber I, Biehl H, Schäfer M (1995) Mannheimer Langzeitstudie der Schizophrenie. Nervenarzt 66:820–827

an der Heiden W, Krumm B, Müller S, Weber I, Biehl H, Schäfer M (1996) Eine prospektive Studie zum Langzeitverlauf schizophrener Psychosen: Ergebnisse der 14-Jahres-Katamnese. ZMP 5:66–75

Angermeyer MC, Kühn L (1988) Gender differences in age at onset of schizophrenia. Eur Arch Psychiatry Neurol Sci 237:351–364

Angermeyer MC, Kühn L, Goldstein JM (1990) Gender and the course of schizophrenia: differences in treated outcomes. Schizophrenia Bull 16:293–307

Behl C (2002) Neuroprotective effects of estrogens in the central nervous system: mechanisms of action. In: Häfner H (ed) Risk and Protective Factors in Schizophrenia. Steinkopff, Darmstadt, pp 263–270

Biehl H, Maurer K, Schubart C, Krumm B, Jung E (1986) Prediction of outcome and utilization of medical services in a prospective study of first onset schizophrenics – results of a prospective 5-year follow-up study. Eur Arch Psychiatry Neurol Sci 236:139–147

Biehl H, Maurer K, Jablensky A, Cooper JE, Tomov T (1989) The WHO Psychological Impairments Rating Schedule (WHO/PIRS). I. Introducing a new instrument for rating observed behaviour and the rationale of the psychological impairment concept. Br J Psychiatry 155:68–70

Bland RC (1977) Demographic aspects of functional psychoses in Canada. Acta Psychiatr Scand 55:369–380

Castle DJ (1999) Gender and age at onset in schizophrenia. In: Howard R, Rabins P, Castle D (eds) Late Onset Schizophrenia. Wrightson Biomedical, Hampshire, pp 147–164

Castle DJ, Murray RM (1993) The epidemiology of late-onset schizophrenia. Schizo-phrenia Bull 4:691–699

Castle DJ, Wessely S, Murray RM (1993) Sex and schizophrenia: effects of diagnostic stringency, and association with premorbid variables. Br J Psychiatry 162:658–664

Choquet M, Ledoux S (1994) Epidémiologie et adolescence. In: Confrontations psychiatriques, vol 27 (no 35). Rhone-Poulenc rorer specia, Paris, pp 287–309

Crow TJ, Done DJ, Sacker A (1995) Birth cohort study of the antecedents of psychosis: ontogeny as witness to phylogenetic origins. In: Häfner H, Gattaz WF (eds) Search for the Causes of Schizophrenia, vol III. Springer, Berlin Heidelberg, pp 3–20

Dalton K (1959) Menstruation and acute psychiatric illness. Br Med J 1:148–149

DeLisi LE, Bass N, Boccio A, Shilds G, Morganti C, Vita A (1994) Age of onset in fa-milial schizophrenia. Arch Gen Psychiatry 51:334–335

DiPaolo T, Falardeau P (1985) Modulation of brain and pituitary dopamine receptors by estrogens and prolactin. Prog Neuro-Psychopharmacol Biol Psychiatry 9:473–480

Döpfner M, Pluck J, Berner W, Fegert JM, Huss M, Lenz K, Schmeck K, Lehmkuhl U, Poustka F, Lehmkuhl G (1997) Psychische Auffälligkeiten von Kindern und Jugend-lichen in Deutschland Ergebnisse einer repräsentativen Studie: Methodik, Alters-, Geschlechts- und Beurteilereffekte (Mental disturbances in children and adoles-cents in Germany. Results of a representative study: age, gender and rater effects). Zeitschrift für Kinder- und Jugendpsychiatrie Psychotherapie 25:218–233

Endo M, Daiguji M, Asano Y, Yanashita I, Lakahashi S (1978) Periodic psychosis oc-curring in association with the menstrual cycle. J Clin Psychiatry 39:456–461

Esser G, Schmidt MH, Blanz B, Fätkenheuer B, Fritz A, Koppe T, Laucht M, Rensch B, Rothenberger W (1992) Prävalenz und Verlauf psychischer Störungen im Kindes- und Jugendalter (Prevalence and follow-up of psychiatric disorders in childhood and adolescence). Z Kinder Jugendpsychiatr 20:232–242

Fields JZ, Gordon JH (1982) Estrogen inhibits the dopaminergic supersensitivity in-duced by neuroleptics. Life Sciences 30:229–234

Fink G, Sumner B, McQueen JK, Wilson H, Rose R (1998) Sex steroid control of mood, mental state and memory. Clin Exp Pharmacol Physiol 25:764–765

Fitzgerald P, Seeman MV (2000) Women and schizophrenia: treatment implications. In: Castle DJ, McGrath J, Kulkarni J (eds) Women and Schizophrenia. Cambridge University Press, Cambridge, pp 95–110

Gattaz WF, Behrens S, De Vrie J, Häfner H (1992) Östradiol hemmt Dopamin-vermit-telte Verhaltensweisen bei Ratten - ein Tiermodell zur Untersuchung der ge-schlechtsspezifischen Unterschiede bei der Schizophrenie. Fortschr Neurol Psychiatr 60:8–16

Goldberg TE, Gold JM, Torrey EF, Weinberger DR (1995) Lack of sex differences in the neuropsychological performance of patients with schizophrenia. Am J Psychia-try 152:883–888

Goldstein JM, Lewine RRJ (2000) Overview of sex differences in schizophrenia: where have we been and where do we go from here? In: Castle DJ, McGrath J, Kulkarni J (eds) Women and Schizophrenia. Cambridge University Press, Cambridge, pp 111–143

Häfner H (1987) Epidemiology of schizophrenia. In: Häfner H, Gattaz WF, Janzarik W (eds) Search for the Causes of Schizophrenia. Springer, Berlin, pp 47–74

Häfner H (1996) The epidemiology of onset and early course of schizophrenia. In: Häfner H, Wolpert EM (eds) New Research in Psychiatry. Hogrefe & Huber Pub-lishers, Seattle Toronto, pp 33–60

Häfner H (1998) Ist es einzig die Krankheit? In: Möller H-J, Müller N (eds) Schizo-phrenie – Moderne Konzepte zu Diagnostik, Pathogenese und Therapie. Springer, Wien, pp 37–59

Häfner H (2000 a) Gender differences in schizophrenia. In: Frank E (ed) Gender and Its Effects on Psychopathology. American Psychopathological Association Series. American Psychiatric Press Inc, Washington, DC, pp 187–228

Häfner H (2000 b) Ist es alles nur die Krankheit? (Schriften der Mathematisch-naturwissenschaftlichen Klasse der Heidelberger Akademie der Wissenschaften Nr. 7). Springer, Berlin Heidelberg New York

Häfner H (2000 c) Methodische Probleme der Forschung am Verlauf der Schizophrenie. In: Maier W, Engel RR, Möller H-J (eds) Methodik von Verlaufs- und Therapiestudien in Psychiatrie und Psychotherapie. Hogrefe Verlag, Göttingen, pp 5–17

Häfner H (2002) Schizophrenia – do men and women suffer from the same disease? Revista de Psiquiatria Clinica 29:267–292

Häfner H, an der Heiden W (1997) Epidemiology of schizophrenia. Can J Psychiatry 42:139–151

Häfner H, an der Heiden W (1999) The course of schizophrenia in the light of modern follow-up studies: the ABC and WHO studies. Eur Arch Psychiatry Clin Neurosci 249 (Suppl 4):IV/14–IV/26

Häfner H, Nowotny B (1995) Epidemiology of early-onset schizophrenia. Eur Arch Psychiatry Clin Neurosci 245:80–92

Häfner H, Behrens S, de Vry J, Gattaz WF, Löffler W, Maurer K, Riecher-Rössler A (1991) Warum erkranken Frauen später an Schizophrenie? Nervenheilkunde 10: 154–163

Häfner H, Riecher-Rössler A, Hambrecht M, Maurer K, Meissner S, Schmidtke A, Fätkenheuer B, Löffler W, an der Heiden W (1992) IRAOS: an instrument for the assessment of onset and early course of schizophrenia. Schizophrenia Res 6:209–223

Häfner H, Maurer K, Löffler W, Riecher-Rössler A (1993 a) The influence of age and sex on the onset and early course of schizophrenia. Br J Psychiatry 162:80–86

Häfner H, Riecher-Rössler A, an der Heiden W, Maurer K, Fätkenheuer B, Löffler W (1993 b) Generating and testing a causal explanation of the gender difference in age at first onset of schizophrenia. Psychol Med 23:925–940

Häfner H, Maurer K, Löffler W, Bustamante S, an der Heiden W, Riecher-Rössler A, Nowotny B (1995) Onset and early course of schizophrenia. In: Häfner H, Gattaz WF (eds) Search for the Causes of Schizophrenia, vol III. Springer, Berlin Heidelberg, pp 43–66

Häfner H, Hambrecht M, Löffler W, Munk-Jorgensen P, Riecher-Rössler A (1998 a) Is schizophrenia a disorder of all ages? A comparison of first episodes and early course over the life-cycle. Psychol Med 28:351–365

Häfner H, an der Heiden W, Löffler W, Maurer K, Hambrecht M (1998 b) Beginn und Frühverlauf schizophrener Erkrankungen. In: Klosterkötter J (eds) Frühdiagnostik und Frühbehandlung psychischer Störungen. Bayer-ZNS-Symposium, Bd. XIII. Springer, Berlin Heidelberg New York, pp 1–28

Häfner H, Löffler W, Maurer K, Riecher-Rössler A, Stein A (1999 a) Instrument für die retrospektive Erfassung des Erkrankungsbeginns und -verlaufs bei Schizophrenie und anderen Psychosen. Huber, Bern

Häfner H, Maurer K, Löffler W, an der Heiden W, Stein A, Könnecke R, Hambrecht M (1999 b) Onset and prodromal phase and determinants of the course. In: Gattaz WF, Häfner H (eds) Search for the causes of schizophrenia. Vol. IV Balance of the century. Springer, Berlin Heidelberg, Steinkopff, Darmstadt, pp 35–58

Häfner H, Löffler W, Maurer K, Riecher-Rössler A, Stein A (2003) IRAOS. Interview for the retrospective assessment of the onset and course of schizophrenia and other psychoses. Hogrefe & Huber, Göttingen

Häfner H, Löffler W, Riecher-Rössler A, Häfner-Ranabauer W (2001) Schizophrenie und Wahn im höheren und hohen Lebensalter. Nervenarzt 72:347–357

Hallonquist JD, Seeman MV, Lang M, Rector NA (1993) Variation in symptom severity over the menstural cycle of schizophrenics. Biol Psychiatry 33:207–209

Hambrecht M, Maurer K, Sartorius N, Häfner H (1992) Transnational stability of gender differences in schizophrenia? An analysis based on the WHO Study on Determinants of Outcome of Severe Mental Disorders. Eur Arch Psychiatry Clin Neurosci 242:6–12

Hambrecht M, Riecher-Rössler A, Fätkenheuer B, Louza MR, Häfner H (1994) Higher morbidity risk for schizophrenia in males: fact or fiction? Compr Psychiatry 35:39–49

Harris MJ, Jeste DV (1988) Late-onset schizophrenia: an overview. Schizophr Bull 14:39–55

Hruska RE (1986) Evaluation of striatal dopamine receptors by estrogen: dose and time studies. J Neurochem 47:1908–1915

Isohanni M, Rantakallio P, Jones P, Järvelin M-R, Isohanni I, Mäkikyrö T, Moring J (1998a) The predictors of schizophrenia in the 1966 Northern Finland Birth Cohort study. Schizophrenia Res 29:11

Isohanni M, Järvelin M-R, Nieminen P, Jones P, Rantakallio P, Jokelainen J, Isohanni M (1998b) School performance as a predictor of psychiatric hospitalization in adult life. A 28-year follow-up in the northern Finland 1966 birth cohort. Psychol Med 28:967–974

Jablensky A (1995) Schizophrenia: the epidemiological horizon. In: Hirsch SR, Weinberger DR (eds) Schizophrenia. Blackwell Science, Oxford, pp 206–252

Jablensky A, Sartorius N, Ernberg G, Anker M, Korten A, Cooper JE, Day R, Bertelsen A (1992) Schizophrenia: manifestations, incidence and course in different cultures. A World Health Organization ten-country study. Psychological Medicine Monograph Suppl 20. Cambridge University Press, Cambridge

Jenkins R, Bebbington P, Brugha T, Farrell M, Gill B, Lewis G, Meltzer H, Petticrew M (1997) The national psychiatric morbidity survey of Great Britain. Psychol Med 27:765–774

Jones PB, Murray RM, Rodgers B (1995) Childhood risk factors for adult schizophrenia in a general population birth cohort at age 43 years. In: Mednick SA, Hollister JM (eds) Neural Development in Schizophrenia. Plenum Press, New York, pp 151–176

Jung E, Krumm B, Biehl H, Maurer K, Bauer-Schubart C (1989) DAS – Mannheimer Skala zur Einschätzung sozialer Behinderung. Beltz, Weinheim

Kandel DB (2000) Gender differences in the epidemiology of substance dependence in the United States. In: Frank E (ed) Gender and Its Effects on Psychopathology. American Psychopathological Association, Washington, DC, pp 231–252

Kendler KS, Walsh D (1995) Gender and schizophrenia: results of an epidemiologically based family study. Br J Psychiatry 167:184–192

Kessler RC, McGonagle KA, Zhao S, Nelson CB, Hughes M, Eshleman S, Wittchen H-U, Kendler KS (1994) Lifetime and twelve month prevalence of DSM-III-R psychiatric disorders in the United States. Arch Gen Psychiatry 51:8–19

Könnecke R, Häfner H, Maurer K, Löffler W, an der Heiden W (2000) Main risk factors for schizophrenia: increased familial loading and pre- and peri-natal complications antagonize the protective effect of oestrogen in women. Schizophrenia Res 44:81–93

Kraak B, Nord-Rüdiger D (1989) Der Fragebogen zu Lebenszielen und zur Lebenszufriedenheit (FLL). Hogrefe, Göttingen

Kraepelin E (1909–1915) Psychiatrie (Vol 1–4) 8th edn. Barth, Leipzig.

Kulkarni J, De Castella A, Downey M, Hammond J, Reidel A, Ward S, White S, Taffe J, Fitzgerald P, Burger H (2002) Clinical estrogen trials in schizophrenia. In: Häfner H, an der Heiden W, Resch F, Schröder J (eds) Risk and Protective Factors in Schizophrenia – Towards a Conceptual Model of the Disease Process. Steinkopff, Darmstadt, pp 271–284

Lehman AF (1983 a) The well-being of chronic mental patients. Arch Gen Psychiatry 40:369–375

Lehman AF (1983 b) The effects of psychiatric symptoms on quality of life assessments among the chronic mentally ill. Evaluation and Program Planning 6:143–151

Lewine RRJ (1988) Gender and schizophrenia. In: Nasrallah HA (ed) Handbook of Schizophrenia, Vol 3. Elsevier, Amsterdam, pp 389–397

Lewine RRJ, Burback D, Meltzer HY (1984) Effect of diagnostic criteria on the ratio of male to female schizophrenic patients. Am J Psychiatry 141:84–87

Lewine R, Haden C, Caudle J, Shurett R (1997) Sex-onset effects on neuropsychological function in schizophrenia. Schizophrenia Bull 23:51–61

Löffler W, Häfner H, Fätkenheuer B, Maurer K, Riecher-Rössler A, Lützhøft J, Skadhede S, Munk-Jørgensen P, Strömgren E (1994) Validation of Danish case register diagnosis for schizophrenia. Acta Psychiatr Scand 90:196–203

Loranger AW (1984) Sex difference in age of onset of schizophrenia. Arch Gen Psychiatry 41:157–161

Maccoby EE, Jacklin CN (1974) The Psychology of Sex Differences. Stanford University Press, Stanford

McGlashan TH, Bardenstein KK (1990) Gender differences in affective, schizoaffective, and schizophrenic disorders. Schizophrenia Bull 16:319–329

McEwen BS, Biegon A, Rainbow TC, Paden C, Snyder L, DeGroff V (1981) The interaction of estrogens with intracellular receptors and with putative neurotransmitter receptors: implications for the mechanisms of activation of regulation of sexual behaviour and ovulaton. In: Fuxe K, Gustafsson JA, Wetterberg L (eds) Steroid Hormone Regulation of the Brain. Pergamon Press, New York, pp 15–29

Mendelson WB, Gillin JC, Wyatt RJ (1977) Sexual physiology and schizophrenia. Acta Scientifica Venezolana 28:417–425

Moldin SO (2000) Gender and schizophrenia: an overview. In: Frank E (ed) Gender and Its Effects on Psychopathology. American Psychiatric Press Inc, Washington, DC, pp 169–186

Mueser KT, Bellack AS, Morrison RL, Wixted JT (1990 a) Social competence in schizophrenia: premorbid adjustment, social skill, and domains of functioning. J Psychiatr Res 24:51–63

Mueser KT, Yarnold PR, Levinson DF, Singh H, Bellack AS, Kee K, Morrison RL, Yadalam KG (1990 b) Prevalence of substance abuse in schizophrenia: demographic and clinical correlates. Schizophrenia Bull 16:31–56

Mueser KT, Yarnold PR, Bellack AS (1992) Diagnostic and demographic correlates of substance abuse in schizophrenia and major affective disorder. Acta Psychiatr Scand 85:48–55

Opjordsmoen S (1991) Long-term clinical outcome of schizophrenia with special reference to gender differences. Acta Psychiatr Scand 83:307–313

Riecher-Rössler A, Häfner H, Stumbaum M, Maurer K, Schmidt R (1994 a) Can estradiol modulate schizophrenic symptomatology? Schizophrenia Bull 20:203–214

Riecher-Rössler A, Häfner H, Dütsch-Strobel A, Oster M, Stumbaum M, van Gülick-Bailer M, Löffler W (1994 b) Further evidence for a specific role of estradiol in schizophrenia? Biol Psychiatry 36:492–495

Rosenfield S (2000) Gender and dimensions of the self: implications for internalizing and externalizing behavior. In: Frank E (ed) Gender and Its Effects on Psychopathology. American Psychopathological Association Series. American Psychiatric Press Inc, Washington, DC, pp 23–36

Rutter M, Tizard J, Whitmore K (1970) Education, Health and Behaviour. Longmans, London

Salokangas RKR, Stengard E, Räkköläinen V, Kaljonen IHA (1987) New schizophrenic patients and their families (English summary). In: Reports of Psychiatria Fennica, No. 78. Foundation for Psychiatric Research in Finland, pp 119–216

Seeman MV (1981) Gender and the onset of schizophrenia: neuro-humoral influences. Psychiatr J Univ Ottawa 6:136–138

Seeman MV (1982) Gender differences in schizophrenia. Can J Psychiatry 27:107–112

Seeman MV (1996) The role of estrogen in schizophrenia. J Psychiatry Neurosci 21:123–127

Shepherd M, Oppenheim B, Mitchell S (1971) Childhood Behaviour and Mental Health. University of London Press, London

Shughrue PJ, Lane MV, Merchenthaler I (1997) Comparative distribution of estrogen receptor and X and B MRNA in the rat central nervous system. J Compr Neurol 388:507–525

Soyka M (1994) Sucht und Schizophrenie. Nosologische, klinische und therapeutische Fragen. 1. Alkoholismus und Schizophrenie. Fortschr Neurologische Psychiatrie 62:71–87

Sumner BEH, Fink G (1995) Oestradiol-17β in its positive feedback mode significantly increases 5-HT2a receptor density in the frontal, cingulate and piriform cortex of the female rat. J Physiology 483:52

Sumner BEH, Grant KE, Rosie R, Hegele-Hartung C, Fritzemeier K-H, Fink G (1999) Effects of tamoxifen on serotonin transporter and 5-hydroxytryptamine$_{2A}$ receptor binding sites and mRNA levels in the brain of ovariectomized rats with or without acute estradiol replacement. Mol Brain Res 73:119–128

Van Os J, Howard R, Takei N, Murray R (1995) Increasing age is a risk factor for psychosis in the elderly. Soc Psychiatry Psychiatr Epidemiol 30:161–164

Walker EF, Weinstein J, Baum K, Neumann CS (1995) Antecedents of schizophrenia: moderating effects of development and biological sex. In: Häfner H, Gattaz WF (eds) Search for the Causes of Schizophrenia, Vol III. Springer, Berlin Heidelberg, pp 21–42

Weber I (1996) Lebenszufriedenheit einer Kohorte Schizophrener 15,5 Jahre nach stationärer Aufnahme. Doctoral thesis for a Doctor scientiarum humanarum of the Mannheim Faculty of Clinical Medicine of the Ruprecht Karls University of Heidelberg

Weiser M, Reichenberg A, Rabinowitz J, Kaplan Z, Mark M, Nahon D, Davidson M (2000) Gender differences in premorbid cognitive performance in a national cohort of schizophrenic patients. Schizophrenia Res 45:185–190

WHO-World Health Organization (1988) Psychiatric Disability Assessment Schedule (WHO/DAS). WHO, Geneva

Wing JK, Cooper JE, Sartorius N (1974) Measurement and classification of psychiatric symptoms: An instruction manual for the PSE and CATEGO program. Cambridge University Press, London

Woolley CS, McEwen BS (1994) Estradiol regulates hippocampal dendritic spine density via an N-Methyl-D-aspartate receptor-dependent mechanism. J Neurosci 14:7680–7687

Section 4
Genetics

Searching for inherited causes for schizophrenia: has progress been made?

Lynn E. DeLisi

Department of Psychiatry, New York University, New York, USA

This book currently outlines the conclusions drawn subsequent to the 5th convening of investigators on "Search for the Causes of Schizophrenia". In all previous such volumes, the prevailing views on genetic causes have been reviewed. In the first, published in 1987, Kringlen concluded that "schizophrenia involves the interaction of biological and environmental factors. However, neither genetically nor environmentally oriented research has yet been able to identify the etiological factors that are necessary and/or sufficient for the disorder ... but are the genes necessary?". In that same year McGuffin and colleagues remained perplexed over which clinical sets of symptoms are inherited and thus valid phenotypes for further genetic studies, and Baron provided cautious optimism to his conclusion that because mathematical genetic modeling confirms the heritable component for schizophrenia, new technology provided by the gene marker strategy will be the way to make progress. In 1991, I too was optimistic in my review of the field and concluded that the "reverse genetics" approach could be applied to studies of families with schizophrenia without knowledge of what a gene for this disorder would be doing, and without a prior working hypothesis (DeLisi and Lovett 1991). In fact, during this period excitement had already been generated by several linkages to regions of the genome being reported for schizophrenia and affective psychoses without ever identifying a clear responsible gene or its mechanism (reviewed in DeLisi et al. 2000). Yet the most recent publications that use this technology to identify candidate genes as ones within regions of linkage (Straub et al. 2002, a 6p locus for dysbindin; Steffanssen et al. 2002, an 8p locus for Neuregulin; and Chumakov et al. 2002 for an unnamed gene on chromosome 13q) have not shown definitive findings, nor do they demonstrate that a mutation in a gene is segregating with schizophrenia within families.

In the last "Search for Causes" meeting, Owen concluded that at least 2 genes, one for the 5HT2a and another for the DRD3 receptors, have been found to at least "confer a small degree of susceptibility" on the basis of DNA sequence association studies (Owen 1999). Yet despite this, 4 years later, when he and Harrison review the literature (2003), these are not among the candidate genes they chose as noteworthy.

Have linkage and association studies proven to be true? And if so, why do they not advance the field further or show consistent patterns across the numerous studies being performed worldwide (see Tables 1a and b and 2)? While statistically significant findings are produced, genes within these candi-

Table 1a. Genome-wide scans: the 4 highest positive chromosomal regions in each independent published report on schizophrenia. n = # of families

Study, et al.	n =	1p	1q	2p	2q	3q	4p	4q	5p	5q	6p	6q	7p	7q	8p	9q	10p
Moises (1995)	5	–	–	+	+	–	+	+	–	–	–	–	–	–	–	–	–
Blouin (1998)	54	–	–	–	–	–	–	–	–	–	–	–	–	–	+	–	–
Faraone (1998)	43	–	–	+	–	–	–	–	–	–	–	+	+	–	–	–	+
Kaufmann (1998)	30	–	–	–	–	–	–	–	–	–	+	–	–	+	+	–	
Levinson (1998)/ Mowry (2000)	71	–	–	–	+	–	–	+	–	–	–	–	–	–	–	+	–
Shaw (1998)/ DeLisi (2002)	301	–	–	+	+	–	–	–	–	–	–	–	–	–	–	–	+
Williams (1999)	138	–	–	–	–	–	+	–	–	–	–	–	–	–	–	–	–
Brzustowicz (2000)	22	–	+	+	–	–	–	–	–	–	–	–	–	+	–	–	–
Garver (2001)	30	+	+	–	–	–	–	–	+	–	–	–	–	–	–	–	–
Gurling (2001)	13	–	+	–	–	–	–	–	–	+	–	–	–	+	–	–	–
Schwab (2000)	72	–	–	–	–	–	–	–	–	+	+	–	–	–	–	–	+
Paunio/Ekelund (2001)	238	–	+	–	+	–	–	–	–	–	+	–	–	–	–	–	–
Bailer (2002)	5	–	–	–	–	++	–	–	–	–	–	+	–	–	–	–	–
Straub (2002)	265	–	–	–	–	–	–	–	–	+	+	–	–	–	+	–	+

date chromosomal regions (including the ones mentioned above) have yet to be identified that convey any moderate susceptibility for psychosis, nor have the studies completed thus far shed any light on how the disorder is transmitted and what is transmitted. The challenge is to now determine the best approach that will lead to progress over the coming years.

If it is as Owen concluded in 1999 that large, "well-characterized patient samples, the meta-analyses of combined data-sets, and combined laboratory analyses" should yield more definitive findings, then examining these specific pursuits should be convincing. Yet they are all as inconsistent as the results from small data sets by themselves. Both Badner and Gershon (2002) and Lewis and colleagues (in press) have conducted meta-analyses on overlapping set of samples using different mathematical methods and obtaining inconsistent results (see Table 3). Levinson additionally has organized two combined consistent laboratory marker studies for multiple independent family cohorts with schizophrenia in an attempt to confirm already significant findings on smaller data sets. Yet these large datasets fail to yield more robust findings or confirm other findings (Levinson et al. 2000, 2002).

An alternative view must be considered. Vallada and Collier (1999) in the last "Search for Causes" unknowingly may have uncovered such a mechanism

Table 1 b. Genome-wide scans: the 4 highest positive chromosomal regions in each independent published report on schizophrenia. n = # of families

Study, et al.	n =	Chromosome Arms										
		10q	11q	12q	13q	14q	15p	18q	20	22q	Xp	Xq
Moises (1995)	5	–	–	–	–	–	–	–	–	–	–	–
Blouin (1998)	54	–	–	–	+	+	–	–	–	+	–	–
Faraone (1998)	43	–	–	–	–	–	–	–	–	–	–	–
Kaufmann (1998)	30	–	–	–	–	–	+	–	–	–	–	–
Levinson (1998)/ Mowry (2000)	71	+	–	–	–	–	–	–	–	–	–	–
Shaw (1998)/ DeLisi (2002)	301	–	–	+	–	–	–	–	–	–	–	–
Williams (1999)	138	–	–	–	–	–	–	+	–	–	+	+
Brzustowicz (2000)	22	–	–	–	+	–	–	–	–	–	–	–
Garver (2001)	21	–	–	–	–	–	–	–	+	–	–	–
Gurling (2001)	13	–	+	–	–	–	–	–	–	–	–	–
Schwab (2001)	72	–	–	–	–	–	–	–	–	+	–	–
Paunio/Ekelund (2001)	238	–	–	–	–	–	–	–	–	–	+	–
Bailer (2002)	5	–	–	+	–	–	–	–	–	–	–	–
Straub (2002)	265	–	–	–	–	–	–	–	–	–	–	–

worth further pursuit. While these authors were led to a possible chromosome 22q locus through linkage, they acknowledged that despite a large combined collaborative cohort to examine this region (Gill et al. 1998), the results remain inconclusive. Based on data from this study showing significantly stronger linkage to maternally inherited than paternally inherited alleles, they posed the hypothesis that genomic imprinting (i.e., epigenetic gene modification of one, but not the other parental alleles) may be involved. Others have also focused on epigenetic gene modification, but none of the hypotheses proposed suggest rules for transmission and modification. The evidence that imprinting may be involved in schizophrenia is weak if at all present (Ohara 2001; McGinnis et al. 1999; DeLisi et al. 2000), but differential parental transmission is not the only evidence that epigenetic modification of gene expression has taken place. It has been suggested that the pattern of weak linkages reported along with a non-Mendelian form of inheritance, may in itself be evidence that epigenetic transmission is occurring (i.e., inheritance of DNA methylation patterns) rather than actual DNA sequence variation (e.g., Raykan et al. 2001).

This current (2003) search for causes, as well as the last (Tsuang et al. 1999; Maier et al. 1999) emphasizes alternative phenotypes that are inherited other than those that make up the clinical manifestations of disease, such as brain structural patterns or cognitive defects. New methods to mathematically per-

Table 2. Schizophrenia genome-wide screens of genetic isolate populations chromosomal arms with reported suggestions of linkage

	n	1p	1q	2p	2q	3q	4q	5q	6p	6q	7q	8p	9q	13q	20p	Xp
(Iceland) Moises et al.	162*	–	–	–	–	–	–	–	–	–	–	+	–	–	–	–
(Finland)** Hovatta et al. (1999)	20	–	+	–	–	–	+	–	–	–	–	–	+	–	–	+
(Finland)*** Ekelund/Paunio et al. (2001)	238	–	+	–	+	–	–	+	–	–	+	–	–	–	+	–
(N Sweden) Wetterberg	1	–	–	–	–	–	–	–	–	–	–	+	–	–	–	–
(N Sweden) Lindholm	1	–	–	–	–	–	–	–	+	–	–	–	–	–	–	–
(Palau) Coon et al. (1998) Camp et al.	7	–	–	+	–	+	–	+	–	–	–	–	–	+	–	–
(Costa Rica) DeLisi et al. (2002)	98	+	–	+	–	–	–	+	–	–	–	+	–	–	–	–
(E Quebec) Maziade et al.	21								–	+				–	–	
(Bantu/S Africa) Riley et al.	16									–				–		
(Azures) Pato et al.												+				

* Parent-child pairs, ** Northeastern Finland, *** All Finland

Table 3. Meta-analyses/multicenter studies of schizophrenia genome-wide scans

Study	# Pedigrees	Linked regions
Gill et al. 1996	445	22q
Levinson et al. 2000	735	6q and 10p, NOT 5q, 13q
Levinson et al. 2002	779	NOT 1q
Badner and Gershon 2002	681	8p, 13q and 22q
Levinson submitted	1208	2p-q, 3p, 11q, 5q, 20p, 8p, 6p and 22q

form genetic linkage studies to such quantitative phenotypes are now also "in vogue" (Almasy and Blangero 2001). However, it is thus far unclear as to whether any of these so-called "intermediate phenotypes" are heritable to the same degree as the diagnosis of schizophrenia. Very few studies of these markers have been completed in families with multiple affected individuals so that it can be determined whether all individuals that have the illness within families also have the putative candidate heritable trait. Most studies are performed to show that siblings of individuals with schizophrenia appear to demonstrate more abnormalities in cognitive functioning particularly than controls, but how these are related to the genetic phenotype for a psychosis is unclear (e.g., Cannon et al. 1994; Shedlack et al. 1997; Freedman et al. 1999; Saoud et al. 2000; Staal et al. 2000; Egan et al. 2001a,b; Krabbendam et al. 2001).

There are two other approaches to finding genes that have been also currently popular. One is to examine animal "models" for specific quantitative traits that are thought to be intermediate phenotypes for schizophrenia, such as evoked potential disturbances (e.g., Simosky et al. 2001). DNA from mice bred to transmit these deficits at a high probability is then examined in a genome-wide search for linkage to the trait. Once a candidate quantitative locus (QTL) is found, the comparable human chromosomal locus can then be examined for linkage to schizophrenia in human studies. While this strategy seems novel, one has to give credence to the notion that an animal model may be relevant to schizophrenia, and this point is certainly refutable.

The final approach currently in its infancy is the application of the new microarray technology to study the expression of a large number of genes at once. Microarrays can be custom made for any set of genes possible, i.e., those for neuronal development and/or neurochemical transmission. Thus far, a handful of microarray studies have been published (Table 4), with conflicting results, partly because these "fishing expeditions" are hard to replicate, each has assembled a different set of gene arrays, and the selection of postmortem brain regions used across studies varied. This seems an informable task to produce results of any significance if one considers that the numbers of postmortem brains used in these studies are small, that there is tremendous human variation and heterogeneity even within those individuals diagnosed as schizophrenia, and that there are likely to be age and sex differences in gene expression.

Where should we go from here? First one needs to reflect on the true facts about schizophrenia and construct an hypothesis about the genetic transmission that is consistent with these facts:

▌ psychosis clearly runs in families, but only weakly so. That is, 50% of monozygotic twins will be discordant for schizophrenia and the risk to secondary relatives of a proband with illness falls off dramatically to only about 2% (Gottesman and Shields 1982). If inheritance is non-Mendelian, there must be other mechanisms other than transmission of a DNA sequence variation that are operative.

▌ Environmental causes have been ruled out as primary (Kety et al. 1982; Crow and Done 1986) despite years of searching.

▌ Schizophrenia is clearly a brain disease, the primary initiation of which is so far unrecognized; but many heterogeneous brain structural and functional changes have been detected in patients with schizophrenia. Cortical abnormalities that are frontal and temporal with asymmetric distribution interacting with the normal human cerebral asymmetries are present, as are non-localized sub-cortical ventricular enlargement. The distribution of these anomalies varies among patients with schizophrenia, but they are de-

Table 4. Published studies of differential brain expression using microarrays

Study	Brain regions	Genes found
Mimmack et al. 2002	Prefrontal cortex Stanley brains Japan/N Zeal	Apo L1, L2 and L4: 22q12 Replicated
Mirnics et al. 2000/2001	Prefrontal cortex	RGS4 (Regulator of G-protein Signaling) decreased: 1q21–22
Hakak et al. 2001	Prefrontal cortex	1) MAL (myelin and lymphocyte protein) 2) Gelsolin (actin-capping protein) 3) MAG (myelin associated glycoprotein) 4) Transferrin 5) Neuroregulin receptor Her-3 + several others
Vawter et al. 2001	Cerebellum, prefrontal cortex, middle temporal gyrus Stanley brains	1) tyrosine 3-monooxygenase/tryptophan 5-monooxygenase activation protein 2) Eta polypeptide 3) Sialyltransferase proteasome subunit alpha type 1 4) Ubiquitin carboyl-terminal esterase L1 5) Solute carrier family 10, member 1
Hemby et al. 2002	Temporal L. EC cortex- layer II stellate neurons	G-protein subunit ialpha 1 Glutamate receptor 3 N-methyl-D-aspartate receptor 1 Synaptophysin Sensory nerve action potentials 23 and 25

scribed early in its course, may be present before the onset of clinical symptoms, and sometimes have a progressive component during some portion of the course of illness (reviewed by Shenton et al. 2001).

- There is a characteristic age of onset of the psychotic symptoms in early adulthood and correlated among sibling pairs; but the course and type of symptoms vary considerably among related individuals and rarely breed true. However, there is some data to show that thought disorder (specifically disorganized language production) is correlated among pairs of ill siblings (e.g., Loftus et al. 1999).
- There is indication from many studies that, despite the early adulthood first recognition of illness, there are subtle childhood traits that can be seen by both retrospective and prospective cohort studies to define vulnerability for later schizophrenia (Walker and Lewine 1990; Walker et al. 1993).
- There are sex differences to many aspects of the above (e.g., as reviewed by DeLisi et al. 1989).

Any hypothesis must then draw on the above facts and develop new approaches in the laboratory. To date, one cannot conclude that the genetic

Table 5. Current reported candidate genes based on initial linkage studies showing linkages to regions containing these genes

Gene	Location
COMT	22q11
DISC 1 and DISC 2	1q42.1
Dysbindin	6p22–24
G72	13q34
Neuregulin	8p21–22
Nicotinic acetylcholine Receptor subunit-alpha 7 (CHRNA7)	15q13–14
Protocadherin X-Y	Xq21.3/Yp11

linkage studies have been profitable and in fact, they may have led us on many false pursuits. But what seems clear is that 1) something is happening early in brain development to cause the normal brain structure to deviate. This is likely to occur differently in males and females and be familial. 2) Epigenetic turning on and off of crucial genes for brain development orchestrated during specific time periods somehow takes place. The control of this process is the subject of much research in neuroscience and is the key to what differentiates the human brain from other non-human primates and other animals, since the majority of genes are quite conserved in DNA structure across species (reviewed in Schwartz 1999).

Although, this may be considered a pessimistic conclusion, I predict that we will be searching for the cause for schizophrenia for many years to come. It seems clear that much more knowledge needs to accrue about the precise differentiation of the normal human brain before we can understand its pathology. However, on a more positive note, if individuals at high risk for schizophrenia can be recognized early in the course of the brain changes, there may be therapeutic modifications that can be developed to prevent the subsequent adverse events.

References

Almasy L, Blangero J (2001) Endophenotypes as quantitative risk factors for psychiatric disease: rationale and study design. American Journal of Medical Genetics 105(1):42–44

Badner JA, Gershon ES (2002) Meta-analysis of whole-genome linkage scans of bipolar disorder and schizophrenia. Molecular Psychiatry 7(4):405–411

Bailer U, Leisch F, Meszaros K, Lenzinger E, Willinger U, Strobl R et al (2002) Genome scan for susceptibility loci for schizophrenia and bipolar disorder. Biological Psychiatry 52(1):40–52

Blouin J-L, Dombroski BA, Nath SW, Lasseter VK, Wolyniec PS, Nestadt G (1998) Schizophrenia susceptibility loci on chromosomes 13q32 and 8p21. Nature Genetics 20:70–73

Brzustowicz LM, Hodgkinson KA, Chow EW, Honer WG, Bassett AS (2000) Location of a major susceptibility locus for familial schizophrenia on chromosome 1q21–q22. Science 288(5466):678–682

Cannon TD, Zorrilla LE, Shrasel D, Gur RE, Gur RC, Marco EJ, Moberg P, Price RA (1994) Neuropsychological functioning in siblings discordant for schizophrenia and healthy volunteers. Arch Gen Psychiatry 51:651–661

Chumakov I, Blumenfeld M, Guerassimenko O, Cavarec L, Palicio M, Abderrahim H et al (2002) Genetic and physiological data implicating the new human gene G72 and the gene for D-amino acid oxidase in schizophrenia. Proceedings of the National Academy of Sciences of the United States of America 99(21):13675–1680

Coon H, Myles-Worsley M, Tiobech J, Hoff M, Rosenthal J, Bennett P et al (1998) Evidence for a chromosome 2p13-14 schizophrenia susceptibility locus in families from Palau, Micronesia. Molecular Psychiatry 3:521–527

Crow TJ, Done DJ (1986) Age of onset of schizophrenia in siblings: a test of the contagion hypothesis. Psychiatry Research 18(2):107–117

DeLisi LE, Craddock NJ, Detera-Wadleigh S, Foroud T, Gejman P, Kennedy JL et al (2000) Update of chromosomal locations for psychiatric disorders: report of the Interim Meeting of Chromosome Workshop Chairpersons from the VIIth World Congress of Psychiatric Genetics. Neuropsychiatric Genetics 96:434–449

DeLisi LE, Lovett M (1991) The reverse genetics approach to the etiology of schizophrenia. In: Häfner H, Gattaz WF (eds) Search for the Causes of Schizophrenia, Issue 2. Springer, Heidelberg, pp 144–170

DeLisi LE, Mesen A, Rodriguez C, Bertheau A, LaPrade B et al (2002b) Genome-wide scan for linkage to schizophrenia in a Spanish-origin cohort from Costa Rica. American Journal of Medical Genetics (Neuropsychiatric Genetics) 114:497–508

DeLisi LE, Razi K, Stewart J, Relja M, Shields G, Smith AB et al (2000) No evidence for a parent-of-Origin effect detected in the pattern of inheritance of schizophrenia. Biological Psychiatry 48:706–709

DeLisi LE, Shaw SH, Crow TJ, Shields G, Smith AB, Larach VW et al (2002a) A Genome-wide scan for linkage to chromosomal regions in 382 sibling pairs with schizophrenia or schizoaffective disorder. American Journal of Psychiatry 159: 803–812

Egan MF, Goldberg TE, Gscheidle T, Weirich M, Rawlings R, Hyde TM, Bigelow L, Weinberger DR (2001a) Relative risk for cognitive impairments in siblings of patients with schizophrenia. Biol Psychiatry 50:98–107

Egan MF, Goldberg TE, Kolachana BS, Callicott JH, Mazzanti CM, Straub RE, Goldman D, Weinberger DR (2001b) Effect of COMT Val108/158 Met genotype on frontal lobe function and risk for schizophrenia. Proceedings of the National Academy of Sciences of the United States of America 98(12):6917–6922

Ekelund J, Hovatta I, Parker A, Paunio T, Varilo T, Martin R et al (2001) Chromosome 1 loci in Finnish schizophrenia families. Human Molecular Genetics 10(15):1611–1617

Faraone SV, Matise T, Svrakic D, Pepple J, Malaspina D, Suarez B et al (1998) Genome scan of European-American schizophrenia pedigrees: results of the NIMH Genetics Initiative and Millenium Consortium. Am J of Medical Genetics (Neuropsychiatric Genetics) 81:290–295

Freedman R, Adler LE, Leonard S (1999) Alternative phenotypes for the complex genetics of schizophrenia. Biological Psychiatry 45(5):551–558

Garver DL, Holcomb J, Mapua FM, Wilson R, Barnes B (2001) Schizophrenia spectrum disorders: an autosomal-wide scan in multiplex pedigrees. Schizophrenia Research 52(3):145–160

Gill M, Vallada H, Collier D, Sham P, Holmans P, Murray R et al (1996) A combined analysis of D22S278 marker alleles in affected sib-pairs: support for a susceptibility locus for schizophrenia at chromosome 22q12. Schizophrenia Collaborative Linkage Group (Chromosome 22). American Journal of Medical Genetics 67:40–45

Gottesman II, Shields J (1982) Schizophrenia: The Epigenetic Puzzle. Cambridge University Press, New York

Gurling HMD, Kalsi G, Brynjolfson J, Sigmundsson T, Sherrington R, Mankoo BS et al (2001) Genome-wide genetic linkage analysis confirms the presence of susceptibility loci for schizophrenia on chromosomes 1q32.2, 5q33.2 and 8p21–22 and provides support for linkage to schizophrenia, on chromosomes 11q23.3–24 and 20q12.1–11.23. Am J of Human Genetics 68:661–673

Hakak Y, Walker JR, Li C, Wong WH, Davis KL, Buxbaum JD, Haroutunian V, Fienberg AA (2001) Genome-wide expression analysis reveals dysregulation of myelination-related genes in chronic schizophrenia. Proceedings of the National Academy of Sciences of the United States of America 98(8):4746–4751

Harrison PJ, Owen MJ (2003) Genes for schizophrenia? Recent findings and their pathophysiological implications. The Lancet 361:417–419

Hemby SE, Ginsberg SD, Brunk B, Arnold SE, Trojanowski JQ, Eberwine JH (2002) Gene expression profile for schizophrenia: discrete neuron transcription patterns in the entorhinal cortex. Archives of General Psychiatry 59(7):631–640

Hovatta I, Varilo T, Suvisaari J, Terwilliger JD, Ollikainen V, Arajarvi R, Juvonen H et al (1999) A genome-wide screen for schizophrenia genes in an isolated Finnish subpopulation, suggesting multiple susceptibility loci. American J of Human Genetics 65:11114–11124

Kaufmann CA, Suarez B, Malaspina D, Pepple J, Svrakic D, Markel PD, Meyer J, Zambuto CT, Schmitt K, Cox D, Matise T, Harkavy-Friedman JM, Hampe C, Lee H, Shore D, Wynne D, Faraone SV, Tsuang MT, Cloninger CR (1998) NIMH genetics initiative millenium schizophrenia consortium: linkage analysis of African-American pedigrees. Am J of Medical Genetics (Neuropsychiatric Genetics) 81:282–289

Kety SS (1983) Mental illness in the biological and adoptive relatives of schizophrenic adoptees: findings relevant to genetic and environmental factors. Am J of Psychiatry 140:720–727

Krabbendam L, Marcelis M, Delespaul P, Jolles J, Van Os J (2001) Single or multiple familial cognitive risk factors in schizophrenia? Am J of Med Genetics 105:183–188

Kringlen E (1987) Contributions of genetic studies on schizophrenia. In: Häfner H, Gattaz WF, Janzarik W (eds) Search for the Causes of Schizophrenia. Springer, Berlin Heidelberg, pp 123–142

Levinson DF, Holmans PA, Laurent C, Riley B, Pulver AE, Gejman PV, Schwab SG et al (2002) No major schizophrenia locus detected on chromosome 1q in a large multicenter sample. Science 296(5568):739–741

Levinson DF, Holmans P, Straun RE, Owen MJ, Wildenauer DB, Gejman PV et al (2000) Multicenter linkage study of schizophrenia candidate regions on chromosomes 5q, 6q, 10p, and 13q: schizophrenia linkage collaborative group III. American Journal of Human Genet 67(3):652–663

Levinson DF, Mahtani MM, Nancarrow DJ, Brown DM, Kruglyak L, Andrew K, Hayward NK (1998) Genome scan of schizophrenia. The American J of Psychiatry 155:741–750

Lewis CM, Levinson DF, Wise LH, DeLisi LE, Straub RE, Hovatta I, Williams NM, Schwab SG, Pulver AE, Faraone SV et al (2003) Genome scan meta-analysis of schizophrenia and bipolar disorder Part II: Schizophrenia. American J of Human Genet 73(1):34–48

Lindholm E, Ekholm B, Shaw S, Jalonen P, Johansson G, Pettersson U, Sherrington R, Adolfsson R, Jazin E (2001) A schizophrenia-susceptibility locus at 6q25, in one of the world's largest reported pedigrees. American Journal of Human Genetics 69(1):96–105

Maier W (1999) Discussion: current status of the search for genes accounting for schizophrenia. In: Gattaz WF, Häfner H (eds) Search for the Causes of Schizophrenia, Vol IV Balance of the Century. Steinkopff, Darmstadt Berlin, pp 215–220

Maziade M, Roy MA, Rouillard E, Bissonnette L, Fournier JP, Roy A, Garneau Y, Montgrain N, Potvin A, Cliché D, Dion C, Wallot H, Fournier A, Nicole L, Lavallee JC, Merette C (2001) A search for specific and common susceptibility loci for schizophrenia and bipolar disorder: a linkage study in 13 target chromosomes. Molecular Psychiatry 6(6):684–693

Maziade M, Fournier A, Phaneuf D, Cliché D, Fournier JP, Roy MA, Merette C (2002) Chromosome 1q12–q22 linkage results in eastern Quebec families affected by schizophrenia. American Journal of Medical Genetics 114(1):51–55

McInnis MG, Crow TJ, McMahon FJ, Ross CA, DeLisi LE (1999) Anticipation in schizophrenia: a review and reconsideration. American Journal of Medical Genetics (Neuropsychiatric Genetics) 88:686–693

Mimmack ML, Ryan M, Baba H, Navarro-Ruiz J, Iritani S, Faull RL, McKenna PJ, Jones PB, Arai H, Starkey M, Emson PC, Bahn S (2002) Gene expression analysis in schizophrenia: reproducible up-regulation of several members of the apolipoprotein L family located in a high-susceptibility locus for schizophrenia on chromosome 22. Proceedings of the National Academy of Sciences of the United States of America 99(7):4680–4685

Mirnics K, Middleton FA, Lewis DA, Levitt P (2001) The human genome: gene expression profiling and schizophrenia. American Journal of Psychiatry 158(9):1384

Mirnics K, Middleton FA, Marquez A, Lewis DA, Levitt P (2000) Molecular characterization of schizophrenia viewed by microarray analysis of gene expression in prefrontal cortex. Neuron 28:53–67

Moises HW, Yang L, Kristbjarnarson H, Wiese C, Byerley W, Macciardi F et al (1995) An international two-stage genome-wide search for schizophrenia susceptibility genes. Nature Genetics 11:321–324

Mowry BJ, Ewen KR, Nancarrow DJ, Lennon DP, Nertney DA, Jones HL et al (2000) Second stage of a genome scan of schizophrenia: study of five positive regions in an expanded sample. American Journal of Medical Genetics 96(6):864–869

Niculescu AB, Segal DS, Kuczenski R, Barrett T, Hauger RL, Kelsoe JR (2000) Identifying a series of genes for mania and psychosis: a convergent functional genomics approach. Physiological Genomics 4:83–91

Ohara K (2001) Anticipation, imprinting, trinucleotide repeat expansions and psychoses. Progress in Neuro-Psychopharmacology & Biological Psychiatry 25(1):167–192

Owen MJ (1999) Searching for susceptibility genes in schizophrenia. In: Gattaz WF, Häfner H (eds) Search for the Causes of Schizophrenia, Vol IV Balance of the Century. Steinkopff, Darmstadt Berlin, pp 169–180

Paunio T, Ekelund J, Varilo T, Parker A, Hovatta I, Turunen JA et al (2001) Genome-wide scan in a nationwide study sample of schizophrenia families in Finland reveals susceptibility loci on chromosomes 2q and 5q. Human Molecular Genetics 10(26):3037–3048

Rakyan VK, Preis J, Morgan HD, Whitelaw E (2001) The marks, mechanisms and memory of epigenetic states in mammals. Biochem Journal 356:1–10

Riley BP, Lin MW, Mogudi-Carter M, Jenkins T, Williamson R, Powell JF, Collier D, Murray R (1998) Failure to exclude a possible schizophrenia susceptibility locus on chromosome 13q14.1–q32 in southern African Bantu-speaking families. Psychiatric Genetics 8(3):155–162

Saoud M, d'Amato T, Gutknecht C, Triboulet P, Bertaud JP, Marie-Cardine M, Dalery J, Rochet T (2000) Neuropsychological deficit in siblings discordant for schizophrenia. Schizophrenia Bulletin 26:893–902

Schizophrenia Collaborative Linkage Group for Chromosome 22 (1998) A transmission disequilibrium and linkage analysis of D22S278 marker alleles in 574 families: further support for a susceptibility locus for schizophrenia at 22q12. Schizophrenia Research 32:115–121

Schwab SG, Hallmeyer J, Albus M, Lerer B, Eckstein GN, Borrmann M et al (2000) A genome-wide autosomal screen for schizophrenia susceptibility loci in 71 families with affected siblings: support for loci on chromosome 10p and 6. Molecular Psychiatry 5:638–649

Shaw SH, Kelly M, Smith AB, Shields G, Hopkins PJ, Loftus J et al (1998) A genome-wide search for schizophrenia susceptibility genes. Am J Med Genetics 81(5):364–376

Shedlack K, Lee G, Sakuma M, Xie SH, Kushner M, Pepple J et al (1997) Language processing and memory in ill and well siblings from multiplex families affected with schizophrenia. Schizophr Research 25(1):43–52

Shenton ME, Dickey CC, Frumin M, McCarley RW (2001) A review of MRI findings in schizophrenia. Schizophrenia Research 49:1–52

Simosky JK, Stevens KE, Kem WR, Freedman R (2001) Intragastric DMXB-A, an alpha7 nicotinic agonist, improves deficient sensory inhibition in DBA/2 mice. Biological Psychiatry 50(7):493–500

Stefansson H, Sarginson J, Kong A, Yates P, Steinthorsdottir V, Gudfinnsson E et al (2003) Association of neuregulin 1 with schizophrenia confirmed in a Scottish population. American Journal of Human Genetics 72(1):83–87

Stefansson H, Sigurdsson E, Steinthorsdottir V, Bjornsdottir S, Sigmundsson T, Ghosh S et al (2002) Neuregulin 1 and susceptibility to schizophrenia. American Journal of Human Genetics 71(4):877–892

Staal WG, Hijman R, Hulshoff PHE, Kahn RS (2000) Neuropsychological dysfunctions in siblings discordant for schizophrenia. Psychiatry Research 95:227–235

Straub RE, Jiang Y, MacLean CJ, Ma Y, Webb BT, Myakishev MV et al (2002) Genetic variation in the 6p22.3 gene DTNBP1, the human ortholog of the mouse dysbindin gene, is associated with schizophrenia. American Journal of Human Genetics 71(2):337–348

Straub RE, MacLean CJ, Ma Y, Webb BT, Myakishev MV, Harris-Kerr C et al (2002) Genome-wide scans of three independent sets of 90 Irish multiplex schizophrenia families and follow-up of selected regions in all families provides evidence for multiple susceptibility genes. Molecular Psychiatry 7(6):542–559

Tsuang MT, Seidman LJ, Faraone SV (1999) New approaches to the genetics of schizophrenia: neuropsychological and neuroimaging studies of nonpsychotic first degree relatives of people with schizophrenia. In: Gattaz WF, Häfner H (eds) Search for the Causes of Schizophrenia, Vol IV Balance of the Century. Steinkopff, Darmstadt Berlin, pp 191–207

Vallada HP, Collier DA (1999) Genetics of schizophrenia – new findings. In: Gattaz WF, Häfner H (eds) Search for the Causes of Schizophrenia, Vol IV Balance of the Century. Steinkopff, Darmstadt Berlin, pp 181–189

Vawter MP, Crook JM, Hyde TM, Kleinman JE, Weinberger DR, Becker KG, Freed WJ (2002) Microarray analysis of gene expression in the prefrontal cortex in schizophrenia: a preliminary study. Schizophrenia Research 58(1):11–20

Vawter MP, Barrett T, Cheadle C, Sokolov BP, Wood WH 3rd, Donovan DM, Webster M, Freed WJ, Becker KG (2001) Application of cDNA microarrays to examine gene expression differences in schizophrenia. Brain Research Bulletin 55(5):641–650

Walker EF, Grimes KE, Davis DM, Smith AJ (1993) Childhood precursors of schizophrenia: facial expressions of emotion. Am J Psychiatry 150(11):1654–1660

Walker E, Lewine RJ (1990) Prediction of adult-onset schizophrenia from childhood home movies of the patients. Am J Psychiatry 147(8):1052–1056

Williams NM, Rees MI, Holmans P, Norton N, Cardno AG, Jones LA et al (1999) A two-stage genome scan for schizophrenia susceptibility genes in 196 affected sibling pairs. Human Molecular Genetics 8:1729–1739

▌Gene expression in psychotic disorders:

dissecting the genetic basis of complex neuropsychiatric disorders

SABINE BAHN

University of Cambridge and Babraham Institute, Cambridge, UK

▌ Introduction

Psychiatric disorders are amongst the most widespread diseases. The major psychotic disorders (schizophrenia and bipolar affective disorder) alone affect about 2% of the population worldwide. Due to their early onset and chronic, debilitating course these illnesses are from a healthcare point of view amongst the costliest in the developed world. The mortality for the disorders is also very high, about 10% commit suicide, nevertheless schizophrenia and bipolar affective disorder do not receive the same attention as other major causes of death and ill-health like heart disease and cancer.

The challenge of "cracking" complex neuropsychiatric disorders

The aetiology of schizophrenia and bipolar disorder remains elusive, despite the fact that there is no shortage of hypotheses. Over the years a wide variety of genes, neurotransmitter systems, enzymes etc. have been implicated and genetic loci reportedly associated with increased risk are scattered all over most chromosomes. However, the crucial ingredient that is lacking is reproducible evidence that would support these hypotheses.

The main problem with psychiatric illnesses is the ominous fact that they are "complex". Several or more likely many genes may predispose an individual to develop schizophrenia or bipolar disorder. To complicate matters further it is now widely believed that epigenetic variables such as environmental factors and risk-conferring behaviours/exposures interact with a predisposing genotype to result in the disease phenotype.

The real challenge is to identify and then disentangle these complex, multifactorial components in order to enhance the biological understanding of the disorders and in turn translate new insights into effective strategies for disease diagnosis, prevention and therapy.

A first and crucial step to enhance the understanding of complex neuropsychiatric disorders is to obtain empirical data. As Lars Terenius put it in his summary of the Nobel Symposium, "Schizophrenia: Pathophysiological Mechanisms" back in October 1998 (Terenius 2000): "Without leading theories the brutal approach to search the total human genome seems the most powerful approach".

The draft of the human genome has now been published and a number of expression profiling studies on schizophrenia postmortem brains have been conducted. Although it is early days, there is already some consensus in the observations obtained by different research groups who work on different brain collections. For example, three independent groups have found abnormalities in the expression levels of some myelin-related genes in schizophrenia using microarray technologies (Hakak et al. 2001; Pongrac et al. 2002; Tkachev et al. 2003).

Most will agree that functional genomics and other "-omics" have become fashionable in the molecular biology world. However, not very long ago such approaches were dismissed as "fishing expeditions" and "non-hypothesis driven research" was close to heresy.

This has now changed … "Fishing" is the thing to do these days, either in the form of global expression profiling or by searching for single nucleotide polymorphisms (SNPs) in disease populations.

Sir John Sulston, Nobel laureate and former director of the Sanger Centre, summarised the optimism and hope associated with the Human Genome Project (HGP), when he stated: "Galileo…took us away from the idea that we were the centre of the universe. The theory of evolution took us away from the conviction that we were a unique life form. And this work [on the human genome] will eventually tell us what makes our brains work and therefore our minds. It will tell us what we are."

We now know that there are far fewer genes in the human genome than was originally thought, somewhere between 30 000–40 000 (which is only two times the number of genes found in the nematode worm). Although, as yet we lack a functional understanding for more than half of these genes, few will doubt that the completion of the HGP is likely to mark the beginning of a new era of molecular research and is likely to transform the field of medicine with respect to disease understanding, diagnosis and therapeutic interventions.

Already, microarray technologies offer opportunities to obtain global profiles of all expressed genes and thus facilitate the investigation for differences in transcript expression in disease and control tissue on a very large scale. However, a big deficiency is that most available microarrays do not distinguish splice variants as yet. More importantly, in order to obtain information on functional effects of gene expression changes we have to look at protein levels. Great efforts are now being directed to develop high-throughput proteomics techniques, but we are far off from a "global" protein profiling methodology (not to mention a high-throughput technique that can distinguish the activity status of proteins). Then there are the above mentioned SNP analyses: SNP databases, documenting variations in the genome, are growing at a staggering pace and ultimately should allow for a genome-wide comparison of the distribution of SNPs in normal and disease population, which in turn may point towards disease genes.

The expectation is that the combined application of these global profiling technologies will help to unravel both the genetic and environmental factors that predispose and precipitate complex neuropsychiatric disorders, thus instilling hope that evidence-based hypotheses will (at last) emerge. In turn, this should lead to a greater understanding of the biological basis of the disorders.

The complex neuropsychiatric disorders represent the ultimate challenge for these technologies. At present, no other approach holds as much promise to – eventually – move psychotic illnesses (the archetype of madness) into the realm of a biologically understandable condition and thus lead to de-stigmatisation of these most destructive disorders.

▌ Gene expression profiling with microarrays

With the working draft of the human genome published, the race is now on to identify the genes involved in pathological processes, determine their functional significance, understand their role in complex functional pathways and figure out the role of environmental factors that act on a given genotype to result in a disease phenotype. Until recently, functional studies were mainly performed on a "one gene at a time" basis. However to understand biological networks and pathways a high-throughput and genome-wide approach is needed. Over the last few years microarray technology has attracted increasing interest in the biological sciences (e.g. Lockhart et al. 1996; Welsh et al. 2001). The technique allows a global examination of (almost) all expressed genes that reside in the human genome on two (credit card sized) chips (the Affymetrix U133a+b chips claim to cover 80% of the human genome). Affymetrix Inc. owns a registered trademark, *GeneChip®*, which refers to its high-density array of synthetic oligonucleotides that are immobilised on a glass surface. The photochemical, solid-phase technology used for the generation of a *GeneChip®* provides a high-resolution and precise probe placement that is essential for the high-throughput analyses (*http://www.affymetrix.com*).

An array is basically an orderly arrangement of samples (oligonucleotides or complementary DNA [cDNA]) that provides a medium for the identification of complementary sequences through base-pairing – i.e. the process of hybridisation (Southern et al. 1999). The difference between macro- and microarrays is the size of the sample spots, macroarray spots are 300 microns or larger and microarray spots are less than 200 microns in size (*GeneChip®* spots are as small as 18 microns; *http://www.affymetrix.com*). Microarrays are fabricated by high-speed robotics, generally on glass but sometimes on nylon membranes. DNA arrays are used for a number of applications that range from genotyping, comparative genomic hybridisation to expression analysis. For gene expression analysis, extracted RNA from say disease and control postmortem brains is labelled and then hybridised to the immobilised DNA sequence probes on the array surface followed by high-stringency washes. The signal of the retained labelled "target" from the postmortem brain extract is then measured and compared to control samples thus providing a measure of the abundance of any given mRNA species in the complex sample hence allowing massively parallel gene expression and gene discovery studies.

▐ Gene expression profiling in the postmortem human brain: potentials and pitfalls

Gene expression studies on human brain require specific considerations and caution in order to provide useful and valid information. For any given experiment to be successful it is imperative that intact mRNA can be extracted and analysed from postmortem tissue. During the last decade concern and pessimism have been expressed about mRNA stability. However, it is now clear that as long as sufficient care is taken with respect to postmortem delay, pH (especially in connection with agonal states) and freezing of tissue, good quality mRNA can be readily obtained. Furthermore, with appropriate tissue fixation the structural integrity of postmortem tissue can be preserved allowing for detailed morphological, morphometrical and ultrastructural investigations (e.g. Benes 1988; Ravid et al. 1992; Waldvogel et al. 1999).

Human brain tissue

Postmortem human brain material is a precious and valuable resource and arguably the only way to investigate the molecular abnormalities in complex neuropsychiatric disorders at the molecular level. However, an important factor in determining mRNA integrity is the processing and freezing of the brain postmortem.

When working with postmortem human brain, two of the most critical factors in selecting cases for inclusion in a study are neuropathological verification of the clinical diagnosis (if possible) and the exclusion of brains exhibiting co-existing pathology. When selecting postmortem brains for direct studies it is important to match "normal" and "disease" samples for several factors including age, gender, ethnicity, medications, agonal state, postmortem interval, disease severity, brain region, laterality of the brain and length of fixation (e.g. Benes et al. 1986). Once these criteria have been satisfied the next step is to extract and evaluate RNA integrity.

mRNA stability

Good quality mRNA is an essential prerequisite for the application of all molecular techniques including *in situ* hybridisation, Northern blot analysis, RT-PCR and high throughput mRNA profiling. The belief that postmortem delay critically influences mRNA stability is still a widely held notion despite overwhelming evidence that mRNAs are stable for long periods, at least up to 48 h, in post-mortem tissue (Barton et al. 1993; Harrison et al. 1997; Leonard et al. 1993; Schramm et al. 1999). It is of note that ante- and peri-mortem factors, especially hypoxia, exert a more profound effect. Several studies have demonstrated that hypoxia due to prolonged agonal states significantly reduces mRNA and protein integrity and conten (Harrison et al. 1991, 1995; Kingsbury et al. 1995; Yates et al. 1990). A simple and reliable, albeit crude, indicator of mRNA integrity is brain tissue pH (Kingsbury et al. 1995). In their study, tissue with low pH had reduced or absent mRNA levels showing a strong correlation between tissue pH and mRNA quality. The correlation was consistent both for control and pathological brain tissue. Harrison et al. (1995) confirmed these findings demonstrating that in human and rat brain postmortem interval had a limited impact on mRNA and protein integrity. Brain tissue pH can thus be used as a reliable indicator, superior to clinical assessment of mode of death and agonal state, of RNA quality; intact mRNA being associated with brain pH measurements in the range of pH 6.1–7. Further, brain tissue pH is stable postmortem, is unaffected during freezer storage and is remarkably consistent across different brain areas (Johnston et al. 1997) allowing the tissue pH of any region to predict the mRNA integrity of all areas. If RNA degradation has occurred, samples can occasionally be used for selective RT-PCR-based methods which do not require full length transcripts: this tissue could not be used for comparative mRNA profiling using cDNA microarrays as most membrane arrays require transcripts with intact 3′ ends. Oligonucleotide-based chip technologies (e.g. Affymetrix) may be more amenable but again intact 3′ mRNA is required for first strand cDNA synthesis.

In our laboratories we routinely evaluate the purity and integrity of human brain RNA using the Agilent "lab on a chip" system.

Specificity and reproducibility of observed expression changes

The specificity of any expression change associated with a given disease will have to be critically evaluated in a number of ways:
▮ Crossvalidation of results with independent technologies (highly sensitive and gene-specific quantitative real-time PCR is probably the most reliable technique to validate microarray-derived gene expression results).
▮ Validation of results on a large sample of well-matched brains to overcome inter-individual variability and to allow for the detection of changes that show only small, but potentially important fold-differences. Ideally, also validation on independent brain collections.
▮ To establish that results are not secondary to confounding factors such as drug treatment requires rigorous and appropriate statistical analysis and a full treatment history of investigated patients (and controls).
▮ It would be of great value to investigate whether expression changes say in the psychotic disorders are also present in for example neurodegenerative disorders such as Alzheimer's disease. This could help to unravel overlapping and distinct pathological processes in different neuropsychiatric disorders.

Potential of expression profiling studies for psychiatric practice include 1) disease gene discovery, 2) disease diagnosis, 3) drug discovery: *Pharmacogenomics*, 4) prediction of genetic vulnerability and 5) prediction of drug responsiveness.

Consistent changes in gene expression in the psychotic disorders may help to unravel the aetiology of these disorders. Expression changes could also implicate downstream gene expression pathways, which could be followed up with other technologies, e.g. SNP analysis. On the basis of such empirical evidence new testable hypotheses will emerge which will require classical molecular biological investigations *in vitro* and in animal models to establish the functional significance of gene expression changes. It is likely that expression data will point towards genetic heterogeneity within the disease categories of schizophrenia and bipolar disorder, which will impact on classification of the disorders. On the other hand, expression studies in our own laboratory showed an overlap of expression changes between schizophrenia (SZ) and bipolar disorder (BD) that may point towards genetic relatedness. Most of all there will be opportunities to discover new drug targets and even personalised therapies could be envisaged on the basis of gene expression profiles. If expression changes in the brain can be reproduced in peripheral tissue, especially blood, diagnostic tools could be developed.

▮ Gene expression profiling studies in bipolar disorder and schizophrenia

We recently generated and screened a customised array comprising 300 candidate genes (Mimmack et al. 2002). The genes selected have previously been either implicated in SZ, make conceptual sense in the light of the current understanding of the disorder or reside on high-susceptibility loci of the genome. The high-density array was screened with radioactive cDNA probes taken from the prefrontal cortex of 10 SZ and 10 control individuals. Amongst the significantly changed genes identified was the apolipoprotein L1 (apo L1), which showed a particularly consistent upregulation on the array. We were able to cross-validate the upregulation by quantitative real-time PCR (Q-PCR) on an independent postmortem brain collection, again focusing on the prefrontal cortex. As the apo L1 gene is a member of a family of related genes, including apo L1 through to apo L6, we decided to investigate the expression profiles of all 6 apo L genes and found that apo L2 was even greater and more consistently upregulated. In a next step, we investigated the expression of apo L1 and L2 transcripts in the prefrontal cortices of BD and major depression patients.

Interestingly, the apo L cluster resides on chromosome 22q, one of the two genome regions linked in the whole-genome meta-analysis by Badner and Gershon (Badner and Gershon 2002) to both BD and SZ. Statistical analysis of Q-PCR data obtained from the Stanley Foundation brain collection comprising 15 SZ, 15 BD, 15 major depression and 15 control brains, showed that the apo L2 gene was not only significantly increased in the SZ sample, but also in the BD sample, which did not correlate with antipsychotic treatment or other potential confounders. A multivariate analysis of prefrontal cortex data from the Stanley Foundation brain collection also found the majority of abnormalities observed in SZ brains also present in BD postmortem brains (Knable et al. 2001).

Whilst we undertook our candidate-array study, Hakak et al. (2001) published results from an Affymetrix gene chip analysis and found down-regulation of several myelin-related genes. As apolipoproteins and myelin-related genes are both associated with lipid metabolism, we tried to cross-validate the findings of Hakak et al. and undertook an extensive study investigating oligodendrocyte-, lipid- and cholesterol-related gene expression. We were able to confirm the downregulation of several of the myelin-related genes reported by Hakak et al. and found several other oligodendrocyte- and myelin-related transcripts altered. A further Affymetrix investigation on yet another brain collection as carried out by Mirnics and colleagues who recently reported downregulation of myelin-related genes (Tkachev et al. 2003). Interestingly in our studies, for both the apo L2 and most of the differentially expressed oligodendrocyte- and myelin-related genes, we found a significant overlap of the data dispersion for BD and SZ (unpublished data). For several genes a subpopulation of the BD group appears to behave like the SZ group and many genes showed a greater dispersion in BD patients.

Conclusion

There has been a paradigm shift in the way biological research is carried out. This shift is in the context of the development of several enabling technologies: genomics, which allows massively parallel gene expression analysis and the advent of other genome-wide experiments that aim at obtaining functional information about as many gene products as possible. Limitations arise from the fact that genomics by itself cannot usually determine the biochemical, cellular and physiological functions of a protein. Furthermore, disease-related processes may not be represented at the transcript level but rather at the post-translational level, then there are splice variants and discrepancies between transcript and protein regulation and so forth.

However, despite the evident shortcomings of the current high-throughput methods, they – for the first time – open new avenues to glimpse at complex gene interactions and without any doubt will change the face of medicine including psychiatry.

Acknowledgment. S.B. gratefully acknowledges support by the Theodore and Vada Stanley Foundation and the donations of the Stanley Foundation Brain Collection courtesy of Drs. Michael B. Knable, E. Fuller Torrey, Maree J. Webster, and Robert H. Yolken, who also provided much encouragement and valued discussions. The Department of Psychiatry gratefully acknowledges centre support from the Stanley Foundation.

References

Badner JA, Gershon ES (2002) Meta-analysis of whole-genome linkage scans of bipolar disorder and schizophrenia. Mol Psychiatry 7:405–411

Barton AJ, Pearson RC, Najlerahim A, Harrison PJ (1993) Pre- and postmortem influences on brain RNA. J Neurochem 61:1–11

Benes FM (1988) Post-mortem structural analyses of schizophrenic brain: study designs and the interpretation of data. Psychiatr Dev 6:213–226

Benes FM, Davidson J, Bird ED (1986) Quantitative cytoarchitectural studies of the cerebral cortex of schizophrenics. Arch Gen Psychiatry 43:31–35

Hakak Y, Walker JR, Li C, Wong WH, Davis KL, Buxbaum JD, Haroutunian V, Fienberg AA (2001) Genome-wide expression analysis reveals dysregulation of myelination-related genes in chronic schizophrenia. Proc Natl Acad Sci USA 98:4746–4751

Harrison PJ, Burnet PW, Falkai P, Bogerts B, Eastwood SL (1997) Gene expression and neuronal activity in schizophrenia: a study of polyadenylated mRNA in the hippocampal formation and cerebral cortex. Schizophr Res 26:93–102

Harrison PJ, Heath PR, Eastwood SL, Burnet PW, McDonald B, Pearson RC (1995) The relative importance of premortem acidosis and postmortem interval for human brain gene expression studies: selective mRNA vulnerability and comparison with their encoded proteins. Neurosci Lett 200:151–154

Harrison PJ, Procter AW, Barton AJ, Lowe SL, Najlerahim A, Bertolucci PH, Bowen DM, Pearson RC (1991) Terminal coma affects messenger RNA detection in post mortem human temporal cortex. Brain Res Mol Brain Res 9:161–164

Johnston NL, Cervenak J, Shore AD, Torrey EF, Yolken RH, Cerevnak J (1997) Multivariate analysis of RNA levels from postmortem human brains as measured by three different methods of RT-PCR. Stanley Neuropathology Consortium [published erratum appears in J Neurosci Methods 1998 Feb 20; 79(2):233]. J Neurosci Methods 77:83–92

Kingsbury AE, Foster OJ, Nisbet AP, Cairns N, Bray L, Eve DJ, Lees AJ, Marsden CD (1995) Tissue pH as an indicator of mRNA preservation in human post-mortem brain. Brain Res Mol Brain Res 28:311–318

Knable MB, Torrey EF, Webster MJ, Bartko JJ (2001) Multivariate analysis of prefrontal cortical data from the Stanley Foundation Neuropathology Consortium. Brain Res Bull 55:651–659

Leonard S, Logel J, Luthman D, Casanova M, Kirch D, Freedman R (1993) Biological stability of mRNA isolated from human postmortem brain collections. Biol Psychiatry 33:456–466

Lockhart DJ, Dong H, Byrne MC, Follettie MT, Gallo MV, Chee MS, Mittmann M, Wang C, Kobayashi M, Horton H, Brown EL (1996) Expression monitoring by hybridization to high-density oligonucleotide arrays. Nat Biotechnol 14:1675–1680

Mimmack ML, Ryan M, Baba H, Navarro-Ruiz J, Iritani S, Faull RL, McKenna PJ, Jones PB, Arai H, Starkey M, Emson PC, Bahn S (2002) Gene expression analysis in schizophrenia: reproducible up-regulation of several members of the apolipoprotein L family located in a high-susceptibility locus for schizophrenia on chromosome 22. Proc Natl Acad Sci USA 99:4680–4685

Pongrac J, Middleton FA, Lewis DA, Levitt P, Mirnics K (2002) Gene expression profiling with DNA microarrays: advancing our understanding of psychiatric disorders. Neurochem Res 27:1049–1063

Ravid R, Van Zwieten EJ, Swaab DF (1992) Brain banking and the human hypothalamus – factors to match for, pitfalls and potentials. Prog Brain Res 93:83–95

Schramm M, Falkai P, Tepest R, Schneider-Axmann T, Przkora R, Waha A, Pietsch T, Bonte W, Bayer TA (1999) Stability of RNA transcripts in post-mortem psychiatric brains. J Neural Transm 106:329–335

Southern E, Mir K, Shchepinov M (1999) Molecular interactions on microarrays. Nat Genet 21:5–9

Terenius L (2000) Schizophrenia: pathophysiological mechanisms – a synthesis. Brain Res Brain Res Rev 31:401–404

Tkachev D, Mimmack ML, Ryan MM, Wayland M, Freeman T, Jones PB, Starkey M, Webster MJ, Yolken RH, Bahn S (2003) Oligodendrocyte dysfunction in schizophrenia and bipolar disorder. Lancet 362:798–805

Waldvogel HJ, Kubota Y, Fritschy J, Mohler H, Faull RL (1999) Regional and cellular localisation of GABA(A) receptor subunits in the human basal ganglia: an autoradiographic and immunohistochemical study. J Comp Neurol 415:313–340

Welsh JB, Zarrinkar PP, Sapinoso LM, Kern SG, Behling CA, Monk BJ, Lockhart DJ, Burger RA, Hampton GM (2001) Analysis of gene expression profiles in normal and neoplastic ovarian tissue samples identifies candidate molecular markers of epithelial ovarian cancer. Proc Natl Acad Sci USA 98:1176–1181

Yates CM, Butterworth J, Tennant MC, Gordon A (1990) Enzyme activities in relation to pH and lactate in postmortem brain in Alzheimer-type and other dementias. J Neurochem 55:1624–1630

Brain morphological abnormalities in first-degree relatives of schizophrenic patients

Peter Falkai[1], Kai Vogeley[2], Thomas Kamer[1], Ralf Tepest[2], Thomas Schneider-Axmann[1], and Wolfgang Maier[2]

[1] Department of Psychiatry and Psychotherapy, University of Saarland, Homburg/Saar, Germany
[2] Department of Psychiatry and Psychotherapy, University of Bonn, Bonn, Germany

Introduction

Based on postmortem and imaging studies there is now consistent evidence for brain morphological abnormalities in schizophrenia (e.g. Wright et al. 2000; Nelson et al. 1998).

The changes comprise a subtle whole brain volume reduction, enlargement of the ventricular system, mainly the lateral ventricles, changes in the frontal as well as temporal lobes especially a bilateral hippocampal volume reduction. However, the origins of these changes might be diverse. Three possible sources have to be taken into account:

Vulnerability-associated changes. These changes can be found in most of the persons with an increased risk to develop schizophrenia. These changes specifically relate to first-degree relatives of schizophrenic patients.

Disease-related changes. Changes prior to the onset of the illness. As we know especially from the ABC study (Häfner et al. 1987) about 4 years prior to the first episode of schizophrenia unspecific prodromal signs occur relating to affective symptoms and cognitive deficits. It is fair to assume that at least part of the changes in schizophrenia develop prior to the manifestation of the full picture of the illness.

Course-related changes. Once the full picture of schizophrenia is present, we know from MRI follow-up studies, that especially in cortical regions there are changes over time (Hulshoff Pol et al. 2001). These changes might be partly due to the course of the illness but, on the other hand, might well be related to individual life style and pharmacological therapy.

The presented data merely focus on changes relating to the risk to develop schizophrenia.

Description of sample

Between 1996 and 2001, all together 294 persons were included in the so-called "Family Study". The sample consisted of 71 patients with schizophrenia based on the ICD10 diagnosis schizophrenia or schizoaffective disorder, 46 first-degree relatives with a psychiatric diagnosis beside schizophrenia, 88

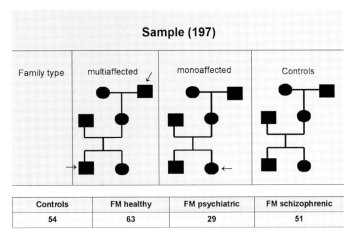

Sample (197)

| Family type | multiaffected | monoaffected | Controls |

Controls	FM healthy	FM psychiatric	FM schizophrenic
54	63	29	51

Fig. 1. Sample description of the Family Study
→ arrow = family member with schizophrenia

family members without any psychiatric diagnosis and 89 control subjects. The schizophrenic index persons came from 48 families of which 28 had more than one member suffering from schizophrenia (multiply affected) and from 20 families only having 1 member with the diagnosis of schizophrenia (uniaffected). Out of this sample a subsample of 197 persons was chosen as for these persons clinical as well as imaging data were completely available (for further details see Fig. 1).

▮ Global or focal changes?

Using an SPM-based algorithm the MRI scans of the 196 persons were examined receiving global measures like whole brain volume, global cerebrospinal fluid space (CSF) volume, grey and white matter volumes. For all subsequent analysis three groups are compared:

▮ the group of control subjects
▮ the group of the first-degree relatives without psychosis, and
▮ the group of family members suffering from schizophrenia.

Using this algorithm no significant changes were found for the whole brain volume comparing schizophrenic patients with the control sample or with their first-degree relatives.

Looking at the global CSF spaces which summarises central (ventricular system) and peripheral cerebral spinal fluid spaces a significant increase of this global measure of atrophy was found in schizophrenics compared to the controls ($p < 0.0005$) and to the first-degree relatives [($p < 0.002$) (Fig. 2 a, b)] while there was no significant difference between controls and first-degree relatives. Therefore, this global measure of atrophy indicates that the most prominent changes can be found in the schizophrenic patients followed by their

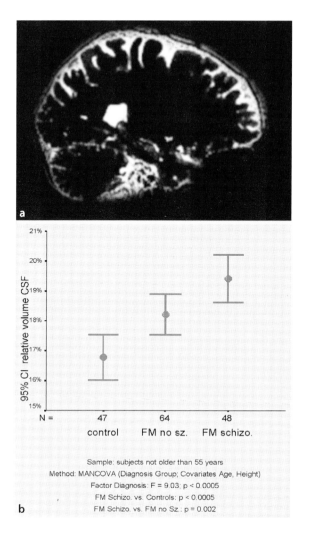

Fig. 2 a, b. a CSF segmentation. b CSF spaces

first-degree relatives. However, as the difference between the first-degree relatives not suffering from schizophrenia and the control subjects was not significant, this parameter does not qualify as a so-called intermediate phenotype. A parameter qualifies as an intermediate phenotype, if it is significantly different from the patient as well as significantly different from the control group.

Looking at the volumes of white and grey matter a quite clear cut result was achieved. All volumes mentioned subsequently are relative values of ratios between absolute volumes and the individual whole brain volume. While there was virtually no change in global white matter volumes (Fig. 3 a, b), a significant reduction of the grey matter volume was revealed in schizophrenic patients compared to controls ($p < 0.001$) and compared to their first-degree relatives [($p < 0.002$) (for further details see Fig. 4 a, b)].

Although there was a clear-cut volume reduction demonstrable in schizophrenics, there was still no difference between first-degree relatives and controls.

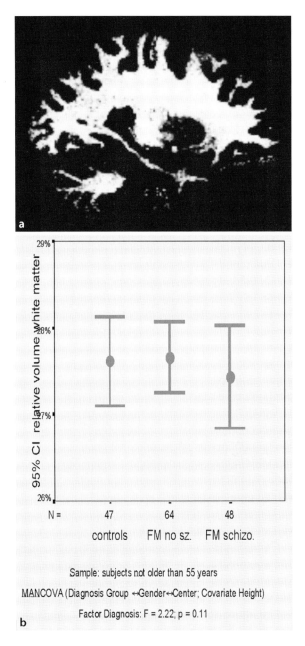

Fig. 3 a, b. a Segmentation of the white matter. **b** Relative volumes of the white matter

▌ Which lobes are involved in cortical grey matter reduction?

Using a specifically developed segmentation algorithm (Kamer et al., manuscript in preparation) we were able to determine grey and white matter volumes of the different lobes including frontal, parietal, occipital, temporal lobes

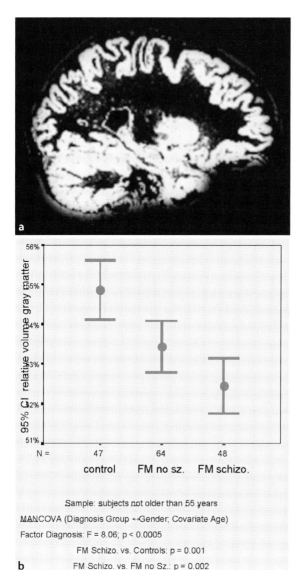

Fig. 4a, b. a Segmentation of the gray matter. **b** Relative volume of the gray matter

and cerebellum. It is interesting to note that there was no change in the parietal or occipital lobe, where there were significant change in temporal and the most pronounced volume reduction in the pre-frontal or frontal lobe bilaterally (factor diagnosis: $F = 12.45$, $p < 0.0005$). As demonstrated in Fig. 5, there was a clear volume reduction in the frontal lobe between controls and schizophrenic patients and between a schizophrenic patient and the first-degree relatives.

However, in the search of an intermediate phenotype once more there was no difference between the first-degree relatives and the control subjects.

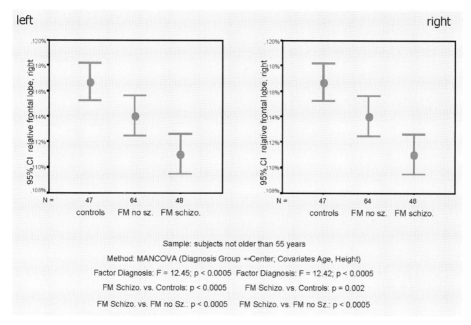

Fig. 5. Relative frontal lobe volumes

▮ Specification of frontal lobe changes

Recently we have demonstrated hypergyrification in the frontal lobe in schizophrenia (Vogeley et al. 2000, 2001). Using the gyrification index (Zilles et al. 1988) the gyrification pattern of the frontal and parietal lobe was determined in the family sample. It was interesting that frontal hypergyrification was confirmed in the family members suffering from schizophrenia compared to the controls and the first-degree relatives (Falkai et al. 2003; for further details see Fig. 6).

Most interestingly there was a significant difference not only between schizophrenics and controls as well as first-degree relatives but in addition a significant difference between first-degree relatives and control subjects was only found for the left frontal gyrification index in the uniaffected families. Therefore, the gyrification index in the frontal lobe qualifies as an intermediate phenotype in the "sporadic form" of schizophrenia. In addition to this it is worthwhile mentioning that there is no diagnostic effect on the gyrification index for the parietal lobe. Coming back to the frontal hypergyrification we subsequently determined the frontal gyrification in healthy monozygotic and dizygotic twin pairs. As suggested by others, the frontal gyrification index was highly significantly correlated between monozygotic twins, while there was less correlation in dizygotic pairs. This pattern is taken as a sign of high degree of heritability and in addition to the so-called intermediate phenotype qualifies the gyrification index as a so-called endophenotype. A biological marker is called an endophenotype, if it shows an intermediate phenotypic

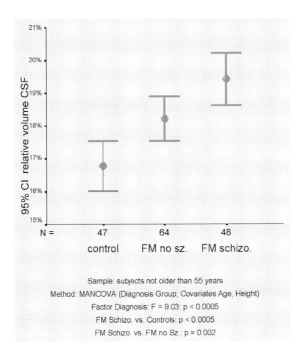

Sample: subjects not older than 55 years
Method: MANCOVA (Diagnosis Group; Covariates Age, Height)
Factor Diagnosis: F = 9.03; p < 0.0005
FM Schizo. vs. Controls: p < 0.0005
FM Schizo. vs. FM no Sz.: p = 0.002

Fig. 6. Gyrification index frontal left

pattern as demonstrated for the gyrification index in uniaffected families and in addition a high degree of heritability. In the literature biological markers qualifying as an endophenotype are assumed to be linked to the molecular bases schizophrenia (Gottesman and Gould 2003).

As the gyrification index is correlated with the thickness of the grey matter [($r = -0.272$, $p < 0.016$) (Fig. 7)], it is fair to suggest that the loss of frontal lobe grey matter volume is related to frontal hypergyrification in schizophrenia.

Temporal lobe pathology

As outlined above beside a clear cut grey matter volume reduction in the frontal lobe, there were similar but less pronounced changes in the temporal lobe. Based on the current literature, volume reduction of the hippocampus (Nelson et al. 1998) and enlargement of the sylvian fissure (e.g. Bogerts et al. 1987; Honer et al. 1996; Falkai et al. 2002) seem to represent prominent findings in the temporal lobe of schizophrenic patients.

The hippocampus

Using a region of interest-based morphometric approach, the volume of hippocampus was determined in the family sample (Fig. 8 a, b). A bilateral volume reduction of this structure in schizophrenics compared to the control subjects (left –14%, $p < 0.013$; right –15%, $p < 0.020$) and compared to the first-degree

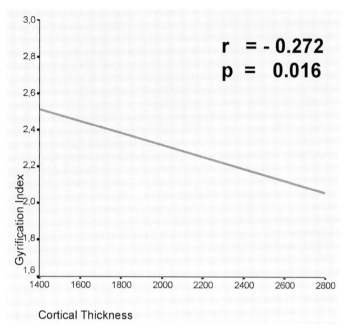

Fig. 7. Gyrification and cortical thickness

relatives (left –10%, p < 0.26; right –6%, p < 0.12) was revealed. Multivariate analysis of variance revealed bilaterally a significant decrease in subjects with documented severe labour and delivery complications (grade 3, McNeal Scale) and a significant interaction between status as well as labour and delivery complications for the left hippocampal volume (F = 5.65, df 1.44, p = 0.022) demonstrating a smaller left hippocampus in the uniaffected group with severe obstetric complications (Ebner et al. 2003). The conclusions from these hippocampal findings are that the reported volume reduction qualify as vulnerability factors with almost an endophenotypic pattern. This is supported by other groups (e.g. Seidman et al. 2002). In addition to that, severe labour and delivery complications, as reported by the mothers on recall, seem to contribute to the hippocampal volume loss in general and especially the changes on the left side in uniaffected (= sporadic) schizophrenia.

In a subgroup of the probands included into the family study the shape of the hippocampus was determined comparing schizophrenic patients with their well siblings as well as controls. The most pronounced shape abnormalities were found in the anterior portion of the hippocampus bilaterally with most pronounced changes in the subicular formation (Tepest et al. 2003). This kind of analysis will be important in the future to determine more focal changes in the hippocampal formation in schizophrenia which should lead to a better understanding of the disturbed neural networks involved in this disorder.

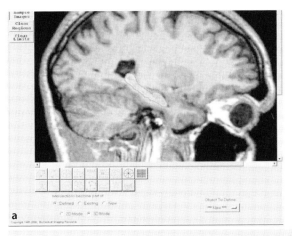

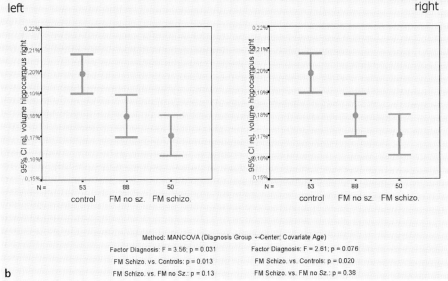

Fig. 8a, b. a Lateral view on the brain. **b** Relative volumes of the hippocampus

The sylvian fissure

Sylvian fissure enlargement is a very prominent finding in schizophrenia, however, completely underresearched. Recent findings point to the importance of the parietal lobe in the beginning of the disorder (Thompson et al. 2001). In a small subset of subjects we have determined the volume of the sylvian fissure on MRI (see Fig. 9a) in all subsequent coronal sections through this structure.

We found a bilateral volume increase of the sylvian fissure comparing siblings with their family members suffering from schizophrenia (see Fig. 9b). The same extent of volume increase was found in schizophrenic subjects lack-

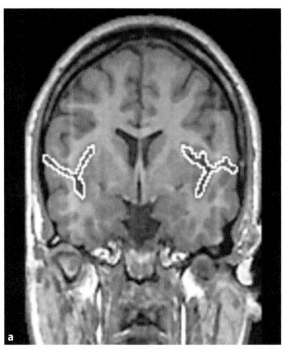

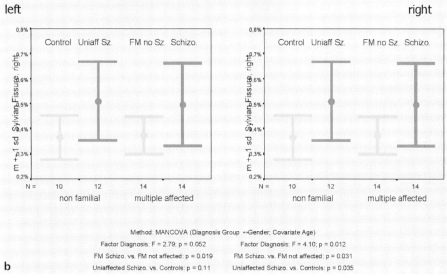

Fig. 9 a, b. a Sylvian fissure. **b** Sylvian fissure volumes

ing the family member with schizophrenia over three subsequent generations. This comparison between "sporadic" schizophrenia and healthy controls reveals a significant volume increase of the right sylvian fissure and a clear cut trend for the left side. Therefore, first-degree relatives of subjects suffering from schizophrenia revealed a normal size of the sylvian fissure which means that there is no sign of increased vulnerability for this brain region. In conclusion, enlargement of the sylvian fissure in schizophrenia is therefore not a result of a genetic vulnerability, but rather reflects the disease process itself. One might possibly conclude that the changes found in this region develop with the onset of the illness and possibly worsen with the course of the disease.

▌ Conclusions

Brain morphological abnormalities in first-degree relatives of schizophrenic patients are frequently found in different brain regions. Beside a global increase of the cerebral spinal fluid spaces there seems to be a more focal volume loss of the grey matter in the frontal as well as temporal lobes. The frontal lobe grey matter loss is associated with increased gyrification in schizophrenia. For the left frontal lobe in uniaffected families with schizophrenia the gyrification index forms a good intermediate phenotype which in addition of high degree of heritability qualifies as a potential endophenotypic marker. Beside frontal lobe grey matter pathology the second region of interest for brain abnormalities in first-degree relatives of schizophrenic patients is the temporal lobe. Of specific interest is the hippocampus showing a bilateral volume reduction in the family members suffering from schizophrenia and to a lesser degree in their first-degree relatives. It is interesting to know that also the volume reduction in first-degree relatives was not significant compared to the controls subjects. However, it almost reached the level of significance for the right side. Therefore, the hippocampal formation is the second structure qualifying as an intermediate phenotype for schizophrenia.

In addition, it is interesting to know that severe obstetric complications as recorded by maternal recall did not influence grey matter volume reduction in the frontal lobe, but did influence the bilateral volume reduction of the hippocampus for all members of the families. In addition to this modulating effect on volume loss, there was a specific significant interaction between the volume reduction of the left hippocampus and the occurrence of severe obstetric complications in uniaffected (= sporadic) schizophrenia.

Therefore, genetic vulnerability for schizophrenia seems to effect brain structure to different degrees. Furthermore, non-genetic environmental factors also seem to contribute to the changes seen in schizophrenics as well as their first-degree relatives. However, this modulating effect seems to be regional-specific and possibly even hemispheric-specific which is interesting on the basis of the cerebral asymmetry discussion related to schizophrenia.

Therefore, left frontal GI as well as left hippocampal volume might be interesting parameters to serve as vulnerability measures to predict an increased risk to develop schizophrenia. Catamnestic studies are needed to evaluate whether persons with changes in these regions are at an increased risk to develop the clinical picture of schizophrenia.

▮ References

Bogerts B, Wurthmann C, Piroth HD (1987) [Brain substance deficit with paralimbic and limbic involvement in computerized tomography studies of schizophrenic patients]. Nervenarzt 58(2):97–106 (German)

Ebner F et al (2004) The hippocampus in families with schizophrenia in relation to genetic loading and obstetric complications. Schiz Research (submitted)

Falkai P et al (2002) Neuropathology of schizophrenia: is there evidence for neurodevelopmental disorder? In: Häfner H et al (eds) Risk and Protective Factors in Schizophrenia. Steinkopff, Darmstadt, pp 61–70

Falkai P, Honer WG, Alfter D, Schneider-Axmann T, Bussfeld P, Cordes J, Blank B, Schonell H, Steinmetz H, Maier W, Tepest R (2002) The temporal lobe in schizophrenia from uni- and multiply affected families. Neurosci Lett 325(1):25–28

Falkai P, Schneider-Axmann T, Honer WG, Vogeley K, Schonell H, Pfeiffer U, Scherk H, Block W, Traber F, Schild HH, Maier W, Tepest R (2003) Influence of genetic loading, obstetric complications and premorbid adjustment on brain morphology in schizophrenia: a MRI study. Eur Arch Psychiatry Clin Neurosci 253(2):92–99

Gottesman II, Gould TD (2003) The endophenotype concept in psychiatry: etymology and strategic intentions. Am J Psychiatry 160(4):636–645 (Review)

Honer WG, Bassett AS, Falkai P, Beach TG, Lapointe JS (1996) A case study of temporal lobe development in familial schizophrenia. Psychol Med 26(1):191–195

Hulshoff Pol HE, Schnack HG, Mandl RC, van Haren NE, Koning H, Collins DL, Evans AC, Kahn RS (2001) Focal gray matter density changes in schizophrenia. Arch Gen Psychiatry 58(12):1118–1125

Nelson MD, Saykin AJ, Flashman LA, Riordan HJ (1998) Hippocampal volume reduction in schizophrenia as assessed by magnetic resonance imaging: a meta-analytic study. Arch Gen Psychiatry 55(5):433–440

Seidman LJ, Faraone SV, Goldstein JM, Kremen WS, Horton NJ, Makris N, Toomey R, Kennedy D, Caviness VS, Tsuang MT (2002) Left hippocampal volume as a vulnerability indicator for schizophrenia: a magnetic resonance imaging morphometric study of nonpsychotic first-degree relatives. Arch Gen Psychiatry 59(9): 839–849

Thompson PM, Vidal C, Giedd JN, Gochman P, Blumenthal J, Nicolson R, Toga AW, Rapoport JL (2001) Mapping adolescent brain change reveals dynamic wave of accelerated gray matter loss in very early-onset schizophrenia. Proc Natl Acad Sci USA 98(20):11650–11655

Thurm I, Haefner H (1987) Perceived vulnerability, relapse risk and coping in schizophrenia. An explorative study. Eur Arch Psychiatry Neurol Sci 237(1):46–53

Vogeley K, Schneider-Axmann T, Pfeiffer U, Tepest R, Bayer TA, Bogerts B, Honer WG, Falkai P (2000) Disturbed gyrification of the prefrontal region in male schizophrenics – a morphometric postmortem study. Am J Psychiatry 157:34–39

Vogeley K, Tepest R, Pfeiffer U, Schneider-Axmann T, Maier W, Honer WG, Falkai P (2001) Right frontal hypergyria differentiates affected from non-affected siblings in families with schizophrenia – a morphometric MRI study. Am J Psychiatry 158:494–496

Wright IC, Rabe-Hesketh S, Woodruff PW, David AS, Murray RM, Bullmore ET (2000) Meta-analysis of regional brain volumes in schizophrenia. Am J Psychiatry 157(1):16–25

Zilles K, Armstrong E, Schleicher A, Kretschmann HJ (1988) The human pattern of gyrification in the cerebral cortex. Anat Embryol (Berl) 179(2):173–179

Genetics of schizophrenia and the impact of neuropsychology

W. Maier[1], M. Wagner[1], P. Falkai[2], and S. G. Schwab[1]

[1] Department of Psychiatry, University of Bonn, Bonn, Germany
[2] Department of Psychiatry, Saarland University, Homburg, Germany

Introduction

As evidenced by a bulk 0of twin and family studies schizophrenia is clearly a genetically influenced disorder, with more than 50% of the etiological variance being due to genetic variation. This genetic diathesis has to be considered together with the preferential onset of the disorder in late adolescence and early adulthood, and the severe associated disability and impairment. On this basis a decline of prevalence over time in all populations has been proposed but not observed; this constellation is called the "paradox of schizophrenia".

The paradox of schizophrenia

Schizophrenia has comparable prevalence rates across all countries and cultures. Schizophrenia is associated with reduced *fertility* because of its early age at onset. How can a genetically driven common disorder with reduced fertility survive given the forces of *selection* and evolution? Two models are feasible:

■ **Alternative 1.** The disorder is *monogenic* or a combination of monogenic diseases which balance selective disadvantages with selective advantages; the classical example is sickle cell anemia, a recessive disorder, which provides an advantage to heterozygotes against malaria. A similar concept has been proposed for schizophrenia: The disorder emerges from the same genetic basis as language capacities which provide an advantage in social attraction and mating behavior (Crow, 1995).

■ **Alternative 2.** The disorder is *polygenic* with common variants at multiple genes impacting on the disorder; each genetic variant only exerts a *small or modest* gene effect by itself; the disorder emerges from combinations of these common genes; only the disorder itself induces reduced fertility; a single common variant alone has no effects in this direction; it occurs – as it is substantially more common than the disease – *most frequently outside* the context of schizophrenia, therefore the disease genes are not under the pressure of selection and survival.

Exploration of the pattern of clustering of cases in families cannot decide between these alternatives. A conclusive decision between these two alternatives is only possible on the DNA-based genetics of schizophrenia.

Recent progress in the molecular genetics of schizophrenia and solutions of the paradox

Recent progress in the molecular genetics of schizophrenia is comparable to other common disorders. A consensus strategy to unravel genes for non-mendelian complex genetic disorders has been elaborated during recent years (Fig. 1). The first step is to conduct *linkage analysis in families with multiple affected* members, and to isolate *candidate regions which are likely to include disease or susceptibility genes, respectively.* If these candidate regions are replicable, fine mapping will finally uncover susceptibility genes. This strategy requires that the effect of a susceptibility gene is of sufficient magnitude. In this respect recent progress in schizophrenia can be reported.

▌ **Progress 1.** Multiple genome-wide scans proposed a variety of candidate regions. However, replications of candidate regions (i.e., regions which are likely to cover susceptibility genes) emerging from a single study were either negative or inconsistent with a mixture of negative and positive results. Not a single candidate region was consistently replicable in all replication tests. However, about 10 candidate regions were at least replicable. *Sample size limitations* and the apparently small effects of each susceptibility gene might explain those inconsistencies.

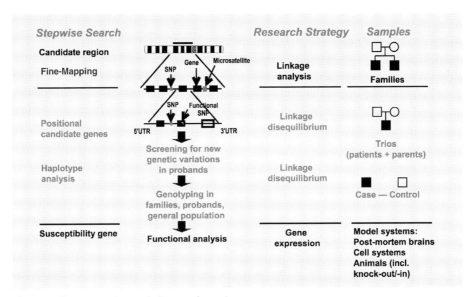

Fig. 1. Finding genes that underlie complex traits

In all linkage studies the magnitude of linkage to any region turned out to be, at best, modest. Thus the following conclusions are possible: Major genes or even a single gene with strong effects on the disease are unlikely because these constellations should induce a higher degree of consistency. A polygenic transmission can therefore be assumed.

Given the inconsistencies skeptical attitudes towards the conclusiveness of linkage analyses were expressed (DeLisi et al., 2000). However, the strategies of metaanalyses or combinations of independent samples were able to reduce ambiguities and to propose more valid results. Several candidate regions (on chromosome 6p, 6q, 8p, 13q and 22q) emerged from these strategies (Fig. 2). These regions are very likely to be "true positives". The results confirm the argument that the single studies were too small in sample size to guarantee the replication of true positive findings (Levinson et al., 2000; Badner and Gershon, 2002).

▮ **Progress 2.** In 2002 five specific polymorphic susceptibility genes were identified by fine mapping in candidate areas emerging from linkage analysis and confirmed by metaanalysis; these genes code for the following products (Fig. 2): dysbindin (chromosome 6p), neuregulin 1 (chromosome 8p), G72 (chromosome 13), COMT (chromosome 22). Although the pathogenic mutations have still to be identified, haplotype associations have turned out to be replicable in independent samples.

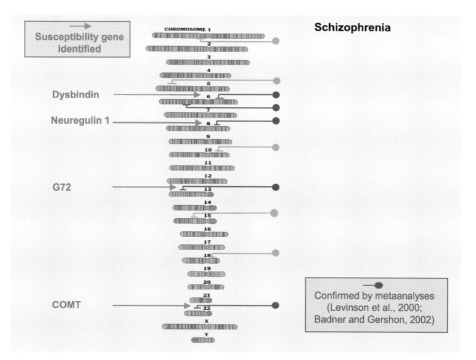

Fig. 2. Schizophrenia: candidate regions and identified susceptibility genes

Recently, a common denominator was proposed for the identified susceptibility genes: All these genes converge in an impact on the glutamatergic system (Harrison and Owen, 2003). However, all these genes serve also other
functions. Therefore, this speculation remains suggestive.

Taken together, there is now sufficient reason to assume 1) that multiple
genes impact on schizophrenia, and 2) that there is not a major gene determining schizophrenia.

Consequences for the clinical phenotype

▌ **Consequence 1: Relationship to bipolar disorder.** Like in schizophrenia multiple candidate regions were identified by genome-wide scans for bipolar disorder. The patterns of inconsistencies are similar to schizophrenia with about 7–
10 regions emerging from at least two genome-wide scans. A metaanalysis by
Badner and Gershon (2002) confirmed two of these regions: one on chromosome 13, one on chromosome 22. Interestingly both of these candidate regions
overlap with confirmed schizophrenia regions (Fig. 3). This coincidence is unexpected and beyond random variations.

Overlap of candidate regions does not guarantee identity of susceptibility
genes. However, Hattori et al. (2003) observed that the susceptibility gene G72
on chromosome 13 for schizophrenia is also a susceptibility gene for bipolar
disorder (Fig. 3). Consequently, comorbidity of both disorders in patients and

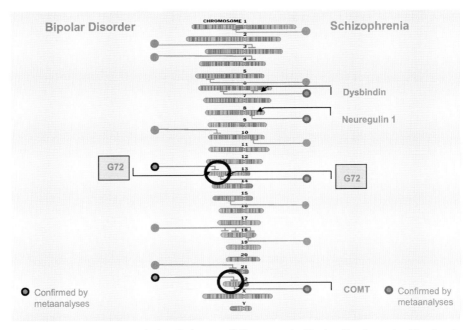

Fig. 3. Candidate regions and identified susceptibility genes in bipolar disorder and schizophrenia
(○ = overlap)

cosegregation in families can be – at least partly – explained by shared genetic basis.

▌ **Consequence 2: Nature of disease gene variants.** Functional disease gene variants with a small or moderate effect are likely to be common (Wright et al., 1999) as shown in Fig. 4. Common genetic variants need a large number of generations to become common; thus they are likely to be of ancient origin (Wright et al., 1999). The contributing genetic variants were probably already present in times when the human population spread out from Africa about 150,000 years ago (Fig. 5). Interestingly this is about the time when humans are believed to have developed their language abilities. The ancient origin of schizophrenia can explain its occurrence in all countries with comparable prevalence (at least under the assumption of low impact of environment).

▌ **Consequence 3: Endophenotypes.** Susceptibility genes for schizophrenia do not directly code for the heterogeneous diagnosis of schizophrenia. Instead, it is very likely that specific susceptibility genes are coding for one or some of the large number of neurobiological features associated with schizophrenia (Fig. 6). Biological features might be closer to the direct influence of genes than the symptoms of the disorder. Quantitative neurobiological factors associated with and genetically linked to the disorder are called *endophenotypes* (Gottesman and Gould, 2003). In this perspective, the clinical profile may be considered as a *"final common pathway"* deriving from different functional and structural brain abnormalities rooted in different multifactorial causal conditions with both genetic and non-genetic components.

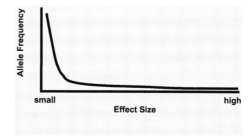

Fig. 4. Hypothetical relationship between effect size and allele frequency

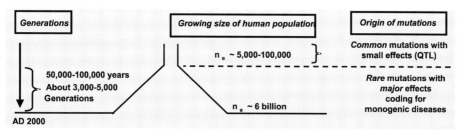

Fig. 5. Evolutionary age of the predisposing gene mutations

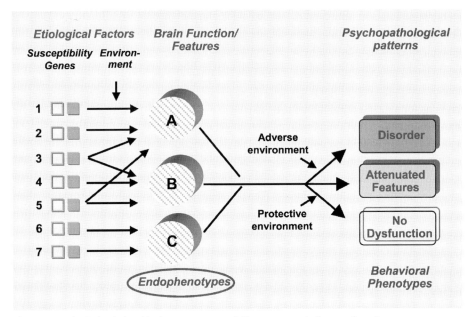

Fig. 6. Hypothetical relationship between susceptibility genes and disease phenotype

Endophenotypes hold the promise that their genetic basis is less complex (e.g., smaller number of genes involved) than that of schizophrenia. This statement is, however, an up to now unproven suggestion. Given this suggestion it is speculated that endophenotypes allow a more efficient unraveling of disease genes than the clinical phenotype. Currently, endophenotypes are more strongly recommended than the unitary phenotypes defined in clinical or biological terms (Fig. 6).

In internal medicine the endophenotype strategy was recently successful (e.g., for the QTc syndrome). Unfortunately, in psychiatry up to now this strategy has not held its promise. In the near future, the study of the genotype-phenotype relationship targeted on identified susceptibility genes will support or reject if endophenotypes are really more directly and more simply related to the susceptibility genes.

▌ **Consequence 4: Attenuated features in family members.** Genetic variants with only moderate or small effects are likely to be common (Wright et al., 1999), and particularly more common than the disease they are influencing. If endophenotypes emerge from only a few or even single disease susceptibility genes, endophenotypes will occur more frequently than the disease in families of patients with schizophrenia.

Indeed, neurobiological and psychological correlates of the disease were observed among unaffected siblings and children of patients more often than expected by chance. Following the tradition of the schizophrenia spectrum, schizophrenia might thus be conceptualized as the iceberg of a substantially broader phenotype including associated neuropsychological and -biological dysfunctions. Under this perspective the concept of schizotaxia has been revitalized in a renewed genetic framework by Tsuang et al. (2002).

From neuropsychology of schizophrenia to the genetics of the cognitive phenotype

Schizophrenia is defined by symptoms of behavior, thought and self-experience. Subsequently, objective cognitive correlates (mainly memory, perceptions, and language) were detected. These features reflect brain functions and are therefore *hypothetical endophenotypes*. They are of particular interest for tracing genes coding for schizophrenia as they are easy to administer.

The criteria for endophenotypes can be formulated as shown in Table 1. At least some of the cognitive correlates of schizophrenia fulfill the majority of requirements listed for endophenotypes:

▮ **Association with schizophrenia.** A large variety of cognitive functions is impaired among patients with schizophrenia as has been demonstrated by a number of investigations. A most comprehensive metaanalysis reveals the highest degree of impairment in language-related functions and in perceptual and motor abilities (Heinrichs and Zakzanis, 1998). Language-related abilities were still most severely impaired in schizophrenia when sensory processing is controlled (Wexler et al., 2002).

▮ **Preceding the emergence of psychotic symptoms.** In order to prove that cognitive dysfunctions present as endophenotypes it has to be excluded that they are exclusively a consequence of the disorder. One possibility is to demonstrate that they precede the emergence of the disorder. Several studies report lower mean cognitive achievements in non-psychotic subjects who later develop schizophrenia. Furthermore, subjects with "prodromal" symptoms who are at immediate risk for schizophrenia reveal lower mean cognitive performance in several domains; the first signs of schizophrenia – attenuated negative symptoms – are already associated with a broad spectrum of cognitive impairments; this pattern can be recognized among the "early prodromal cohort" in

Table 1. Endophenotype criteria

▮ Association with the disorder
▮ Preceding the disorder/not only consequence of the disorder
▮ Aggregation in unaffected family members
▮ Genetic influence
▮ Genetically mediated link to the disorder
▮ Reliable measurement

Optional: Stable over time
         No influence of medication

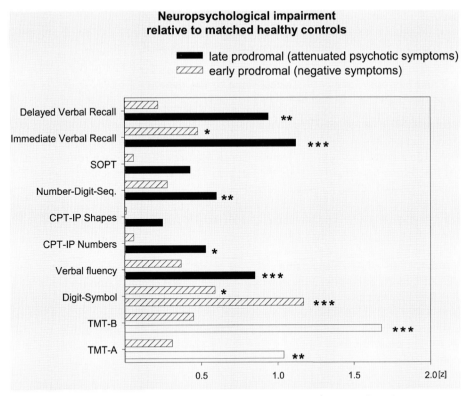

Fig. 7. Neuropsychological deficits precede schizophrenia: associations with prodromal states

a preliminary analysis of probands recruited in Bonn (Wagner et al., 2002) for the German Early Recognition project (KNS) as displayed in Fig. 7.

Familial relationship with schizophrenia. Non-affected first-degree biological relatives reveal reduced cognitive performance in some but not all domains which are also dysfunctional in schizophrenia; the amount of impairment is always lower than among patients with psychosis; cognitive domains with maximal impairment among relatives refer to working memory, attention and verbal abilities, mainly fluency. Our family study is in agreement with others demonstrating that *particularly working memory* deficits (here: "recurrent digit") are characteristic for an elevated risk for schizophrenia among unaffected relatives (Faraone et al., 1995); verbal fluency is also reduced but less so.

Genetic influences on cognition. As displayed in Table 2 cognitive functions are under genetic control. Substantial genetic influences have been demonstrated on the variation of cognitive abilities in the general population: A *general cognitive factor* shows maximal genetic impact. *Specific cognitive functions* are also under genetic control to a lower degree; among the more specific cognitive functions particularly *verbal abilities* reveal high heritabilities (50–

Table 2. Heritability of selected cognitive abilities (non-patient samples)

▌ Global cognitive factor/IQ	55–89%
▌ Verbal abilities	50–65%
▌ Performance abilities	40–55%
▌ Working memory	40–48%
▌ Attentional function	10–50%

65%); *working memory* is apparently the most heritable memory function; recent twin studies report heritabilities of 40–48% for working memory; some evidence of heritability is observed for components of attention. Recently, the genetic influence on working and episodic memory functions was directly demonstrated for variants of the BDNF and the COMT genes (Egan et al. 2001, 2003).

Interestingly, the most heritable cognitive correlate of schizophrenia (verbal abilities) does not present as the most discriminative feature between unaffected relatives of schizophrenia patients and controls (according to most recent studies: working memory is most discriminative).

▌ **Genetically mediated link to schizophrenia.** The link between cognitive impairments and schizophrenia may be secondary to the disorder or may be due to environmental forces. Thus, in order to establish a genetic link between cognitive dysfunctions and symptoms of schizophrenia it is essential to disentangle the direct impact of the disease and of the environment from the genetic effects on the cognition.

The optimal design to explore this hypothesis is a discordant twin design comparing unaffected monozygotic twins (MZ) and unaffected dizygotic twins (DZ) of index cases with schizophrenia; unaffected control twins might present as a third comparator. These three groups of healthy subjects define a *liability dimension graded by genetic load for schizophrenia* with
- ▌ a maximal (100%) sharing of genes with a schizophrenic MZ co-twin,
- ▌ an elevated (50%) sharing of genes with a schizophrenic DZ co-twin, and
- ▌ a baseline level of genetically defined risk for schizophrenia.

Cannon et al. (2000) were up to now the only group to perform this crucial analysis for the genetic relationship between schizophrenia and cognition. They used a battery of neurocognitive measures. A compound neurocognitive global indicator was able to distinguish between these three vulnerability groups.

Which specific cognitive dysfunctions contribute most to the discrimination of different levels of genetic vulnerability to schizophrenia? Very similar to inquiries in unaffected family members the most discriminative dysfunction is (spatial) *working memory* together with divided attention; *episodic verbal memory* and the most tested language-related dysfunctions are more related to the *environmental* influences on the disorder; this result is unexpected as we have seen that language functions are under substantial genetic influence; a plausible explanation is that the genetic underpinnings of schizophrenia and of language abilities do not reveal major overlaps.

Thus, all criteria of the endophenotype (Table 1) are fulfilled for specific cognitive correlates of schizophrenia, at least for working memory functions (mainly spatial modality).

Conclusions

Taken together, despite of serious doubts in the etiological and pathophysiological validity of the clinical diagnosis of schizophrenia some consistency of linkage analyses was attained through metaanalyses, and several disease-associated susceptibility genes have recently been detected. The endophenotype strategy might present an alternative for defining the phenotype in the future search for disease genes. Cognitive endophenotypes, particularly working memory, are particularly promising in this respect. Cognitive endophenotypes might also help to explain the associations of schizophrenia with risk haplotypes.

‖ **Acknowledgment.** This paper was written within the framework of the German Research Networks on "Schizophrenia" and on "Depression/Suicidality" and was funded by the German Federal Ministry for Education and Research BMBF (grants: 01GI9934/2 and 01GI0229).

References

Badner JA, Gershon ES (2002) Meta-analysis of whole-genome linkage scans of bipolar disorder and schizophrenia. Mol Psychiatry 7:405–411

Cannon TD, Huttunen MO, Lonnqvist J, Tuulio-Henriksson A, Pirkola T, Glahn D, Finkelstein J, Hietanen M, Kaprio J, Koskenvuo M (2000) The inheritance of neuropsychological dysfunction in twins discordant for schizophrenia. Am J Hum Genet 67:369–382

Crow TJ (1995) A Darwinian approach to the origins of psychosis. Br J Psychiatry 167:12–25

DeLisi LE, Craddock NJ, Detera-Wadleigh S, Foroud T, Gejman P, Kennedy JL, Lendon C, Macciardi F, McKeon P, Mynett-Johnson L, Nurnberger JI jr, Paterson A, Schwab S, Van Broeckhoven C, Wildenauer D, Crow TJ (2000) Update on chromosomal locations for psychiatric disorders: report of the interim meeting of chromosome workshop chairpersons from the VIIth World Congress of Psychiatric Genetics, Monterey, California, October 14–18, 1999. Am J Med Genet 96:434–449

Egan MF, Goldberg TE, Kolachana BS, Callicott JH, Mazzanti CM, Straub RE, Goldman D, Weinberger DR (2001) Effect of COMT Val108/158 Met genotype on frontal lobe function and risk for schizophrenia. Proc Natl Acad Sci USA 98:6917–6922

Egan MF, Kojima M, Callicott JH, Goldberg TE, Kolachana BS, Bertolino A, Zaitsev E, Gold B, Goldman D, Dean M, Lu B, Weinberger DR (2003) The BDNF val66met polymorphism affects activity-dependent secretion of BDNF and human memory and hippocampal function. Cell 112:257–269

Faraone SV, Seidman LJ, Kremen WS, Pepple JR, Lyons MJ, Tsuang MT (1995) Neuro-psychological functioning among the nonpsychotic relatives of schizophrenic patients: a diagnostic efficiency analysis. J Abnorm Psychol 104:286–304

Gottesman II, Gould TD (2003) The endophenotype concept in psychiatry: etymology and strategic intentions. Am J Psychiatry 160:636–645

Harrison PJ, Owen MJ (2003) Genes for schizophrenia? Recent findings and their pathophysiological implications. Lancet 361:417–419

Hattori E, Liu C, Badner JA, Bonner TI, Christian SL, Maheshwari M, Detera-Wadleigh SD, Gibbs RA, Gershon ES (2003) Polymorphisms at the G72/G30 gene locus, on 13q33, are associated with bipolar disorder in two independent pedigree series. Am J Hum Genet 72:1131–1140

Heinrichs RW, Zakzanis KK (1998) Neurocognitive deficit in schizophrenia: a quantitative review of the evidence. Neuropsychology 12:426–445

Levinson DF, Holmans P, Straub RE, Owen MJ, Wildenauer DB, Gejman PV, Pulver AE, Laurent C, Kendler KS, Walsh D, Norton N, Williams NM, Schwab SG, Lerer B, Mowry BJ, Sanders AR, Antonarakis SE, Blouin JL, DeLeuze JF, Mallet J (2000) Multicenter linkage study of schizophrenia candidate regions on chromosomes 5q, 6q, 10p, and 13q: schizophrenia linkage collaborative group III. Am J Hum Genet 67:652–663

Tsuang MT, Stone WS, Tarbox SI, Faraone SV (2002) An integration of schizophrenia with schizotypy: identification of schizotaxia and implications for research on treatment and prevention. Schizophr Res 54:169–175

Wagner M, Frommann I, Schröder C, Matuschek E, Pukrop R (2002) Neurocognitive performance in presumed prodromal stages of schizophrenia. Schizophr Res 53 (Suppl 3):35–36

Wexler BE, Donegan N, Stevens AA, Jacob SA (2002) Deficits in language-mediated mental operations in patients with schizophrenia. Schizophr Res 53:171–179

Wright AF, Carothers AD, Pirastu M (1999) Population choice in mapping genes for complex diseases. Nat Genet 23:397–404

Human genome and the perspectives for schizophrenia

ELIDA P. B. OJOPI [1], SHEILA PASSOS GREGORIO [1,2], PEDRO EDSON MOREIRA GUIMARÃES [1], CINTIA FRIDMAN [1], and EMMANUEL DIAS NETO [1]

[1] Laboratory of Neurosciences (LIM27), Institute of Psychiatry, HCFMUSP, São Paulo, SP – Brazil
[2] Chemistry Institute – IQ-USP, São Paulo, SP – Brazil

Introduction

The first attempts to comprehend biology are probably as old as language and conscious thought. Mankind has been always driven to understand his origins as well as to influence the mechanics of life, death, and disease. While we have seen dramatic discoveries in this area, particularly over the last 50 years, in the past three years the field has taken a significant leap due primarily to breakthroughs enabled by genomic sequencing processes. The laser-based, semi-automated DNA sequencing technology (a technique that allows a fast accumulation of genetic information, the genetic blueprint for a given organism) has fundamentally changed our knowledge of biology, and many associated fields. The implementation of this technique enabled the accomplishment of one of the most important scientific achievements ever made: the sequencing of the human genome.

The human genome sequencing represents a pivotal step for understanding human biology and for the rational planning of biomedical research. The completion of a working draft of our genetic material has generated enthusiasm for genetic approaches for assessing disease risk and individualizing therapy. However, it is important to note that the sequencing of a particular genome is not in and of itself the significant piece of the puzzle. The genomic information should be used as a map, and it is with this "map" that we can begin to understand the basis of disease and genetic variation through the analysis of complexity and behaviour of regulatory regions, genes and proteins, gene functions, and systems at a cellular level. However, it is crucial to the cross genetic information with clinical, ethnical and environmental information to permit a full view of the scenario. As the genetic map unfolds, for example, we should be able to create databanks of genetic variations, and in the future a set of customized drugs and therapies targeted specifically at a disease for individuals with different genetic backgrounds. Medicine will know why one patient has a propensity for a particular disease while another does not. We may also expect to be able to predict how a disease is likely to progress and how can we block this progress by using more adequate drugs and other interventions. The bioscience era will change our lives in such fundamental ways — some subtle, some overt — that we can only begin to grasp the enormity of this new age (McLeod and Evans 2001; Evans and Relling 1999).

Table 1. Genes or genomic regions possibly associated with schizophrenia

Chromosomal locus	Candidate gene	Description	Gene function	Marker	Reference
1q21–q22	KCNN3	potassium intermediate/small conductance calcium-activated channel, subfamily N, member 3	The encoded protein is an integral membrane protein that forms a voltage-independent calcium-activated channel with three other calmodulin-binding subunits	D1S1653–D1S1679	Brzustowicz et al. (2000)
1q23	RGS4	regulator of G-protein signaling 4	Regulator of G protein signaling (RGS) family members are regulatory molecules that act as GTPase activating proteins (GAPs) for G alpha subunits of heterotrimeric G proteins		Brzustowicz et al. (2000) Mirnics et al. (2001)
1q23.3	–	–	–	D1S196	Gurling et al. (2001)
2p13–p14	–	–	–	D2S358	Camp et al. (2001)
2q12–q13	–	–	–	D2S135	Moises et al. (1995)
2q37	–	–	–	D2S427	Paunio et al. (2001)
3q13.3	DRD3	dopamine receptor D3	This gene encodes the D3 subtype of the dopamine receptor. It inhibits adenylyl cyclase through inhibitory G-proteins and is expressed in brain regions involved with emotion and cognitive functions.		Jonsson et al. (2003)

Table 1 (continued)

Chromosomal locus	Candidate gene	Description	Gene function	Marker	Reference
4p16.1-p15.3	DRD5	dopamine receptor D5	This gene encodes the D5 subtype of the dopamine receptor, a G-protein coupled receptor which stimulates adenylyl cyclase. This receptor is expressed in neurons of the limbic regions of the brain	D4S615	Muir et al. (2001)
5p14.1–13.1	–	–	–	D5S111	Silverman et al. (1996)
5q32-q33	–	–	–	D5S422	Gurling et al. (2001)
6p21.3	NOTCH4	Notch homolog 4 (Drosophila)	Members of this Type 1 trans-membrane protein family share structural characteristics including an extracellular domain consisting of multiple epidermal growth factor-like (EGF) repeats, and an intracellular domain consisting of multiple, different domain types. Notch genes are involved in a variety of developmental processes by controlling cell fate		Wassink et al. (2003) Skol et al. (2003)
6p23	–	–	–	D6S309–D6S1578	Lindholm et al. (1999)
6q25	–	–	–	D6S253	Lindholm et al. (2001)

Table 1 (continued)

Chromosomal locus	Candidate gene	Description	Gene function	Marker	Reference
8p21-p12	NRG1	neuregulin 1	Neuregulin 1 (NRG1) was originally identified as a 44-kD glycoprotein that interacts with the NEU/ERBB2 receptor tyrosine kinase increasing its phosphorylation on tyrosine residues. Through interaction with ERBB receptors, NRG1 isoforms induce the growth and differentiation of epithelial, neuronal, glial, and other types of cells		Stefansson et al. (2002)
11p15.5	DRD4	dopamine receptor D4	This gene encodes the D4 subtype of the dopamine receptor, a G-protein coupled receptor which inhibits adenylyl cyclase		Seeman et al. (1993) Lung et al. (2002)
11q23	DRD2	dopamine receptor D2	Encodes the D2 subtype of the dopamine receptor, a G-protein coupled receptor that inhibits adenylyl cyclase activity		Noble (2003)
12q24	DAO	D-amino-acid oxidase	This gene encodes the peroxisomal enzyme D-amino acid oxidase. Its biological function is not known; it may be involved in acid-base balance in the kidney, or it may be a fossil enzyme		Chumakov et al. (2002)

Table 1 (continued)

Chromosomal locus	Candidate gene	Description	Gene function	Marker	Reference
13q12-22	–	–	–	D13S894	Camp et al. (2001)
13q32	–	–	–	D13S174	Blouin et al. (1998)
13q33.1	G72	putative protein LG72	G72 and DAO can interact, resulting in the activation of DAO. DAO is expressed in human brain, where it oxidizes D-serine, a potent activator of N-methyl-D-aspartate-type glutamate receptor		Chumakov et al. (2002)
15q14	CHRNA7	cholinergic receptor, nicotinic, alpha polypeptide 7	The nicotinic acetylcholine receptors (nAChRs) are members of a superfamily of ligand-gated ion channels that mediate fast signal transmission at synapses	D15S118	Freedman et al. (2001)
15q15	–	–	–	D15S1042–D15S659	Stober et al. (2000) Stober et al. (2002)
18p	GNAL	guanine nucleotide binding protein (G protein), alpha activating activity polypeptide, olfactory type	G-protein alpha subunit; component of heterotrimeric G-protein complexes, heterotrimer signals from G protein-coupled receptors to intracellular effectors		Lara et al. (2001)

Table 1 (continued)

Chromosomal locus	Candidate gene	Description	Gene function	Marker	Reference
21q22.3	S100β	S100 calcium binding protein, beta (neural)	S100B protein, a calcium binding protein produced and released by glial cells, has been used as a sensitive marker of brain damage		Lara et al. (2001)
22q11.21	PRODH	proline dehydrogenase (oxidase) 1	PRODH2 encodes proline dehydrogenase, a mitochondrial enzyme that converts proline to Δ^1-pyrroline-5-carboxylate and is involved in transfer of redox potential across the mitochondrial membrane		Liu et al. (2002)
	DGCR6	DiGeorge syndrome critical region gene 6	The gene product is similar to the Drosophila gonadal protein, which participates in gonadal and germ cell development, and with the human laminin gamma-1 chain, which upon polymerization with alpha- and beta-chains forms the laminin molecule. Laminin binds to cells through inter-action with a receptor and has functions in cell attachment, migration, and tissue organization during development		Liu et al. (2002)

Table 1 (continued)

Chromosomal locus	Candidate gene	Description	Gene function	Marker	Reference
22q11.21	COMT	catechol-O-methyltransferase	Catechol-O-methyltransferase catalyzes the transfer of a methyl group from S-adenosylmethionine to catechol-amines, including the neurotransmitters dopamine, epinephrine, and norepinephrine. This O-methylation results in one of the major degradative pathways of the catecholamine transmitters	D22S315	Shifman et al. (2002)
22q11–q13	–	–	–	D22S278 D22S279–D22S276	Schwab and Wildenauer (1999) Jorgensen et al. (2002)

The most important biomedical challenge that we have is the comprehension of the complex diseases that affects our species. Complex diseases have such a huge and multi-factorial origins that sometimes appear to be different disorders wrongly classified as the same. After obtaining the genome sequence, the study of such diseases will benefit more. Genetic associations were found in diverse chromosomes in all the complex diseases that affect us. Many studies have focused in genomic regions involved in many diseases, but up to now it has been very difficult and timely (expensive) to find the critical genes. Now we have the opportunity to look carefully to all these regions and to pinpoint the collection of alterations that may elucidate the origins of the important clinical findings in all these diseases.

In this chapter we will discuss some of the research opportunities created after the human genome sequencing, and new alternatives of analysis that can be performed to approach the associations of the human genome and schizophrenia.

▌ The draft of the human genome

"The human genome contains the genetic code that sits at the core of every one of the 10 trillion cells in each human being. It profoundly influences our bodies, our behaviour and our minds; it will help the study of non-genetic influences on human development; it will unlock new insights into our origins and history as a species; and it points to new ways of combating disease" (Nature 2001). With these phrases, the Nature magazine editors opened the edition of the historical issue that has published on February 15, 2001, the articles describing the findings derived from the human genome sequencing. This seminal issue launched the era of post-genomic science.

The articles in this issue Nature indicate that our genome is formed of 2.9 to 3.2 billion nucleotides. Of that, over 50% consists of repetitive, or "parasite" elements of unknown function and only 1.1 to 1.4% is known to code proteins. About 5% of our genome consists of large DNA segments that have been recently duplicated, and these include a number of genes. The public initiative produced a list of approximately 22 000 human genes while the private publication found about 26 000 (IHGSC 2001; Venter et al. 2001). This compares with 6 000 genes for yeast, 13 000 for a fly (*Drosophila melanogaster*), 18 000 for a worm (*Caenorhabditis elegans*) and 26 000 for a plant (*Arabidopsis thaliana*). The number of predicted human genes was at the lower end of previous estimates, which had ranged between about 30 000 and 120 000 (Fields et al. 1994; Dunham et al. 1999; Ewing and Green 2000; Liang et al. 2000; Roest Crollius et al. 2000; Lander et al. 2001; Venter et al. 2001). The list of predicted genes should enlarge after the development of more adequate software for gene identification or the accumulation of further experimental evidence. The analysis of gene content does not explain our complexity over other organisms, and the understanding of our complexity will remain a challenge for the future.

In the years to come we will have to unveil the presence and functional relevance of alternatively processed forms of human transcripts that are derived from different transcription initiation sites, alternative exon splicing, and multiple polyadenylation sites (Gong et al. 2001; Yi et al. 2000; Edwalds-Gilbert et al. 1997). Determining the various transcript forms and investigating the purpose of these complex mixtures of instructions will be the next great endeavour toward understanding human biology.

▌ Genetic variation and its relation to human disease

One of the most important findings of the human genome project was to determine the nucleotide diversity between different individuals. Every individual on the planet – with the exception of identical twins — has a unique genome, and even though any two genomes are roughly 99.9% identical, that still leaves millions of differences among the 3.2 billion base pairs of nucleotides. The level of identity between any two genomes is about the same, independent of the ethnical origins of the individuals. Genetic differences between two white Europeans or between a white European and an Asiatic are the same. This is valid for all ethnical backgrounds and has destroyed, at the DNA level, the concept of races.

It is these subtle differences that account for heritable variation among individuals, including susceptibility to disease and response to pharmaceuticals. Most of the differences take the form of substitutions at a single base pair, or SNPs (single nucleotide polymorphisms). The high frequency of variations within most, if not all, human genes (Lander and Weinberg 2000) constitute the backbone of genetic predisposition of human diseases. About 90% of variations are SNPs, and over 1.42 million SNPs were already identified at the time of the first draft of the human genome available (International SNP Map Working Group 2001). This number has increased dramatically and strategies are now unfolding to compile comprehensive libraries of all phenotypically relevant SNPs (Brookes 1999; Cargill et al. 1999). Databases of polymorphisms are a boon to pharmacogeneticists and other clinical scientists, particularly those without access to genomic and informatics technology for SNP discovery and evaluation on their genes of interest.

While the most frequent SNPs (those with a minimal allele frequency of 40%) appear in every 3280 nucleotides of our genome (with a calculated number of SNPs close to one million), rare alleles are more common in our DNA. Around eleven million bases of our genome have a small variation index (alleles have a minimal frequency of 1%), but occur once in every 290 nucleotides of our genome. The combination of these SNPs form the genotypes. Genotypes are unique for each individual, and this same genetic combination will never occur again.

A key element of the puzzle of genetic disease is the understanding of genetic variation in the genome. The good thing of SNPs, specially in neuropsychiatric disorders, is its ease use. Every nucleated cell of our body contains the same DNA content, and it is stable independent of age, use of drugs, presence or absence of a crisis. There is no need to have access to the diseased tissue in order to evaluate the presence of a SNP and a simple collection of a small volume of blood permits the evaluation of thousands of polymorphisms.

In the database of SNPs (dbSNP) we saw a recent explosion in the number of polymorphisms registered. From January 2002 to February 2003, the number of registered SNPs has increased in about 2 million entries (going from 4 119 087 to 6 107 661 – *www.ncbi.nlm.nih.gov/SNP/snp_summary.cgi*). However, this database reflects the early days of SNPs. The majority of these SNPs have not been experimentally validated or classified yet, and only 39 480 (or 0.6%) have genotype frequencies available. The mapping of some SNPs to more than one chromosome location is also frequent and sometimes the SNP databases can be confusing and difficult to use. This also raises concern that there are an undetermined number of additional SNPs, many of them located within genes relevant to human therapy and disease, that are waiting to be found and will not be identified by *in silico* analysis alone. This may reflect the focus on EST (Expressed Sequence Tags) libraries (which are biased toward 3′ regions) and Human Genome Project output (which use DNA from a limited number of individuals, with resulting reduced power to observe variants). In addition to this, there is a high degree of variation present in SNP frequencies between different world populations. EST sequences do not provide yet an accurate representation of all possible variations. This suggests that sequencing-based strategies for DNA SNP discovery and validation, especially using sources from different ethnic groups, are still essential in order to achieve the goal of comprehensive analysis of clinically relevant polymorphisms. Indeed, validation of SNPs discovered by *in silico* analysis should be the main focus of future work.

Impact of genomics in the study of schizophrenia

It is expected that genomic information will have a broad range of applications in medicine. Hundreds of projects are using genetic information for drug discovery, pharmacogenomics, targeted gene therapy, studies of ageing, design of viral vectors, disease management, regenerative biology, cloning, diagnostics, prognostics, disease research, reproduction, nutriceuticals and the list go on.

The human genome sequence is an important piece in the puzzle of complex diseases such as hypertension, cancer, Alzheimer's disease or schizophrenia. However, the genetic approaches to investigate such complex diseases should not be solely based on SNPs or on the investigation of differential expression of a few genes. The full exploitation of the genomic intricacy has to include alternative splicing, comparative genomics, protein-protein interaction, and haplotypes collected in a large set of SNPs, accumulated in the same large set of patients.

Schizophrenia (SZ), as a complex disease, seems to be caused by a series of factors, including environmental and genetic. Twin and adoption studies have revealed that SZ has an important genetic component. However, it is clear that SZ is not a single disease entity but it reflects a common symptomatology caused by several distinct genetic abnormalities. As many cancers, SZ may require more than one genetic "hit" to be manifested clinically (Sawa and Snyder 2002). The genes that have to be hit are distributed over vast regions of our genome, and according to this, genetic loci that appear to confer susceptibility to SZ have been mapped to several chromosomes, including 1q21-22, 6p25, 8p21, 10p14, 13q32, 18p11, and 22q11-13 (Berrettini 2000; Brzustowics et al. 2000; Straub et al. 1995; Blouin et al. 1998; Ekelund et al. 2001). However, while the lists of candidate genes currently available accumulate, no highly reliable candidate SZ gene has yet emerged. Moreover, in some genomic regions there are no candidate genes identified yet.

Linkage and association strategies have been applied in the search of DNA sequence variations that may be responsible for the development of the disease. Linkage studies from the very beginning of SZ studies some 15 years ago (Sherrington et al. 1988; Kennedy et al. 1988) as well as more recent studies (Hovatta et al. 1999; Kendler et al. 2000; Baron 2001) have been marked with numerous controversial findings. Numerous genomic regions have been suspected to carry the genes predisposing to the disease; however, such regions of putative susceptibility vary significantly from study to study, from pedigree to pedigree, suggesting a large degree of genetic heterogeneity of the disease. After the sequencing of the human genome and its interpretation through studies that are focused in determining gene function, we are living a period where many data from different sources can be evaluated simultaneously.

The rational selection of candidate genes for genetic association studies in SZ were usually based on pharmacological, neurochemical, and clinical evidence that points at specific receptors, enzymes or any other molecules that might be involved in thc etiopathogenesis of the disease. Examples are the genes encoding dopamine and serotonin receptors that exhibit high affinity to antipsychotic agents. Several gene variants of these receptors have been studied; however, the results were also contradictory. This selection can now be improved if it incorporates genomic DNA sequences that were not available previously. When both approaches are undertaken we can obtain a list of genes of interest that can be mapped to important genomic regions for SZ (Table 1).

A good example is the search for expansion of trinucleotide repeats that may associated with the intriguing anticipation phenomena, repeatedly suggested in SZ (McInnis et al. 1999). Up to now, tremendous efforts have been made in the search for these repeats using several techniques including Repeat Expansion Detection (RED; Schalling et al. 1993) and others, but thus far the results of this search are controversial and could not identify a repeat unequivocally associated with SZ anticipation. The human genome sequence now offers a map where virtually all repeats can be located, selected according to aspects of interest (chromosomal location, proximity to genes of interest, etc.) and studied by amplification techniques, using minute amounts of DNA as a template.

Other approaches can include investigation of regions that demonstrated association of SZ with chromosomal rearrangements, such as translocations and deletions. A good example is a ~ 3 Mb deletion on the long arm of chromosome 22 that causes velocardiofacial syndrome (VCFS) and often leads to psychotic symptoms very similar to SZ. This finding indicates that genes located in the deletion region could modulate the risk to SZ. The genes or polymorphisms from this region, associated with SZ, have not been identified yet, and the huge number of ESTs available today, together with SAGE (Serial Analysis of Gene Expression) tags, LongSAGE tags (Saha et al. 2002) and genomic sequences of other organisms, offers the possibility of identifying genomic conserved blocks in this deleted region, which are likely to contain physiologically conserved DNA sequences.

Despite the huge efforts for finding susceptibility genes, the results of the molecular genetic studies of SZ, thus far, have been quite modest. This can be explained by many reasons. It should be always clear that environmental factors have a tremendous impact in the establishment of the disease. The impact of environment is as strong as those posed by genetics, and may dramatically disturb the genetic associations. The inheritance pattern of SZ is still unclear and usually does not follow a Mendelian mode, and the majority of cases of the disease are sporadic (Gottesman and Shields 1976). In addition, the clinical variation we see in SZ and the currently available diagnostic tools, based on questionnaires and presence/absence of a series of symptoms, may not be optimal and precise as molecular genetic studies may require.

As we see progress of neurochemistry and imaging in the analysis of SZ, we can count on new approaches derived from genomic studies. The proper use of genomics may help to unravel the causes of schizophrenia, and the approaches to be undertaken can include a series of aspects, such as:

▌ Gene discovery: large genomic regions, possibly involved with the disease, have already been sequenced. However, gene finding using *in silico* methods are not reliable, and a careful study of coding potential, comparative genomics and EST mapping is required for a better analysis of gene content in the human genome and for the identification of genes and regulatory regions potentially involved. Comparative genomics with DNA of other primates should unravel important regulatory regions, key for regulation of expression in our genome.

▌ Understanding of genetic variation: SNPs.

▌ Analysis of alternative spliced isoforms: new splicing isoforms are being revealed in many different human genes. The study of splicing in SZ is a very promising approach, if, as other expression analysis, samples from specific regions of fresh brains, controlled for age, use of drugs etc., are used.

▌ Analysis of differential gene expression: These techniques (such as DNA microarrays, RDA and SAGE) have been shown to be powerful in the evaluation of complex diseases such as cancer and hypertension. The use of these techniques is just starting in SZ.

▌ Dissection of metabolic pathways of interest: the selection of genes belonging to pathways such as phospholipid metabolism, neurogenesis or synaptogenesis, together with mapping information, should permit the selection of candidate genes for association studies, based in sums of criteria.

One of the main problems found in the actual biomedical investigation, and this is also true for SZ, is that the populations studied may consist of different ethnic backgrounds with different allele frequencies across various genetic polymorphisms. This ethnic variation also influences haplotype studies, as genomic blocks may vary dramatically between ethnic groups. In addition, allele frequencies may be different in males and females as well as in different age groups. When controls are not well matched to cases for their ethnic background, age, and sex, there is a good chance that evidence for genetic association may be a false negative. On the other hand, it is possible that true associations are not valid for the disease in a different ethnic background. After the economic globalization and the immigration flux that occurs all around the globe, the definition of a precise ethnic background is becoming more and more difficult, if not artificial. While there is an immense value in the identification of associations specific to certain pedigrees, the definition of robust association markers that are valid for any population should be considered as one of the most important targets in the modern biomedical research.

▌ Crossing information for selecting candidate genes

It is well recognised today that, in schizophrenia, the primary disorder is neurodevelopmental rather than neurodegenerative. An analysis of the human genome using the Gene Ontology bank (February 2003 – *http://www.godatabase. org/cgi-bin/go.cgi*) indicates the presence of 366 human genes related to neurogenesis (GO:0007399). On the other hand, an analysis of the literature shows that at least 27 genomic regions could be associated with SZ by different studies (Table 1). An approach that is being undertaken in our laboratory is to cross gene mapping information and gene function in order to obtain candidate genes for association studies. After crossing the list of genes involved with neurogenesis with genomic regions associated with SZ, we ended up with a list of at least 100 genes involved with neurodevelopment and that could be mapped to important SZ regions. Using this set of genes, we performed searches in databases in order to identify putative polymorphic sites such as SNPs or DNA microsatellites in a portion of these genes, focusing in alterations that would modify the protein. After confirming the polymorphic nature of the selected site, by using EST and genomic sequences, the most confident loci were used for experimental validation in a set of 200 DNA samples (400 alleles). All the first 18 putative polymorphisms that we choose for validating this approach showed to be true variations based in DNA alignment with other sequences. For 11 of these 18 polymorphisms we were able to design primers and all these could be experimentally confirmed. These 11 polymorphisms are ready to be used in all our DNA samples.

Together with the search for new polymorphisms we are committed with the expansion of our DNA bank, the polymorphisms are being continuously investigated to form a more detailed picture. Meanwhile, software for the identification of polymorphisms was developed in a collaboration between our laboratory and a Brazilian company (*www.scylla.com.br*). We have also designed a detailed system for storing clinical and molecular information from cases and controls together with data from sample collection, DNA extraction, quantification, quality and storage, as well as the cumulative genotyping obtained from every DNA sample. Our aim is to have a collection of DNA where genotype information is continuously added for an increasing number of loci. This set of samples and polymorphisms will be open for collaboration with colleagues in other studies.

A large set of patients in this bank ensures that the most diverse clinical phenotypes shall be well represented. This permits the stratification of patients without loosing statistical power due to a reduction in sampling. Stratification will be important to cover different forms of the disease as well as to provide samples for pharmacogenetic studies. The main advantage of having a large set of genes to be evaluated in the same set of patients is that we can have the accumulative effect of a series of genes of a small effect. New genes can easily be added to this system, using information derived from cDNA microarrays or SAGE tags that suggest a regulated expression of some genes.

∎ Futurology

Although there are likely to be many surprises in the future, the convergence of biochemical, imaging, neuroanatomy, psychopharmacology, clinical and genetic studies let us predict that we may be coming much closer to understanding the biological basis of SZ. What can we expect in the field of genetics for the 15–20 years to come? While all the possibilities are far too broad to discuss here, a few things appear to be relatively certain:

- ∎ A fairly comprehensive list of human gene products will provide a vast range of potential human-based drugs (similar to human insulin, interferons or growth hormone).
- ∎ Future medical records shall include a fair amount of genetic information, and eventually the person's complete genome and the status of a long list of polymorphic loci that can be used to predict responses to certain drugs, chemical and environmental substances, and the individual's propensity to certain diseases.
- ∎ Unravelling the genetic basis of complex disease will enable the development of prevention strategies to impede the establishment of the disease, and the design of drugs for a most efficient treatment.
- ∎ A growing industry will develop in pharmacogenomics and personalised medicine in which drugs are geared to the specific genetic traits of groups or individuals.

The availability of these achievements will have a dramatic impact on the SZ research, and we can expect better years to come. In order to cover the vast aspects of SZ, it would be extremely desirable to create an international network of researchers that could contribute with samples and data including the vast aspects related with the disease. A common depository of data derived from the many disciplines mentioned, and a DNA bank of these individuals, from diverse ethnic backgrounds shall permit a quantum leap in schizophrenia research.

▌ **Acknowledgments.** The authors thank Drs. Juliana Yacubian and Paulo Sallet for providing clinical samples and clinical data, and Prof. Wagner Gattaz for his continuous support. The Laboratory of Neurosciences (LIM27) receives financial support from Associação Beneficente Alzira Denise Hertzog Silva (ABADHS), Fundação de Amparo à Pesquisa do Estado de São Paulo (FA-PESP) and Conselho Nacional de Pesquisas (CNPq). The authors wish to thank Applied Biosystems for their collaboration with our group.

▌ References

Baron M (2001) Genetics of schizophrenia and the new millennium: progress and pitfalls. Am J Hum Genet 68(2):299–312

Berrettini WH (2000) Are schizophrenic and bipolar disorders related? A review of family and molecular studies. Biol Psychiatry 48(6):531–538

Blouin JL, Dombroski BA, Nath SK et al (1998) Schizophrenia susceptibility loci on chromosomes 13q32 and 8p21. Nat Genet 20:70–73

Brookes AJ (1999) The essence of SNPs. Gene 234:177–186

Brookes AJ, Lehvaslaiho H, Siegfried M, Boehm JG, Yuan YP, Sarkar CM, Bork P, Ortigao F (2000) HGBASE: a database of SNPs and other variations in and around human genes. Nucleic Acids Res 28:356–360

Brzustowicz LM, Hodgkinson KA, Chow EW, Honer WG, Bassett AS (2000) Location of a major susceptibility locus for familial schizophrenia on chromosome 1q21-q22. Science 288(5466):678–682

Buetow KH, Edmonson MN, Cassidy AB (1999) Reliable identification of large numbers of candidate SNPs from public EST data. Nat Genet 21:323–325

Camp NJ, Neuhausen SL, Tiobech J et al (2001) Genomewide multipoint linkage analysis of seven extended Palauan pedigrees with schizophrenia, by a Markov-Chain Monte Carlo method. Am J Hum Genet 69:1278–1289

Cargill M, Altshuler D, Ireland J, Sklar P, Ardlie K, Patil N, Shaw N, Lane CR, Lim EP, Kalyanaraman N, Nemesh J, Ziaugra L, Friedland L, Rolfe A, Warrington J, Lipshutz R, Daley GQ, Lander ES (1999) Characterization of single-nucleotide polymorphisms in coding regions of human genes. Nat Genet 22:231–238

Chumakov I, Blumenfeld M, Guerassimenko O, Cavarec L, Palicio M, Abderrahim H et al (2002) Genetic and physiological data implicating the new human gene G72 and the gene for D-amino acid oxidase in schizophrenia. Proc Natl Acad Sci 99(21):13675–13680

Dunham I, Shimizu N, Roe BA, Chissoe S, Hunt AR, Collins JE et al (1999) The DNA sequence of human chromosome 22. Nature 402:489–495

Edwalds-Gilbert G, Veraldi KL, Milcarek C (1997) Alternative poly(A) site selection in complex transcription units: means to an end? Nucleic Acids Res 25:2547–2561

Ekelund J, Hovatta I, Parker A, Paunio T, Varilo T, Martin R et al (2001) Chromosome 1 loci in Finnish schizophrenia families. Hum Mol Genet 10(15):1611–1617

Evans WE, Relling MV (1999) Pharmacogenomics: translating functional genomics into rational therapeutics. Science 286:487–491

Ewing B, Green P (2000) Analysis of expressed sequence tags indicates 35 000 human genes. Nat Genet 25:232–234

Fields C, Adams MD, White O, Venter JC (1994) How many genes are in the human genome? Nat Genet 7:345–346

Freedman R, Leonard S, Gault JM, Hopkins J, Cloninger CR, Kaufmann CA, Tsuang MT, Farone SV, Malaspina D, Svrakic DM, Sanders A, Gejman P (2001) Linkage disequilibrium for schizophrenia at the chromosome 15q13-14 locus of the alpha7-nicotinic acetylcholine receptor subunit gene (CHRNA7). Am J Med Genet 105(1):20–22

Gong QH, Cho JW, Huang T, Potter C, Gholami N, Basu NK, Kubota S, Carvalho S, Pennington MW, Owens IS et al (2001) Thirteen UDP glucuronosyltransferase genes are encoded at the human UGT1 gene complex locus. Pharmacogenetics 11(4):357–368

Gottesman II, Shields J (1976) A critical review of recent adoption, twin, and family studies of schizophrenia: behavioral genetics perspectives. Schizophr Bull 2(3): 360–401

Gurling HM, Kalsi G, Brynjolfson J, Sigmundsson T, Sherrington R, Mankoo BS, Read T, Murphy P, Blaveri E, McQuillin A, Petursson H, Curtis D (2001) Genome-wide genetic linkage analysis confirms the presence of susceptibility loci for schizophrenia, on chromosomes 1q32.2, 5q33.2, and 8p21-22 and provides support for linkage to schizophrenia, on chromosomes 11q23.3-24 and 20q12.1-11.23. Am J Hum Genet 68(3):661–673

Hewett M, Oliver DE, Rubin DL, Easton KL, Stuart JM, Altman RB, Klein TE (2002) PharmGKB: the pharmacogenetics knowledge base. Nucleic Acids Res 30:163–165

Hirakawa M (2002) HOWDY: an integrated database system for human genome research. Nucleic Acids Res 30:152–157

Hovatta I, Varilo T, Suvisaari J, Terwilliger JD, Ollikainen V, Arajarvi R, Juvonen H, Kokko-Sahin ML, Vaisanen L, Mannila H, Lönnqvist J, Peltonen L (1999) A genomewide screen for schizophrenia genes in an isolated Finnish subpopulation, suggesting multiple susceptibility loci. Am J Hum Genet 65(4):1114–1124

International Human Genome Sequencing Consortium (2001) Initial sequencing and analysis of the human genome. Nature 409:860–921

International SNP Map Working Group (2001) A map of human genome sequence variation containing 1.42 million single nucleotide polymorphisms. Nature 409: 928–933

Irizarry K, Kustanovich V, Li C, Brown N, Nelson S, Wong W, Lee CJ (2000) Genome-wide analysis of single-nucleotide polymorphisms in human expressed sequences. Nat Genet 26:233–236

Jonsson EG, Flyckt L, Burgert E, Crocq MA, Forslund K, Mattila-Evenden M, Rylander G, Asberg M, Nimgaonkar VL, Edman G, Bjerkenstedt L, Wiesel FA, Sedvall GC (2003) Dopamine D3 receptor gene Ser9Gly variant and schizophrenia: association study and meta-analysis. Psychiatr Genet 13(1):1–12

Jorgensen TH, Borglum AD, Mors O, Wang AG, Pinaud M, Flint TJ, Dahl HA, Vang M, Kruse TA, Ewald H (2002) Search for common haplotypes on chromosome 22q in patients with schizophrenia or bipolar disorder from the Faroe Islands. Am J Med Genet 114(2):245–252

Kendler KS, Myers JM, O'Neill FA, Martin R, Murphy B, MacLean CJ, Walsh D, Straub RE (2000) Clinical features of schizophrenia and linkage to chromosomes 5q, 6p, 8p, and 10p in the Irish Study of High-Density Schizophrenia Families. Am J Psychiatry 157(3):402–408

Kennedy JL, Giuffra LA, Moises HW, Cavalli-Sforza LL, Pakstis AJ, Kidd JR, Castiglione CM, Sjogren B, Wetterberg L, Kidd KK (1988) Evidence against linkage of schizophrenia to markers on chromosome 5 in a northern Swedish pedigree. Nature 336(6195):167–170

Kruglyak L, Nickerson DA (2001) Variation is the spice of life. Nature Genetics 27:234–236

Lander ES, Weinberg RA (2000) Genomics: journey to the center of biology. Science 287:1777–1782

Lander ES, Linton LM, Birren B, Nusbaum C, Zody MC, Baldwin J, Devon K, Dewar K, Doyle M, FitzHugh W et al (2001) Initial sequencing and analysis of the human genome. Nature 409:860–921

Lara DR, Gama CS, Belmonte-de-Abreu P, Portela LV, Goncalves CA, Fonseca M, Hauck S, Souza DO (2001) Increased serum S100B protein in schizophrenia: a study in medication-free patients. J Psychiatr Res 35(1):11–14

Liang F, Holt I, Pertea G, Karamycheva S, Salzberg SL, Quackenbush J (2000) Gene index analysis of the human genome estimates approximately 120 000 genes. Nat Genet 25:239–240

Lindholm E, Ekholm B, Balciuniene J, Johansson G, Castensson A, Koisti M, Nylander PO, Pettersson U, Adolfsson R, Jazin E (1999) Linkage analysis of a large Swedish kindred provides further support for a susceptibility locus for schizophrenia on chromosome 6p23. Am J Med Genet 88(4):369–377

Lindholm E, Ekholm B, Shaw S, Jalonen P, Johansson G, Pettersson U, Sherrington R, Adolfsson R, Jazin E (2001) A schizophrenia-susceptibility locus at 6q25, in one of the world's largest reported pedigrees. Am J Hum Genet 69(1):96–105

Liu H, Heath SC, Sobin C, Roos JL, Galke BL, Blundell ML, Lenane M, Robertson B, Wijsman EM, Rapoport JL, Gogos JA, Karayiorgou M (2002) Genetic variation at the 22q11 PRODH2/DGCR6 locus presents an unusual pattern and increases susceptibility to schizophrenia. Proc Natl Acad Sci 99(6):3717–3722

Lung FW, Tzeng DS, Shu BC (2002) Ethnic heterogeneity in allele variation in the DRD4 gene in schizophrenia. Schizophr Res 57(2-/3):239–245

Marsh S, Kwok P, McLeod HL (2002) SNP databases and pharmacogenetics: great start, but a long way to go. Human Mutation 20:174–179

McInnis MG, McMahon FJ, Crow T, Ross CA, DeLisi LE (1999) Anticipation in schizophrenia: a review and reconsideration. Am J Med Genet 88(6):686–693

McLeod HL, Evans WE (2001) Pharmacogenomics: unlocking the human genome for better drug therapy. Ann Rev Pharmacol Tox 41:101–121

Mirnics K, Middleton FA, Stanwood GD, Lewis DA, Levitt P (2001) Disease-specific changes in regulator of G-protein signaling 4 (RGS4) expression in schizophrenia. Mol Psychiatry 6(3):293–301

Moises HW, Yang L, Kristbjarnarson H, Wiese C, Byerley W, Macciardi F, Arolt V, Blackwood D, Liu X, Sjogren B et al (1995) An international two-stage genome-wide search for schizophrenia susceptibility genes. Nat Genet 11(3):321–324

Muir WJ, Thomson ML, McKeon P, Mynett-Johnson L, Whitton C, Evans KL, Porteous DJ, Blackwood DH (2001) Markers close to the dopamine D5 receptor gene (DRD5) show significant association with schizophrenia but not bipolar disorder. Am J Med Genet 105(2):152–158

Nature (2001) Human genomes, public and private. Nature 409:745

Noble EP (2003) D2 dopamine receptor gene in psychiatric and neurologic disorders and its phenotypes. Am J Med Genet 116(1 Suppl):103–125

Ohnishi Y, Tanaka T, Yamada R, Suematsu K, Minami M, Fujii K, Hoki N, Kodama K, Nagata S, Hayashi T, Kinoshita N, Sato H, Sato H, Kuzuya T, Takeda H, Hori M, Nakamura Y (2000) Identification of 187 single nucleotide polymorphisms (SNPs) among 41 candidate genes for ischemic heart disease in the Japanese population. Hum Genet 106:288–292

Paunio T, Ekelund J, Varilo T et al (2001) Genome-wide scan in a nationwide study sample of schizophrenia families in Finland reveals susceptibility loci on chromosomes 2q and 5q. Hum Mol Genet 10:3037–3048

Roest Crollius H, Jaillon O, Bernot A, Dasilva C, Bouneau L, Fischer C, Fizames C, Wincker P, Brottier P, Quetier F, Saurin W, Weissenbach J (2000) Estimate of human gene number provided by genome-wide analysis using *Tetraodon nigroviridis* DNA sequence. Nat Genet 25:235–238

Sawa A, Snyder SH (2002) Schizophrenia: diverse approaches to a complex disease. Science 296(5568):692–695

Saha S, Sparks AB, Rago C, Akmaev V, Wang CJ, Vogelstein B, Kinzler K, Velculescu V (2002) Using the transcriptome to annotate the genome. Nature Biotechnology 19:508–512

Schalling M, Hudson TJ, Buetow KH, Housman DE (1993) Direct detection of novel expanded trinucleotide repeats in the human genome. Nat Genet 4(2):135–139

Schwab SG, Wildenauer DB (1999) Chromosome 22 workshop report. Am J Med Genet 88:276–278

Seeman P, Guan HC, Van Tol HHM (1993) Dopamine D4 receptors elevated in schizophrenia. Nature 365:441–445

Sherrington R, Brynjolfsson J, Petursson H, Potter M, Dudleston K, Barraclough B, Wasmuth J, Dobbs M, Gurling H (1988) Localization of a susceptibility locus for schizophrenia on chromosome 5. Nature 336(6195):164–167

Sherry ST, Ward MH, Kholodov M, Baker J, Phan L, Smigielski EM, Sirotkin K (2001) dbSNP: the NCBI database of genetic variation. Nucleic Acids Res 29:308–311

Shifman S, Bronstein M, Sternfeld M, Pisante-Shalom A, Lev-Lehman E, Weizman A, Reznik I, Spivak B, Grisaru N, Karp L, Schiffer R, Kotler M, Strous RD, Swartz-Vanetik M, Knobler HY, Shinar E, Beckmann JS, Yakir B, Risch N, Zak NB, Darvasi A (2002) A highly significant association between a COMT haplotype and schizophrenia. Am J Hum Genet 71(6):1296–1302

Silverman JM, Greenberg DA, Altstiel LD, Siever LJ, Mohs RC, Smith CJ, Zhou G, Hollander TE, Yang XP, Kedache M, Li G, Zaccario ML, Davis KL (1996) Evidence of a locus for schizophrenia and related disorders on the short arm of chromosome 5 in a large pedigree. Am J Med Genet 67(2):162–171

Skol AD, Young KA, Tsuang DW, Faraone SV, Haverstock SL, Bingham S, Prabhudesai S, Mena F, Menon AS, Yu CE, Rundell P, Pepple J, Sauter F, Baldwin C, Weiss D, Collins J, Keith T, Boehnke M, Schellenberg GD, Tsuang MT (2003) Modest evidence for linkage and possible confirmation of association between NOTCH4 and schizophrenia in a large veterans affairs cooperative study sample. Am J Med Genet 118B(1):8–15

Smigielski EM, Sirotkin K, Ward M, Sherry ST (2000) dbSNP: a database of single nucleotide polymorphisms. Nucleic Acids Res 28:352–355

Stefansson H, Sigurdsson E, Steinthorsdottir V, Bjornsdottir S, Sigmundsson T, Ghosh S et al (2002) Neuregulin 1 and susceptibility to schizophrenia. Am J Hum Genet 71(4):877–892

Stober G, Saar K, Ruschendorf F, Meyer J, Nürnberg G, Jatzke S et al (2000) Splitting schizophrenia: periodic catatonia-susceptibility locus on chromosome 15q15. Am J Hum Genet 67:1201–1207

Stober G, Seelow D, Ruschendorf F, Ekici A, Beckmann H, Reis A (2002) Periodic catatonia: confirmation of linkage to chromosome 15 and further evidence for genetic heterogeneity. Hum Genet 111(4/5):323–330

Straub RE, Maclean CJ, O'Neill FA, Burke J, Murphy B, Duke F, Shinkwin R, Webb BT, Zhang J, Walsh D et al (1995) A potential vulnerability locus for schizophrenia on chromosome 6p24-22: evidence for genetic heterogeneity. Nature Genet 11:287

Venter JC, Adams MD, Myers EW, Li PW, Mural RJ, Sutton GG, Smith HO, Yandell M, Evans CA, Holt RA et al (2001) The sequence of the human genome. Science 291:1304–1351

Wassink TH, Nopoulos P, Pietila J, Crowe RR, Andreasen NC (2003) NOTCH4 and the frontal lobe in schizophrenia. Am J Med Genet 118B(1):1–7

Yamada R, Tanaka T, Ohnishi Y, Suematsu K, Minami M, Seki T et al (2000) Identification of 142 single nucleotide polymorphisms in 41 candidate genes for rheumatoid arthritis in the Japanese population. Hum Genet 106:293–297

Yi X, White DM, Aisner DL, Baur JA, Wright WE, Shay JW (2000) An alternate splicing variant of the human telomerase catalytic subunit inhibits telomerase activity. Neoplasia 2:433–440

Discussion: The genetics of psychosis is the genetics of the speciation of Homo sapiens

T. J. Crow

SANE POWIC, Warneford Hospital, Oxford, OX3 7JX, UK

If we agree that the one conclusion that we can be sure of in the aetiology of psychosis is that there is a genetic contribution the identification of the relevant gene or genes overrides anything else. The contributions to this session illustrate a diversity of approaches; do they approach the core of the problem?

Emmanuel Diaz Neto has given us a masterly overview of present knowledge of the human genome. We now know a lot about its constitution and size. Given the vast number of single nucleotide polymorphisms that have now been identified Emmanuel puts his faith, as many others have done, in the linkage approach as the sure route to identifying the genetic contribution. With this hypothesis-free method it has been suggested it will be possible to "drain the pond dry".

But already much data has been collected. One can ask how consistent are the findings across analyses? In his table Neto includes no fewer than 27 positive linkages and 16 candidate genes that have been identified from these linkages. Wolfgang Maier in his chapter specifies 5 linkages and identifies 5 candidate genes. This sounds like progress but how much can these findings be relied upon?

Although there have been claims for replication of linkages across genome scans the number of positive claims has been large [(DeLisi and Crow, 1999; DeLisi et al., 2000) – see Introductory chapter by Lynn DeLisi] and in collations of the findings it has been unclear that these represent more than a co-incidence of peaks within chromosomal arms. However there have now been two meta-analyses of the genome scans in relation to schizophrenia and two in relation to bipolar disorder (Table 1).

Taken together the findings are instructive:

- Of the two meta-analyses in schizophrenia one draws attention to three and the other to nine possible loci of significance. Badner and Gershon (2002) pointed to 8p, 13q and 22q as the regions of greatest significance whilst by the method they adopted (Lewis, 2003) the strongest finding was on 2p with significant evidence for linkage on 3p, 11q, 5q, 20p, all yielding stronger evidence than the strongest candidate (8p) in the first study. Thus the two meta-analyses applied to a material with an overlap of approximately 500 pedigrees out of a total of 681 (Badner and Gershon, 2002) or 1208 (Lewis et al., 2003) agree only on two out of ten chromosome arms identified as candidates to harbour a locus for schizophrenia. The strongest finding in one study (Lewis et al., 2003; linkage to 2p) was not detected in the other

Table 1. Meta-analyses of genome scans for linkage in psychosis

Study	Badner and Gershon (2002) schizophrenia	Lewis et al. (2003) schizophrenia	Badner and Gershon (2002) bipolar disorder	Segurado et al. (2003) bipolar disorder
No. of families	681	1,208	353	347
Affected individuals	1,929	2,945	1,228	959
Core phenotype	Schizophrenia, schizo affective disorder	Schizophrenia, schizo affective disorder (rank order in brackets)	Bipolar, schizo-affective, unipolar depression	Bipolar, schizo-aff ective disorder
Genome-wide, or by-bin, significance reported by bin or locus	8p 13q 22q	2p (1) 2q (8) 3p (2) 5q (4) 6p (7) 8p (6) 11q (3) 20p (5) 22q (9)	13q 22q	9p 10q 14q 18q

analysis. The reason for this is that this locus emerged from a large study (DeLisi et al., 2002; n = 380 sib pairs) that was included only in the second meta-analysis.

▮ While the second meta-analyses of schizophrenia (Lewis et al., 2003) and of bipolar disorder (Badner and Gershon, 2002) were conducted with an identical methodology the conclusions that the authors draw are quite different. Whereas the schizophrenia meta-analysis concluded that there were eight bins that yielded genome-wide evidence of linkage, the bipolar meta-analysis revealed no such evidence of linkage (the locations given in the table for this study are the nominal 5% by-bin significances) and those locations that yielded the largest rank sums showed no overlap with the bins identified for schizophrenia. This is surprising to those who expected that there would be some genetic commonality between these major phenotypes (Stassen et al., 1988; Gershon et al., 1988; Maier et al., 1993). It is the more surprising when it is appreciated that the core phenotype in both meta-analyses included schizo-affective diagnoses.

▮ The two findings in the first analysis of bipolar disorder (Badner and Gershon, 2002) of 353 families were not replicated in the second meta-analysis (Segurado et al., 2003) that included 347 families from essentially the same published literature but identified four different locations as of interest.

Where does this leave the search for genes for psychosis? At the very least it is clear that no strong signal is emerging, and more importantly there is no obvious criterion for distinguishing signal from noise. Given these difficulties none of the linkages or candidate genes identified by Neto and Maier can be taken seriously as relating to the disease process. One possible conclusion, that favoured by Maier, is that many genes of small effect are relevant, that significant heterogeneity across populations is present, and that samples much larger than those currently available (1208 pedigrees and 2945 affected individuals in the second schizophrenia meta-analysis) will be required to detect reliable linkage. The second possibility is that the genetic contribution is of a nature that is intrinsically invisible to the linkage strategy. One interpretation of the findings of the linkage literature is that the pond is dry and no genes have been found!

Microarrays as an alternative to linkage

An alternative hypothesis-free approach is that followed by Sabine Bahn – the micro-array strategy applied to post-mortem RNA. Sabine gives a clear and spirited account of the endeavour – as was said of the linkage method it is "bound to succeed" – and there are a number of significant differences between the brains of patients with psychosis and the comparison series (Tkachev et al., 1972). How are we to interpret the findings? It is true that changes in ApoE proteins may be associated with changes in white matter. It can be argued that these and other changes seen in micro-array studies are real and reflect a myelin-based pathophysiology, perhaps a primary change of oligodendrocytic function. In a general way this might be seen as consistent with the concept that in psychosis there is a disorder of connectivity. But if the primary change is at the level of the oligodendrocyte or myelin synthesis surely what would be expected would be deficits in long tract function rather than the rather subtle failures of "higher cognitive" functions that psychotic symptoms represent. For an account of pathophysiology to be convincing it needs to provide some explanation of the selectivity of the disease process and the nature of symptoms. Some of the other changes reported in micro-array studies – for example deviations in glutamate-related indices, in N-acetyl aspartate, lysophosphatidic acid and mitochondrial function – seem likewise to be of too general a nature to be directly related to the primary disturbance.

Sabine Bahn presents data to answer the sceptic who wonders whether neuroleptic or other medication may have something to do with the schizophrenic-control differences observed. These findings are generally reassuring but two case histories from the schizophrenia literature of the past are worth recollecting. The large literature that was generated by the observation of Murphy and Wyatt (1972) that the activity of the enzyme mono-amine oxidase was reduced in the platelets of patients with schizophrenia was only finally brought into perspective by studies that showed that, for reasons that are as yet unclear, mono-amine oxidase activity in the platelet declines slowly over weeks and months after patients are started on neuroleptic medication (DeLisi et al., 1981; Owen et al., 1981) and that a reduction is not seen in those who have never been on such medication (Owen et al., 1976).

The second case history relates to the reduction of glutamic acid decarboxylase that was reported in a large series of cases of schizophrenia and "schizophrenia-like" psychoses by Bird et al. (1977). This also, it was suggested, was a correlate of the disease process. But later careful studies by the same group (Spokes, 1979) established that the level of glutamic acid decarboxylase in post-mortem brain tissue is a function of hypoxic mode of death, and that such modes of death are often more common in patients with psychosis than in control series.

Relating to an even earlier literature Seymour Kety's masterly reviews (Kety, 1959a;b) of the difficulty of establishing that any hypothesised biochemical anomaly is indeed associated with the disease rather than with its treatment or the circumstances in which patients with the condition find themselves can still be regarded as required reading for those in the field.

The nature of changes in the cerebral cortex

What is the nature of the genetic contribution? Perhaps the strongest clue that we have to pathophysiology are the structural brain changes – there is a degree of ventricular enlargement (Johnstone et al., 1976) that is replicable across studies and relatively uniform in magnitude – the variance is not increased in the patient group relative to controls (Daniel et al., 1991; Vita et al., 2000). The disease is at least in part structural and the genetic contribution must relate to this. What is the meaning of the ventricular change? That it reflects some change in subcortical structures has often been suggested, but those structures that have been examined, e.g. hippocampus (Heckers et al., 1990; Walker et al., 2002), amygdala (Chance et al., 2002), dorso-medial nucleus of the thalamus (Cullen et al., 2003), in post-mortem brain have shown no change. On the other hand there is evidence of change at the level of the cerebral cortex. The obvious conclusion is that the relevant gene is one that influences the development of the cortex. If some aspect of cortical development is delayed or anomalous this may be reflected in increased ventricular volume. But exactly which aspect of cortical development?

Peter Falkai presents data from a family study that attempts to address this issue. These workers have focussed on two aspects of the morphological problem – gyrification of the cortex and changes in the temporal lobe, specifically in the hippocampus. They have adopted the strategy of contrasting patients with unaffected relatives and with normal controls as a method of examining the genetic influence. Falkai et al write that –

"Based on post-mortem and imaging studies there is now consistent evidence for brain morphological abnormalities in schizophrenia"

but there is much less agreement on exactly what these changes are. They continue

"The changes comprise a subtle whole brain volume reduction, enlargement of the ventricular system, mainly the lateral ventricles, changes in the frontal as well as temporal lobes especially a bilateral hippocampal volume reduction."

These statements illustrate the difficulty. As noted above while there is some agreement between imaging and post-mortem studies on the presence of ventricular enlargement, and evidence from imaging studies that this is a relatively uniform change, this is not the case for a reduction in hippocampal volume (Heckers et al., 1990; Walker et al., 2002) and the nature of the change at the level of the cerebral cortex is obscure. As the accumulating body of literature on the application of "voxel-based morphometry" to the problem makes clear attempts to identify specific cortical structures that are selectively affected has led to inconsistent conclusions.

It is plausible as Falkai et al. suggest that there is some general deviation in the formation of the gyri and that this may be the clue to the pathophysiology. But here also the results of different studies are inconsistent. At this meeting Sallet et al. (2003) presented evidence for significant bilateral reduction of gyral folding in 40 patients with schizophrenia by comparison with 20 controls with the greatest reductions in those with disorganisation, and confined to the left side in those with a paranoid syndrome.

By contrast with these studies a recent attempt (Highley et al., 2003) to apply stereological principles to the assessment of gyrification in the cortex as a whole revealed no differences between patients and controls. Rather there was a sex-dependent effect on white matter in the occipito-parietal regions with a decrease in females and an increase in males relative to controls. That there may be changes in gyrification but that these are subtle is suggested by a study in adolescent onset psychosis (White et al., 2003) – on global measures the gyri were found to be slightly more pointed and the depths of the sulci flattened in patients relative to controls. Application of the same technique to a large series of adult onset psychoses (Nopoulos et al., 2003) revealed changes that were sex-specific and related to symptoms. Patients tended to have more 'peaked' gyri and flatter or wider sulci. In male patients the more abnormal the shape (peaked gyri and shallower sulci) the greater the severity of symptoms; in female patients the greater the severity of psychosis the lesser the area of cortex.

It may be that some such change at the level of cortex reflected in an alteration in gyral structure is a constant accompaniment of the disease process and the proximal cause of the enlargement of the ventricles. But the question remains what is the cause of the gyral change and what is its relation to the genetic predisposition?

Language and the origin of the species

Wolfgang Maier draws attention to the consistency and magnitude of the psychological deficits as summarised by Heinrichs and Zakzanis (1998).

"A most comprehensive meta-analysis reveals the highest degree of impairment in language-related functions and to perceptual and motor abilities… Language-related abilities were still most severely impaired in schizophrenia when sensory processing is controlled".

This opens up a new perspective on the disease, and one that leads to quite different evolutionary and genetic conclusions. If language is the function that is most affected why do we not consider that this is the primary abnormality and that the impairments of other measurable dimensions of psychological ability are secondary? Arguably the first rank symptoms are disorders of language (Crow, 1998). Language after all is the defining characteristic of *Homo sapiens* as a species. It has features that the communicative systems of other primates do not share. Its origins are a problem for evolutionary theory (Bickerton, 1990; Crow, 2002).

The question has been asked (Crow, 1995 b; Crow 1997) how old is the genetic variation relating to schizophrenia? Given the relative uniformity of incidence across populations as demonstrated in the World Health Organization Ten-Country study (Jablensky et al., 1992) as well as the earlier studies (Murphy, 1976) that showed that schizophrenic symptoms are seen with similar features in populations that are widely separated geographically and in culture [the "anthropoparity principle" (Crow, 1995 a)] the problem can be cast in the context of the Out of Africa hypothesis, the theory that modern *Homo sapiens* arose as a species perhaps between 100 and 150,000 years ago somewhere in Africa and that all subsequent populations are derived from this origin (Stringer and McKie, 1996). If schizophrenic illnesses (and psychotic illnesses more generally) are seen with similar characteristics and incidences in each of these populations and they are genetic in origin then it is implausible to suggest that the genetic variation arose after the separation of these populations – it must have been present at the origin of the species (Fig. 1).

This conclusion relates the problem to the large issue of the nature of the species origin and its genetic and neural basis. What was it that changed 100 to 150,000 years ago? Attaching the label of a "speciation event" to the transition focuses attention on the genetic and evolutionary implications. Was this a single event or did it occur in a population? Was it a response to an environmental change or an intrinsic genetic mutation that conferred an advantage that was independent of the immediate environment? Was its survival ensured by an advantage in the process of mate choice? If so to which sex was the ad-

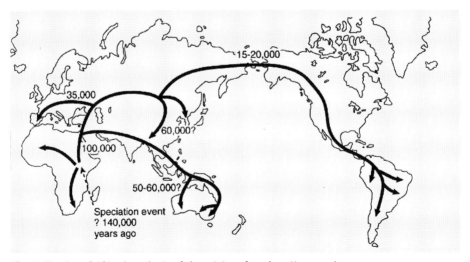

Fig. 1. The Out of Africa hypothesis of the origins of modern *Homo sapiens*

vantage, and how did it generalise? The identification of the transition as genetic (as indeed it must have been) draws attention to fundamental and unresolved issues in evolutionary theory. When these issues are related to the singular capacities of the species – its biological success in terms of population numbers relative to any other primate species, its tolerance and exploitation of a wide range of environmental habitats, its ability to mould the environment to its survival – the peculiarity and significance of the speciation event become apparent.

This genetic change brought about a modification of brain function that transformed the survival ability of the species. What was the change and with what function was it associated?

To the second part of this question Isocrates 2,300 years ago had an answer:

> "because there is born in us the power to persuade each other and to show each other whatever we wish, we not only have escaped from living as brutes, but also by coming together have founded cities and set up laws and invented arts, and speech has helped us attain practically all of the things we have devised" (quoted in Harris and Talbot, 1997).

Language, that is to say the capacity for symbolic representation, is what characterises the species. But with what neural change was this capacity associated? How can this capacity have originated so abruptly as the archaeological record (Noble and Davidson, 1996; Mellars, 2002) suggests?

After he had convinced himself (Broca, 1861) that the earlier observation of Marc Dax – that some aspect of the motor control of speech is located in the frontal lobe on the left side of the brain – is correct, in 1877 Broca formulated the following further concept:

> "Man is, of all the animals, the one whose brain in the normal state is the most asymmetrical. He is also the one who possesses the most acquired faculties. Among these faculties…the faculty of articulate language holds pride of place. It is this that distinguishes us most clearly from the animals."

Cerebral lateralization and the speciation event

Was Broca right? The concept that lateralization is the characteristic that defines the human brain, that it is the correlate of language and that it has a genetic basis has been pursued particularly by Marian Annett (1985, 2002). From her work three generalisations can be drawn: 1) a single gene will account for asymmetry as manifest in handedness; 2) directional handedness is specific to man; 3) cerebral asymmetry is the major determinant of cognitive ability.

Concerning the first there is now little disagreement (see e.g. McManus, 1991). On the second Annett is in agreement with Broca. The conclusion that population-based directional asymmetry is specific to *Homo sapiens* is substantially reinforced by the studies of Marchant and McGrew (1996) of chimpanzees in the Gombe National Park [and by the subsequent careful cross-species comparisons in a series of primates by Holder (1999)] who concluded that "No species level left- or right-handedness was found for any of the five *species (common chimpanzee, red colobus, redtail monkey, grey-checked manga-bey, and mountain gorilla) studied"*. In reviewing the primate literature, McGrew and Marchant (1997) wrote that *"non-human primate hand function has not been shown to be lateralized at the species level – it is not the norm for any species, task or setting, and so offers no easy model for the evolution of human handedness"*.

The anatomical correlate of directional asymmetry for handedness is what is described as the Yakovlevian torque from the right frontal to left occipital lobes of the brain, a bias that is reflected in the asymmetry to the left of the planum temporale (Geschwind and Levitsky, 1968). Evidence that this torque is specific to *Homo sapiens* has recently been presented (Buxhoeveden et al., 2001). These authors describe asymmetries of the minicolumn structure of the planum temporale that are present in man but absent in the chimpanzee and rhesus monkey.

If asymmetry is specific to man and the substrate of language, as Broca suggested, to unravel its genetic basis becomes a priority. Two independent items of evidence support the hypothesis (Crow, 1993) that the gene for asymmetry is in a region of homology between the X and the Y chromosomes:

∥ in a series of 15,000 families direction of handedness was found to be significantly more often associated with sex than would be expected by chance (Corballis et al., 1996).

∥ Sex chromosome aneuploidies (Turner's syndrome, Klinefelter's and XXX syndromes) are associated with relative hemispheric deficits on neuropsychological tests – Turner's (XO) individuals have right hemisphere and Klinefelter's and XXX syndrome individuals have left hemisphere or verbal deficits (Crow, 1994).

These findings directed attention to a region of homology that has been created in the course of hominid evolution – a block of 4 mB reduplicatively translocated from the Xq21.3 region to the Y chromosome short arm, and the block on the Y was subject to at least four deletions and a paracentric inversion. What selective force was responsible for the retention of these sequences on the Y and for their subsequent modification? The gene content of the homologous block is now established. Three genes are present but one of these (PABPC5) has been eliminated from the Y by one of the deletions. Of the remaining two (TGIFLX/Y and PCDHX/Y) the first is expressed mainly if not exclusively in the testis while the latter Protocadherin X and Y is of interest because the two "gametologues" code for cell surface adhesion molecules that are each expressed in the brain (Blanco et al., 2000). Comparisons of the two sequences in man with the single sequence (PcdhX) that is present on the X chromosome in each of the great apes and the mouse establishes that the PCDHX ectodomain and the PCDHY cytodomain have been subject to positive selective pressure (pressure for change) in the course of hominid evolution. These selective pressures are a consequence of the presence of the gene on the Y and are likely to reflect the interaction of the two forms of the protein. A possible sequence of events is that the original translocation (that occurred approximately 3MYA) is that Y gene was selected by the doubling of

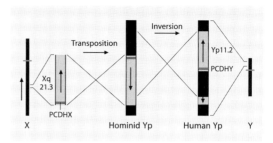

Fig. 2. The reduplicative translocation and subsequent paracentric inversion that generated the Xq21.3/Yp block of homology and its orientation in modern *Homo sapiens*. Vertical arrows indicate the orientation of the gene sequence. *Yp* Y chromosome short arm; cross bars indicate the centromers on the X and Y chromosomes; *PCDHX* ProtocadherinX, *PCDHY* ProtocadherinY (adapted from Schwartz et al., 1998)

dosage that occurred in the first male that carried the translocated block. The spread of the new Y within the population may be the initial event in the *Australopithecus/Homo* transition (Williams and Crow, 2002). Subsequently changes occurred in the Y ectodomain. These may have occurred rapidly although they do not reveal the signature of positive selection, perhaps because the accumulation of subsequent synonymous base changes has obscured the signal. The consequence of these changes was to create a new extracellular environment for the X ectodomain – the presence of a new protein sequence expressed from PCDHY – to which the change in the X ectodomain was the response. These changes in the X sequence, because they affect females as well as males, probably were critical in determining the cerebral characteristics (perhaps including asymmetry) of the new hominid species (Fig. 2).

Later there were changes in the Y cytodomain that presumably entailed new effector interactions in the male. At some stage there were also deletions from the translocated block on the Y chromosome, one of which removed the small exons 7 and 8 from the Y coding sequence and another of which may have affected the expression of the PCDHY gene. Each of these changes might have been relevant to differences between the sexes and may also relate to one of the transitions between hominid species. Although such changes on the Y chromosome will have had a primary effect in males there are two ways in which they will also have had an influence on the X chromosome in females – first as noted above through selective effects on the X ectodomain sequence through the interaction of the molecules at the cell surface, and second through an influence on the process of X inactivation. There is a general rule that genes that are also present on the Y chromosome are protected from X inactivation although the mechanism is unclear. If as seems likely some sort of pairing between the X and Y sequences in male meiosis is involved then the orientation of the sequence on the Y is relevant. Thus the paracentric inversion that reversed the orientation of most, including the PCDHY sequence, of the translocated block on the Y may have played a critical role. It is a candidate for the transition from the immediate precursor hominid species (perhaps *Homo heidelbergensis*) to modern *Homo sapiens*.

The epigenetics of cerebral dominance and psychosis

These considerations have implications for the genetic basis of individual differences because they raise the possibility that the variation is epigenetic rather than sequence based. If the expression of the Protocadherin sequence from the X, and possibly also the Y, is in part dependent upon the pairing of the X and Y sequences in male meiosis a source of variation is present that relates to the core characteristic of the species, here assumed to be cerebral asymmetry, that is independent of the DNA sequence.

The findings of psychosis genetics are more compatible with an epigenetic influence than is often appreciated. The fact that identical twins are no more than 50% concordant for psychosis in the absence of any environmental explanation for the discordance (Torrey et al., 1994) suggests that the course of development differs between the twins and that the origin of the difference is at some stage determined by a stochastic influence and that that influence is mediated by a difference in gene expression. There is further evidence from twin studies that the relevant dimension is anatomical asymmetry. In the NIMH twin study (Suddath et al., 1990) there was a deficit in volume of grey matter in the temporal lobe in the ill twin relative to his well co-twin that was present in the left but not on the right. A subsequent study (Bartley et al., 1993) examined the morphology of the Sylvian fissure. Again although not emphasised in the primary publication there was a loss of asymmetry of the posterior segment of the Sylvian fissure – the ill twin was closer to symmetry and the well twin more asymmetrical than pairs of control twins both of whom were well (Crow, 1999). These findings are consis-

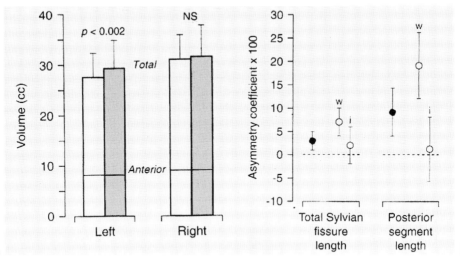

Fig. 3. Deviations in cerebral asymmetry in the NIMH discordant monozygotic twin study. **a** Decrease in volume of grey matter in the posterior temporal lobe on the left side (open columns – ill twin; filled columns – well twin). The horizontal bars indicate the volume of grey matter in the anterior segment of the temporal lobe that is unchanged (from Suddath et al., 1990). **b** Asymmetry coefficients [(L–R)/(L+R)×100] of total and posterior segment Sylvian fissure lengths. Open circles represent values in pairs discordant for schizophrenia: *i* ill, *w* well. Filled circles – values in control pairs of twin pairs, both well (data from Bartley et al., 1993)

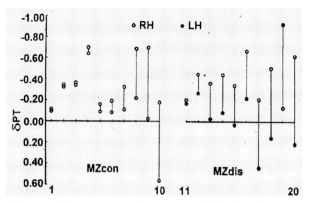

Fig. 4. Distribution of direction and degree of planum temporale asymmetry in 20 pairs of monozygotic twins: MZ concordant; twin pairs 1–10 concordant for right handedness: MZ discordant; twin pairs 11–20 discordant for handedness (X-axis), Y-axis – negative values indicate leftward and positive values rightward planum temporale asymmetry (from Steinmetz et al., 1995)

tent with the conclusion of an earlier CT scan twin study that suggested that ill and well twins differed with respect to asymmetry (Reveley et al., 1987). Together these studies indicate that cerebral asymmetry is the key variable for understanding the genetics of psychosis and that the relevant variation is epigenetic (Fig. 3).

The findings of these twin studies can be placed in the context of a twin study (Steinmetz et al., 1995) that demonstrated that when MZ twins are discordant for handedness they are more likely to be discordant for asymmetry of the planum temporale, left handers showing less asymmetry of this structure than right handers. This study thus reinforces that for this crucial dimension that underlies the defining capacity of the species for language the important variation that distinguishes individuals is epigenetic (Fig. 4).

The central paradox

Armed with this knowledge we can re-contemplate the paradox first clearly identified by Huxley et al. (1964) – that schizophrenia is a condition that is genetic in origin and is associated with a substantial fecundity disadvantage. Why are these genes not selected out of the population? The answer that Huxley et al. gave – that the disadvantage is somehow balanced by an advantage to the individual in terms of resistance to wound shock and stress – is obviously in error, as Kuttner et al. (1967) were quick to point out. It makes more sense to suppose that the balancing advantage relates to some human capacity – Kuttner et al. suggested as alternatives complex social ability, intelligence and language. But these three are not independent and of the three language is most distinctively the species-defining characteristic, and one that as Broca indicated has an identifiable neural basis. The notion that psychosis is a *Homo sapiens*-specific condition and that its genetic origin relates to the change (the "speciation event") that gave birth to the species puts Huxley *et al.'s* paradox in a new context. Schizophrenia is "the price that *Homo sapiens* pays for language" (Crow 1997, 2000) in the sense that the relevant genetic variation was generated in the sequence of chromosomal changes that gave the species its distinctive biological advantage – the ability to encode and decode symbolic representations. The variation is approximately uniform across populations and appears to be unrelated to variations in the DNA sequence (thus accounting for the apparent failure of the linkage approach). It may be supposed that it relates to other individual differences, for example the sex differences in the acquisition of words and spatial ability and the sex difference in degree and direction of handedness that are related to the core characteristic of the species and are probably relatively constant across populations.

What is the nature of this species-specific variation? One can only suppose that it arises as a consequence of the chromosomal changes outlined above and in their subsequent epigenetic modification. It can be argued that the sex chromosomes are particularly relevant to species transitions and to inter-species differences. The X chromosome is remarkably constant across mammalian species but the Y chromosome is variable. One concept of speciation is that this takes place through an initial change in a feature in one sex, generally the male, that is then selected by individuals of the other sex (Kaneshiro, 1980; Carson, 1997) and modified by a process of sexual selection to create a new "mate identification system" (Paterson, 1985). It is plausible that this process reflects primary changes in sex chromosomal structure and their subsequent modification by sequence changes and epigenetic processes in the genes that have thus been selected. If this is so the case of the Xq21.3 translocation and the subsequent changes in the translocated block on the Y chromosome together with their associated genetic and epigenetic modulations exemplify a process that has more general significance in speciation theory.

Summary – the way ahead

In conclusion the failure of the linkage strategy to identify genes that can be reliably related to the genetic predisposition to psychosis has been salutary. Taken in the context of the nature of the morphological changes and more general considerations of the nature of the condition (uniformity of incidence across populations, fecundity disadvantage, the sex difference in age of onset) this failure can now be seen to be instructive in relation to the nature of the genetic predisposition and its evolutionary significance. Schizophrenia is a condition the manifestations of which [e.g. the first rank symptoms (Crow, 1998)] can be conceived as disorders of the human capacity for language and the primary pathophysiology as a deviation or spectrum of deviations in the specific trajectory of development (the cerebral torque) on which this capacity depends. The morphological changes cannot be understood except on the basis of an understanding of the torque and its influence on the structure of the cerebral cortex and cortico-cortical connexions. The genetic predisposition cannot be understood except on the basis that it relates to the chromosomal changes and the subsequent modifications that gave rise to the torque and the human capacity for language.

References

Annett M (1985) Left, Right, Hand and Brain: The Right Shift Theory. Lawrence Erlbaum, London

Annett, M (2002) Handedness and Brain Asymmetry: The Right Shift Theory. Psychology Press, Hove, Sussex

Badner J, Gershon ES (2002) Meta-analysis of whole-genome linkage scans of bipolar disorder and schizophrenia. Molecular Psychiatry 7:405–411

Bartley AJ, Jones DW, Torrey EF et al (1993) Sylvian fissure asymmetries in monozygotic twins: a test of laterality in schizophrenia. Biological Psychiatry 34:853–863

Bickerton, D (1990) Language and Species. University of Chicago, Chicago

Bird ED, Spokes EG, Barnes J et al (1977) Increased brain dopamine and reduced glutamic acid decarboxylase and choline acetyl transferase activity in schizophrenia and related psychoses. Lancet 2:1157–1158

Blanco P, Sargent CA, Boucher C et al (2000) Conservation of PCDHX in mammals; expression of human X/Y genes predominantly in the brain. Mammalian Genome 11:906–914

Broca P (1861) Remarques sur la siegé de la faculté du langue. Bulletin de la Société Anatomique de Paris (2nd series) 6:330–357

Buxhoeveden D, Switala AE, Litaker M et al (2001) Lateralization of minicolumns in human planum temporale is absent in nonhuman primate cortex. Brain Behavioural Evolution 57:349–358

Carson HL (1997) Sexual selection: a driver of genetic change in Hawaiian Drosophila. Journal of Heredity 88:343–352

Chance SA, Esiri MM, Crow TJ (2002) Amygdala volume in schizophrenia: post-mortem study and review of magnetic resonance imaging findings. British Journal of Psychiatry 180:331–338

Corballis MC, Lee K, McManus IC et al (1996) Location of the handedness gene on the X and Y chromosomes. American Journal of Medical Genetics (Neuropsychiatric Genetics) 67:50–52

Crow TJ (1993) Sexual selection, Machiavellian intelligence and the origins of psychosis. Lancet 342:594–598

Crow TJ (1994) The case for an X-Y homologous determinant of cerebral asymmetry. Cytogenetics and Cell Genetics 67:393–394

Crow TJ (1995 a) A continuum of psychosis, one human gene and not much else – the case for homogeneity. Schizophrenia Research 17:135–145

Crow TJ (1995 b) Constraints on concepts of pathogenesis: language and the speciation process as the key to the etiology of schizophrenia. Archives of General Psychiatry 52:1011–1014

Crow TJ (1997) Is schizophrenia the price that Homo sapiens pays for language? Schizophrenia Research 28:127–141

Crow TJ (1998) Nuclear schizophrenic symptoms as a window on the relationship between thought and speech. British Journal of Psychiatry 173:303–309

Crow TJ (1999) Commentary on Klaening: twin studies of psychosis and the genetics of cerebral asymmetry. British Journal of Psychiatry 175:399–401

Crow TJ (2000) Schizophrenia as the price that Homo sapiens pays for language: a resolution of the central paradox in the origin of the species. Brain Research Reviews 31:118–129

Crow TJ (2002) Introduction. In: Crow TJ (ed) The Speciation of Modern Homo Sapiens. Oxford University Press, Oxford, pp 1–20

Cullen TJ, Walker MA, Parkinson N et al (2000) A postmortem study of the mediodorsal nucleus of the thalamus in schizophrenia. Schizophrenia Research 60:157–166

Daniel DG, Goldberg TE, Gibbons RD et al (1991) Lack of a bimodal distribution of ventricular size in schizophrenia: a Gaussian mixture analysis of 1056 cases and controls. Biological Psychiatry 30:886–903

DeLisi LE, Craddock N, Detera-Wadleigh SD et al (2000) Update on chromosomal locations for psychiatric disorders: report of the Interim Meeting of Chromosome Workshop Chairpersons from the VIIth World Congress of Psychiatric Genetics, Monterey, California, October 14–18, 1999. American Journal of Medical Genetics (Neuropsychiatric Genetics) 96:434–449

DeLisi LE, Crow TJ (1999) Chromosome Workshops 1998: current state of psychiatric linkage. American Journal of Medical Genetics (Neuropsychiatric Genetics) 88:215–218

DeLisi LE, Shaw S, Crow TJ et al (2002) A genome-wide scan for linkage to chromosomal regions in 382 sibling pairs with schizophrenia or schizoaffective disorder. American Journal of Psychiatry 159:803–812

DeLisi LE, Wise CD, Bridge TP et al (1981) A probable neuroleptic effect on platelet monamine oxidase in chronic schizophrenic patients. Psychiatry Research 4:95–107

Gershon ES, DeLisi LE, Hamovit J et al (1988) A controlled family study of chronic psychoses: schizophrenia and schizo-affective disorder. Archives of General Psychiatry 45:328–336

Geschwind N, Levitsky W (1968) Human brain: left-right asymmetry in temporal speech region. Science 161:186–187

Harris R, Talbot TJ (1997) Landmarks in Linguistic Thought 1. Routledge, London

Heckers S, Heinsen H, Heinsen YC et al (1990) Limbic structures and lateral ventricle in schizophrenia. A quantitative postmortem study. Archives of General Psychiatry 47:1016–1022

Heinrichs RW, Zakzanis KK (1998) Neurocognitive deficit in schizophrenia: a quantitative review of the evidence. Neuropsychology 12:426–445

Highley JR, DeLisi LE, Roberts N et al (2003) Sex-dependent effects of schizophrenia: an MRI study of gyral folding, and cortical and white matter volume. Psychiatry Research Neuroimaging 124:11–23

Holder MK (1999) Influences and constraints on manual asymmetry in wild African primates: reassessing implications for the evolution of human handedness and brain lateralization (Dissertation Abstracts International Section A). Humanities and Social Sciences 60:470

Huxley J, Mayr E, Osmond H et al (1964) Schizophrenia as a genetic morphism. Nature 204:220–221

Jablensky A, Sartorius N, Ernberg G et al (1992) Schizophrenia: manifestations, incidence and course in different cultures. A World Health Organization Ten Country Study. Psychological Medicine 22 (Suppl 20):1–97

Johnstone EC, Crow TJ, Frith CD et al (1976) Cerebral ventricular size and cognitive impairment in chronic schizophrenia. Lancet 1992 ii:924–926

Kaneshiro KY (1980) Sexual isolation, speciation and the direction of evolution. Evolution 34:437–444

Kety SS (1959a) Biochemical theories of schizophrenia (part 1). Science 129:1528–1532

Kety SS (1959b) Biochemical theories of schizophrenia (part 2). Science 129:1590–1596

Kuttner RE, Lorincz AB, Swan DA (1967) The schizophrenia gene and social evolution. Psychological Reports 20:407–412

Lewis CM, Levinson DF, Wise LH et al (2003) Genome scan meta-analysis of schizophrenia and bipolar disorder II: schizophrenia. American Journal of Human Genetics 73:34–48

Maier W, Lichtermann D, Minges J et al (1993) Continuity and discontinuity of affective disorders and schizophrenia. Archives of General Psychiatry 50:871–883

Marchant LF, McGrew WC (1996) Laterality of limb function in wild chimpanzees of Gombe National Park: comprehensive study of spontaneous activities. Journal of Human Evolution 30:427–443

McGrew WC, Marchant LF (1997) On the other hand: current issues in and meta-analysis of the behavioral laterality of hand function in nonhuman primates. Yearbook of Physical Anthropology 40:201–232

McManus IC (1991) The inheritance of left-handedness. In: Bock GR, Marsh J (eds) Biological Asymmetry and Handedness (CIBA Foundation Symposium 162). Wiley, Chichester, pp 251–281

Mellars P (2002) Archaeology and the origins of modern humans: European and African perspectives. In: Crow TJ (ed) The Speciation of Modern Homo Sapiens. Oxford University Press, Oxford, pp 31–48

Murphy DL, Wyatt RJ (1972) Reduced MAO acitivity in blood platelets from schizophrenic patients. Nature 238:225–226

Murphy JM (1976) Psychiatric labelling in a cross-cultural perspective. Science 191:1019–1028

Noble W, Davidson I (1996) Human Evolution, Language and Mind. Cambridge University Press, Cambridge

Nopoulos PC, Magnotta V, O'Leary D et al (2003) Cortical surface abnormalities in patients with first episode schizophrenia. Schizophrenia Research 60:203

Owen F, Bourne RC, Crow TJ et al (1981) Platelet monoamine oxidase activity in acute schizophrenia: relationship to symptomatology and neuroleptic medication. Brit J Psychiatry 139:16–22

Owen F, Bourne RC, Crow TJ et al (1976) Platelet monoamine oxidase in schizophrenia. An investigation in drug-free chronic hospitalized patients. Archives of General Psychiatry 33:1370–1373

Paterson HEH (1985) The recognition concept of species. In: Vrba ES (ed) Species and Speciation. Transvaal Museum Monograph, Pretoria, pp 21–29

Reveley MA, Reveley AM, Baldy R (1987) Left hemisphere hypodensity in discordant schizophrenic twins: a controlled study. Archives of General Psychiatry 44:625–632

Sallet PC, Elkis H, Alves TM et al (2003) Reduced cortical folding in schizophrenia: an MRI morphometric study. American Journal of Psychiatry 160:1606–1613

Schwartz A, Chan DC, Brown LG et al (1998) Reconstructing hominid Y evolution: X-homologous block, created by X-Y transposition, was disrupted by Yp inversion through LINE-LINE recombination. Human Molecular Genetics 7:1–11

Segurado R, Detera-Wadleigh SD, Gill M et al (2003) Bipolar disorder geonome scan meta-analysis. American Journal of Human Genetics 73:49–62

Spokes EG (1979) An analysis of factors influencing measurements of dopamine, noradrenaline, glutamate decarboxylase and choline acetylase in human post-mortem brain tissue. Brain 102:333–346

Stassen HH, Scharfetter C, Winokur G et al (1988) Familial syndrome patterns in schizophrenia, schizoaffective disorder, mania, and depression. European Archives of Psychiatry and Neurological Science 237:115–123

Steinmetz H, Herzog A, Schlaug G et al (1995) Brain (a)symmetry in monozygotic twins. Cerebral Cortex 5:296–300

Stringer C, McKie R (1996) African Exodus: the Origins of Modern Humanity. J Cape, London

Suddath RL, Christison GW, Torrey EF et al (1990) Anatomical abnormalities in the brains of monozygotic twins discordant for schizophrenia. New England Journal of Medicine 322:789–794

Tkachev D, Mimmack ML, Ryan MM et al (1972) Oligodendrocyte dysfunction in schizophrenia and bipolar disorder. Lancet 362:798–805

Torrey EF, Bowler AE, Taylor EH et al (1994) Schizophrenia and Manic-Depressive Disorder. Basic Books, New York

Vita A, Dieci M, Silenzi C et al (2000) Cerebral ventricular enlargement as a generalized feature of schizophrenia: a distribution analysis on 502 subjects. Schizophrenia Research 44:25–34

Walker MA, Highley JR, Esiri MM et al (2002) Estimated neuronal populations and volumes of the hippocampus and its subfields in schizophrenia. American Journal of Psychiatry 150:821–828

White T, Andreasen NC, Nopoulos P et al (2003) Gyrification abnormalities in childhood and adolescent onset schizophrenia. Biological Psychiatry 54:418–426

Williams NA, Crow TJ (2002) Domain-specific positive selection on gametologues Protocadherin Y and X in hominid evolution (submitted)

Section 5
Controversies in schizophrenia

Criminal and antisocial behaviours and schizophrenia: a neglected topic

SHEILAGH HODGINS

Institute of Psychiatry, King's College, University of London, UK

Introduction

This chapter reviews current findings of antisocial and violent behaviour among persons who develop schizophrenia. Initially, the evidence indicating that persons who develop schizophrenia are at increased risk for both non-violent and violent crime is briefly reviewed. Next, the current understanding of criminality in the general population is presented demonstrating the importance of studying sub-groups of offenders defined by age of onset of criminal activities. Part 3 of the chapter presents data describing a sample of 224 men with schizophrenia, 58 non-offenders and 116 offenders divided by age at first crime. Part 4 synthesises what is known about possible aetiological factors contributing to antisocial behaviour in persons who develop schizophrenia. The final section of the chapter concludes by suggesting that research aimed at identifying the aetiology of schizophrenia will be enriched, and perhaps moved closer towards its goal, by taking account of antisocial behaviour among those who develop schizophrenia and their relatives.

Part 1: Criminality of persons who develop schizophrenia

In the last decade, several epidemiological studies of large unbiased birth cohorts and population cohorts conducted in a number of different countries have compared the criminality of individuals with schizophrenia to that of the general population. All have found that persons with schizophrenia are at increased risk for nonviolent offending and at even higher risk for violent offending (Arseneault et al. 2000; Brennan et al. 2000; Mullen et al. 2000; Swanson et al. 1990; Tiihonen et al. 1997). These investigations likely underestimate the criminality of persons with, or who will develop, schizophrenia. All but one (Arseneault et al. 2000) examined treated cases, thereby underestimating the prevalence of schizophrenia, and official criminality, thereby underestimating antisocial and aggressive behaviours that have not led to criminal convictions.

Further, studies in jurisdictions in which all persons accused of homicide undergo a psychiatric assessment have found that persons with schizophrenia, as compared to the general population, are at increased risk to commit homicide. These studies indicate that persons with schizophrenia are responsible for anywhere between 6% and 28% of homicides (for reviews see Erb et al. 2001).

Consistent with these findings are the results of studies reporting that persons with schizophrenia living in the community are convicted for more nonviolent and violent offences than their non-disordered neighbours (Belfrage 1998; Lindqvist 1986). Diagnostic studies of representative samples of convicted offenders have documented rates of schizophrenia between 2 and 7 times higher than those for age- and gender-matched samples of the general population (see for example, Brinded et al. 1999; Brink et al. 2001; Gunn 2000; Hodgins and Côté 1995). The proportion of persons with, or who will develop schizophrenia, that are convicted of crimes vary from one country to another and parallel the rates of criminality in the general population (see for example, Hodgins and Janson 2002; Mullen et al. 2000).

While the increase in the risks of nonviolent offending and particularly of violent offending for persons with schizophrenia reported in various studies are similar (Hodgins 1998), the proportions of persons with this disorder who offend differ. These differences result from many factors including the crime rate in the region being studied, the rate of resolution of criminal offences, the era under study, and the age of the subjects when the criminal data were obtained. For example, the criminality of a Danish cohort that included more than 358 000 persons was examined in 1991 when the cohort members were in their forties. Men with schizophrenia were found to be 4.6 times (95% confidence interval 3.8–5.6) more likely to be convicted of a violent offence than the men who had never been admitted to a psychiatric ward. The women with schizophrenia were 23.2 times (95% confidence interval 14.4–37.4) more likely to have a conviction for a violent offence than women with no psychiatric admissions (Brennan et al. 2000). However, only 11.3% of the men and 2.3% of the women who developed schizophrenia committed violent offences. In the 1953 Stockholm birth cohort, when cohort members were aged 30, 50% of the men and 19% of the women with a major mental disorder had been convicted of at least one offence (Hodgins 1992). In the Dunedin birth cohort, 15.4% of the cohort members with a schizophrenia spectrum disorder had at least one criminal conviction between their 20th and 21st birthdays (Arseneault et al. 2000). Among the patients with schizophrenia in the state of Victoria, Australia, 26.3% were reported to have a record of criminal convictions as compared to 8.6% of the matched control subjects (Mullen et al. 2000). With compelling evidence demonstrating that some persons who develop schizophrenia are at increased risk to engage in serious criminal activities, the challenge now is to understand how the offenders with schizophrenia differ from those with the same disorder who do not offend.

Part 2: A description of criminal offenders with schizophrenia

In order to understand the criminality of persons who develop schizophrenia, it is helpful to briefly review what is known about criminality among persons without this disorder.

Criminality among persons with no major mental disorders

Investigations conducted in many different countries have consistently found that the age at first crime identifies groups of offenders that differ as to the frequency, diversity, and types of crimes that they commit and the factors that are associated with criminal offending:

- life-course persistent offenders display antisocial behaviour from a young age that escalates in frequency and severity over time leading to convictions in criminal court by adolescence;
- adolescent-limited offenders, most of whom terminate offending in adolescence;
- individuals with no childhood or adolescent history of antisocial behaviour who commit their first crimes as adults; and
- discontinuous offenders (Moffitt 1994; Moffitt et al. 1994).

Life course persistent offenders have been identified in a number of prospective longitudinal investigations conducted in different countries. Despite differences in culture and the health, education, and justice systems in these countries, the prevalence of such offenders is surprisingly similar, approximately 5% among men and less than 1% among women (for a review, see Hodgins 1994). Life-course persistent offenders are responsible for most of the crimes that are committed. For example, we examined a cohort that included all 15 117 persons born in Stockholm in 1953 and followed to age 30. Of the male cohort members, 6.2% of the men and 0.4% of the women were classified as life-course persistent offenders. The life-course persistent males were responsible for 70% of all the offences and for 71% of the violent offences committed by the men in the cohort. Life-course persistent females were responsible for 33% of all offences and 30% of the violent offences (Kratzer and Hodgins 1999). Other prospective longitudinal investigations have obtained similar results (Moffitt and Caspi 2001; Stattin and Magnusson 1991).

In the general population, life-course persistent offenders present distinct characteristics from an early age. For example, in a prospective study of a population cohort from Dunedin, New Zealand, the distinguishing features have been found to include:

- neurocognitive risk measured as neurological and developmental abnormalities at age 3, lower than average verbal abilities at age 5, working memory impairments;
- low heart rate; and
- extremes of temperament measured as difficult at age 2 and undercontrolled at age 3.

As children, disobedience, antisocial and aggressive behaviour are displayed early and escalate in severity over time. Children who display such behaviours are subjected to inconsistent and harsh discipline, and rejection by both parents and peers (Moffitt and Caspi 2001; Moffitt et al. 2002). Their parents often have themselves been convicted of criminal offences, mothers are young at the child's birth, and poor (see for example, Farrington 2002).

By contrast, adolescent-limited offenders are distinguished largely by social and relationship factors rather than by individual characteristics (Moffitt 1993, 1997). They do not present antisocial or aggressive behaviour in childhood, and their intelligence, reading abilities, and personality traits have been found to be well within normal limits (Moffitt and Caspi 2001). During adolescence, however, they become involved with delinquent peers and commit multiple non-violent offences. Despite the name of this group, recent data from the Dunedin project at age 26 indicate that 34% had been convicted of an offence in adult court (Moffitt et al. 2002). Individuals who commit their first criminal offence as adults are rare, more often female than male, and very little is known about them (Kratzer and Hodgins 1999).

Criminality among persons who develop schizophrenia

Similar to offenders in the general population, those with schizophrenia constitute a population that is heterogeneous, with respect to both criminal offending and the correlates of offending. Knowledge about the origins of criminal offending in the general population has exploded since investigations began to focus on the sub-groups described above that are defined by age at onset of antisocial behaviour. Available data suggest that a similar approach to the study of offenders with schizophrenia may prove useful for beginning to unravel the aetiology of both the violence and the schizophrenia and for the development of effective treatment programmes[1].

Surprisingly, as in the general population, age at first offence identifies groups of offenders with schizophrenia that differ as to both patterns of criminal activities and the factors that influence criminal offending. Among those who develop schizophrenia, as in the general population, many more men than women commit criminal offences and consequently, much more is known about male than female offenders.

Among men with schizophrenia, a group who resemble life-course persistent offenders have been identified in several investigations. (To distinguish them from the offenders with no major mental disorders, they are referred to as early-starters.) Two lines of evidence suggest that the prevalence of early-starters within the population of men who develop schizophrenia is higher than the prevalence of life-course persistent offenders in the general male population. One, the epidemiological investigations of birth and population co-

---

[1] Comparisons of offenders and non-offenders with schizophrenia do not advance understanding of criminal offending and schizophrenia. This is largely because the offenders constitute a very heterogeneous group. The most prolific offenders are those we have described as early-start offenders. In multi-variate analyses comparing offenders and non-offenders, the characteristics of these early-start offenders are identified as the variables that significantly distinguish the offenders from the non-offenders. However, these variables do not characterise many of the offenders who begin engaging in antisocial behaviour after the onset of schizophrenia. A second reason why comparisons of offenders and non-offenders do not shed much light on the aetiology of offending relates to sample bias. Depending on the proportion of the sample who are early-starters, the results vary.

horts, identify greater proportions of early-start offenders among those who develop psychotic disorders than life-course persistent offenders among those with no major mental disorders (Hodgins and Janson 2002). Two, the prevalence of antisocial personality disorder (APD) that includes by definition a history of conduct problems by at least age 15 is higher among both men and women with schizophrenia than those without (Robins et al. 1991; Robins 1993)). For example, in a sample of well functioning individuals with schizophrenia living in the community, 23% of the men and 17% of the women were diagnosed with DSM-III-R APD, in a sample of men with schizophrenia found not guilt by reason of insanity for a criminal offence 27% met DSM-III-R criteria for APD, and in a representative sample of men with schizophrenia who were convicted for a criminal offence 62% met similar criteria for APD (Hodgins et al. 1996). These findings are consistent with the hypothesis that there is an association between schizophrenia and antisocial behaviour that emerges in childhood and is stable across the life-span.

Offenders with schizophrenia: an analysis by age of first crime

In order to describe offenders with schizophrenia and to illustrate the heterogeneity of this population, data are presented from the Comparative Study of the Prevention of Crime and Violence by Mentally Ill Persons[2] (Hodgins et al. in press). Two hundred and twenty-four men with schizophrenia or schizo-

---

[2] "The comparative study of the Prevention of Crime and Violence by Mentally Ill Persons" is being conducted by S. Hodgins, Ph. D., Institute of Psychiatry, King's College, UK, A. Tengström, Ph. D., Maria-Ungdom Research Centre, Karolinska Institute, Sweden, D. Eaves, M. D., Vancouver, Canada, S. Hart, Ph. D., Simon Fraser University, Canada, R. Kronstrand, Ph. D., Rättsmedicinalverket and Linköping University, Sweden, S. Levander, M. D., Ph. D., University Hospital, MAS, Malmö, Sweden, R. Müller-Isberner, Dr. med., Klinik für forensische Psychiatrie Haina, Germany, J. Tiihonen, M. D., Ph. D., University of Kuopio, Finland, C. D. Webster, Ph. D., Simon Fraser University and University of Toronto, Canada, M. Eronen, M. D., Vanha Vaasa Hospital, Finland, R. Freese, M. D., Klinik für forensische Psychiatrie Haina, Germany, A. Grabovac, M. D., Riverview Hospital, Vancouver, Canada, Dr. Jöckel, D. med., Klinik für forensische Psychiatrie Haina, Germany, A. Kreuzer, Dr. jur., Justus Liebig University, Germany, A. Levin, M. D., Forensic Psychiatric Hospital, British Columbia, Canada, S. Maas, Klinik für forensische Psychiatrie Haina, Germany, E. Repo-Tiihonen, M. D., Ph. D., Niuvanniemi Hospital, Finland, D. Ross, M. Sc., Riverview Hospital, Vancouver, Canada, E. Tuninger, M. D., University Hospital, MAS, Malmö, Sweden, I. Kotilainen, M. D., University of Kuopio, Finland, K. Väänänen, Vanha Vaasa Hospital, Finland, P. Toivonen, M. D., Vanha Vaasa Hospital, Finland, H. Vartiainen, M. D., Ph. D., A. Vokkolainen, Niuvanniemi Hospital, Finland.

Grants to support this study have been awarded by the BIO-MED-II programme of the European Union; Canada: the Forensic Psychiatric Services Commission of British Columbia, the Mental Health, Law and Policy Institute, Simon Fraser University, Riverview Hospital; Finland: Niuvanniemi and Vanha Vaasa State Mental Hospitals; Germany: Deutsche Forschungsgemeinschaft, Institut für forensische Psychiatrie Haina; Sweden: Medicinska Forskningrådet, Vårdalstiftelsen, National Board of Forensic Medicine, Forensic Science Centre, Linköping University, and Linköping University.

affective disorder discharged from general and forensic psychiatric hospitals in Canada, Finland, Germany, and Sweden were examined. Each site of this study is responsible for all of the mentally ill persons who commit crimes within a large catchment area[3]. Consecutive discharges of patients with a diagnosis of a major mental disorder from the forensic psychiatric hospitals serving the catchment areas were invited to participate. Patients with same sex and diagnoses and similar age being discharged from a general psychiatric hospital in the same geographic region were also recruited into the study. In the weeks preceding discharge exhaustive assessments were undertaken that included diagnostic interviews using the Structured Clinical Interview for DSM-IV (Spitzer et al. 1992), symptom assessments, and measures of personality traits by research team psychiatrists, and documenting social, criminal, and psychiatric histories from official files and interviews with patients and family members. The men with schizophrenia were divided into five groups, one group with no record of criminal activity and four groups of offenders classified by age at first crime. As can be seen in Table 1, the groups differ by age and this difference is important to consider throughout the following discussion.

▌ **Criminal history.** As can be seen in Table 1, the five groups differ as to the number and the types of crimes that they have committed. While 100% of those who began offending before age 18 and 83% of those whose first offence was committed between the ages of 18 and 23 had been convicted of non-violent offences, this was true of only half of those who began offending at later ages. The average number of non-violent offences decreased dramatically with the age of first crime. This association between age at first crime and frequency and persistence of non-violent offending has been observed in other samples of men with schizophrenia (Tengström et al. 2001, in press) and in samples of non-mentally ill offenders (Hodgins and Côté 1993 a,b). Other studies have also reported that early-onset, frequent non-violent offending characterises a sub-group of men with schizophrenia who meet criteria for APD, have criminal careers similar to men with APD and no psychotic disorder, and are often not seen by psychiatric services (Hodgins and Côté 1993 a,b).

While almost all the offenders had committed a violent offence, the average numbers of violent offences decreased with the age of first offence. This was not true for homicide. The highest prevalence (37%) of homicide offenders was found among those who began offending after age 30, as compared to 17% of those who began offending before age 18 and 15% of those who began offending between 18 and 22 years of age. Other studies have also found that homicide offenders with schizophrenia often have no history of antisocial behaviour prior to the onset of the disorder. Some homicide offenders with schizophrenia have a long history of illness before the homicide during which time

---

[3] Sites were selected for inclusion in the study where it is highly likely that all mentally ill persons accused of criminal offences would undergo a thorough psychiatric assessment and if diagnosed with a major mental disorder would be placed in a forensic hospital for treatment.

Table 1. Comparisons of five groups of men with schizophrenia based on age at first crime

	No crime[a] (n=58)	<18 years[b] (n=35)	18–22 years[c] (n=45)	23–30 years[d] (n=46)	31 and older[e] (n=40)	
Mean age (in years)	34.9 (SD=10.4)	35.3 (SD=9.6)	36.1 (SD=11.9)	38.6 (SD=8.10)	47.7 (SD=10.9)	$F_{(4224)}=10.3$, $p=0.000$ $e>a,b,c,d$
Co-morbid diagnoses						
% Alcohol abuse/dependence	40.7%	68.6%	63.8%	56.3%	62.5%	$\chi^2(n=229)=9.71$, $p=0.046$
% Drug abuse/dependence	27.1%	57.1%	66.0%	45.8%	22.5%	$\chi^2(n=229)=26.08$, $p=0.000$
% Antisocial personality disorder	10.2%	57.1%	31.9%	10.4%	10.0%	$\chi^2(n=229)=40.018$, $p=0.000$
Psychosocial functioning						
Mean GAF score	43.7 (SD=11.0)	48.6 (SD=11.6)	49.5 (SD=14.9)	53.4 (SD=11.6)	53.0 (SD=13.6)	$F_{(4217)}=4.802$, $p=0.001$
% Never employed	10.2%	20.0%	6.4%	4.2%	2.5%	$\chi^2(n=229)=9.64$, $p=0.047$
% had intimate partner	39.0%	31.4%	23.4%	47.9%	62.5%	$\chi^2(n=229)=16.07$, $p=0.003$
% successfully completed obligatory military service	45.7%	11.1%	28.6%	41.7%	64.5%	$\chi^2(n=136)=15.83$, $p=0.003$
Psychiatric history						
Mean age at prodrome (years)	20.0 (SD=6.14)	19.1 (SD=5.11)	18.2 (SD=3.94)	19.8 (SD=7.08)	25.3 (SD=9.30)	$F_{(494)}=2.61$, $p=0.040$

Table 1 (continued)

	No crime[a] (n=58)	<18 years[b] (n=35)	18–22 years[c] (n=45)	23–30 years[d] (n=46)	31 and older[e] (n=40)	
Mean age at onset of schizophrenia (years)	23.0 (SD=6.99)	21.3 (SD=7.04)	21.3 (SD=4.79)	23.4 (SD=6.54)	31.6 (SD=9.78)	$F_{(4188)}=10.11$, $p=0.000$
Mean age at first hospitalisation (years)	24.1 (SD=7.39)	21.5 (SD=6.02)	22.6 (SD=7.75)	24.7 (SD=6.54)	32.7 (SD=10.42)	$F_{(4223)}=11.73$, $p=0.000$ e>a,b,c,d
Mean number of admissions	7.5 (SD=6.18)	8.1 (SD=7.32)	8.6 (SD=8.22)	7.1 (SD=5.07)	9.3 (SD=9.11)	$F_{(4224)}=0.10$, $p=0.981$
Mean length of all hospitalisations (months)	2.7 (SD=3.1)	14.7 (SD=14.6)	11.3 (SD=11.9)	16.2 (SD=22.2)	21.5 (SD=31.3)	$F_{(4224)}=7.20$, $p=0.000$ a<b,c,d,e
% with at least one self harm attempt	50.8%	48.6%	53.2%	54.2%	40.0%	$\chi^2_{(n=229)}=2.17$, $p=0.705$
Criminal history						
% with at least one non-violent offence		100.0%	83.0%	56.3%	52.5%	$\chi^2_{(n=170)}=29.716$, $p=0.000$
Mean number of non-violent offences		22.0 (SD=27.7)	11.7 (SD=20.9)	4.7 (SD=9.7)	2.0 (SD=3.0)	$F_{(3166)}=9.88$, $p=0.000$ b>c,d,e
% with at least one violent offence		88.6%	80.9%	91.7%	90.0%	$\chi^2_{(n=170)}=2.95$, $p=0.399$
Mean number of violent offences		5.6 (SD=6.16)	4.5 (SD=8.09)	2.6 (SD=2.69)	1.9 (SD=1.91)	$F_{(366)}=3.85$, $p=0.011$ b>e
% who committed at least one homicide		17.1%	14.9%	20.8%	37.5%	$\chi^2_{(n=170)}=7.41$, $p=0.060$

Table 1 (continued)

	No crime[a] (n=58)	<18 years[b] (n=35)	18–22 years[c] (n=45)	23–30 years[d] (n=46)	31 and older[e] (n=40)	
Aggressive behaviour						
% hurt victim so badly that in hospital treatment was required	23.2%	57.1%	46.5%	52.1%	42.5%	χ^2(n=222)=13.65, p=0.009
Parents and Siblings						
% with a mentally ill father or brother(s)	36.6%	34.8%	48.5%	27.6%	28.1%	χ^2(n=158)=4.01, p=0.404
% with a mentally ill mother or sister(s)	38.0%	25.8%	57.1%	52.6%	38.2%	χ^2(n=188)=8.87, p=0.065
% with a criminal father or brother(s)	30.8%	42.3%	46.9%	17.9%	16.7%	χ^2(n=155)=10.47, p=0.033
% with a criminal mother or sister(s)	7.0%	12.5%	10.3%	6.5%	7.7%	χ^2(n=167)=2.34, p=0.674
% with father or brother(s) with substance abuse	48.9%	74.1%	64.7%	57.6%	55.2%	χ^2(n=168)=5.10, p=0.278
% with a mother or sister with substance abuse	26.1%	22.6%	36.4%	34.3%	15.2%	χ^2(n=178)=5.09, p=0.278
Childhood and adolescence						
% below average in elementary school	26.3%	28.6%	41.9%	21.3%	12.8%	χ^2(n=221)=9.75, p=0.045
% with conduct disorder	11.9%	54.3%	31.9%	12.5%	12.5%	χ^2(n=229)=31.332, p=0.000
Mean number of CD symptoms	1.02 (SD=1.84)	3.21 (SD=2.86)	2.22 (SD=2.11)	1.28 (SD=2.47)	0.84 (SD=1.95)	F(4216)=7.56, p=0.000 b>a,d,e; c>e
Substance abuse	39.0%	80.0%	60.9%	54.2%	15.4%	χ^2(n=227)=36.57, p=0.000

Table 1 (continued)

	No crime[a] (n = 58)	< 18 years[b] (n = 35)	18–22 years[c] (n = 45)	23–30 years[d] (n = 46)	31 and older[e] (n = 40)	
% treatment	42.6%	43.3%	56.8%	40.9%	38.9%	χ^2nN = 201) = 3,03, p = 0.552
% successfully completed obligatory military service	45.7%	11.1%	28.6%	41.7%	64.5%	χ^2(n = 136) = 15.83, p = 0.003
Psychopathy traits						
Mean score PCL	9.95 (SD = 5.71)	20.30 (SD = 7.20)	15.41 (SD = 7.23)	13.88 (SD = 8.27)	9.72 (SD = 6.64)	$F_{(4222)}$ = 14.54, p = 0.000 b > a,d,e; c > a,e; d > e
Mean score history of criminality	0.58 (SD = 0.76)	4.19 (SD = 1.39)	1.95 (SD = 1.85)	1.53 (SD = 1.64)	0.72 (SD = 0.93)	$F_{(4222)}$ = 44.66, p = 0.000 b > a,c,d,e; c > a; d > e
Mean score antisocial behaviour	2.80 (SD = 2.12)	5.29 (SD = 2.33)	4.39 (SD = 2.49)	3.76 (SD = 2.70)	2.83 (SD = 2.60)	$F_{(4222)}$ = 7.86, p = 0.000 b > a,d,e; c > a,e
Mean score impulsivity	2.40 (SD = 1.81)	3.60 (SD = 1.67)	3.28 (SD = 1.86)	2.96 (SD = 1.90)	2.20 (SD = 1.80)	$F_{(4222)}$ = 4.35, p = 0.002 b > a,e; c > e
Defective emotional experience	2.65 (SD = 2.06)	4.91 (SD = 2.15)	4.04 (SD = 2.24)	3.76 (SD = 2.17)	2.85 (SD = 2.03)	$F_{(4222)}$ = 8.01, p = 0.000 b > a,e; c > a
Arrogant and deceitful interpersonal behaviour	1.52 (SD = 1.56)	2.31 (SD = 2.04)	1.74 (SD = 1.57)	1.87 (SD = 2.04)	1.13 (SD = 1.62)	$F_{(4222)}$ = 1.86, p = 0.118

they received no treatments that targeted their aggressive or antisocial behaviours, while others develop schizophrenia at a relatively late age, fail to receive care until after the murder, and then respond well to neuroleptic treatment (see for example, Beaudoin et al. 1993; Erb et al. 2001). In the present study, based on reports by collaterals and the patients themselves, almost one-quarter of those with no criminal history and half of the offenders had assaulted at least one person so badly that they required inpatient medical care. In a British study of over 700 patients with schizophrenia in community treatment, approximately 20% assaulted another person during the two year study period (Walsh et al. 2001).

❙ **Childhood and adolescence.** As has been observed in the general population, among men who develop schizophrenia, those whose criminal career begins in adolescence have a history of conduct problems from an early age. More than half of the offenders with a conviction before age 18 and 32% of those with a first conviction from age 18 to 22 met DSM-IV criteria for conduct disorder as compared to 12% of the non-offenders and 13% of the offenders who began their criminal careers at later ages. While the proportions of patients with poor academic performance in elementary school and who received treatment before age 18 are similar, they likely reflect different problems. Those who began offending at a young age, we hypothesise, did poorly in school and received professional help because of their behaviour problems, while those who began offending later in life, may have presented cognitive difficulties sufficient to warrant interventions. Thus, among male offenders with schizophrenia, as among offenders with no major mental disorder, there is a sub-group who display a stable pattern of antisocial behaviour from a young age. This sub-group of men with schizophrenia have been identified in other prospective investigations (Arseneault et al. 2000; Hodgins et al. 1998) and in clinical samples (Schanda et al. 1992; Tengström et al. 2001, in press). Furthermore, as among non-mentally ill life-course persistent offenders (Farrington et al. 2001; Moffitt and Caspi 2001; Moffitt et al. 2002), the parents and siblings of early-start offenders with schizophrenia present multiple problems including criminality and substance abuse (Tengström et al. 2001). By age 18, the men in this study were already displaying difficulties, as evidenced by the low proportions who were allowed to complete obligatory military service.

❙ **Personality traits.** Among offenders with no major mental disorder, the Psychopathy Checklist Revised[4] (PCL-R) (Hare 1991) identifies a sub-group who commit the most offences and who fail to respond to rehabilitation. The PCL can be divided into five facets: two personality traits, Arrogant and Deceitful Interpersonal Behaviour and Deficient Emotional Experience (Cooke and Michie 2001), and a history of criminality and antisocial behaviour, and impulsivity. As can be seen in Table 1, the earlier the age at first crime, the higher the total

---

[4] While psychopathy is not included in the DSM-IV or the ICD-10, reviewers have commented favourably on the PCL-Rs psychometric properties and its criterion- and constructrelated validities (Fulero 1995; Stone 1995).

score on the PCL and the higher the scores on all the facets except the trait of Arrogant and Deceitful Interpersonal Behaviour. The offenders who began their criminal careers by age 22 obtained higher ratings than the other offenders and than the non-offenders for a history of antisocial behaviour and for impulsivity, while the late-start offenders obtained ratings similar to the non-offenders. The early-start offenders with schizophrenia obtained higher scores for Deficient Emotional Experience than did the other offender groups despite having similar scores for negative symptoms. This finding has also been observed in other samples of offenders with schizophrenia (Hodgins et al. 1998; Tengström et al, in press). Thus, the traits of psychopathy characterize early-start offenders who develop schizophrenia as they do life-course persistent offenders (Loeber et al. 2001). These differences in traits are reflected in the different proportions of patients who meet DSM-IV criteria for APD. While 57% of the offenders who began their criminal careers by age 18 and 32% of those who first offender between the ages of 18 and 22 received this diagnosis, this was true of only 10% of the other offenders and of the non-offenders.

As among the non-mentally ill, among men with schizophrenia the traits of psychopathy and also the diagnosis of APD are strongly associated with:

- patterns of criminality – age of onset, frequency, diversity, and severity of offences;
- patterns of substance use disorders – age of onset, severity, and types of drugs;
- intoxication at the time of the offence;
- unemployment and homelessness;
- a lower prevalence of homicide than among men with schizophrenia who do not present these traits;
- denial of having committed specific offences;
- a childhood history of conduct problems and poor academic performance; and
- parents with criminal records and substance use disorders (Hodgins et al. 1998; Tengström and Hodgins 2002; Tengström et al. in press).

Behavioural genetic studies suggest that these traits precede and underlie antisocial behaviour, including substance misuse (Krueger et al. 2002). Further, conduct problems usually onset before substance misuse (Armstrong and Costello 2002) and are associated with early exposure to alcohol and drugs (Costello et al. 1999; Robins and McEvoy 1990). Our recent work supports this view. We found that among men with schizophrenia who obtained high scores on the traits of psychopathy, the addition of substance abuse/dependence did not increase the risk of offending. By contrast, among men with schizophrenia and low ratings on these traits, substance misuse was associated with criminal offending (Tengström et al. in press).

Substance abuse. As can be seen in Table 1, considerable proportions of all patients were abusing alcohol and/or drugs before age 18. Among the offenders, the proportions decrease dramatically with age at first crime, from 80% among those who first offended by age 18 to 15% among those who first offended after age 30. In a prospective longitudinal investigation, substance abuse in childhood or early adolescence increased the risk of criminality among the mentally ill to a far greater extent than did substance abuse in adulthood (Hodgins and Janson 2002, ch. 5). Offending is not always associated with substance misuse, 19%, 22%, 25%, and 33%, respectively, of the offender groups did not receive diagnoses of alcohol or drug abuse or dependence. Those who first offended after age 30 differ from the other offender groups: 46% met criteria for alcohol abuse/dependence only and one-quarter for drug abuse/dependence. These men with schizophrenia who develop alcoholism and begin to commit offences, usually violent ones, in their thirties, resemble non-mentally ill men with alcoholism who begin engaging in violence towards others at the same age (see for example, Hodgins et al. 1996).

Among those who first offended between the ages of 23 and 30, 29% met criteria only for an alcohol use disorder, 4% for amphetamines, 42% for cannabis, and one-quarter for no substance use disorder. Among those who first offended between the ages of 18 and 23, 13% met criteria for only an alcohol use disorder, 15% for amphetamines, 44% for cannabis, and 22% for no substance use disorder. Among those who first offended before age 18, 29% met criteria for an alcohol use disorder only, 16% for amphetamines, 38% for cannabis, and only 19% for no substance use disorder. Among the non-offenders, 27% met criteria for an alcohol use disorder, 2% for amphetamines, 20% for cannabis, and 46% had no history of a substance use disorder.

Co-morbid drug abuse/dependence and drug plus alcohol abuse/dependence are strongly associated with antisocial behaviour that emerges in childhood and is stable across the life-span. Of those with a diagnosis of drug abuse/dependence, 67% met criteria for APD. By contrast, among those with no drug use disorder, 14% met criteria for APD. Again these results suggest that conduct problems in childhood are associated with drug use disorders. These results also suggest that the aetiology of substance use disorders and the treatments likely to be effective in reducing abuse, differ for those with and without APD.

▌ **Psychiatric history.** Using information from the patients, family members, and files, we estimated ages of onset of the prodrome. This is the first study to our knowledge to examine the relation of the onset of prodromal symptoms and offending. Onset was not easy to establish retrospectively. As can be seen in Table 2, almost half of those whose first offence occurred by age 18 had committed an offence at least two years before the onset of the prodrome, whereas this was true of only 18% of those who first offended between the ages of 18 and 22, 17% of those who first offended between the ages of 22 and 30, and none of those who offended after age 30. There is a positive association between the development of prodromal symptoms and offending (r = 0.42, p = 0.01). This result could be interpreted as suggesting that even for the early-starters, the onset of symptoms is associated with criminal offending. Alternately, this association may be reported by offenders to justify or excuse their criminal activities or it could merely be a coincidental association relating to legal age for criminality and the age at which schizophrenia develops.

Table 2. Temporal relationships between first crime, first admission, and symptom onset

	<18 years	18–22 years	23–30 years	31 years and older	
1st Judgement and 1st admission					
1st judgement before 1st admission	88.6%	48.9%	31.3%	15.0%	
1st judgement after 1st admission	2.9%	38.3%	66.7%	77.5%	$\chi^2(n=170)$ $=55.393,$ $p=0.000$
1st judgement at the same time as 1st admission	8.6%	12.8%	2.1%	7.5%	
1st Crime and onset of schizophrenia					
Crime 2 or more years before	71.9%	34.2%	25.0%	6.7%	
Crime within one year	21.9%	39.5%	15.0%	23.3%	
Crime 2 years or more after	6.3%	26.3%	60.0%	70.0%	$\chi^2(n=140)$ $=47.005,$ $p=0.000$
1st Crime and onset of prodromal symptoms					
Crime 2 or more years before	46.7%	18.2%	16.7%	0	
Crime within one year	46.7%	31.8%	8.3%	8.3%	$\chi^2(n=73)$ $=26.248,$ $p=0.000$
Crime 2 years or more after	6.7%	50.0%	75.0%	91.7%	

There is even a stronger association between age at onset of schizophrenia and age at first crime (r=0.59, p=0.01). This association likely reflects the fact that in at least three of the study sites, persons accused of crimes who were displaying odd or abnormal behaviours would likely undergo a psychiatric assessment. The proportions of patients who committed a criminal offence before first admission to hospital decrease with age at first crime from 89% in the group first convicted by age 18 to 15% in the group first convicted after age 30. Thus, as would be expected, the younger the age at first conviction, the more likely it is that official criminality begins before hospital treatment for psychosis.

Conclusion. The findings described here, as well as those from several other studies, concur in demonstrating that offenders with schizophrenia constitute a population that is heterogeneous with respect to criminal activities and to factors associated with antisocial behaviours. Surprisingly, among male offenders with schizophrenia, there are sub-groups identified by age-related patterns of offending similar to those observed among non-mentally ill offenders. Compelling data continue to accumulate suggesting that both among non-mentally ill offenders and offenders who develop schizophrenia these sub-groups differ as to aetiology and response to interventions. The sub-groups present remarkably different developmental histories, and in adulthood they are well distinguished by behaviour patterns, emotional states and reactions, and attitudes. Yet, findings to date have failed to identify any differences in the acute episodes of psychosis and the course of the disorder.

The relation between the symptoms of schizophrenia and illegal behaviours is not clear. As the above findings illustrate, a sub-group of males who develop schizophrenia begin committing criminal offences even before the onset of the prodrome. In others, initial criminal activities appear to coincide with the on-set of prodromal symptoms, and yet in others, antisocial behaviours emerge for the first time long after the onset of the disorder. Consequently, there is no single answer to this long-running debate about symptoms and violence and/or criminal behaviour, but rather the association differs by sub-groups of offenders. Recent data suggest that the association also differs by treatment circumstances. In the study described above, patients were followed in the community. Most were under court-order to participate in community treatment programmes and they were being carefully supervised and monitored. Consequently, as has been found in other studies, the rate of aggressive behaviour was low, 7% in the first six months after discharge and 10% during the second six months after discharge. The number and severity of positive symptoms of psychosis and threat-control-override symptoms[5], and recent increases in these symptoms, assessed prospectively, predicted aggressive behaviour in the subsequent six months (Hodgins et al. 2003). These findings do concur with results from some studies in which symptoms at the time of an offence were estimated after the offence had occurred (Bjørkley 2000 a, b). Many investigations indicate, however, that the best predictor of offending among persons with schizophrenia is the total score on the Psychopathy Checklist (Bonta et al. 1998). The schizophrenic offenders in this multi-site study had spent three or four years in hospital during which time optimal medication regimes were identified. Consequently, at discharge they presented very low levels of both positive and negative symptoms (Hodgins et al. in press). Surprisingly, we have now observed that severe positive symptoms of psychosis are positively associated with the traits of psychopathy (Andershed and Hodgins, submitted). Thus, in well medicated men with schizophrenia, these findings suggest that there is an association between residual positive symptoms and the personality traits associated with criminal offending.

Care provided to persons with schizophenia who engage in criminal and/or violent behaviour

In the study described above, 79% of the offenders with schizophrenia had already been hospitalised in general psychiatry before committing the offence that lead to admission to a forensic hospital (Müller-Isberner 2001). Of these

---

[5] Threat-control-override symptoms are identified using three questions from the Psychiatric Epidemiological Research Interview (Link and Stueve 1994). 1) "How often have you felt that your mind was dominated by forces beyond your control?"; 2) "How often have you felt that thoughts were put into your head that were not your own?"; and 3 "How often have you felt that there were people who wished to do you harm?".

79%, 40% had committed an offence before first admission to a general psychiatric hospital and the other 60% committed an offence after the first admission but before the offence that led to their becoming a forensic patient. This is similar to what is reported for the state of Victoria, Australia (Mullen et al. 2000). These findings indicate that the escalation in severity of offending that led to admission to a high security hospital may have been avoided. The use of structured and validated risk assessment tools could have identified patients at high risk of offending (see for example, Dolan and Doyle 2000; Douglas et al. 1999). Interventions that specifically target antisocial attitudes and behaviours, aggressive behaviours, and substance abuse, as well as monitoring compliance with all aspects of treatment may have prevented the escalation of violent behaviour (see for example, Hodgins and Müller-Isberner 2000). Once a serious violent crime is committed and patients are admitted to high security or forensic hospitals, in the study sites, they receive more interventions that specifically target their multiple problems than the general psychiatric patients. When they are discharged to the community, they are much less symptomatic than the general psychiatric patients and receive more treatment and monitoring.

▮ Part 3: The aetiology of antisocial behaviour among persons who develop schizophrenia

Little is known of factors that influence antisocial behaviours among persons who develop schizophrenia.

Hereditary factors

Antisocial behaviour, defined in different ways, has been reported to be elevated among the relatives of persons with schizophrenia as compared to relatives of non-disordered persons (Bleuler 1978; Kety et al. 1971; Landau et al. 1972; Lewis and Balla 1970; Lindelius 1970; Robins 1966). Kay (1990) found that it was the relatives of persons with predominately positive symptom schizophrenia who have criminal records. Similarly, Kendler and colleagues (1993) reported an elevated rate of antisocial personality disorder among the relatives of schizophrenic probands. In the Copenhagen High Risk Project, 35% of the mothers with schizophrenia and only 5% of the non-disordered mothers had criminal records, while equal proportions of the fathers of both groups had prior criminal convictions. Criminal records were screened when the offspring were aged 21 to 31. While 31% of the high risk offspring had been convicted of criminal offences, this was true of only 18% of the low risk offspring (Silverton 1985). In a study of 9182 consecutive births in Copenhagen, more of the offspring of the parents with schizophrenia than the offspring of non-disordered parents had been convicted for criminal offences (Silverton 1985). The male offspring of the schizophrenic mothers examined in the Copenhagen high risk project were also found to have elevated rates of criminality (Mednick et al. 1987). Those who became offenders had been described by their care-givers as infants as having "shorter attention spans" and as being "irritable and nasty" (Silverton 1985).

In Heston's study (1966) of offspring adopted away at birth from mothers with schizophrenia, 11% developed schizophrenia and 23% were convicted of violent criminal offences. Similarly, in the much larger study of Danish adoptees, it was found that schizophrenia in the biological parents significantly increased the risk of criminality among offspring adopted away shortly after birth (Silverton 1985).

The elevated rates of criminality and stable antisocial behaviour among relatives of persons with schizophrenia and more importantly the results of the adoption studies support the hypothesis that the hereditary factors associated with schizophrenia also confer a vulnerability for antisocial behaviour. This hypothesis is further supported by the consistent results showing that persons who develop schizophrenia are at increased risk, as compared to those who do not develop this disorder, to display a stable pattern of antisocial behaviour from childhood throughout adulthood that includes substance abuse.

It may be, however, that the sub-group of persons with schizophrenia who do display a stable pattern of antisocial behaviour have inherited some of the genes that are specifically associated with this pattern of behaviour in the general population. Hereditary factors are associated with a stable pattern of antisocial behaviour across the life-span among persons who do not develop mental illness. A recent meta-analysis of twin and adoption studies reported that the heritability of stable antisocial behaviour was approximately 0.41 (Rhee and Waldman 2002). Several investigations have noted that these hereditary factors confer a propensity for a stable pattern of antisocial behaviour that includes substance abuse (Krueger et al. 2002). The traits of impulsivity (Gottesman and Goldman, 1994) and novelty seeking (Ebstein et al. 1996) that characterise the early-start offenders with schizophrenia are determined to a large extent by genes. Further, the low activity-MAOA genotype has been identified as conferring a susceptibility for stable antisocial behaviour in the presence of severe child abuse (Caspi et al. 2002).

To conclude, the small amount of evidence that is available suggests that hereditary factors associated with antisocial behaviour among persons who develop schizophrenia may differ depending on the age of onset and stability of this behaviour pattern. While the easiest explanation for the early-start offenders would be to suggest that they inherit vulnerabilities both for schizophrenia and for stable antisocial behaviour, this explanation fails to take account of the compelling evidence that stable antisocial behaviour, and the associated substance misuse problems, are more common among persons who develop schizophrenia than in the general population.

Obstetrical factors (OCs)

To our knowledge, there has only been one study of OCs and antisocial or violent behaviour among persons with schizophrenia. We examined the 81 men and 79 women from the 1953 Stockholm birth cohort who developed a major mental disorder by age 30. Information was extracted from obstetric files, health, social and work records, and official criminal records. Among men who developed major mental disorders (mainly schizophrenia), having experienced complications in the neo-natal period increased the risk of offending two-fold, the risk of violent offending 2.5 times, and the risk of early-start offending 3 times. Among these men who developed major mental disorders, those who had experienced complications in the neonatal period committed, on average, more offences (M = 18.00, SD = 23.96) than those who had not experienced such complications (M = 6.26, SD = 13.94; MW z = 3.0, p < 0.003). Of the 12 offenders who had experienced complications in the neo-natal period, eight were convicted of their first criminal offence before the age of 18. Neither complications during pregnancy or at birth, nor inadequate parenting or low SES of the family of origin increased the risk for offending. Among females, none of these factors were found to be statistically associated with offending (Hodgins et al. 2002 a). These results suggest that OCs may play a more important role in the offending of persons who develop schizophrenia than among those without this disorder (Hodgins et al. 2001). Consistent with these findings are the results indicating that maternal exposure to the influenza epidemic during the end of the six month of pregnancy significantly increased the risk of convictions for violent crimes in adulthood, as it did the risk of schizophrenia (Tehrani and Mednick 2000).

Evidence has accumulated in recent years indicating that maternal smoking during pregnancy is associated with conduct problems in childhood and adolescence, and with early onset, persistent and violent offending in adulthood among male offspring (Wakschlag et al. 1997). Three investigations have examined population cohorts and gathered information about the pregnancy, prospectively (Brennan et al. 1999; Fergusson et al. 1998; Räsänen et al. 1999). The results of these investigations are remarkably similar in demonstrating an independent association between maternal smoking during pregnancy and antisocial and criminal behaviour among male offspring in childhood, adolescence, and adulthood. Taken together, the evidence suggests that maternal smoking during pregnancy is associated specifically with early onset, persistent behaviour problems which develop into violent offending and that it is not related to other types of disorders or symptoms (Hodgins et al. 2002 b). The link between maternal smoking and stable antisocial behaviour appears to be direct, for it remains once many other factors such as parental criminality, antisocial behaviour, and substance abuse, maternal alcohol consumption during pregnancy, maternal characteristics such as age at child's birth, poverty, and parenting practices have been controlled. It combines additively with other factors known to increase the risk of stable antisocial behaviour (Hodgins et al. 2002 b; Räsänen et al. 1999). Persons with schizophrenia are more likely than those without these disorders to smoke (Lasser et al. 2000). If this is also true of their relatives, maternal smoking during pregnancy could be one factor contributing to the development of stable antisocial behaviour among men who develop schizophrenia.

Early childhood

A recent analysis of the participants in the prospective, longitudinal investigation of a Dunedin birth cohort found that motor delays, neurological signs, receptive language deficits, and lower IQ specifically characterised those who developed schizophreniform disorder by age 26 (Cannon et al. 2002). Surprisingly, these impairments resemble those presented by both males and females who developed a stable pattern of antisocial behaviour into adulthood (Moffitt and Caspi 2001). Both groups were also reported to be rejected by their peers (Cannon et al. 2002; Moffitt and Caspi 2001). In an analysis of the 1953 Stockholm birth cohort, we found that low marks at elementary and high school, behaviour problems, and family adversity greatly increased the risk of early start offending and mental illness (mainly schizophrenia). Family problems, below average intelligence and academic performance, were associated with late-start offending and mental illness (Hodgins 2000).

Analyses of several longitudinal investigations suggest that aggressive behaviour decreases from early childhood onwards (Tremblay 2000). From infancy onwards, the challenge for the child is to learn not to engage in physical aggression. This is usually accomplished by acquiring verbal skills to negotiate with others. Children who will later develop schizophrenia and those with stable antisocial behaviour present verbal and other cognitive deficits that hinder learning the skills necessary to reduce aggressive behaviour. Further, the traits that characterise early-start offenders, such as impulsivity, sensation seeking, and insensitivity to the feelings of others, would likely be present at this early age (Caspi 2000) and would further inhibit learning prosocial behaviours. Prospective longitudinal investigations of children of parents with schizophrenia have identified a sub-group, larger among the males than the females, that presented disruptive, aggressive behaviour from a young age (Asnarow 1988). In the Copenhagen High Risk project, such behaviours in childhood were found to be an antecedent of schizophrenia characterised primarily by positive symptoms (Cannon et al. 1990). Aggressive behaviour is very stable over the life-span. Interestingly, two prospective investigations of population cohorts have reported that aggressive behaviour in childhood is also strongly predictive of thought disorder in early adulthood (Ferdinand and Verlust 1995) and cluster A personality disorders (Bernstein et al. 1996). Similarly, the risk of schizophrenia increases in a linear fashion with the number of conduct disorder symptoms present before age 15 (Robins and Price 1991).

Repetitive aggressive behaviour and disobedience on the part of a child is often accompanied by harsh and inconsistent discipline from parents, and within a few years rejection (Loeber et al. 1998). Rejection by parents compounds the rejection by peers and deprives the vulnerable child of valuable learning experiences. Thus, with reduced cognitive and verbal abilities, traits of sensation seeking, impulsivity, and callousness, and a lack of prosocial skills, these youth who are vulnerable for schizophrenia make decisions about experimenting with alcohol and drugs.

Parental characteristics such as criminality, and mental disorders have been found to be important risk factors for stable antisocial behaviour (Moffitt et al. 2002). In the study reported above and, more strongly in others, parental criminality and substance abuse have been associated with early-start offending among men who developed schizophrenia (Tengström et al. 2001). These characteristics may be associated with increased risk for antisocial behaviour via genes, and with increased risk due to inappropriate modelling of prosocial behaviours and of the use of alcohol and drugs. Furthermore, the importance of assortative mating in increasing the risks for offspring has not been well studied, but it is known that both those with antisocial personalities (Krueger et al. 1998) and with schizophrenia tend to mate with individuals with similar disorders (Parnas 1988). There is also some evidence that women with schizophrenia disproportionately mate with antisocial men (Parnas 1988). Interestingly, in 1972, in Gottesman and Shield's volume *Schizophrenia and Genetics*, preliminary findings are reported indicating that among the offspring of mothers with schizophrenia, those with "psychopathic" fathers showed fewer skin conductance and other abnormalities than those of other fathers (pp. 336–337).

▌ Part 4: Conclusions

The suffering of persons with schizophrenia and their families is amplified by antisocial behaviours that often accompany this disorder. In addition, stigma attached to schizophrenia is greatly increased by sensational, even if rare, cases of violent crimes by persons with this disorder. Violent offences committed by persons with schizophrenia seriously limit efforts to obtain funding for community treatment programmes and housing. Further, the presence of antisocial behaviours reduces the effectiveness of treatments for schizophrenia and may even contribute to the aetiology of schizophrenia. For example, adolescents with a history of conduct problems are at increased risk to abuse cannabis during adolescence, thereby increasing the risk of schizophrenia (Arseneault et al. 2002; Zammit et al. 2002). Unravelling the aetiology of the antisocial behaviours that characterise a sub-group of persons who develop schizophrenia, and other spectrum disorders, would provide valuable information for establishing intervention programmes for children and adolescents. Such programmes would aim at reducing antisocial behaviour, including substance abuse, before the onset of schizophrenia. The challenge is to adapt programmes with demonstrated efficacy in the general population for children and adolescents who may be at risk for schizophrenia. Furthermore, understanding the differences in aetiology of the various sub-groups of offenders with schizophrenia may be relevant for developing effective treatments for the early-starters, those with alcohol problems, those with drug but no other antisocial behaviours, and for those who avoid treatment services and hurt others when actively psychotic.

The body of literature described in this chapter has implications for research on the aetiology of schizophrenia. As noted above, the presence of conduct problems among children already at risk for schizophrenia via genes and perinatal factors may further contribute to the development of the disorder.

As these children are exposed early to alcohol and drugs, and have traits of impulsivity and sensation seeking, and many have parents who themselves are antisocial and/or abuse alcohol and drugs, they would be more likely than other children at risk for schizophrenia to abuse substances, like cannabis, that appear to play a role in the aetiology of the disorder.

Current knowledge about the aetiology of schizophrenia may be imprecise because antisocial behaviours and personality traits have been largely ignored.

■ The high risk studies have contributed substantially to the current understanding of the causes of schizophrenia. Yet, even though one of these studies showed that almost one-third of the schizophrenic mothers, as compared to only 5% of the non-disordered mothers, had criminal records, the implication of this result for the development of schizophrenia among the offspring has been ignored.

■ The behavioural genetic studies of schizophrenia have failed to take account of the influence of hereditary factors associated with antisocial behaviour and various forms of substance abuse. As described above, current evidence suggests that such factors may well characterise a significant proportion of parents of individuals who develop schizophrenia, as well as the offspring. Yet, the studies of schizophrenia ignore the findings indicating that the genes associated with antisocial behaviours and substance abuse may be more common among families genetically loaded for schizophrenia spectrum disorders than in the general population.

■ Studies of obstetrical complications and schizophrenia ignore the role of parental antisocial behaviours. For example, mothers with antisocial behaviour engage in activities during pregnancy – smoking, drinking, inadequate prenatal care, exposure to infections, inadequate and/or inappropriate nutrition – known to harm the developing foetal brain. If the foetus carries the genes associated with schizophrenia spectrum disorders, the damage caused by these factors may be enhanced. Antisocial men engage in many behaviours, for example, smoking and taking drugs, that may alter the genes that they transmit to their offspring. The role of such non-hereditary mutations has largely been ignored, but recent evidence showing that advanced paternal age increases the risk of schizophrenia (Brown et al. 2002) underlines the importance of investigating these factors.

■ Parents who engage in antisocial behaviours themselves are unlikely to provide optimal parenting for children who are vulnerable for schizophrenia. Little research is undertaken to investigate the role of these factors in the development of schizophrenia.

■ Finally, it is possible that research undertaken in an effort to further understanding of the brain abnormalities that are central to schizophrenia would benefit from taking account of antisocial behaviour patterns. For example, there is some evidence from small numbers of subjects indicating that antisocial men with schizophrenia may show less generalised brain abnormalities than non-antisocial men with schizophrenia (Hodgins et al. 1998; Joyal et al. 2003). It is possible that the biological characteristics associated with stable antisocial behaviour, such as low heart rate and low brain serotonergic activity (Ishikawa and Raine 2002), somehow attenuate the brain abnormalities associated with schizophrenia. Generally, it may be important to take account of antisocial behaviours, personality traits associated with these behaviours, and the duration and severity of substance abuse in order to distinguish brain abnormalities that are specific to schizophrenia. This may be especially true during adolescence and early adulthood when brain structures that play critical roles in schizophrenia and in antisocial behaviour are still developing.

▮ **Acknowledgement.** I would like to thank Drs. Louise Arseneault and Elisabeth Walsh for their helpful comments on this manuscript.

▮ References

Andershed H, Hodgins S (2002) Can psychopathy (PCL-R) be assessed in men with schizophrenia? Manuscript submitted for publication

Armstrong T, Costello EJ (2002) Community studies on adolescent substance use, abuse, or dependence and psychiatric comorbidity. Journal of Consulting and Clinical Psychology 70:1224–1239

Arseneault L, Cannon M, Poulton R, Murray R, Caspi A, Moffitt TE (2002) Cannabis use in adolescence and risk for adult psychosis: longitudinal prospective study. British Medical Journal 325:1212–1213

Arseneault L, Moffitt TE, Caspi A, Taylor PJ, Silva PA (2000) Mental disorders and violence in a total birth cohort. Archives of General Psychiatry 57:979–986

Asnarow JR (1988) Children at risk for schizophrenia: converging lines of evidence. Schizophrenia Bulletin 14:613–631

Beaudoin MN, Hodgins S, Lavoie F (1993) Homicide, schizophrenia, and substance abuse or dependency. Canadian Journal of Psychiatry 38:541–546

Belfrage H (1998) New evidence for a relation between mental disorder and crime. British Journal of Criminology 38:145–154

Bernstein DP, Cohen P, Skodol A, Bezirganian S, Brook JS (1996) Childhood antecedents of adolescent personality disorders. American Journal of Psychiatry 153:907–913

Bjørkley S (2002a) Psychotic symptoms and violence towards others – a literature review of some preliminary findings: Part 2. Hallucinations. Aggression and Violent Behavior 7:617–631

Bjørkley S (2002b) Psychotic symptoms and violence towards others – a literature review of some preliminary findings: Part 2. Hallucinations. Aggression and Violent Behavior 7:605–615

Bleuler M (1978) The Schizophrenic Disorders: Long-term Patient and Family Studies. Yale University Press, New Haven

Bonta J, Law M, Hanson K (1998) The prediction of criminal and violent recidivism among mentally disordered offenders: a meta-analysis. Psychology Bulletin 123:123–142

Brennan PA, Grekin ER, Mednick SA (1999) Maternal smoking during pregnancy and adult male criminal outcomes. Archives of General Psychiatry 56:215–219

Brennan PA, Mednick SA, Hodgins S (2000) Major mental disorders and criminal violence in a Danish birth cohort. Archives of General Psychiatry 57:494–500

Brinded MJ, Stevens I, Mulder RT, Fairley N, Malcom F, Wells JE (1999) The Christchurch prisons psychiatric epidemiology study: methodology and prevalence rates for psychiatric disorders. Criminal Behaviour and Mental Health 9:131–143

Brink J, Doherty D, Boer A (2001) Mental Disorder in Federal Offenders: A Canadian Prevalence Study. University of British Columbia and Regional Health Centre, Department of Psychiatry, Abbotsford, British Columbia

Brown AS, Schaefer CA, Wyatt RJ, Begg MD, Goetz R, Bresnahan MA et al (2002) Paternal age and risk of schizophrenia in adult offspring. American Journal of Psychiatry 159:1528–1533

Cannon M, Caspi A, Moffitt TE, Harrington H, Taylor A, Murray RM et al (2002) Evidence for early-childhood, pan-developmental impairment specific to schizophreniform disorder. Archives of General Psychiatry 59:449–456

Cannon TD, Mednick SA, Parnas J (1990) Antecedents of predominantly negative and predominantly positive symptom schizophrenia in a high risk population. Archives of General Psychiatry 47:622–632

Caspi A (2000) The child is father of the man: personality continuities from childhood to adulthood. Journal of Personality & Social Psychology 78:58–72

Caspi A, McClay J, Moffitt TE, Mill J, Martin J, Craig IW et al (2002) Role of genotype in the cycle of violence in maltreated children. Science 297:851–853

Cooke DJ, Michie C (2001) Refining the construct of psychopathy: towards a hierarchical model. Psychological Assessment 13:171–188

Costello EJ, Erkanli A, Federman E, Angold A (1999) Development of psychiatric comorbidity with substance abuse in adolescents: effects of timing and sex. Journal of Clinical Child Psychology 28:298–311

Dolan M, Doyle M (2000) Violence risk prediction. Clinical and actuarial measures and the role of the psychopathy checklist (review). British Journal of Psychiatry 177:303–311

Douglas KS, Ogloff JR, Nicholls TL, Grant I (1999) Assessing risk for violence among psychiatric patients: the HCR-20 violence risk assessment scheme and the psychopathy checklist: screening version. Journal of Consulting & Clinical Psychology 67(6):917–930

Ebstein RP, Novick O, Umansky R, Priel B, Osher Y, Blaine et al (1996) Dopamine D_4 receptor (D_4DR) exon 111 polymorphism associated with the human personality trait of novelty seeking. Nature Genetics 12:78–82

Erb M, Hodgins S, Freese R, Müller-Isberner R, Jöckel D (2001) Homicide and schizophrenia: maybe treatment does have a preventive effect. Criminal Behaviour and Mental Health 11:6–26

Farrington DP (2002) Key results from the first forty years of the Cambridge study in delinquent development. In: Thornberry TP, Krohn MD (eds) Taking Stock of Delinquency: An Overview of Findings from Contemporary Longitudinal Studies. Kluwer Academic/Plenum, New York, pp 137–183

Farrington DP, Jolliffe D, Loeber R, Stouthamer-Loeber M, Kalb LM (2001) The concentration of offenders in families, and family criminality in the prediction of boys' delinquency. Journal of Adolescence 24(5):579–596

Ferdinand RF, Verlust FC (1995) Psychopathology from adolescence into young adulthood: an 8-year follow-up study. American Journal of Psychiatry 152:1586–1594

Fergusson DM, Woodward LJ, Horwood LJ (1998) Maternal smoking during pregnancy and psychiatric adjustment in late adolescence. Archives of General Psychiatry 55:721–727

Fulero SM (1995) Review of the Hare Psychopathy Checklist-Revised. In: Conoley JC, Impara JC (eds) Twelfth Mental Measurement Yearbook. Buros Institute, Lincoln, pp 453–454

Gottesman II, Goldman HH (1994) Developmental psychopathology of antisocial behavior: inserting genes into its ontogenesis and epigenesis. In: Nelson CA (ed) Threats to Optimal Development. Erlbaum, Hillsdale, NY, pp 69–104

Gottesman II, Shields J (1972) Schizophrenia and Genetics: a Twin Study Vantage Point. Academic Press, New York

Gunn J (2000) Future directions for treatment in forensic psychiatry. British Journal of Psychiatry 176:332–338

Hare RD (1991) The Hare Psychopathy Checklist Revised. Multi-Health Systems Inc, Toronto

Heston LL (1966) Psychiatric disorders in foster-home reared children of schizophrenics. British Journal of Psychiatry 112:819–825

Hodgins S (1994) Status at age 30 of children with conduct problems. Studies of Crime and Crime Prevention 3:41–62

Hodgins S (1998) Epidemiological investigations of the associations between major mental disorders and crime: methodological limitations and validity of the conclusions. Social Psychiatry and Epidemiology 33(1):29–37

Hodgins S (2000) The etiology and development of offending among persons with major mental disorders. In: Hodgins S (ed) Violence among the Mentally Ill Effective Treatments and Management Strategies. Kluwer Academic Publishers, Dordrecht, The Netherlands, pp 89–116

Hodgins S, Côté G (1993a) The criminality of mentally disordered offenders. Criminal Justice and Behavior 28:115–129

Hodgins S, Côté G (1993b) Major mental disorder and APD: a criminal combination. Bulletin of the American Academy of Psychiatry and the Law 21:155–160

Hodgins S, Côté G (1995) Major mental disorder among Canadian penitentiary inmates. In: Stewart L, Stermac L, Webster C (eds) Clinical Criminology: Toward Effective Correctional Treatment. Solliciteur général et Service correctionnel du Canada, Toronto, pp 6–20

Hodgins S, Côté G, Toupin J (1998) Major mental disorders and crime: an etiological hypothesis. In: Cooke D, Forth A, Hare RD (eds) Psychopathy: Theory, Research and Implications for Society. Kluwer Academic Publishers, Dordrecht, Netherlands, pp 231–256

Hodgins S, Hiscoke UL, Freese R (2003) The antecedents of aggressive behavior among men with schizophrenia: a prospective investigation of patients in community treatment. Behavioral Sciences and the Law 21:523–546

Hodgins S, Janson C-G (2002) Criminality and Violence among the Mentally Disordered: The Stockholm Metropolitan Project. Cambridge University Press, Cambridge

Hodgins S, Kratzer L, McNeil TF (2001) Obstetrical complications, parenting, and risk of criminal behavior. Archives of General Psychiatry 58:746–752

Hodgins S, Kratzer L, McNeil TF (2002a) Obstetrical complications, parenting practices and risk of criminal behavior among persons who develop major mental disorders. Acta Psychiatrica Scandinavica 105:179–188

Hodgins S, Kratzer L, McNeil TF (2002b) Are pre and perinatal factors related to the development of criminal offending? In: Corrado RR, Roesch R, Hart SD, Gierowski JK (eds) Multi-problem Violent Youth: A Foundation for Comparative Research on Needs, Interventions, and Outcomes. IOS Press, Amsterdam, pp 58–80

Hodgins S, Mednick SA, Brennan P, Schulsinger F, Engberg M (1996) Mental disorder and crime: evidence from a Danish birth cohort. Archives of General Psychiatry 53:489–496

Hodgins S, Müller-Isberner R (eds) (2000) Violence, Crime and Mentally Disordered Offenders: Concepts and Methods for Effective Treatment and Prevention. John Wiley & Sons, Chichester, UK

Hodgins S, Tengström A, Östermann R, Eaves D, Hart S, Konstrand R, Levander S, Müller-Isberner R, Tiihonen J, Webster CD, Eronen M, Freese R, Jöckel D, Kreuzer A, Levin A, Maas S, Repo E, Ross D, Tuninger E, Kotilainen I, Väänänen K, Vartianen H, Vokkolainen A (2003) An international comparison of community treatment programs for mentally ill persons who have committed criminal offences. Criminal Justice and Behavior (in press)

Hodgins S, Toupin J, Côté G (1996) Schizophrenia and antisocial personality disorder: a criminal combination. In: Schlesinger LB (ed) Explorations in Criminal Psychopathology: Clinical Syndromes with Forensic Implications. Charles C Thomas Publisher, Springfield, IL, pp 217–237

Ishikawa SS, Raine A (2002) Behavioral genetics and crime. In: Glickson J (ed) The Neurobiology of Criminal Behaviour. Kluwer Academic Publishers, Dordrecht, Netherlands, pp 81–110

Joyal C, Hallé P, Hodgins S, Lapierre D (2003) Drug abuse and/or dependence and better neuropsychological performance in patients with schizophrenia. Schizophrenia Research 63(3):297–299

Kay SR (1990) Significance of the positive-negative distinction in schizophrenia. Schizophrenia Bulletin 16:635

Kendler KS, McGuire M, Gruenberg AM, O'Hare A, Spellman M, Walsh D (1993) The Roscommon Family Study III. Schizophrenia-related personality disorders in relatives. Archives of General Psychiatry 50:781–788

Kety SS, Rosenthal D, Wender PH, Schulsinger F (1971) Mental illness in the biological and adoptive families of adopted schizophrenics. American Journal of Psychiatry 128(3):302–306

Kratzer L, Hodgins S (1999) A typology of offenders: a test of Moffitt's theory among males and females from childhood to age 30. Criminal Behaviour and Mental Health 9:57–73

Krueger RF, Hicks BM, Patrick CJ, Carlson SR, Iacono WG, McGue M (2002) Etiologic connections among substance dependence, antisocial behavior, and personality: modeling the externalizing spectrum. Journal of Abnormal Psychology 111:411–424

Krueger RF, Moffitt TE, Caspi A, Bleske A, Silva PA (1998) Assortative mating for antisocial behavior: developmental and methodological implications. Behavior Genetics 28:173–186

Landau R, Harth P, Othany N, Sharfhertz C (1972) The influence of psychotic parents on their children's development. American Journal of Psychiatry 129:38

Lasser K, Boyd JW, Woolhandler S, Himmelstein DU, McCormick D, Bor DH (2000) Smoking and mental illness: a population-based prevalence study. Journal of the American Medical Association 284(20):2606–2610

Lewis DO, Balla DA (1970) Delinquency and Psychopathology. Grune & Stratton, New York

Lindelius R (ed) (1970) A study of schizophrenia: a clinical prognostic and family investigation. Acta Psychiatrica Scandinavica (Suppl 216):1–122

Lindqvist P (1986) Criminal homicide in Northern Sweden 1970–1981: alcohol intoxication, alcohol abuse and mental disease. International Journal of Law and Psychiatry 8:19–37

Link BG, Stueve A (1994) Psychotic symptoms and the violent/illegal behavior of mental patients compared to community controls. In: Monahan J, Steadman H (eds) Violence and Mental Disorders. University of Chicago Press, Chicago, pp 137–159

Loeber R, Farrington DP, Stouthamer-Loeber M, Moffitt TE, Caspi A (1998) The development of male offending: key findings from the first decade of the Pittsburgh youth study. Studies on Crime and Prevention 7(2):141–171

Loeber R, Farrington DP, Stouthamer-Loeber M, Moffitt TE, Caspi A, Lynam D (2001) Male mental health problems, psychopathy, and personality traits; key findings from the first 14 years of the Pittsburgh Youth Study. Clinical Child & Family Psychology Review 4(4):273–297

Mednick SA, Parnas J, Schulsinger F (1987) The Copenhagen high-risk project 1962–1986. Schizophrenia Bulletin 13:485

Moffitt TE (1993) "Life-course-persistent" and "adolescence-limited" antisocial behavior: a developmental taxonomy. Psychological Review 100:674–701

Moffitt TE (1994) Natural histories of delinquency. In: Weitekamp E, Kerner HJ (eds) Cross-national Longitudinal Research on Human Development and Criminal Behaviour. Kluwer Academic, Dordrecht, Netherlands, pp 3–61

Moffitt TE (1997) Adolescence-limited and life-course-persistent offending: a complementary pair of developmental theories. In: Thornberry T (ed) Advances in Criminological Theory: Developmental Theories of Crime and Delinquency. Transaction Press, London, pp 11–54

Moffitt TE, Caspi A (2001) Childhood predictors differentiate life-course persistent and adolescence-limited antisocial pathways among males and females. Development and Psychopathology 13:355–375

Moffitt TE, Caspi A, Harrington H, Milne BJ (2002) Males on the life-course-persistent and adolescence-limited antisocial pathways: follow up at age 26 years. Development and Psychopathology 14:179–207

Moffitt TE, Silva PA, Lynam DR, Henry B (1994) Self-reported delinquency at age 18. In: Junger-Tas J, Terlouw GJ (eds) The International Self-report Delinquency Project. Ministry of Justice of the Netherlands, The Hague, pp 356–371

Mullen PE, Burgess P, Wallace C, Palmer S, Ruschena D (2000) Community care and criminal offending in schizophrenia. Lancet 355:614–617

Müller-Isberner R (2001) Criminality of mentally ill patients in general psychiatry (abstract). European Psychiatry 17(1):26

Parnas J (1988) Assortative mating in schizophrenia: results from the Copenhagen High-Risk Study. Psychiatry 51:58–64

Räsänen P, Hakko H, Isohanni M, Hodgins S, Järvelin M-R, Tiihonen J (1999) Maternal smoking during pregnancy and the risk of criminal behavior among adult male offspring in the Northern Finland 1966 birth cohort. American Journal of Psychiatry 156:857–862

Rhee SH, Waldman ID (2002) Genetic and environmental influences on antisocial behavior: a meta-analysis of twin and adoption studies. Psychological Bulletin 128:490–529

Robins LN (1966) Deviant Children Grown Up. Williams and Wilkins, Baltimore

Robins LN (1993) Childhood conduct problems, adult psychopathology, and crime. In: Hodgins S (ed) Mental Disorder and Crime. Sage Publications Inc, Newbury Park, CA, pp 173–207

Robins LN, McEvoy L (1990) Conduct problems as predictors of substance abuse. In: Robins LN, Rutter M (eds) Straight & Deviant Pathways from Childhood to Adulthood. Cambridge University Press, Cambridge, pp 182–204

Robins LN, Price RK (1991) Adult disorders predicted by childhood conduct problems: results from the NIMH epidemiologic catchment area project. Psychiatry 54:116–132

Robins LN, Tipp J, Przybeck T (1991) Antisocial personality. In: Robins LN, Regier D (eds) Psychiatric Disorders in America: the Epidemiologic Catchment Area study. Macmillan/Free Press, New York, pp 258–290

Schanda H, Födes P, Topitz A, Knecht G (1992) Premorbid adjustment of schizophrenic criminal offenders. Acta Psychiatrica Scandinava 86:121–126

Silverton L (1985) Crime and the Schizophrenia Spectrum: A Study of Two Danish Cohorts. Doctoral dissertation, University of Southern California

Spitzer RL, Williams JBW, Gibbon M, First MB (1992) The structured clinical interview for DSM-III-R (SCID) I: history, rationale, and description. Archives of General Psychiatry 49:624–629

Stattin H, Magnusson D (1991) Stability and change in criminal behaviour up to age 30: findings from a prospective, longitudinal study in Sweden. British Journal of Criminology 31:327–346

Stone GL (1995) Review of the Hare Psychopathy Checklist-Revised. In: Conoley JC, Impara JC (eds) Twelfth Mental Measurement Yearbook. Buros Institute, Lincoln, pp 454–455

Swanson JW, Holzer CED, Ganju VK, Jono RT (1990) Violence and psychiatric disorder in the community: evidence from the Epidemiologic Catchment Area surveys. Hospital and Community Psychiatry 41:761–770

Tehrani JA, Mednick SA (2000) Etiological factors linked to criminal violence and adult mental illness. In: Hodgins S (ed) Violence among the Mentally Ill Effective Treatments and Management Strategies. Kluwer Academic Publishers, The Netherlands, pp 59–75

Tengström A, Hodgins S (2002) Assessing psychopathic traits among persons with schizophrenia: a way to improve violence risk assessment. In: Blaauw E, Sheridan L (eds) Psychopaths Current International Perspective. Elsevier, Holland, pp 81–111

Tengström A, Hodgins S, Grann M, Långström N, Kullgren G (2003) Schizophrenia and criminal offending: the role of psychopathy and substance misuse. Criminal Justice and Behavior (in press)

Tengström A, Hodgins S, Kullgren G (2001) Men with schizophrenia who behave violently: the usefulness of an early versus late starters typology. Schizophrenia Bulletin 27:205–218

Tiihonen J, Isohanni M, Räsänen P, Koiranen M, Moring J (1997) Specific major mental disorders and criminality: a 26 year prospective study of the 1966 Northern Finland birth cohort. American Journal of Psychiatry 154:840–845

Trembley RE (2000) The development of aggressive behaviour during childhood: what have we learned in the past century? International Journal of Behavioural Development 24:129–141

Wakschlag LS, Lahey BB, Loeber R, Green SM, Gordon RA, Leventhal BL (1997) Maternal smoking during pregnancy and the risk of conduct disorder in boys. Archives of General Psychiatry 54:670–676

Walsh E, Gilvarry C, Samele C, Harvey K, Manley C, Tyrer P, Creed F, Murray R, Fahy T (2001) Reducing violence in severe mental illness: randomised controlled trial of intensive case management compared with standard care. British Medical Journal 323(10):1–5

Zammit S, Allebeck P, Andreasson S, Lundberg I, Lewis G (2002) Self reported cannabis use as a risk factor for schizophrenia in Swedish conscripts of 1969: historical cohort study. British Medical Journal 325:1199–1201

The aetiological continuum of psychosis

INEZ MYIN-GERMEYS [1,2], JANNEKE SPAUWEN [1], NELE JACOBS [1],
ROSELIND LIEB [3], HANS-ULRICH WITTCHEN [3], and JIM VAN OS [1,4]

[1] Dept. Psychiatry and Neuropsychology, European Graduate School of Neuroscience,
Maastricht University, Maastricht, The Netherlands
[2] Mondriaan Zorggroep, Section Social Cognition, Heerlen, The Netherlands
[3] Max Planck Institute of Psychiatry, Clinical Psychology and Epidemiology Unit, Munich,
Germany
[4] Division of Psychological Medicine, Institute of Psychiatry, London, UK

Introduction

In clinical practice, psychosis usually is conceived of as an all-or-none phenomenon, reflecting the necessarily dichotomous medical decision to either treat or not treat. Thus conceptually one either suffers from psychosis, indicating that one is in need of care, or one is healthy and symptom-free. While it is only natural that the binary decision to treat is reflected in clinical formulations of categories of mental illness, there is a growing body of research, conducted outside the realm of the psychiatric clinic, that suggests that the psychosis phenotype is expressed differently in Nature. Thus, there is evidence that the phenotype exists as a continuous distribution of psychotic experiences in the general population, the extreme of which constitutes psychotic disorder as seen in the clinic. Psychotic symptoms such as hallucinations and delusions are commonly reported in non-clinical population samples and the experiences resembling negative symptoms also appear to be distributed. Studies using structured diagnostic interviews have demonstrated that large proportions of the general population report psychosis-like experiences. In the National Comorbidity Study, 28.4% of all individuals from the general population reported one or more psychosis-like experience (Kendler et al. 1996). In the Dutch NEMESIS study, 17.5% of all general population subjects endorsed at least 1 of 17 Composite International Diagnostic Interview positive psychotic items (Van Os et al. 2000). Poulton et al. (2000) demonstrated in a birth cohort that 20.1% of the subjects reported delusions and 13.2% reported hallucinations at age 26. Olfson et al. (2002) reported that 20.9% of the clients in a large, urban, general medicine practice reported one or more psychotic symptoms. In the Acquitaine Sentinel Network of GPs, 16% of the subjects with no psychiatric history reported on a self-report questionnaire that they had experienced verbal hallucinations and 10% reported paranoid ideation (Verdoux and Van Os 2002). These data suggest that there is a symptomatic continuum between "normal" subjects and subjects with psychotic disorder.

However, the question then arises whether the psychosis-like experiences that are prevalent in non-clinical, general population samples, are on a true quantitative continuum with psychotic disorders, or whether they are qualitatively different and therefore not directly related to disorders such as RDC, ICD or DSM constructs of schizophrenia. If psychotic disorder really differed qualitatively from psychosis-like experiences, its ontogeny could in all likelihood be traced to causal influences with a low prevalence in the general population, linked in a specific way to the disorder. However, if it were possible to demonstrate that psychotic disorder is related to the same aetiological influences as psychosis-like experiences, i.e. if aetiological continuity can be demonstrated, it becomes much more likely that both phenomena are on a quantitative continuum. The continuity hypothesis may subsequently be further refined to include either a fully dimensional view, or alternatively a semi-continuous one indicating that psychotic disorder is in part the result of unique causal factors related to disorder per se (see Section 1, Chapter 4 in this volume: Krabbendam et al. 2004) and in part caused by shared risk factors. Therefore, the continuity hypothesis of psychotic disorder and psychosis-like experiences allows for both quantitative and qualitative differences occurring simultaneously. In the present chapter, we will investigate the existence of an aetiological continuity (either fully or semi-dimensional) and we will describe several studies that have provided evidence in favour of such continuity.

▌ Part 1: demographic risk factors associated with a psychosis continuum

In the first part, we will investigate whether demographic variables that are known to be associated with the clinical expression of psychosis, are similarly associated with subtler, non-clinical but much more frequent psychotic experiences. If the relationship between the demographic factors and the clinical disorder is qualitatively different from the relationship between these factors and the non-clinical psychotic experiences, it is unlikely that they play a causal role in the expression of a continuity of psychosis. Instead, they may merely facilitate the influence of a rare cause resulting in disorder.

Samples of patients who receive a diagnosis of schizophrenia for the first time (incident cases) show, as a group, a characteristic pattern of associations with a range of demographic variables. Thus, incident patients are more likely to be young, single, unemployed, and of lower educational level. Van Os et al. (2000) reported similar associations with non-clinical psychotic and psychosis-like symptoms.

Additionally, the expression of schizophrenia has been reported to differ between the sexes (Crow 1993). A number of studies have found men to display more negative symptoms than women (Roy et al. 2001; Schultz et al. 1997; Shtasel et al. 1992), while women may have a higher prevalence of positive symptoms. These sex differences in psychotic expression were also reported in the wider range of psychotic experiences along a continuum from normality through to stressful psychotic experiences (Crow 1986; Kendell and Brockington 1980; Maier et al. 1993; Van Os et al. 2000). Male sex was associated with more negative psychotic experiences, while positive psychotic experiences were more prevalent in women (Maric et al. 2002). Below, these sex-related differences in the realm of both psychotic disorder and non-clinical psychotic experiences will be explored in more detail (Spauwen et al. in press).

Study 1: sex differences in psychosis: evidence for an aetiological continuity?

In addition to sex differences related to the expression of symptoms, it is also known that the age during which these symptoms become apparent is different in both sexes. In fact, this finding is among the most robust of epidemiological findings in the field of schizophrenia research. The dramatic increase in the incidence of schizophrenia after puberty occurs at an earlier age in boys than in girls, causing the prevalence of the disorder to be higher in boys than in girls during adolescence (Konnecke et al. 2000; WHO 1992). This epidemiological imbalance is thought to reflect sex differences in the timing of maturational events that facilitate the onset of psychotic disorder (Galdos et al. 1993; Kraepelin 1919) (Fig. 1). If a similar age-related difference exists in the expression of subtler, non-clinical psychotic experiences and the non-clinical psychotic experiences increase differentially with age in boys and girls in the same fashion as the clinical disorder schizophrenia, a likely explanation would be that a normal, sex-related maturational event after puberty causes expression of psychosis along a continuum of severity. However, if the sex differences in age of onset of schizophrenia are not reflected in similar sex differences in the age of onset of non-clinical psychotic experiences, a plausible explanation is that maturational events themselves are not directly implicated but merely facilitate the causal influence of a rare, early brain abnormality that is more common in males and remained "dormant" until after puberty. This latter theory is commonly referred to as the neurodevelopmental hypothesis of schizophrenia (Murray and Lewis 1988; Waddington et al. 1999; Weinberger 1987).

Method

The Early Developmental Stages of Psychopathology (EDSP) study (Lieb et al. 2000) collected data on the prevalence, incidence, risk factors, comorbidity and course of mental disorders in a random representative population sample of adolescents and young adults (age range 14–24 years) in the Munich area (Germany). The overall design of the study is prospective, consisting of a baseline survey (n=3021), two follow-up surveys and a family supplement. Fourteen to 15-year-olds were sampled at twice the probability of persons 16–

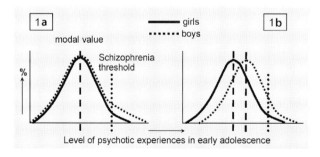

Fig. 1. Models explaining higher prevalence of schizophrenia in boys during adolscence

21 years of age, and 22- to 24-year-olds were sampled at half this probability. A complete and detailed description of design, sample, instruments, procedures and statistical methods of the EDSP is given elsewhere (Wittchen et al. 1998). The baseline sample was drawn in 1994 from the government registries in Munich, Germany, of registrants expected to be 14 to 24 years of age at the time of the baseline interview in 1995. A total of 3021 interviews were completed at baseline (T0; response rate, 71%). The first follow-up study (T1) was conducted only for respondents aged 14 to 17 years at baseline, whereas the second follow-up study was conducted for all respondents. The current results are based on the second follow-up. From the 3021 respondents of the baseline study, a total of 2548 interviews were completed at the second follow-up (T2), which occurred at an average of 42 months after baseline (response rate, 84%). Respondents were assessed with the computer-assisted version of the Munich-Composite International Diagnostic Interview (M-CIDI) (Wittchen and Pfister 1997), an updated version of the World Health Organization's Composite International Diagnostic Interview version 1.2 (Atakan and Cooper 1989). The ratings from the 15 M-CIDI core psychosis sections on delusions (11 items) and hallucinations (4 items) were used (items G3–G5, G7–G14, G17, G18, G20, G21). These concern classic psychotic symptoms involving, for example, persecution, thought interference and auditory hallucinations. All of these items can be rated in two ways: 1, no and 5, yes. The presence of positive psychotic experiences was broadly defined as any rating of 5 on any of the 15 M-CIDI core psychosis items.

Results

15.7% reported having had at least one delusional experience and 4.6% reported having had at least one hallucinatory experience. In those who reported at least one psychotic experience, the mean age was lower in boys (21.3 years, SD = 3.3) than in girls (22.4 years, SD 3.5, $t = -2.9$, df = 440, $P = 0.0042$). Logistic regression indicated that there was no main effect of age (in years) or sex on the presence of at least one positive symptom (OR 1.00, 95% CI 0.97–1.03 and OR 0.92, 95% CI 0.75–1.13, respectively). However, a significant interaction between age and sex was present (likelihood ratio test: 2 = 6.7, p = 0.0097). Stratified analysis revealed that in the younger half of the cohort (split around the median age of 21 years) the risk of having a positive psychotic symptom was higher for males than for females (OR = 0.70, 95% CI 0.52–0.95), while no sex difference was found in the older cohort (OR = 1.18, 95% CI 0.89–1.58).

Conclusion

Non-clinical experiences of psychosis showed differential age distributions by sex that resembled those reported for the clinical disorder schizophrenia. This suggests that sex differences in psychosis may reflect differential age-related variation of a continuous phenotype, rather than differential expression of a rare causal pathological risk factor.

Conclusion part 1

The present data demonstrate that at least some demographic variables show a qualitatively similar pattern of association with both clinical disorder and psychosis-like experiences, suggestive of an aetiological continuity.

▌ Part 2: social and environmental risk factors associated with a psychosis continuum

Similar to the argument for the demographic variables, the social and environmental risk factors for psychotic illness should also contribute to a larger pool of preclinical psychotic experiences, which exist in the general population. If this were true, populations who report higher levels of disorder due to more exposure to certain social and environmental risk factors should show a similar increase in the level of psychosis-like symptoms (Fig. 2).

There is evidence that environmental factors such as childhood trauma or discrimination are associated with psychotic disorder. Studies have demonstrated a high incidence of trauma in the lifetimes of patients with psychosis and immigrant groups have higher incidence rates of psychotic disorder, which has been hypothesised to be related to their much greater level of exposure to discrimination. A series of studies in Maastricht provided evidence that these environmental risk factors were also associated with psychosis-like experiences. Janssen et al. (in press) demonstrated that childhood abuse was significantly associated with both psychosis-like experiences and with psychotic disorder. The same authors reported that discrimination was associated with higher levels of psychosis-like experiences in the general population (Janssen et al. 2003).

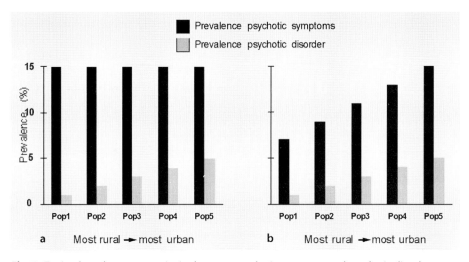

Fig. 2. Testing hypotheses on continuity between psychotic symptoms and psychotic disorders

Another environmental risk factor associated with psychotic disorder is urban birth and upbringing. In the next study, the association between urbanicity and psychotic disorder and psychosis-like experiences will be investigated in more detail (Van Os et al. 2001).

Study 2:
prevalence of psychotic disorder and community level of psychotic symptoms

Urban birth, upbringing or residence is a risk factor for psychotic disorder, suggesting that urban and rural populations have different lifetime risks (Lewis et al. 1992; Marcelis et al. 1998, 1999; Mortensen et al. 1999). It would be interesting to investigate to what degree the increase in risk for psychotic disorder associated with urban life is reflected in similar increases in the mean number of psychotic and psychosis-like symptoms. In the current study (Van Os et al. 2001), it was hypothesised that the mean level of symptoms would increase with the rate of disorder across increasingly urbanised areas. In addition, it was hypothesised that the association between symptoms and disorder would be constant across the populations in the different strata, suggesting variation of susceptibility between populations rather than within populations.

Method

The current report is based on data pertaining to the Netherlands Mental Health Survey and Incidence Study (NEMESIS), a longitudinal study of the prevalence, incidence and consequences of psychiatric disorders in the Dutch general population (Bijl et al. 1998 a, b). Subjects were interviewed on three occasions: in 1996 (T0), in 1997 (T1 – assessing the 12 month-period between T0 and T1), and in 1999 (T2 – assessing the 24 month-period between T1 and T2). A comprehensive description of the project objectives, sample procedure, response, diagnostic instruments, quality control procedures and analyses is provided in previous publications (Bijl et al. 1998 a, b). NEMESIS is based on a multistage, stratified, random sampling procedure in which 90 municipalities, a sample of private households within each municipality, and members with the most recent birthday within each household were selected. Subjects were aged 18–64 years and sufficiently fluent in Dutch to be interviewed. A total of 7076 individuals provided informed consent and were interviewed at T0, (response rate = 69.7%). The current report is based on the baseline data.

Subjects were interviewed at home using the Composite International Diagnostic Interview (CIDI) version 1.1 (Robins and Guze 1970; Smeets and Dingemans 1993; WHO 1990) for all three measurements. The CIDI generates *Diagnostic and Statistical Manual of Mental Disorders,* Third Edition, Revised (DSM-III-R) diagnoses and is designed for trained interviewers who are not clinicians. Ninety interviewers experienced in systematic data collection collected the data, having received 3 day training course in recruiting and interviewing, followed by a 4 day course at the WHO-CIDI training centre in Amsterdam. Extensive monitoring and quality checks took place throughout the entire data collection period.

Lifetime ratings from the 17 CIDI core psychosis sections on delusions (13 items) and hallucinations (4 items) were used (items G1-G13, G15, G16, G20, and G21). All of these items can be rated in 6 ways: "1" – No symptom, "2" – Symptom present but not clinically relevant (not bothered by it and not seeking help for it), "3" – Symptom result of ingestion of drugs, "4" – Symptom result of somatic disease, "5" – True psychiatric symptom, "6" – Symptom may not really be a symptom because there appears to be some plausible explanation for it. Because psychotic symptoms may be difficult to diagnose in a structured interview (Anthony et al. 1985; Cooper et al. 1998; Helzer et al. 1985), clinical re-interviews were conducted by telephone by an experienced psychiatric trainee for all subjects who had evidence of significant psychosis at baseline (at least one rating of "5" or "6"). The re-interviews were conducted by using questions from the Structured Clinical Interview for DSM-III-R (SCID), an instrument with proven reliability and validity in diagnosing schizophrenia (Spitzer et al. 1992). If the clinician's CIDI psychotic symptom rating did not coincide with that of the lay interviewer, the rating of the lay interviewer was replaced with that of the clinician. These corrected CIDI ratings were then entered into the CIDI diagnostic program. The DSM-III-R diagnoses of psychotic disorder at baseline were thus based on the Structured Clinical Interview for DSM-III-R data from these clinical re-interviews.

Psychotic disorder was defined as any DSM-III-R affective or nonaffective psychotic diagnosis. *Psychotic symptom* was defined as any CIDI rating of 2,3,4,5, or 6 on any of the 17 CIDI core psychosis items. Five levels of *urbanisation* were defined based on the density of addresses per square kilometre in an area (less than 500, 500 to 999, 1000 to 1499, 1500 to 2499, and 2500 or more).

Results

The lifetime prevalences of DSM-III-R psychotic disorder, and psychotic symptoms increased in a monotonic fashion with level of urbanicity (see Table 1). Psychotic symptoms were strongly associated with psychotic disorder (sum-

Table 1. Sample prevalences of psychotic disorder and psychotic symptoms in relation to urbanicity

	No. interviewed	Psychotic disorder		Psychotic symptoms	
		No (%)	OR (95% CI)	No (%)	OR (95% CI)
<500	1185	7 (0.59)	1*	163 (13.76)	1*
500–999	1610	15 (0.93)	1.58 (0.64–3.89)	223 (13.85)	1.01 (0.81–1.25)
1000–1499	1541	23 (1.49)	2.55 (1.09–5.96)	262 (17.00)	1.28 (1.04–1.59)
1500–2499	1497	28 (1.87)	3.21 (1.40–7.37)	303 (20.24)	1.59 (1.29–1.96)
≥2500	1242	34 (2.74)	4.74 (2.09–10.73)	286 (23.03)	1.88 (1.52–2.32)
OR linear trend**		1.44 (1.42–1.68), $p < 0.001$		1.19 (1.14–1.25), $p < 0.001$	

* Reference category
** The summary increase in risk with 1-unit change in address density

mary OR over 6 levels, 3.59; 95% CI, 3.17–4.06). There was no evidence that this association differed as a function of urbanicity (χ^2 4 = 4.20, p = 0.38).

Conclusion

Lifetime level of psychotic and psychosis-like symptoms independently increased with level of urbanicity in the same manner as did DSM-III-R psychotic disorder. At all levels of urbanicity, psychosis-like symptoms were strongly associated with psychotic disorder. These findings therefore suggest that the increased prevalence of psychotic disorder in urban environments should be interpreted in the light of increased levels of "psychosis proneness" in urban populations. Populations with higher mean levels of psychosis produce more psychotic disorder, suggesting underlying between-population aetiological differences in the prevalence of risk factors that impact on whole populations rather than a small segment of a population being "hit" by a rare risk factor.

Conclusion part 2

Several environmental risk factors have been identified that are related both to clinical psychosis and non-clinical psychosis-like experiences. It was shown that populations who live in more urban areas have higher levels of psychotic disorder and also have higher levels of psychosis-like experiences. The mean level of psychosis-like experiences in a population is directly associated with the prevalence of disorder: the prevalence of psychotic disorder, therefore, is a reflection of the mean level of "psychosis" of the source population and cannot be seen to occur in isolation as a "rare" disorder. These data strengthen the hypothesis that both clinical and non-clinical psychotic experiences are situated on an aetiological continuum.

▮ Part 3: personality traits and the continuum of psychosis

Personality trait profiles of patients with psychotic disorder tend to differ from normal controls. For instance, they report higher levels of peculiarity and neuroticism, while they report lower levels of conscientiousness and extraversion (Berenbaum and Fujita 1994; Gurrera et al. 2000). Myin-Germeys et al. (2001) used a structured diary technique, the Experience Sampling Method, to show that subjects who suffer from psychotic disorder are more emotionally reactive to small stressors in their daily life, compared to healthy controls. In addition, the first-degree relatives of these patients reported a significantly stronger emotional reaction to daily life stress, compared to the healthy controls. As the personality profile of the healthy relatives was found to be different from that of control subjects, it can be hypothesised that personality characteristics, such as altered stress-sensitivity, reflect an underlying vulnerability to schizophrenia.

If psychosis-like experiences are quantitatively rather than qualitatively different from psychotic disorder, one would expect them to be associated with the same personality profiles that characterise patients with psychotic disorder.

Below, the relationship between the personality trait neuroticism, and psychosis-like experiences will be explored in more detail (Krabbendam et al. 2002).

Study 3: neuroticism and the continuum of psychosis in the general population

Neuroticism, a personality trait related to stress reactivity, anxiety proneness and autonomic lability (Horwood and Fergusson 1986; Ormel et al. 1989), is known to be related to psychotic disorder. Patients with psychotic disorder show increased levels of neuroticism (Berenbaum and Fujita 1994; Gurrera et al. 2000) and it has been suggested that neuroticism is a maintaining factor in psychosis (Freeman and Garety 1999). Recent longitudinal data from a national birth cohort yielded evidence that childhood neuroticism is a risk factor for the onset of psychosis in adult life, independent of its (better known) association with depression (Van Os and Jones 2001). The present study investigated the relationship between neuroticism and psychosis-like experiences in a general population sample (Krabbendam et al. 2002).

Method

For this study, data from the NEMESIS study were used (for description: see study 2). At T2, two items of the Brief Psychiatric Rating Scale (BPRS; (Overall and Gorham 1962)) that represent the positive symptoms for psychosis, "unusual thought content", and "hallucinations" were scored by a clinician. The range of the scores for each symptom was from 1, "absent" to 7, "very severe". Ratings of 2–3 indicate non-pathological intensities of symptoms, 4–7 indicate a pathological intensity of symptoms (Lukoff et al. 1986). The two BPRS psychosis ratings were used in the analyses in two ways: i) any rating >1 on either "unusual thought content" or "hallucinations" (hereafter: psychosis broadly defined) and ii) any rating >3 on either "unusual thought content" or "hallucinations" (hereafter: psychosis narrowly defined). In order to skew the sample at T2 towards individuals with lifetime first-ever occurrence of symptoms, only individuals were included who i) at baseline interview (T0) had a rating of lifetime absence on all the individual items in the CIDI psychosis section and ii) at T1 interview also had a rating of lifetime absence on all the individual items in the CIDI psychosis section. The additional exclusion of individuals at T1 was added to make sure that any prevalent psychosis cases that were missed at baseline were still excluded. At every measurement occasion, subjects also completed the 14-item Groningen Neuroticism Scale (Ormel 1980).

Logistic regression (StataCorp 2001) was carried out to examine the associations between T0 baseline neuroticism and incident psychotic symptoms broadly and narrowly defined at T2. Associations were expressed as odds ratios (ORs) with their 95% confidence intervals (CIs). To examine dose-response relationships between neuroticism and later risk for psychotic symptoms, the sample was divided into three groups according to their tertile group level on the continuous neuroticism scores (±33% subjects with lowest score on neuroticism; ±33% subjects with middle score on neuroticism; ±33% subjects with highest score on neuroticism).

Results

Neuroticism at T0 was positively associated with presence of psychosis, broadly defined, at T2 (OR 1.16, 95% CI 1.09, 1.23). The strength of the association increased with increasing levels of neuroticism (summary OR over three groups 2.21, 95% CI 1.36, 3.60; middle scores, OR 1.80, 95% CI 0.43, 7.54; high scores, OR 3.89, 95% CI 1.03, 14.71; low scores used as reference category with OR = 1). Level of neuroticism at baseline also significantly predicted narrowly defined psychosis at T2 (OR 1.20, 95% CI 1.05, 1.36).

Conclusion

The findings suggest that baseline neuroticism contributes to the risk of psychosis-like symptoms at 3-year follow-up, and therefore confirm that neuroticism may constitute a vulnerability factor to develop psychosis-like experiences. Given the fact that neuroticism was conceived as a measure tapping into sensitivity to stress or trait anxiety, the findings lend credence to the earlier suggestion that the expression of psychosis is facilitated by higher levels of sensitivity to stressors in daily life (Myin-Germeys et al. 2001).

Conclusion part 3

Personality traits that constitute an underlying vulnerability to schizophrenia seem to be similarly related to the development of non-clinical psychosis-like symptoms in the general population. These results are compatible with the hypothesis of aetiological continuity underlying the expression of psychosis at all levels.

▌ Part 4: familial transmission and the continuum of psychosis

Several studies provide evidence for an important genetic contribution to the development of psychotic disorder. Using twin-studies comparing monozygotic and dizygotic twin probands, Cardno et al. (1999) demonstrated that psychotic disorder was transmitted in families, and the genetic contribution to the variance in liability was estimated between 82% and 85%. However, in order to compare levels of familial and genetic transmission of psychotic disorder with psychosis-like symptoms, the investigation needs to focus on familial clustering of symptom dimensions, as subjects in the general population may have psychosis-like symptoms in the absence of a formally diagnosable disorder. In the next study, the patterns of familial transmission of symptom dimensions in the general population will be investigated (Jacobs et al. submitted).

Study 4: familial transmission of psychotic symptom dimensions in the general population

Twin studies of probands with psychosis and studies investigating familial clustering of psychopathology in multiply affected families have shown significant familiality and genetic transmission of the psychomotor poverty or nega-tive symptom dimension, of the manic dimension and of the disorganisation dimension (Cardno et al. 2001; Van Os et al. 1997; Wickham et al. 2001). In addition, twin studies of affected probands showed a pattern of familial aggre-gation of a general psychotic dimension and a significant heritability (71%) of the nuclear syndrome, characterised by one or more Schneiderian first-rank symptoms (Cardno et al. 2002). These results were replicated, albeit at the non-clinical level of psychosis, in a large general population twin-study inves-tigating 3685 individuals including 1438 complete twin pairs. In this general population sample, Hay et al. (2001) found evidence for familial resemblance and a genetic effect for positive and negative psychosis-like "schizotypy" di-mensions measured with the Chapman scales.

One criticism that can be brought to bear on these findings is that dimen-sions of psychosis are strongly correlated with each other (Stefanis et al. 2002), and that showing patterns of familial transmission and heritability of separate dimensions should take into account their considerable co-variation so that true specificity and independence can be demonstrated. Fanous et al. (2001) reported that positive symptoms in probands with non-affective psy-chosis were predictive of positive schizotypy in the relatives, while negative symptoms in the probands were predictive of negative schizotypy in the rela-tives, which is suggestive for familial and possibly genetic homotypy of these psychosis dimensions. In the current study, the specificity and relative inde-pendence of familial transmission of positive and negative symptom dimen-sions will be investigated in a general population twin study (Jacobs et al. sub-mitted).

Method

The sample consisted of 250 female twin pairs collected from the East Flan-ders Prospective Twin Survey (EFPTS). The EFPTS has recorded multiple births in the province of East Flanders (Belgium) since 1964. Basic perinatal data such as birth weight, gestational age, mode of delivery, and placentation are collected. The zygosity of the twins is determined by sex, placentation, blood groups and, since 1982, by examination of five highly polymorphic DNA markers. Unlike-sex twins and same-sex twins with at least one different genetic marker were classified as dizygotic; monochorionic twins were classi-fied as monozygotic. For all same-sex dichorionic twins with the same genetic markers, a probability of monozygosity was calculated using a lod-score meth-od (Vlietinck 1986). After DNA fingerprinting, a probability of monozygosity of 0.999 was reached. To be included in the analysis, dichorionic MZ pairs had to reach a probability of monozygosity of at least 95%. So far, the register has collected information on more than 5600 pairs of twins (Loos et al. 1998).

All subjects in the current study were female and in the age range of 18 to 45 years. The sample consisted of 150 monozygotic twin pairs and 100 dizygotic twin pairs. The subclinical symptoms were assessed with the CAPE (Stefanis et al. 2002). The Cape is a 42-item self-report questionnaire, constructed to measure (sub)-clinical psychotic experiences in the general population. The

CAPE uses two dimensional scales. The first scale scores the frequency of the experience (measured on a four-point scale from "never" to "nearly always") and the second scale scores the degree of distress (measured on a four-point scale from "not distressed" to "very distressed"). The CAPE consists of 20 positive symptom items, two hallucination items and 16 items derived from the PDI, a self-report instrument to measure delusional ideation in the general population. In addition, there are 14 negative symptom items, which are derived from the SANS (Andreasen 1989), and an instrument of subjective experience of negative symptoms, the SENS (Selten et al. 1998). Finally, 8 depression items are assessed. As it is difficult to discriminate between negative and depressive symptoms, items of depressive symptoms that are most specific for depression, i.e. cognitive symptoms of depression (e.g. sadness, pessimism, hopelessness, feeling a failure, feeling guilty) (Kibel et al. 1993) were used. The CAPE provides an overall total score and additionally two scores per dimension by i) adding up the number of positive answers to the frequency question yielding a frequency score, and ii) adding up the scores of the distress questions yielding a distress score. Data showing the validity of the CAPE were presented previously (Stefanis et al. 2002).

The familial transmission of the positive and negative symptom dimensions was analysed using a regression analysis with for each symptom dimension, the frequency score of twin 1 as the dependent variable and the frequency score of twin 2 as the independent variable. In order to investigate specificity, a cross-sib within-trait analysis was conducted with as covariates the frequency of symptoms on the other dimensions of the co-twin. In order to investigate independence, the proband symptom dimension scores other than the dependent variable were also included together in the analysis. For example, we modelled the positive symptom score in the proband twins as a function of the positive symptom score of the co-twin, adjusting for the negative and depressive scores of both the proband (independence) and the co-twin (specificity).

Results

There was cross-twin, within trait resemblance for both positive and negative psychotic experiences. Thus, presence of positive psychotic experiences in one twin was associated with positive psychotic experiences in the other (B = 0.20; SE = 0.07; p = 0.01). The same result was apparent for negative psychotic experiences (B = 0.27; SE = 0.06; p = 0.00). In addition, there was no significant cross-sib cross-trait resemblance. Thus, the presence of positive psychotic symptoms in one twin was not associated with negative psychotic and depressive experiences in the other twin, and the same was true for negative psychotic experiences. These results are therefore indicative of the specificity of familial transmission of dimensions of psychosis which in turn is suggestive of genetic homotypy. In addition, the effects were independent from the other symptom dimensions because they remained significant when controlled for the other symptom dimensions, both within and cross-sib.

Conclusion

In addition to the evidence for a genetic transmission of both positive and negative symptoms in patients with disorder and in the general population, the present results demonstrated that the familial and possibly genetic homotypy found in patients and their relatives could also be replicated in twins from the general population. Although the current sample was not large enough to provide the required statistical power for traditional twin modeling, a future analysis with an extended sample will be able to shed light on this issue. It is likely, however, that the sibling resemblance seen in this study is to a large part attributable to shared genetic factors.

Conclusion part 4

The present data demonstrate that the dimensions of psychosis-like experiences show similar patterns of genetic and familial transmission as reported for dimensions of psychotic disorder. In addition, the same familial and possibly genetic homotypy was found for both phenomena. This again is supportive for an aetiological continuity.

▌ Part 5: the case for gene-environment interaction

In the previous parts of this chapter, we have shown that psychosis-like experiences and psychotic disorder seem to be aetiologically continuous, both genetically and in terms of demographic and environmental risk factors. In the case of multifactorial disorders such as schizophrenia and other psychotic disorders, however, it is often thought that environmental risk factors interact with personal vulnerability factors, such as familial liability (Cannon et al. 1993; Tienari et al. 1985; Van Os and Marcelis 1998). If psychosis and psychosis-like experiences are situated on an aetiological continuum, one would hypothesise similar patterns of biological synergism between genetic liability and environmental risk (Van Os et al. in press).

Study 5: biological synergism between urbanicity and familial liability

It is thought that urbanicity is a proxy environmental risk factor for schizophrenia and psychosis-like experiences (Mortensen et al. 1999). In addition, it has been reported that there is familial liability to psychosis which is thought to largely represent the influence of shared genes rather than shared environment (Cardno et al. 1999; Kety et al. 1994). The question then arises as to what degree the environmental risk, i.e. urbanicity, interacts with the personal vulnerability factor of familial liability to psychosis. In this study, we will investigate to what degree urbanicity and familial liability for psychosis co-participate in producing psychosis outcomes, using recently specified models to examine biological synergism between two causes (Darroch 1997).

Method

For this study, data from the NEMESIS study were used (for description: see study 2). *Psychotic disorder outcome* at T0 was defined as any DSM-III-R affective or non-affective psychotic diagnosis. *Psychotic experiences* at T0 were defined as any CIDI rating of 2, 3, 4, 5, or 6 on any of the 17 CIDI core psychosis items. *Psychotic experiences narrowly defined* at T0 included a clinical reinterview rating of 5 on any of the CIDI psychosis items. Again five levels of urbanicity were defined (see study 2). For the assessment of familial liability, probands were asked separately for each first-degree relative whether he or she had ever had delusions or hallucinations, at T1. In addition, probands were asked if any first-degree relative or half-sib had ever received treatment from a psychiatrist or had ever been admitted to a psychiatric hospital for a mental health problem. There were 310 probands (5.6%) who indicated that a first-degree relative had had delusions or hallucinations, and 201 (3.6%) indicated that they had such relatives who had received psychiatric treatment as defined above. These two groups were designated, respectively, family history of psychosis broadly and narrowly defined. The number of probands with a family history of psychiatric treatment other than for delusions or hallucinations was 804 (14.5%).

Recent progress in the study of interactions indicates that the most frequently used statistical models of interaction are not suitable to identify biological synergism. For example, the commonly used statistical models in which genes and environment multiply each other's effects (multiplicative models) assume that individuals who are exposed to both the genetic and the environmental factor cannot have contracted the illness because the effect of genes alone or the environment alone (Darroch 1997). It has been shown that the true degree to which two causes co-participate in producing an outcome can be estimated from (but is not the same as) the additive statistical interaction (see Darroch 1997). We calculated the statistical additive interaction and estimated from that the population amount of biological synergism between urbanicity and family history (see Darroch 1997). This was done using the calculations developed by Darroch (1997). For these latter analyses, a dichotomised measure of urbanicity was used (1, 2, 3 = 0 and 4, 5 = 1). In order to calculate the statistical interaction under an additive model, the BINREG procedure in STATA (StataCorp 2001), which fits generalised linear models for the binomial family estimating risk differences (Hardin and Cleves 1999; Wacholder 1986), was used to model interactions between urbanicity and family history. Statistical significance of the interactions was assessed by Wald test (Clayton and Hills 1993).

Results

There was a significant positive interaction on the additive scale between urbanicity and family history in their effects on psychotic disorder in the proband, in that the effect size of urbanicity differed between those with and without a family history by approximately a factor 8 (Table 2 – broadly defined: $\chi^2 = 15.4$, df = 1, P<0.001; narrowly defined: $\chi^2 = 9.1$, df = 1, P = 0.003).

The risk of psychotic disorder in the population exposed to neither urbanicity (using the dichotomised measure of urbanicity as described above) or family history, broadly defined was 0.85% (28/3294). The risk of psychotic disorder in the population exposed to urbanicity alone was 1.59% (31/1946), the risk in those exposed to family history, broadly defined, alone was 3.01% (5/166), and the risk in those exposed to both was 9.72% (14/144). Filling in these risks in the formulae provided by Darroch (1997) revealed that synergism was between 0.0588 and 0.0662, which represents respectively 61% and 68% of the risk in those exposed to both urbanicity and family history (0.0588/0.0972 = 61% and 0.0662/0.0972 = 68%). Thus, between 60% and 70% of the individuals exposed to both urbanicity and family history had developed psychotic disorder because of the synergistic action of the two proxy causes (Table 2).

A similar result, though of a smaller effect size, was apparent for narrowly and broadly defined psychotic experiences. Thus, the summary risk of urbanicity on narrowly defined psychotic symptoms on the additive scale was 2.8% (P = 0.012) in those with a family history broadly defined, but only 0.8% (P < 0.001) in those without family history (test for interaction: $\chi^2 = 3.08$, df = 1, P = 0.079). Similarly, the summary risk of urbanicity on broadly defined psychotic symptoms on the additive scale was 5.1% (P = 0.004) in those with a family history broadly defined, but only 1.9% (P < 0.001) in those without family history (test for interaction: $\chi^2 = 2.98$, df = 1, P = 0.085). Thus, while the effects of urbanicity in those with and without family history differed by a factor of 8 for the psychotic disorder outcome (see Table 2), for the narrowly and broadly defined symptom outcome they differed by approximately a factor of 3.

Conclusion

The risk-increasing effect of urbanicity on the occurrence of psychotic disorder was greater in those with higher levels of familial liability for psychosis. Around 60–70% of the psychosis outcome in probands exposed to both familial liability and urbanicity was attributable to the synergistic action of these two factors. A similar pattern of interaction, though less marked, was apparent for the attenuated psychosis outcomes.

Conclusion part 5

The study presented demonstrated a significant biological synergism between a hypothesised proxy factor for genetic risk and a proxy factor for environmental risk in the occurrence of psychotic disorder. A similar interaction pattern was identified for psychosis-like symptoms. The fact that the reported interactions were of smaller effect size for the attenuated psychosis outcomes indicates that the effect size associated with the combined effect of urbanicity and familiality is not the same along the hypothesised continuum. Thus, the mental states at the lower end of the continuum may represent variation that

Table 2. Interactions between family history (FH) and urbanicity on the additive scale (risk difference)

Urbanicity		Family history Number of psychosis cases per population in urbanicity stratum (%)		Risk difference FH
		FH present (n=310)	FH absent (n=5240)	
Family history broadly defined	Level 1	0/34 (0.00)	5/937 (0.53)	-0.53% (-1.00, -0.07)
	Level 2	1/55 (1.82)	9/1215 (0.74)	1.08% (-2.49, 4.64)
	Level 3	4/77 (5.19)	14/1142 (1.23)	3.96% (-1.03, 8.97)
	Level 4	7/64 (10.94)	11/1101 (1.00)	9.94% (2.27, 17.61)
	Level 5	7/80 (8.75)	20/845 (2.37)	6.38% (0.11, 12.66)
	Summary risk difference urbanicity[a]	2.65% (1.51%, 3.78%)	0.34% (0.14, 0.54)	
	Additive interaction[b]	$\chi^2=15.4$, df=1, p<0.001		
	Approximate amount of biological synergism[c] between urbanicity[d] and family history	61% – 68%		
		FH present (n=201)	FH absent (n=5349)	
Family history narrowly defined	Level 1	0/25 (0.00)	5/946 (0.53)	-0.53% (-0.99, -0.07)
	Level 2	1/32 (3.13)	9/1238 (0.73)	2.39% (-3.65, 8.45)
	Level 3	2/49 (4.08)	16/1170 (1.37)	2.71% (-2.87, 8.29)
	Level 4	4/44 (9.09)	14/1121 (1.25)	7.84% (-0.68, 16.4)
	Level 5	5/51 (9.80)	22/874 (2.52)	7.29% (-0.94, 15.51)
	Summary risk difference urbanicity[a]	2.58% (1.18%, 3.97%)	0.40% (0.19, 0.60)	
	Additive interaction[b]	$\chi^2=9.1$, df=1, p=0.003		
	Approximate amount of biological synergism[c] between urbanicity[d] and family history	61%–70%		

[a] Summary increase in risk with one unit change in urbanicity
[b] Tests whether increase in risk in "Family History Absent" group is significantly greater than increase in risk in "Family History Present" group
[c] The proportion of individuals exposed to both urbanicity and family history who developed psychosis because of the synergistic action of the two causes
[d] For these analyses, a dichotomised measure of urbanicity was used (1/3=0 and 4/5=1)

is the result of the effect of familial risk or urbanicity alone, whereas more severe states may be more specifically associated with synergistic co-actions of risk factors.

▌ Part 6: a consequence of the continuity view: redefining schizophrenia?

The existence of both a symptomatic and an aetiological continuum of psychosis may have consequences for concepts that have long been accepted. For example, the concept of schizophrenia has been defined as a unitary concept based on clinical observations of patients. However, as the evidence above suggests that the psychosis phenotype may at least in part be continuous across the general population, the question becomes whether the observations from clinical samples reflect the true nature of the phenomenon. In the next study, we will therefore investigate to what degree the concept of schizophrenia as a unitary disorder is the result of biases arising out of the skewed perception of mental state phenomena in the psychiatric clinic (Maric et al. submitted).

Study 6: schizophrenia: a matter of Berkson's bias?

Experienced clinicians such as Kraepelin and Bleuler identified schizophrenia as a unitary concept based on observations of patients. However, given the fact that factor analyses of psychotic psychopathology have shown that the symptoms related to schizophrenia cluster into several symptom dimensions (Andreasen 1982; Berman et al. 1997; Bilder et al. 1985; Crow 1980; Cuesta and Peralta 1995; Liddle et al. 1989; Strauss et al. 1974; Young et al. 1991), and these symptom dimensions reveal itself as continuous in nature, one can speculate to what degree the concept of schizophrenia, as we know it today, is the result of Berkson's bias.

According to Berkson, high rates of comorbidity seen in clinical practice, such as the comorbidity between the positive and negative features of schizophrenia, may be in part an artifact if both positive and negative features independently influence help-seeking behaviour and need for care at the level of the general population (Berkson 1950). This phenomenon will therefore result in a higher estimate of the comorbidity between these two dimensions in clinical samples than would be the case if non-clinical cases had been investigated – a selection bias known as a treatment seeking bias or Berkson's bias (Fig. 3).

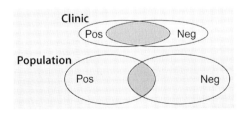

Fig. 3. The comorbidity between positive and negative symptom dimensions in clinical samples is higher compared to that seen in the general population, if both dimensions independently contribute to patient status

Since the concept of schizophrenia is based on observations of patients by clinicians, the association between positive and negative dimensions might be spuriously high, obscuring the fact that positive and negative dimensions may be relatively independent dimensions of psychopathology that appear much more "concentrated" in clinical settings (Fig. 3). In the present study, we will explore to what degree the concept of schizophrenia may be the result of Berkson's bias by investigating whether positive and negative psychosis dimensions independently contribute to patient status at the level of the general, non-clinical population (Maric et al. submitted).

Method

Data were part of the Netherlands Mental Health Survey and Incidence Study (NEMESIS) (see study 2 for description). Positive psychotic experience (PPE) was defined as any CIDI rating of 2, 3, 4, 5 or 6 on any of the 17 CIDI core psychosis items at the baseline assessment. They were joined together into a single broad rating of PPE (rated "1"=present or "0"=absent), for the purposes of the current study. Negative psychotic experience (NPE) were based on the three CIDI ratings of observed negative symptoms at baseline. These were:

▌ blunted affect (n = 24, 0.3%),
retardation of movement (n = 13, 0.2%) and
retardation of speech (n = 49, 0.7%).

A dichotomous rating of NPE was constructed with score "1 = present" if any of these three items had been rated by the trained lay interviewer. Mental health care rated at baseline (MHC_{T0}) was defined as any lifetime contact with:

▌ a community mental health centre,
▌ a psychiatric outpatient clinic,
▌ a private psychiatrist,
▌ a psychologist,
▌ a psychotherapist, or any
▌ psychiatric admission or
▌ day treatment.

The rating thus covered the lifetime history of mental health care up to the moment of T0 interview. In addition, mental health care was investigated at T1 and T2 (MHC_{T2}). MHC_{T2} was defined as receiving mental health care for any kind of psychological disturbance between T0 and T2 (measured at T1 and T2). In order to examine the association between PPE, NPE and MHC_{T0}, logistic regression models yielding odds ratios were estimated. First the associations between PPE and MHC_{T0}, and between NPE and MHC_{T0} were calculated in separate models, in order to assess whether both dimensions were separate predictors of MHC_{T0}. In addition, the effect of both PPE and NPE on MHC_{T0} was calculated in one multivariate model so as to assess the independent effect of one corrected for the other. As MHC_{T0}, PPE and NPE were all lifetime retrospective assessments, it is difficult to untangle the direction of causation. Therefore, the effect of PPE and NPE on prospective MHC_{T2} was calculated in a model of the association between PPE, NPE and MHC_{T2}. The multivariate model including both PPE and NPE were also calculated.

Results

The rating of MHC was strongly associated with NPE (OR = 8.6 95% CI 5.3, 14.0). The association of MHC and PPE was significant as well (OR = 2.7 95% CI 2.3, 3.1). The effects of both NPE and PPE remained strong and significant in the multivariate analysis with both variables entered simultaneously in the equation (see Table 3), illustrating that both psychosis dimensions independently contributed to mental health care consumption. In the models predicting MHC_{T2} with the baseline assessment of PPE and NPE, similar associations were found. Both PPE (OR = 2.3 95% CI 2.1, 2.9) and NPE (OR = 5.4 95% CI 2.9, 10.1) had large and significant effects on MHC_{T2}. These associations remained significant when entered jointly in the multivariate model including both PPE and NPE (Table 3).

Conclusion

Both the positive dimension and the negative dimension were independently associated with mental health care use. These results, therefore, suggest that the concept of schizophrenia, as a unitary entity, is in part the result of Berkson's bias or artificial morbidity concentration. The association between both dimensions in clinical samples may be spuriously high due to the fact that both positive and negative dimensions independently contribute to patient status. Their independently increased risks will therefore lead to an increase in the number of patients in clinical samples with dimensional comorbidity.

Overall conclusion

There is credible evidence that is compatible with the suggestion of a continuity model of psychosis. Several studies have already shown that there is a symptomatic continuum between normal subjects and patients with psychotic

Table 3. Association between PPE, NPE, and MHC

	PPE	NPE
	MHC_{T0}	
OR (95% CI)	2.6 (2.3, 3.0)	7.2 (4.3, 11.8)
	MHC_{T2}	
OR (95% CI)	2.4 (2.0, 2.8)	4.5 (2.4, 8.5)

OR – Odds ratio on multivariate model including both PPE and NPE

disorder. The current chapter has provided further validity to this hypothesis as the studies described have suggested that psychosis-like symptoms and psychotic disorder are related to the same demographic, personality, (proxy) environmental and (proxy) genetic risk factors. These associations have been found across several general population samples, from young adolescents in the ESDP study in Munich, to subjects from the general population in the NEMESIS study in the Netherlands, and twins collected in the context of the EFPTS study. Therefore, it is attractive to conclude that both psychosis-like experiences and psychotic disorders are situated, at least in part, on an aetiological continuity underlying the symptomatic continuity discussed in the introduction. This chapter, however, did not provide evidence to differentiate between a true or a semi-continuous distribution. Although it is most likely that there are unique factors that specifically contribute to the development of disorder and need for care (see (Krabbendam et al. 2003), this volume), this chapter has provided evidence suggesting that both psychotic disorder and psychosis-like experiences are at least in part related to shared environmental and genetic risk factors.

The notion of a psychosis continuum has important implications. As we have discussed in part 5 of this chapter, the existence of a symptomatic and aetiological continuum of psychosis questions the validity of traditional diagnostic systems, in which disorders are classified as all-or-none phenomena based on observations of patients admitted to psychiatric hospitals. The continuity of several symptom dimensions supports a dimensional rather than a categorical approach of psychiatric nosology in which patients can have more or less psychopathology rated on several dimensions, rather than being classified as having a binary disorder. Several studies have shown that the diagnostic *usefulness* of a dimensional representation of psychosis is better than its categorical counterpart (McGorry et al. 1998; Van Os et al. 1996, 1999).

The continuum hypothesis also has important implications for research. Firstly, it provides the opportunity to measure underlying mechanisms that drive variation along the continuum. Secondly, the study of symptom dimensions is important in the search for the causes of psychopathology. Symptom dimensions may be interesting phenotypes for molecular genetic studies and the study of within-person lifetime dimensional comorbidity may prove to be an essential instrument for consistent results in molecular genetic studies of psychosis. Thirdly, the study of more attenuated experiences in the general population provides the opportunity to identify clearer relationships between putative risk factors, mediating factors and symptomatology without the contamination of hospitalisation, medication and a range of other variables associated with patient status. From the methodological point of view, much larger samples can be recruited compared to studies with clinical populations, and more precision may be obtained by analysing variation along a continuous scale rather than differences between arbitrary categories with the ensuing loss of information.

References

Andreasen NC (1982) Negative symptoms in schizophrenia: definition and reliability. Arch Gen Psychiatry 39:784–788

Andreasen NC (1989) The Scale for the Assessment of Negative Symptoms (SANS): conceptual and theoretical foundations. Br J Psychiatry Suppl:49–58

Anthony JC, Folstein M, Romanoski AJ, Von Korff MR, Nestadt GR, Chahal R, Merchant A, Brown CH, Shapiro S, Kramer M et al (1985) Comparison of the lay Diagnostic Interview Schedule and a standardized psychiatric diagnosis. Experience in eastern Baltimore. Arch Gen Psychiatry 42:667–675

Atakan Z, Cooper JE (1989) Behavioural Observation Schedule (BOS), PIRS 2nd edition: a revised edition of the PIRS (WHO, Geneva, March 1978). Symposium: Negative symptoms in schizophrenia (1987, London, England). Br J Psychiatry 155:78–80

Berenbaum H, Fujita F (1994) Schizophrenia and personality: exploring the boundaries and connections between vulnerability and outcome. J Abnorm Psychol 103:148–158

Berkson J (1950) Are there two regressions? J Am Stat Ass 45:164–180

Berman I, Viegner B, Merson A, Allan E, Pappas D, Green AI (1997) Differential relationships between positive and negative symptoms and neuropsychological deficits in schizophrenia. Schizophr Res 25:1–10

Bijl RV, Ravelli A, Van Zessen G (1998a) Prevalence of psychiatric disorder in the general population: results of The Netherlands Mental Health Survey and Incidence Study (NEMESIS). Soc Psychiatry Psychiatr Epidemiol 33:587–595

Bijl RV, Van Zessen G, Ravelli A, de Rijk C, Langendoen Y (1998b) The Netherlands Mental Health Survey and Incidence Study (NEMESIS): objectives and design. Soc Psychiatry Psychiatr Epidemiol 33:581–586

Bilder RM, Mukherjee S, Rieder RO, Pandurangi AK (1985) Symptomatic and neuropsychological components of defect states. Schizophr Bull 11:409–419

Cannon TD, Mednick SA, Parnas J, Schulsinger F, Praestholm J, Vestergaard A (1993) Developmental brain abnormalities in the offspring of schizophrenic mothers. I. Contributions of genetic and perinatal factors. Arch Gen Psychiatry 50:551–564

Cardno AG, Marshall EJ, Coid B, Macdonald AM, Ribchester TR, Davies NJ, Venturi P, Jones LA, Lewis SW, Sham PC, Gottesman, II, Farmer AE, McGuffin P, Reveley AM, Murray RM (1999) Heritability estimates for psychotic disorders: the Maudsley twin psychosis series. Arch Gen Psychiatry 56:162–168

Cardno AG, Sham PC, Farmer AE, Murray RM, McGuffin P (2002) Heritability of Schneider's first-rank symptoms. Br J Psychiatry 180:35–38

Cardno AG, Sham PC, Murray RM, McGuffin P (2001) Twin study of symptom dimensions in psychoses. Br J Psychiatry 179:39–45

Clayton D, Hills M (1993) Wald tests. In: Clayton D, Hills M (Eds) Statistical Models in Epidemiology. Oxford: Oxford Science Publications, pp 101–102

Cooper L, Peters L, Andrews G (1998) Validity of the Composite International Diagnostic Interview (CIDI) psychosis module in a psychiatric setting. J Psychiatr Res 32:361–368

Crow TJ (1980) Molecular pathology of schizophrenia: more than one disease process? BMJ 280:66–68

Crow TJ (1986) The continuum of psychosis and its implication for the structure of the gene. Br J Psychiatry 149:419–429

Crow TJ (1993) Sexual selection, Machiavellian intelligence, and the origins of psychosis. Lancet 342:594–598

Cuesta MJ, Peralta V (1995) Psychopathological dimensions in schizophrenia. Schizophr Bull 21:473–482

Darroch J (1997) Biological synergism and parallelism. Am J Epidemiol 145:661–668

Fanous A, Gardner C, Walsh D, Kendler KS (2001) Relationship between positive and negative symptoms of schizophrenia and schizotypal symptoms in nonpsychotic relatives. Arch Gen Psychiatry 58:669–673

Freeman D, Garety P (1999) Worry, worry processes and dimensions of delusions: an exploratory investigation of a role for anxiety processes in the maintenance of delusional distress. Behav Cogn Psychotherapy 27:47–62

Galdos PM, Van Os JJ, Murray RM (1993) Puberty and the onset of psychosis. Schizophr Res 10:7–14

Gurrera RJ, Nestor PG, O'Donnell BF (2000) Personality traits in schizophrenia: comparison with a community sample. J Nerv Ment Dis 188:31–35

Hardin J, Cleves M (1999) seb29: Generalized linear models: extensions to the binomial family. Stata Technical Bulletin 50:21–25

Hay DA, Martin GM, Foley D, Treloar SA, Kirk KM, Heath AC (2001) Phenotypic and genetic analyses of a short measure of psychosis-proneness in a large-scale Australian twin study. Twin Research 4:30–40

Helzer JE, Robins LN, McEvoy LT, Spitznagel EL, Stoltzman RK, Farmer A, Brockington IF (1985) A comparison of clinical and diagnostic interview schedule diagnoses. Physician reexamination of lay-interviewed cases in the general population. Arch Gen Psychiatry 42:657–666

Horwood LJ, Fergusson DM (1986) Neuroticism, depression and life events: a structural equation model. Soc Psychiatry 21:63–71

Jacobs N, Myin-Germeys I, Derom C, Van Os J (2003) Familial transmission of psychotic dimensions in the general population. (submitted)

Janssen I, Hanssen M, Bak M, Bijl RV, de Graaf R, Vollebergh W, McKenzie K, Van Os J (2003) Discrimination and delusional ideation. Br J Psychiatry 182:71–76

Janssen I, Krabbendam L, Bak M, Hanssen M, Vollebergh W, de Graaf R, Van Os J (2004) Childhood abuse as a risk factor for psychotic experiences. Acta Psychiatr Scand 109:38–45

Kendell RE, Brockington IF (1980) The identification of disease entities and the relationship between schizophrenic and affective psychoses. Br J Psychiatry 137:324–331

Kendler KS, Gallagher TJ, Abelson JM, Kessler RC (1996) Lifetime prevalence, demographic risk factors, and diagnostic validity of nonaffective psychosis as assessed in a US community sample. The National Comorbidity Survey. Arch Gen Psychiatry 53:1022–1031

Kety SS, Wender PH, Jacobsen B, Ingraham LJ, Jansson L, Faber B, Kinney DK (1994) Mental illness in the biological and adoptive relatives of schizophrenic adoptees. Replication of the Copenhagen Study in the rest of Denmark. Arch Gen Psychiatry 51:442–455

Kibel DA, Laffont I, Liddle PF (1993) The composition of the negative syndrome of chronic schizophrenia. Br J Psychiatry 162:744–750

Konnecke R, Häfner H, Maurer K, Loffler W, Van der Heiden W (2000) Main risk factors for schizophrenia: increased familial loading and pre- and peri-natal complications antagonize the protective effect of oestrogen in women. Schizophr Res 44:81–93

Krabbendam L, Hanssen M, Bak M, Van Os J (2004) Psychotic experiences in the general population: risk factors for what? In: Gattaz WF, Häfner H (Eds) Search for the Causes of Schizophrenia. Steinkopff, Darmstadt, pp 54–78

Krabbendam L, Janssen I, Bak M, Bijl RV, de Graaf R, Van Os J (2002) Neuroticism and low self-esteem as risk factors for psychosis. Soc Psychiatry Psychiatr Epidemiol 37:1–6

Kraepelin E (1919) Dementia Preacox and Paraphrenia (translated by M Barclay). Churchill Livingstone, Edinburgh

Lewis G, David A, Andreasson S, Allebeck P (1992) Schizophrenia and city life. Lancet 340:137–140

Liddle PF, Barnes TR, Morris D, Haque S (1989) Three syndromes in chronic schizophrenia. Br J Psychiatry Suppl:119–122

Lieb R, Isensee B, Von Sydow K, Wittchen HU (2000) The Early Developmental Stages of Psychopathology Study (EDSP): a methodological update. Eur Addict Res 6:170–182

Loos R, Derom C, Vlietinck R, Derom R (1998) The East Flanders Prospective Twin Survey (Belgium): a population-based register. Twin Research 1:167–175

Lukoff D, Nuechterlein KH, Ventura J (1986) Manual for the Expanded Brief Psychiatric Rating Scale. Schizophr Bull 12:594–602

Maier W, Lichtermann D, Minges J, Hallmayer J, Heun R, Benkert O, Levinson DF (1993) Continuity and discontinuity of affective disorders and schizophrenia. Results of a controlled family study. Arch Gen Psychiatry 50:871–883

Marcelis M, Navarro-Mateu F, Murray R, Selten JP, Van Os J (1998) Urbanization and psychosis: a study of 1942–1978 birth cohorts in The Netherlands. Psychol Med 28:871–879

Marcelis M, Takei N, Van Os J (1999) Urbanization and risk for schizophrenia: does the effect operate before or around the time of illness onset? Psychol Med 29:1197–1203

Maric N, Krabbendam L, Vollebergh W, de Graaf R, Van Os J (2003) Sex differences in symptoms of psychosis in a non-selected, general population sample. Schizophr Res 63:89–95

McGorry PD, Bell RC, Dudgeon PL, Jackson HJ (1998) The dimensional structure of first episode psychosis: an exploratory factor analysis. Psychol Med 28:935–947

Mortensen PB, Pedersen CB, Westergaard T, Wohlfahrt J, Ewald H, Mors O, Andersen PK, Melbye M (1999) Effects of family history and place and season of birth on the risk of schizophrenia. N Engl J Med 340:603–608

Murray RM, Lewis SW (1988) Is schizophrenia a neurodevelopmental disorder? Br Med J (Clin Res Ed) 296:63

Myin-Germeys I, Van Os J, Schwartz JE, Stone AA, Delespaul PA (2001) Emotional reactivity to daily life stress in psychosis. Arch Gen Psychiatry 58:1137–1144

Olfson M, Lewis-Fernandez R, Weissman MM, Feder A, Gameroff MJ, Pilowsky D, Fuentes M (2002) Psychotic symptoms in an urban general medicine practice. Am J Psychiatry 159:1412–1419

Ormel J (1980) Moeite met Leven of een Moeilijk Leven? Groningen, University of Groningen

Ormel J, Stewart R, Sanderman R (1989) Personality as modifier of the life change-distress relationship. A longitudinal modelling approach. Soc Psychiatry Psychiatr Epidemiol 24:187–195

Overall JE, Gorham DR (1962) The brief psychiatric rating scale (BPRS). Psychol Rep 10:799–812

Poulton R, Caspi A, Moffitt TE, Cannon M, Murray R, Harrington H (2000) Children's self-reported psychotic symptoms and adult schizophreniform disorder: a 15-year longitudinal study. Arch Gen Psychiatry 57:1053–1058

Robins E, Guze SB (1970) Establishment of diagnostic validity in psychiatric illness: its application to schizophrenia. Am J Psychiatry 126:983–987

Roy MA, Maziade M, Labbe A, Merette C (2001) Male gender is associated with deficit schizophrenia: a meta-analysis. Schizophr Res 47:141–147

Schultz SK, Miller DD, Oliver SE, Arndt S, Flaum M, Andreasen NC (1997) The life course of schizophrenia: age and symptom dimensions. Schizophr Res 23:15–23

Selten JP, Gernaat HB, Nolen WA, Wiersma D, Van den Bosch RJ (1998) Experience of negative symptoms: comparison of schizophrenic patients to patients with a depressive disorder and to normal subjects. Am J Psychiatry 155:350–354

Shtasel DL, Gur RE, Gallacher F, Heimberg C, Gur RC (1992) Gender differences in the clinical expression of schizophrenia. Schizophr Res 7:225–231

Smeets RMW, Dingemans PMAJ (1993) Composite International Diagnostic Interview (CIDI) Version 1.1. Amsterdam/Geneva, World Health Organization

Spauwen J, Krabbendam L, Lieb R, Wittchen HU, Van Os J (2003) Sex differences in psychosis: normal or pathological? Schizophr Res 62:45–49

Spitzer RL, Williams JB, Gibbon M, First MB (1992) The Structured Clinical Interview for DSM-III-R (SCID), I: history, rationale, and description. Arch Gen Psychiatry 49:624–629

StataCorp (2001) STATA Statistical Software: Release 7.0. Texas, College Station

Stefanis NC, Hanssen M, Smirnis NK, Avramopoulos DA, Evdokimidis IK, Stefanis CN, Verdoux H, Van Os J (2002) Evidence that three dimensions of psychosis have a distribution in the general population. Psychol Med 32:347–358

Strauss JS, Carpenter WT, Jr, Bartko JJ (1974) The diagnosis and understanding of schizophrenia. Part III. Speculations on the processes that underlie schizophrenic symptoms and signs. Schizophr Bull:61–69

Tienari P, Sorri A, Lahti I, Naarala M, Wahlberg KE, Pohjola J, Moring J (1985) Interaction of genetic and psychosocial factors in schizophrenia. Acta Psychiatr Scand Suppl 319:19–30

Van Os J, Fahy TA, Jones P, Harvey I, Sham P, Lewis S, Bebbington P, Toone B, Williams M, Murray R (1996) Psychopathological syndromes in the functional psychoses: associations with course and outcome. Psychol Med 26:161–176

Van Os J, Hanssen M, Bak M, Bijl RV, Vollebergh W (2003) Do urbanicity and familial liability co-participate in causing psychosis? Am J psychiatry 160:477-482

Van Os J, Hanssen M, Bijl RV, Ravelli A (2000) Strauss (1969) revisited: a psychosis continuum in the general population? Schizophr Res 45:11–20

Van Os J, Hanssen M, Bijl RV, Vollebergh W (2001) Prevalence of psychotic disorder and community level of psychotic symptoms: an urban-rural comparison. Arch Gen Psychiatry 58:663–668

Van Os J, Jones PB (2001) Neuroticism as a risk factor for schizophrenia. Psychol Med 31, 1129–1134

Van Os J, Marcelis M (1998) The ecogenetics of schizophrenia: a review. Schizophr Res 32:127–135

Van Os J, Marcelis M, Sham P, Jones P, Gilvarry K, Murray R (1997) Psychopathological syndromes and familial morbid risk of psychosis. Br J Psychiatry 170:241–246

Van Os J, Verdoux H, Bijl RV, Ravelli A (1999) Psychosis as an extreme of continuous variation in dimensions of psychopathology. In: Gattaz WF, Häfner H (Eds) Search for the Causes of Schizophrenia. Steinkopff, Darmstadt, vol. 4, pp 59–79

Verdoux H, Van Os J (2002) Psychotic symptoms in non-clinical populations and the continuum of psychosis. Schizophr Res 54:59–65

Vlietinck R (1986) Determination of the zygosity of twins. Leuven, Katholieke Universiteit Leuven (PhD)

Wacholder S (1986) Binomial regression in GLIM: estimating risk ratios and risk differences. Am J Epidemiol 123:174–184

Waddington JL, Lane A, Larkin C, O'Callaghan E (1999) The neurodevelopmental basis of schizophrenia: clinical clues from cerebro-craniofacial dysmorphogenesis, and the roots of a lifetime trajectory of disease. Biol Psychiatry 46:31–39

Weinberger DR (1987) Implications of normal brain development for the pathogenesis of schizophrenia. Arch gen psychiatry 44:660–669

WHO (1990) Composite International Diagnostic Interview (CIDI); Version 1.0 Geneva

WHO (1992) International Classification of Diseases, 10th edn. Geneva, WHO

Wickham H, Walsh C, Asherson P, Taylor C, Sigmundson T, Gill M, Owen MJ, McGuffin P, Murray R, Sham P (2001) Familiality of symptom dimensions in schizophrenia. Schizophr Res 47:223–232

Wittchen H-U, Pfister H (1997) DIA-X-Interviews: Manual für Screening-Verfahren und Interview; Interviewheft Längsschnittuntersuchung (DIA-X-Lifetime); Ergänzungsheft (DIA-X-Lifetime); Interviewheft Querschnittsuntersuchung (DIA-X-12 Monats-Version); Ergänzungsheft (DIA-X-12 Monats-Version); PC-Programm zur Durchführung der Interviews (Längs und Querschnittsuntersuchung). Auswertungsprogramm. Swets & Zeitlinger, Frankfurt

Wittchen HU, Perkonigg A, Lachner G, Nelson CB (1998) Early developmental stages of psychopathology study (EDSP): objectives and design. Eur Addict Res 4:18–27

Young AH, Blackwood DH, Roxborough H, McQueen JK, Martin MJ, Kean D (1991) A magnetic resonance imaging study of schizophrenia: brain structure and clinical symptoms. Br J Psychiatry 158:158–164

When does structural brain change appear in schizophrenia and is it clinically relevant?

Lynn E. DeLisi

Department of Psychiatry, New York University, New York, USA

Despite Kraepelin's descriptions in the early 1900's of structural brain pathology at the cellular level in patients with dementia praecox (Kraepelin 1919), little acceptance of this notion was present among 20th century psychiatrists who were focused on perfecting psychoanalytic techniques even for schizophrenia (Fromm-Reichmann 1943). Great care was taken to separate psychoses into those that were "organic" (i.e. a brain disease) and those that were functional (i.e. due to psychological factors; Davison 1987). Although early pneumoencephalographic studies clearly showed evidence that brain ventricular enlargement was present in patients with chronic schizophrenia (Haug et al. 1963, 1982; Huber 1957, 1979; Jacobi and Winkler 1927), it was not until Johnstone et al. (1976) and then Weinberger et al. (1979) demonstrated with CT that this finding was widely present in populations of patients with schizophrenia, that researchers began to accept its presence and attempt to uncover its relevance. When magnetic resonance imaging was available for human medical imaging, numerous brain scans of subjects with schizophrenia were examined further for both cortical and subcortical structural changes, and a large array of findings about brain structure, other than ventricular enlargement, emerged (reviewed in Shenton et al. 2001). Without any clear indication that duration of illness or any treatments had an effect on these findings, various brain developmental hypotheses about schizophrenia were proposed (Weinberger 1987; Murray et al. 1991; Feinberg 1982/83) and consideration was also given to a lifetime trajectory of deviant brain change that is likely to be genetically controlled (DeLisi 1997), or at least have both a developmental and degenerative component (Woods 1998; Waddington et al. 1997). In addition, what has emerged relatively consistently across studies is that some changes are asymmetrical and sometimes only relate to differences in asymmetry rather than absolute differences in one side of the brain, leading Crow and colleagues (1989) to propose that the primary defect in schizophrenia relates to the anomalous development of normal cerebral asymmetries.

However, in an attempt to refute the notion that only early brain developmental anomalies lead to later susceptibility to schizophrenia rather than an adult progressive degenerative process, or at least to show that a lifetime active process is occurring (DeLisi 1997), a series of longitudinal MRI studies have been independently conducted. To date, they have produced diverse findings that together suggest that some patients have non-localized brain structural changes that progress after the onset of a first psychotic episode and far beyond normal human age-related variation (reviewed by DeLisi 1999a,b; Tables 1 and 2). Even the

Table 1. Brain change over time in patients with chronic schizophrenia

Study et al.	#Subjects	Time (yrs)	Finding
Davis (1998) CT	53 male pts 13 controls	5	Ventricles increased left > right, poor outcome patients only
Illowsky (1988) CT	13 pts	7–9	No change in ventricles
Kemali (1989) CT	18 pts 8 controls	3	1/3 pts greater increase in ventricles than controls
Mathalon (2001) MRI	24 male pts 25 controls	0.7–7.5	Right hemisphere decrease, gray matter decrease bilaterally, superior temporal gyrus decreased bilaterally, CSF increased bilaterally
Nair (1997) MRI	18 pts 5 controls	1.1–3.8	Ventricles increased in poor outcome pts only
Nasrallah (1986) CT	11 pts	3	No change in ventricles
Rapaport (1997) MRI Jacobsen (1998)	16 adol. pts 24 controls	1.5–4	Hemispheres decreased bilaterally, ventricles increased, striatum decreased, thalamus decreased, temporal lobes and superior, temporal gyrus decreased bilaterally, left hippocampus decreased
Vita (1988) CT	15 pts	2–5	No change in ventricles
Woods (1990) CT	9 pts	1–4.5	8/9 ventricles increased

early pneumoencephalographic studies showed that on follow-up spanning from a few months to up to 5 years, some patients had further ventricular enlargement over time (Moore et al. 1935; Huber 1957; Haug 1963). In addition, the two recent independent brain MRI high-risk studies published, thus far, have shown longitudinal change, particularly in the temporal lobe, in those individuals who go on to develop a psychotic illness (Table 3). Nevertheless, it should be noted that the changes seen in these studies are not only inconsistent with each other, but inconsistent with the changes reported in longitudinal studies of first episode patients with schizophrenia. For example, the Pantelis et al. study (2003) reported reduced left parahippocampal and other gyri over time in high-risk individuals when they become psychotic, while in a similar group, Lawrie et al. (2002) reported a change in the right temporal lobe. Yet, none of the longitudinal studies beginning with first-episode psychotic patients show similar structural changes, but rather report non-localized progression, such as overall cortical volume reduction and ventricular enlargement over time, or in the case of the

Table 2. Brain change over time in 1st episode patients with schizophrenia

Study et al.	#Subjects	Time (yrs)	Finding
Degreef (1991) MRI Lieberman (2001)	13 1st ep pts 8 controls	1–2	No change in ventricles. Increase associated with poor outcome
DeLisi (1995, 1997) MRI	50 1st ep pts 20 controls	4–5	Hemispheres decreased, left ventricles increased, right cerebellum decreased, no change in temporal lobe
Gur (1998) MRI	20 1st ep pts 20 chronic pts 17 controls	2–3	Frontal lobes decreased in 1st ep only, no change in temporal lobe, no change in total volume, no change in CSF, frontal lobe change correlated with good outcome
Kasai (2003) MRI	13 1st ep SZ pts 15 1st ep Aff Dis 14 controls	1.5	Left superior temporal gyrus decrease in 1st ep SZ only
Jaskiw (1994) CT	7 1st ep pts	5–8	No change in ventricles
Sponheim (1991) CT	15 1st ep pts	1–3	No change in ventricles
Vita (1994) CT	9 1st ep pts	2–4	No change in ventricles
Wood (2001) MRI	30 1st ep pts 26 controls	0.5–4.2	No change in hippocampus or temporal lobe, decrease in whole brain volume
Cahn (2002) MRI	34 1st ep pts 36 controls	1	Total gray matter decreased, total brain volume decreased, ventricular volume increased, changes associated with poor outcome and amount of medication
James (2002) MRI	16 1st ep pts 16 controls adolescents	2.7 pts 1.7 controls	No changes over time.

Gur et al. (1998) study, frontal lobe reduction (reviewed in Tables 1 and 2), but not temporal.

Some investigators have concluded that brain change is associated with degeneration in specifically a poor prognosis subgroup (Lieberman 1999; Davis et al. 1998; Garver et al. 2000), yet others find that it is unrelated to prognosis, or if anything, related to better outcome (Gur et al. 1998; DeLisi et al. 1998) and this issue is yet unresolved.

Table 3. Findings from high-risk longitudinal brain imaging studies

Study	# Subjects	Follow-up time	Follow-up Dx	Findings initially	Findings on follow-up
Pantelis et al. (2003)	21 HR	>1 year	10 Psychosis 11 No psychosis	Psychotic vs Non-psychotic: decreased gray in right medial & lateral temporal, and inferior frontal cortex, decreased gray in cingulate bilateral	Psychotic: decrease in left parahippocampal, fusiform, orbital frontal and cerebellar cortices and cingulate gyri, Non-psychotic: only decrease in cerebellum.
Lawrie et al. (2002)	66 HR 20 C	2 years	19 Psychosis 47 No psychosis		Psychotic: decrease in right temporal lobe
Johnstone et al. (2002)	66 HR 20 C	–	–	HR: decreased prefrontal lobes and thalamus bilaterally	

HR = High Risk; *C* = control

Table 4. Ten-year follow-up study of first-episode schizophrenia: percent change in ventricle volume as measured by MRI over time

	Patients (n = 26)	Controls (n = 10)	Mann-Whitney U (p<)
Years 1–10			
█ Left ventricle	2.32 ± 3.67	0.46 ± 0.81	83 (0.08)
█ Right ventricle	1.93 ± 3.86	0.09 ± 1.31	87 (0.11)
Years 5–10			
█ Left ventricle	3.31 ± 4.96	0.82 ± 1.40	74 (0.05)
█ Right ventricle	2.24 ± 5.01	0.04 ± 2.91	106 (0.14)

In general, the studies of first-episode patients show more inconsistencies in specific brain regional volume changes than those of chronic patients. However, studies of chronic patients may be biased by over sampling patients at the more severe end of the illness spectrum.

In one of the longest follow-up MRI studies (10 years: DeLisi et al. (in press)), 26 patients and 10 controls were evaluated 10 years subsequent to the first episode, some patients continued to have further ventricular enlargement between the 5th and 10th year that was outside the normal range, but despite several measures of outcome, this did not appear to be associated with clinical state (see Table 4 and Figs. 1 and 2).

R 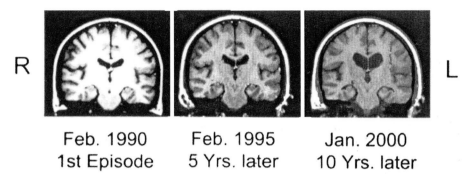 L

Feb. 1990   Feb. 1995   Jan. 2000
1st Episode   5 Yrs. later   10 Yrs. later

Fig. 1. Illustration of MRI scans showing progressive ventricular enlargement in a 34-year-old female patient whose illness is characterized by chronic negative symptoms with positive symptoms stabilized and responsive to maintenance neuroleptic treatment. In addition, she has a sibling with chronic schizophrenia

Most longitudinal MRI studies have begun with adult onset cases of schizophrenia. However, two investigative groups examined patients with illness onset before age 18. An NIMH group (Rapoport et al. 1997; Giedd et al. 1999; Jacobsen et al. 1998; Table 1) studied chronic poor-outcome patients who were adolescents with a childhood onset of illness, while UK researchers (James et al. 2002; Table 2) studied adolescents beginning at their first episode of illness. Thus, both cohorts were adolescents when studied, but one group was further along in the course of illness than the other. The NIMH study of adolescents reported dramatic changes in the patients compared with controls, whereas the UK study reported no differences.

A possible explanation for these inconsistencies is that brain change takes place in schizophrenia, but at a rate that varies between individuals, just as clinical course and behavioral manifestation of the illness vary. It is possible that abnormal brain change might correspond to a process initiating the onset of symptoms. The process, in a majority of cases, might slow or halt after a few years of degeneration. In some patients, however, the brain change may continue long into the illness, and perhaps may re-emerge after a period of quiescence. Thus, differences in study results could be explained by differences in when the cohorts are sampled during the lifetime course of illness (from first pre-morbid signs onward) and variation among individuals in the total time course for the development of brain pathology. However, despite this heterogeneity, most studies appear to find that brain changes are present early in the course of illness and may even be occurring for a period of time in association with subtle behavioral changes prior to the onset of psychotic symptoms. The latter is consistent with the earlier observations that ventricular enlargement at the first episode is correlated with a poor pre-morbid history (implying that a subclinical illness has been occurring for some time; De-Lisi et al. 1983) and that initial ventricular size at the first-episode of illness is inversely correlated with the amount of later change (DeLisi et al. 1997).

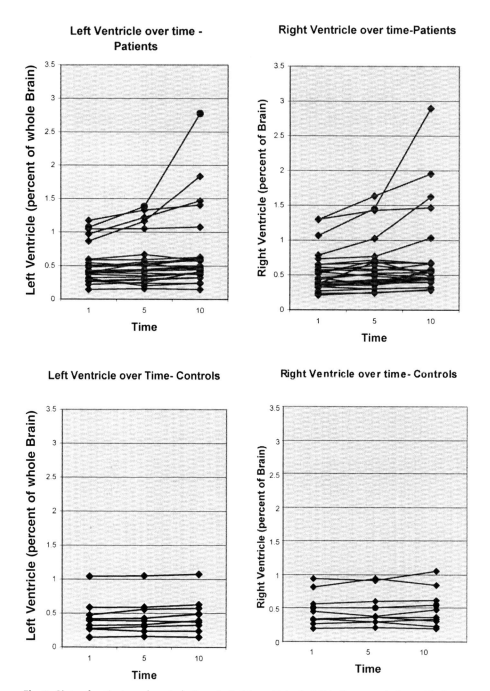

Fig. 2. Plots of patients and controls time 0, 5, 10 yrs. Note that this figure controls ventricular expansion for whole brain size. If brain size is reduced over time, then the ventricular expansion may not be detected.

In summary, several, but not all, pneumoencephalographic, CT, MRI and postmortem studies of chronic patients with schizophrenia have shown lateral and third ventricular enlargement, and temporal cortex, frontal lobe, cingulate gyrus, thalamus, hippocampal, parahippocampal gyrus, uncinate bundle and non-localized gray matter reductions, as well as anomalous changes in normal cerebral asymmetries. Many of these changes, when present, can be shown in first-episode patients and even in those at high risk for schizophrenia. Progressive ventricular enlargement and possible cortical reduction is occurring in some patients (and possibly all patients to varying degrees) over time and likely explains the extensive past literature describing several brain structural differences between chronic patients and controls. These brain changes are variable in time of onset and time period of change among individuals. Progression is also likely not to be the same for each deficit. There do not appear to be clear clinical correlates of the progression, although more studies show a correlation with poor outcome than the reverse, and it is unclear whether neuroleptics affect brain structure. Thus it is unknown at present whether the observed progressive change is an epiphenomenon or primary to the illness process. While we do not know the cause for any of these structural deviations (genetic, virus, other brain developmental insults; secondary to medication use, drug abuse, physiological change, or scanning and measurement errors; Table 5), the eventual delineation of the normal course and variation in human brain development throughout the human lifespan, and genetic or envi-

Table 5. Significance of structural brain change in schizophrenia as detected by MRI

Subject changes
- Neuronal degeneration
- Deficit growth & repair
- Glial cell deficiency
- Hydration/body weight/fat change
- Change in clinical condition: e.g., medication, substance abuse
- Age
- Chronic viral infection

Scanner changes
- Software upgrade
- Pixel/voxel size
- TE/TR's
- Head tilt
- Slice alignment
- Slice thickness

Image analysis problems
- Reliability and validity of measurements
- Field inhomogeneity
- Partial voluming effects
- Software errors
- Inaccurate anatomical boundaries
- Intensity changes

ronmental causes for its deviation, will clarify the mechanism for development and progression of brain pathology in schizophrenia. While the non-localization and lack of consistent correlation to symptoms of the documented brain structural changes make their clinical relevance to schizophrenia questionable at present, they might provide clues to the underlying basis for schizophrenia.

Acknowledgments. The author acknowledges the continual advice and encouragement to pursue this topic received from Richard Jed Wyatt. She regrets that he passed away before its conclusion and the search for the causes of schizophrenia is complete. This work was partially supported by NIMHR01 44233 and The Stanley Institute for Medical Research.

References

Cahn W, Hulshoff P, Hilleke E, Lems EBTE, van Haren NEM, Schnack HG, van der Linden JA, Schothorst PF, van Egeland H, Kahn RS (2002) Brain volume changes in first-episode schizophrenia: a 1-year follow-up study. Archives General Psychiatry 59:1002–1010

Crow TJ, Ball J, Bloom SR, Brown R, Bruton CJ, Colter N, Frith CD, Johnstone EC, Owens DG, Roberts GW (1989) Schizophrenia as an anomaly of development of cerebral asymmetry. A postmortem study and a proposal concerning the genetic basis of the disease. Archives of General Psychiatry 46(12):1145–1150

Davis KL, Buchsbaum MS, Shihabuddin L, Spiegel-Cohen J, Metzger M, Frecska E, Keefe RS, Powchick P (1998) Ventricular enlargement in poor-outcome schizophrenia. Biological Psychiatry 43:783–793

Davison K (1987) Organic and toxic concomitants of schizophrenia: association or chance? In: Helmchen H, Henn FA (eds) Biological Perspectives of Schizophrenia. Life Sciences Research Reports 40. John Wiley and Sons, Chichester New York, pp 139–161

DeGreef G, Ashtari M, Wu H, Borenstein M, Geisler S, Lieberman J (1991) Follow-up MRI study in first-episode schizophrenia. Schizophrenia Research 5:204–206

DeLisi LE (1999a) Defining the course of brain structural growth and plasticity in schizophrenia. Psychiatry Research, Neuroimaging 92(1):1–9

DeLisi LE (1999b) Regional brain volume change over the life-time course of schizophrenia. Journal of Psychiatric Research 33:535–541

DeLisi LE (1997) Is schizophrenia a lifetime disorder of brain plasticity, growth and aging? Schizophrenia Research 23:119–129

DeLisi LE, Grimson R, Sakuma M, Tew W, Kushner M, Hoff AL (1997) Schizophrenia as a chronic active brain process: a study of progressive brain structural change subsequent to the onset of schizophrenia. Psychiatry Research (Neuroimaging) 74:129–140

DeLisi LE, Sakuma M, Kushner M (1998) Association of brain structural change with the heterogeneous course of schizophrenia from early childhood through five years subsequent to a first hospitalization. Psychiatry Research (Neuroimaging) 84:75–88

DeLisi LE, Sakuma M, Maurizio A, Relja M, Hoff AL (2003) Structural Brain Changes over the first 10 years after the onset of Schizophrenia. (Submitted for publication)

DeLisi LE, Schwartz CC, Targum SD, Byrnes SM, Cannon-Spoor E, Weinberger DR, Wyatt RJ (1983) Prediction of outcome in acute schizophreniform disorder. Psychiatry Research 9:169–171

DeLisi LE, Tew W, Xie S-H, Hoff AL, Sakuma M, Kushner M, Lee G, Shedlack K, Smith AM, Grimson R (1995) A prospective follow-up study of brain morphology and cognition in 1st episode schizophrenic patients. Biological Psychiatry 38:349–360

DeLisi LE, Sakuma M, Maurizio A, Hoff AL (2004) Ten year follow-up of ventricular enlargement in first-episode patients with schizophrenia. Psychiatry Research, Neuroimaging (in press)

Feinberg I (1982/1983) Schizophrenia: caused by a fault in programmed synaptic elimination during adolescence? J Psychiatric Research 17:319–334

Fromm-Reichmann F (1943) Psychoanalytic psychotherapy with psychotics; the influence of the modifications in technique on present trends in psychoanalysis. Journal for the Study of Interpersonal Processes 6 (1943):277–279

Garver DL, Nair TR, Christensen JD, Holcomb JA, Kingsbury SJ (2000) Brain and ventricle instability during psychotic episodes of the schizophrenias. Schizophrenia Research 44(1):11–23

Giedd JN, Jeffries NO, Blumenthal J, Castellanos FX, Vaituzis AC, Fernandez T, Hamburger SD, Liu H, Nelson J, Bedwell J, Tran L, Lenane M, Nicolson R, Rapoport JL (1999) Childhood-onset schizophrenia: progressive brain changes during adolescence. Biological Psychiatry 46(7):892–898

Gur RE, Cowell P, Turetsky BI, Gallacher F, Cannon T, Bilker W, Gur RC (1998) A follow-up magnetic resonance imaging study of schizophrenia. Relationship of neuroanatomical changes to clinical and neurobehavioral measures. Archives of General Psychiatry 55(2):145–152

Haug JO (1963) Pneumoencephalographic studies in mental disease. Acta Psych and Neurol Scand Suppl 165, 38:11–104

Haug JO (1982) Pneumoencephalographic evidence of brain atrophy in acute and chronic schizophrenic patients. Acta Psychiatrica Scandinavica 66(5):374–383

Huber G (1957) Pneumoencephalographische und psychopathologische Bilder bei endogen Psychosen. Springer, Berlin

Huber G (1979) Pure defect and its meaning for a somatosis hypothesis of schizophrenia. In: Obiols J, Ballus C, Gonzales E, Pugol J (eds) Biological Psychiatry Today. Elsevier, Amsterdam, pp 345–350

Illowski BP, Juliano DM, Bigelow LBG, Weinberger DR (1988) Stability of C.T. scan findings in schizophrenia: results of an 8 year follow-up study. Journal of Neurology, Neurosurgery and Psychiatry 51:209–213

Jacobi W, Winkler H (1927) Encephalographische Studien an chronische Schizophrenen. Archiv Psychiat Nervenkrankheiten 81:299–332

Jacobsen LK, Giedd JN, Castellanos X, Vaituzis AC, Hamberger SD, Kumra S, Lenane MC, Rapoport JL (1998) Progressive reduction of temporal lobe structures in childhood-onset schizophrenia. American J of Psychiatry 155:678–685

James AC, Javaloyes A, James S, Smith DM (2002) Evidence for non-progressive changes in adolescent-onset schizophrenia: follow-up magnetic resonance imaging study. British Journal of Psychiatry 180:339–344

Jaskiw GE, Juliano DM, Goldberg TE, Hertzman M, Urow-Hamell E, Weinberger DR (1994) Cerebral ventricular enlargement in schizophreniform disorder does not progress: a seven year follow-up study. Schizophrenia Research 14:23–28

Johnstone EC, Crow TJ, Frith CD, Husband J, Kreel L (1976) Cerebral ventricular size and cognitive impairment in chronic schizophrenia. Lancet 2:924–926

Johnstone EC, Lawrie SM, Cosway R (2002) What does the Edinburgh high-risk study tell us about schizophrenia? Am J of Medical Genetics (Neuropsychiatric Genetics) 114:906–912

Kasai K, Shenton ME, Salisbury DF, Hirayasu Y, Lee CU, Ciszewski AA, Yurgelun-Todd D, Kikinis R, Jolesz FA, McCarley RW (2003) Progressive decrease of left superior temporal gyrus gray matter volume in patients with first-episode schizophrenia. Am J Psychiatry 160(1):156–164

Kemali D, Maj M, Galderisi S, Milici N, Salvati A (1989) Ventricle-to-brain ratio in schizophrenia: a controlled follow-up study. Biological Psychiatry 26:753–756

Kraepelin E (1919) Dementia Praecox and Paraphrenia. Barclay RM (trans) 1971 edition. Krieger, New York

Lawrie SM, Whalley H, Kestelman JN, Abukmeil SS, Byrne M, Hodges A, Rimmington JE, Best JJ, Owens DG, Johnstone EC (1999) Magnetic resonance imaging of brain in people at high risk of developing schizophrenia. Lancet 353(9146):30–33

Lawrie SM, Whalley HC, Abukmeil SS, Kestelman JN, Miller P, Best JJ, Owens DG, Johnstone EC (2002) Temporal lobe volume changes in people at high risk of schizophrenia with psychotic symptoms. British Journal of Psychiatry 181:138–143

Lieberman JA (1999) Is schizophrenia a neurodegenerative disorder? A clinical and neurobiological perspective. Biological Psychiatry 46(6):729–739

Lieberman JA, Chakos M, Wu H, Alvir J, Hoffman E, Robinson D, Bilder R (2001) Longitudinal study of brain morphology in first episode schizophrenia. Biol Psychiatry 49(6):487–499

Mathalon DH, Sullivan EV, Lim KO, Pfefferbaum A (2001) Progressive brain volume changes and the clinical course of schizophrenia in men: a longitudinal magnetic resonance imaging study. Arch Gen Psychiatry 58(2):148–157

Moore MD, Nathan AR, Elliot G, Laubach (1935) Encephalographic studies in mental disease. Am J of Psychiatry 92:43–67

Murray RM, Jones P, O'Callaghan E (1991) Fetal brain development and later schizophrenia. Ciba Foundation Symposium 156:155–163

Nair TR, Christensen JD, Kingsbury SJ, Kumar NG, Terry WM, Garver DL (1997) Progression of cerebral ventricular enlargement and the subtyping of schizophrenia. Psychiatry Research 74:141–150

Nasrallah HA, Olson SC, McCalley-Whitters M, Chapman S, Jacoby CG (1986) Cerebral ventricular enlargement in schizophrenia: a preliminary follow-up study. Archives General Psychiatry 43:157–159

Pantelis C, Velakoulis D, McGorry PD, Wood SJ, Suckling J, Phillips LJ, Yung AR, Bullmore ET, Brewer W, Soulsby B, Desmond P, McGuire PK (2003) Neuroanatomical abnormalities before and after onset of psychosis: a cross-sectional and longitudinal MRI comparison. Lancet 361(9354):281–288

Rapoport JL, Giedd JN, Kumra S, Jacobsen L, Smith A, Lee P, Nelson J, Hamberger S (1997) Childhood schizophrenia: progressive ventricular change during adolescence. Archives General Psychiatry 54:897–903

Shenton ME, Dickey CC, Frumin M, McCarley RW (2001) A review of MRI findings in schizophrenia. Schizophrenia Research 49(1/2):1–52

Sponheim SR, Iacono WG, Beiser M (1991) Stability of ventricular size after the onset of psychosis in schizophrenia. Psychiatry Research (Neuroimaging) 40:21–29

Vita A, Giobbio GM, Dieci M, Garbarini M, Morganti C, Comazzi M, Invernizzi G (1994) Stability of cerebral ventricular size from the appearance of the first psychotic symptoms to the later diagnosis of schizophrenia. Biological Psychiatry 35:960–962

Vita A, Sacchetti E, Valvassori G, Cazullo CL (1988) Brain morphology in schizophrenia: a 2–5 year CT scan follow-up study. Acta Psychiatrica Scandinavica 78: 618–621

Waddington JL, Scully PJ, Youssef HA (1997) Developmental trajectory and disease progression in schizophrenia: the conundrum, and insights from a 12-year prospective study in the Monaghan 101. Schizophrenia Research 23(2):107–118

Weinberger DR (1987) Implications of normal brain development for the pathogenesis of schizophrenia. Archives General Psychiatry 44:660–669

Weinberger DR, Torrey EF, Neophytides A, Wyatt RJ (1979) Lateral cerebral ventricular enlargement in chronic schizophrenia. Archives General Psychiatry 36:735–738

Wood SJ, Velakoulis D, Smith DJ, Bond D, Stuart GW, McGorry PD, Brewer WJ, Bridle N, Eritaia J, Desmond P, Singh B, Copolov D, Pantelis C (2001) A longitudinal study of hippocampal volume in first episode psychosis and chronic schizophrenia. Schizophr Res 52(1/2):37–46

Woods BT (1998) Is schizophrenia a progressive neurodevelopmental disorder? Toward a unitary pathogenetic mechanism. American Journal of Psychiatry 155(12):1661–1667

Woods BT, Yurgelun-Todd D, Benes FM, Frankenburg FR, Pope HC, McSparren J (1990) Progressive ventricular enlargement in schizophrenia: comparison to bipolar affective disorder and correlation to clinical course. Biological Psychiatry 27:341–352

Schizophrenia: developmental, degenerative or both?

JANICE R. STEVENS

Oregon Health Sciences University, Portland, Oregon

Introduction

The fundamental cause or causes of schizophrenia are unknown in a majority of cases. As accepted by most neurologists, *developmental* disorders include a diversity of developmental malformations and diseases acquired during the intrauterine period of life (Adams and Victor 1977). In contrast, *degenerative disorders* include "an inexplicable decline from a previous level of normalcy to a lower level of function" (Adams and Victor 1977). A change in our understanding of the etiology of many genetic, metabolic, toxic, and nutritional disorders has changed the definition of some disorders formerly deemed degenerative to one or more of these designations. What about schizophrenia? Clinical and pharmacological data suggest that schizophrenia results from an imbalance between specific excitatory and inhibitory systems in specific brain regions that occurs most frequently but not exclusively during adolescence and young adult life (Stevens 2002).

Symptoms of schizophrenia include intrusions into consciousness of intermittent or persistent changes in perception such as hallucinations and delusions, disturbances in thinking, and unusual, sometimes bizarre, speech and behavior. These symptoms are often accompanied by progressive social withdrawal, abnormal emotional responses and decline of intellectual faculties. The most frequent age of onset for first symptoms is between 19 and 21 years for males and between 21 and 24 years for females (Häfner 1998) (Fig. 1). In distinction from delirium and from most epilepsies, conscious awareness of external events is retained. In further contrast to the epilepsies, the electroencephalogram (EEG), a record of electrical activity of the brain from the surface of the head, is normal or nearly normal in most schizophrenic patients. However, electrodes placed in subcortical structures such as the septal area or amygdala reportedly revealed abnormal spike activity in these regions during acute psychotic periods. Unlike the multiple rhythmic spikes recorded on the EEG during epileptic seizures, however, the spikes recorded from the depth of the brain in schizophrenia did not coalesce into prolonged or propagated discharges (Heath 1959; Sem Jacobsen et al. 1955).

The current American Psychiatric Association requirements for diagnosis of schizophrenia in the Diagnostic and Statistic Manual IV (1994) are that a 6 month duration of symptoms should occur. However, shorter periods of psychosis with identical symptoms lasting hours, days, weeks or several months

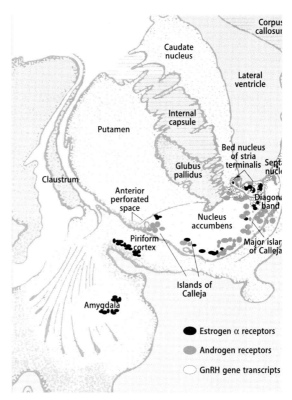

Fig. 1. Frontal section through basal ganglia and basal forebrain showing location of islands of Calleja (I/C) (adapted from Stevens 2002). *Acb* N. accumbens db diagonal band, *Cd* Caudate nucleus, *CC* corpus callosum, *Cl* Claustrum, *GP* globus pallidus, **I/C** Islands of Calleja, *I/Cm* Island of Calleja major, *LV* lateral ventricle, *Pir C* pyriform cortex, *Put* Putamen, *S* septum, *VP* ventral pallidum

also occur and may share similar pathophysiologic substrates with the somewhat arbitrarily defined six month-plus disorder. After onset, schizophrenia may remit, persist or wax and wane for many months, years or a lifetime.

Effective modern treatment of schizophrenia employs a number of antipsychotic agents, which block cerebral receptors for neurotransmitters generally considered inhibitory, e.g., dopamine (DA), serotonin (5HT), norepinephrine (NE), gamma-amino butyric acid (GABA), or that enhance the activity of the excitatory transmitter glutamate. Although infection, trauma or brain neoplasm precede the onset of some typical schizophrenic illnesses, in a majority of cases the cause remains unknown (Stevens 1999). Schizophrenia-like psychoses may be precipitated in susceptible individuals by pharmacological agents that potentiate inhibitory factors, e.g., the excitatory amino acid antagonists phencyclidine (PCP), MK801, and monoamine agonists such as the amphetamines and lysergic acid diethylamide (LSD) (Javitt and Zukin 1991; Angrist et al. 1980; Varidy and Kays 1983; Tamminga 1998). Modern treatment of schizophrenia employs a variety of agents that block inhibitory receptors and may cause convulsive seizures. Although modern treatment often greatly improves schizophrenic symptoms, a majority of individuals diagnosed schizo-phrenia by current U.S. criteria (Diagnos) do not return to their previous level of function (Jablensky 1993).

▮ Neuropathology and pathophysiology

A variety of different anatomic, chemical and molecular deviations from nor-mal controls have been reported in the brain and body fluids of subgroups of individuals with schizophrenia. However, in a majority of individuals with this disorder, the brain appears normal to gross and microscopic inspection and no biochemical, anatomic or molecular anomaly has been discerned that is pathognomonic or universal. Enlargement of lateral ventricles (20–25%) and the third ventricle (30–50%) or reduced size of one or more cortical or sub-cortical areas (10–15%) are reported in varying percentages of individuals with schizophrenia by different investigators (Leonard et al. 1999; Cotter et al. 2000; Rosoklija et al. 2000; Arnold et al. 1991; Staal et al. 2001 and hundreds more!). When repeated imaging studies are performed in the early months of a schizophrenic illness and repeated over a 2–4 year period on the same groups of patients and age and gender-matched controls, progressive enlarge-ment of the ventricles has been reported for a percentage of individuals with schizophrenia (DeLisi et al. 1997). Increased or decreased expression of excita-tory or inhibitory neurotransmitters or receptors, decreased dendritic spines, synaptic density or mRNA for these elements have been reported in the cere-bral cortex, thalamus, hippocampus or cingulate gyrus in subgroups of indivi-duals diagnosed with schizophrenia (Danos et al. 2002; Byne et al. 2002; Staal et al. 2001; Cahn et al. 2002). Reduction in volume, neuron number or specific synaptic markers in the thalamus have also been reported in some individuals (Kock and Friedman 2001). Several but by no means all studies report a de-crease in thalamic volume in subgroups, a finding consistent with the enlarge-ment of the lateral and third ventricles reported in 1/4 to 1/2 of schizophrenic patients. Statistically significant differences are reported between patients and controls for a variety of these measures. However, when individual findings are presented, as for the other measures, there is generally considerable over-lap of schizophrenics and controls in the distribution of whatever is being measured. This suggests that, as with epilepsy, a variety of single or multiple factors may contribute to the precipitation of similar clinical presentations in different individuals.

▮ Pharmacology

Before the introduction of modern pharmacological treatment, patients with schizophrenia were treated by incarceration, restraints, wet cold packs and even application of "cupping" or leeches to the scalp. However, the symptoms of this psychosis first yielded, remarkably enough, to induction of epileptic seizures, induced first by intravenous camphor, then by insulin causing hypoglycemia, later by pentylenetetrazol or application of brief electrical current to the head. Although treatment by inducing epileptic seizures with these methods could be effective in relieving many symptoms of the psychosis for days or weeks, relapse was common. Then came the phenothiazines. Introduced for treatment of psychosis by Delay and Denicker (1952), this class of drugs blocks receptors for DA and other inhibitory transmitters in the brain.

Use of these agents inaugurated a revolution in psychiatric theory and practice. The most florid symptoms and signs of schizophrenia or schizophreniform psychoses were ameliorated or arrested in many (but not all) patients following treatment. Mental hospitals soon discharged thousands of patients to their communities to continue their medications. However, as defined by current DSM IV criteria, which require 6 months of symptoms for diagnosis, fewer than half of those so affected return to their previous level of school, work or social activity even if they continued taking the prescribed drugs (Jablensky 1999). Shorter periods of psychosis with identical symptoms, lasting days, weeks or months are designated brief psychotic reaction or schizophreniform psychosis but may well share a similar pathology and pathophysiology.

The most effective agent against symptoms of schizophrenia resistant to other antipsychotics is the "atypical" antipsychotic clozapine (Kane 2000). Unlike the "typical" earlier antipsychotics, which have a high affinity for DAD_2 receptors, clozapine has greater affinity for the DAD_3 and DAD_4 receptors, specific serotonin, NE, GABA, histamine and acetylcholine receptors and blocks NMDA antagonists (Ackenheil 1989; Guo et al. 1998; Van Tol et al. 1991). Although all neuroleptics can cause convulsions when given in high doses or in susceptible individuals, it is interesting, given the previous use of convulsive therapies, that clozapine is the most proconvulsive of these agents (Devinsky et al. 1991). Unlike the other antipsychotics we have tested in rats, clozapine did not induce generalized convulsions but induced dose-related myoclonic jerks in partially restrained rats (Denney and Stevens 1995). In contrast to other antipsychotics, clozapine blocks DAD_3 receptors in N. accumbens more than DAD_2 receptors in caudate putamen (Guo et al. 1998), does not produce the extrapyramidal side effects associated with all of the earlier typical and by the newer atypical antipsychotics. Increased expression of DAD_3 receptors in N. Accumbens, the gateway from amygdala and hippocampus to the thalamus, hypothalamus and frontal lobes, has been reported in brains from some schizophrenic patients (Gurevich et al. 1997). Although clozapine also has a high affinity for DAD_4 receptors, which are maximally expressed in striatum, cortex and hippocampus, and for 5HT2A receptors, unlike the effectiveness of DAD_2 and DAD_3 antagonists against the symptoms of schizophrenia, DAD_4 and 5HT2A antagonists are not effective (Truffinet et al. 1999; Kramer et al. 1997).

▌ Schizophrenia and the reproductive cycle

Maximum age of onset of schizophrenia during the reproductive period suggests a relationship of this disorder to the physiologic events that occur in the brain during adolescence and young adult life. This in turn focuses attention on the anatomy and physiology of those parts of the brain that are associated with sexual and reproductive activity. The essential role of the amygdala, hippocampus, hypothalamus and their afferent and efferent pathways for reproduction, defense, flight and feeding has been known for decades (Bard 1928; MacLean 1957). It is then of special interest that amygdala and hippocampus have a lower threshold for epileptic discharge than any other brain region (MacLean 1957). Why? This is a risk nature has taken that has important implications for normal and abnormal physiology. Circumscribed episodic rapid rhythmic neuronal discharges occur as part of normal physiology in amygdala, hippocampus, bed nucleus of stria terminalis, septum and other limbic nuclei during coition, ovulation and other critical events of the reproductive cycle (Kawakami and Sawyer 1959; Kawakami et al. 1982; Andrew and Dudek 1984; O'Byrne et al. 1991; Knobil 1992; Wilson et al. 1984). Receptors for estrogen, testosterone and luteinizing releasing hormone (LHRH) are also located in amygdala and in basal forebrain projection sites of both hippocampus and amygdala. Release of neurotransmitters and reproductive hormones during discretely localized pulsatile discharges in this region indicates the physiologic importance of synchronous bursts of rapid neuronal discharge for delivery of critical messages in specific systems, including the neuroendocrine network (Kawakami et al. 1982). Neuroleptics, focal seizures of amygdala, hippocampus and generalized seizures that involve these structures induce elevation of serum prolactin and LH in both males and females (Parra et al. 1980). But propagation of electrical discharge from these critical low seizure threshold brain areas to hypothalamic centers that regulate endocrine secretion must also be well protected from the spread of such activity to cortical areas that regulate consciousness and behavior. This is where the inhibitory systems of DA and other inhibitory neurotransmitters must increase function.

Pulses or bursts of rapid neuronal discharge confined to specific subcortical nuclei are an effective mode for relaying imperative messages (including release of specific hormones) over background "noise" and to prevent neuronal fatigue without triggering seizures. Glutamate and acetylcholine are the principal neurotransmitters responsible for excitatory discharge. Estrogen is also excitatory (McEwen 1999; Becker et al. 1999). Changes in estrogen level during the menstrual cycle correlate with occurrence of seizures in susceptible girls and women (Herzog 1999). Estrogen alpha and beta receptors, progesterone and testosterone (which is converted to estrogen in the brain) receptors are widely distributed in brain of both males and females (Pfaff et al. 1976; Keefer and Stumpf 1975). In addition to hypothalamus, these receptors are maximally expressed in amygdala, lateral septum, Islands of Calleja, bed nucleus of stria terminalis, nucleus of diagonal band and periaqueductal gray (Pfaff et al. 1976; Keefer and Stumpf 1975). Changes in dendritic spine number, density of pyramidal neurons and excitatory amino acid binding have been demonstrated in the highly epileptogenic CA1 area of the hippocampus of the rat in response to estrogen and during the reproductive cycle (Wooley et al. 1997).

Propagation of physiologic rapid neuronal pulsed discharge beyond regions of physiologic utility could lead to seizures but is opposed by inhibitory pathways and transmitters that are widely distributed in brain. These include DA,

NE, 5HT, GABA, specific peptides and the multiple receptors for these agents. Dopamine D2 (DAD_2) receptors are maximally expressed in neostriatum (caudate-putamen) on which excitatory (glutamate) axons from neocortex and thalamus converge. Caudate-putamen project to globus pallidus, thalamus, brainstem and cerebral cortex. DAD_3 receptors predominate in ventral striatum (N. accumbens and associated basal forebrain nuclei) (Guo et al. 1998) where axons from amygdala and hippocampus, the regions which physiologically demonstrate the lowest threshold for epileptic discharge in the brain, project (Stevens 1973). Accumbens projects to ventral pallidum and thence to hypothalamus, dorsomedial thalamus and orbital and medial frontal lobes (Heimer et al. 1997; Groenwegen and Russchen 1984).

The Islands of Calleja (IC) are discrete clusters of small granular neurons surrounded by medium-sized neurons around a cell sparse core embedded in ventral striatum (N. accumbens in man, as olfactory tubercle has largely disappeared). These islands, loosely joined by a syncytium of axons and dendrites, form an arc along the subpial border of ventral striatum anterior to the substantia innominata (Fallon 1983). The largest (major) I/C lies between N. accumbens laterally, vertical limb of the diagonal band and lateral septal nucleus medially. Unlike neostriatum and ventral striatum, some of the larger neurons of the I/C contain LHRH receptors, concentrate estradiol and express estrogen and testosterone receptors in greater density than any other forebrain area (Meyer et al. 1989). DAD_3 receptors are maximally expressed on neurons of the Island of Calleja complexes which express 2 1/2 times the density of DAD_3 receptors as the next highest areas, N. accumbens and the dentate gyrus of the hippocampus (Suzuki et al. 1998).

I/C are present in all species and attain maximum development and dispersion in man (Fallon et al. 1993). The ventral group of I/C lie in the highly vascularized *substantia perforata anterior* in close relation to blood vessels suggesting possible humoral inputs from serum endocrine factors. Principal neural afferents to the larger neurons of the I/C of the rat are from the septal nuclei, nuclei of the diagonal band, cortical nuclei of amygdala, intralaminar nuclei, midline nuclei of the thalamus and from DA neurons from ventral tegmental area and substantia nigra via medial forebrain bundle. Reciprocal efferents project to most of the same structures including ventral pallidum, septum, and midline thalamic nuclei. Axons from larger I/C neurons project, in parallel to ventral striatum, to dorsomedial nucleus of thalamus and could thus influence activity from thalamus projected to frontal lobes. The I/C are the only major projection to the dorsomedial thalamic nucleus that contain more than rare gonadal hormone binding cells (Meyer et al. 1989; Pfaff and Keiner 1973). Surrounded by a dense plexus of DAergic and cholinergic fibers from adjacent substantia innominata, I/C neurons also express neurotensin and the highest concentration of muscarinic receptors in the brain (Talbot et al. 1988a,b). On the basis of anatomic and histochemical data, Fallon et al. (1983) proposed that the I/C form an extra-hypothalamic neuroendocrine-thalamo-cortical interface parallel to the neostriatal and limbic (ventral) striatal systems that regulate sensorimotor and appetitive activities, respectively.

Schizophrenia most often occurs during the fertility period. The peculiar olfactory, tactile and sexual hallucinations and delusions frequently experienced by individuals with this disorder may relate to the flood of gonadal steroids and the concentration of receptors for these hormones in the basal forebrain. A target for projections from amygdala and hippocampus, the septal area is also the brain area in which, if implanted with stimulating electrodes, rats will press a lever hundreds of times per minute for electric stimulation up to the point of provoking seizures (Olds and Milner 1954). The I/C are surrounded by a dense DAergic projection from medial forebrain bundle and express DAD_3 receptors that may limit propagation of physiologic excitatory discharges critical to sexual and reproductive function from extending beyond areas of physiologic utility. If over-expressed in schizophrenia, as mostly cortical excitatory systems are in epilepsy, the special value of clozapine for treatment of schizophrenia could relate to the particularly high affinity of this and related agents for the DAD_3 receptors that are maximally expressed in this area of the brain and are reportedly overly expressed in at least some schizophrenic individuals (Gurevich et al. 1999).

There is other evidence for pathologic change in excitability of neurons in these brain areas in schizophrenia. Many years ago Robert Heath (1959) and Sem-Jacobsen et al. (1955) reported "seizure-like activity" on the EEG recorded from the "septal area" of normal men during orgasm or during orgasmic sensations induced by electrical or cholinergic stimulation of the "septal" region. Heath (1959) and other investigators also recorded episodic spike activity on the EEG from electrodes implanted in the same region in patients with active symptoms of schizophrenia. Similar isolated spike activity is often observed from EEGs recorded over or within an epileptic focus during seizure-free periods in patients with epilepsy, suggesting an excitatory focus under suppression. The antipsychotic agents used in treatment of psychosis block receptors for one or more inhibitory transmitters and may thus decrease pathologic extension of inhibition beyond areas of physiologic utility.

▌ Conclusions

Although a variety of abnormalities have been reported in the brain of individuals with schizophrenia, no single site that is pathognomonic for or essential to schizophrenia has been identified. In addition to the maximum occurrence of schizophrenia at the onset and throughout the reproductive period, there is pharmacological evidence for excessive dopaminergic inhibition in the brain. These facts draw attention to the interaction sites between DA receptors and receptors for the reproductive hormones in basal forebrain. Susceptibility to schizophrenia may be associated with pathologic extension of physiologic inhibition to limit spread of excitation from the flood of excitatory hormones affecting gonadotropic receptors in basal forebrain and amygdala-hippocampus during this period.

References

Ackenheil M (1989) Clozapine – pharmacokinetic investigations and biochemical effects in man. Psychopharmacology 99:S 32–37

Adams RD, Victor M (1967) Principles of Neurology, 5th ed. McGraw Hill, NY, p 957

Andrew DA, Dudek FE (1984) Analysis of intracellularly recorded phasic bursting by mammalian neuroendocrine cells. J of Neurophysiology 51:453–468

Becker JB, Rudick CN, Jenkins WJ (2001) The role of dopamine in the nucleus accumbens and striatum during sexual behavior in the female rat. J Neuroscience 21:3231–3236

Byne W, Buchsbaum MS, Mattiace LA, Hazlett EA, Kemether E, Elhakem SL, Purohit DP, Haroutunian V, Jones L (2002) Postmortem assessment of thalamic nuclear volumes in subjects with schizophrenia. Am J Psychiatry 159:59–65

Danos P, Baumann B, Bernstein HG, Stauch R, Krell D, Falkai P, Bogerts B (2002) The ventral lateral posterior nucleus of the thalamus in schizophrenia. A post mortem study. Psychiatry Res 114:1–9

Cahn W, Pol He, Lems EB, van Heren NE, Schnack HG, Van der Linden JA, Schothorst PF, Van Engelend H, Kahn RS (2002) Brain volume changes in first episode schizophrenia: a 1 year follow-up study. Arch Gen Psychiatry 59:1002–1010

Cotter D, Wilson S, Roberts E, Kerwin R, Everall IP (2000) Increased dendritic MAP2 expression in the hippocampus in schizophrenia. Schiz Research 41:313–323

Delay J, Deniker P (1952) Comptes rendus du 50eme congres des medicins alienistes et neurologistes du France et des pays de langue Francaise

DeLisi LE, Sakuma M, Tew W, Kushner M, Hoff AL, Grimson R (1997) Schizophrenia as a chronic active brain process: a study of progressive brain structural change subsequent to the onset of schizophrenia. Psychiatry Res 74:129–140

Denney D, Stevens JR (1995) Clozapine and Seizures. Biol Psychiatry 37:427–433

Devinsky O, Honigfeld G, Patin J (1991) Clozapine-related seizures. Neurology 41:369–371

Diagnostic and Statistical Manual of Mental Disorders IV (1994) American Psychiatric Association Press, Washington, DC

Fallon JH, Loughlin SE, Ribak CE (1983) The islands of Calleja complex of rat basal forebrain. III. Histochemical evidence for a striatopallidal system. J Comp Neurol 218:91–120

Fallon JH (1983) The islands of Calleja complex of rat basal forebrain II connections of medium and large sized cells. Brain Res Bull 10:775–793

Groenewegen HJ, Russchen FT (1984) Organization of the efferent projections of the nucleus accumbens to pallidal, hypothalamic, and mesencephalic structures: a tracing and immunohistochemical study in the cat. J Comp Neurol 223:347–367

Guo N, Vincent SR, Fibiger HC (1998) Phenotypic characteristics of neuroleptic-sensitive neurons in the forebrain: contrasting targets of haloperidol and clozapine. Neuropsychopharmacology 19:133–145

Gurevich EV, Bordelon Y, Shapiro RM, Arnold SE, Gur RE, Joyce JN (1997) Mesolimbic dopamine D3 receptors and use of antipsychotics in patients with schizophrenia. A postmortem study. Arch Gen Psychiat 54:225–232

Häfner H (1998) Causes and consequences of the gender difference in age at onset of schizophrenia. Schizophrenia Bull 24:99–113

Heath RG (1972) Pleasure and brain activity in man. Deep and surface electroencephalograms during orgasm. J Nerv Ment Dis 154:3–18

Heath RG (1959) Studies in Schizophrenia Cambridge Mass. Harvard University Press

Heckers S (1997) Neuropathology of schizophrenia: cortex, thalamus, basal ganglia, and neurotransmitter-specific projection systems. Schizoph Bull 23:403–421

Heimer L, Alheid GF, de Olmos JS, Groenewegen HJ, Haber SN, Harlan RE, Zahm DS (1997) The accumbens: beyond the core-shell dichotomy. J Neuropsychiatry Clin Neurosci 9:354–381

Heimer L, DeOlmos JS, Alheid GF, Pearson J, Sakamoto N, Shinoda K, Marsteiner J, Switzer RC (1999) In: Bloom FE, Bjorklund A, Hokfelt T (eds) The human basal forebrain Part II. Handbook of Chemical Neuroanatomy. Elsevier, Amsterdam, pp 257–225

Herzog AG (1999) Psychoneuroendocrine aspects of temporal lobe epilepsy. Part Epilepsy and reproductive steroids. Psychosomatics 48:102–108

Honer WG, Falkai P, Chen C, Arango V, Mann JJ, Dwork AJ (1999) Synaptic andplasticity-associated proteins in anterior frontal cortex in severe mental illness. Neuroscience 91:1247–1255

Jablensky A (1999) The conflict of the nosologists: views on schizophrenia and manic depressive illness in the early part of the 20th century. Schiz Res 39:95–100

Javitt DC, Zukin SR (1991) Recent advances in the phencyclidine model of schizophrenia. Am J Psychiatry 148:1301–1308

Kane J (2000) Pharmacologic treatment of schizophrenia. Biol Psychiatry 46:1396–1408

Kawakami M, Sawyer CH (1959) Induction of behavioral and electroencephalographic changes in the rabbit by hormone administration of brain stimulation. Endocrinology 65:631–643

Kawakami M, Terasawa E, Ibuki T (1970) Changes in multiple unit activity of the brain during the estrous cycle. Neuroendocrinology 6:30–48

Kawakami M, Uemura T, Hayashi R (1982) Electrophysiological correlates of pulsatile gonadotropin release on rats. Neuroendocrinology 35:63–67

Keefer DA, Stumpf WE (1975) Atlas of estrogen-concentrating cells in the central nervous system of the squirrel monkey. J Comp Neurol 160:419–442

Knobil E (1992) Remembrance: the discovery of the hypothalamic gonadotropin-releasing hormone pulse generator and of its physiological significance. Endocrinology 131:1005–1006

Kramer MS, Last B, Getson A, Reines SA (1997) The effects of a selective D4 Dopamine receptor antagonist in acutely psychotic inpatients with schizophrenia. Arch Gen Psychiat 54:567–572

Leonard CM, Kuldau JM, Breier JI, Zuffante PA, Gauteir ER, Heron DC, Lavery EM, Packing J, Williams SA, DeBose CA (1999) Cumulative effects of anatomical risk factors for schizophrenia: an MRI study. Biol Psychiat 46:374–382

Meyer G, Gonzalez-Hernandez T, Carrillo-Padilla F, Ferres-Torres R (1989) Aggregations of granule cells in the basal forebrain (islands of Calleja): Golgi and cytoarchitectonic study in different mammals, including man. J Comp Neurol 284: 405–428

O'Byrne KT, Thalabard JC, Grosser PM, Wilson RC, Williams CL, Chen MD, Ladendorf D, Hotchkiss J, Knobil E (1991) Radiotelemetric monitoring of hypothalamic gonadotropin-releasing hormone pulse generator activity throughout the menstrual cycle of the rhesus monkey. Endocrinology 129:1207–1214

Olds J, Milner P (1954) Positive reinforcement produced by electrical stimulation of septal areas and other regions of the rat brain. J Comp Physiol Psychol 47:419–427

Ordog T, Chen MD, Nishihara M, Connaughton MA, Goldsmith JR, Knobil E (1997) On the role of gonadotropin-releasing hormone (GnRH) in the operation of the GnRH pulse generator in the rhesus monkey. Neuroendocrinology 65:307–313

Parra A, Velasco M, Cervantes C, Munoz H, Cerbon MA, Velasco F (1980) Plasma prolactin increase following electric stimulation of the amygdala in humans. Neuroendocrinology 31:60–65

Rosoklija G, Toomayan G, Ellis SP, Keilp J, Mann J, Latov N, Hays AP, Dwork AJ (2000) Structural abnormalities of subicular dendrites in subjects with schizophrenia and mood disorders. Arch Gen Psychiat 57:349–356

Staal WG, Hulshoff Pol HE, Schnack HG, Van Haren NEM, Seifer N, Kahn RS (2001) Structural brain abnormalities in chronic schizophrenia at the extremes of the outcome spectrum. Am J Psychiat 158:1140–1142

Sem-Jacobson CW, Petersen MC, Lazarte JA et al (1955) Intracerebral electrographic recordings from psychotic patients during hallucinations and agitation: preliminary report. Am J Psychiatry 112:278–288

Stevens JR (1973) An anatomy of schizophrenia? Arch Gen Psychiat 29:177–189

Stevens JR (1999) Epilepsy, schizophrenia and the extended amygdala. Ann NY Acad Sci 877:548–561

Stevens JR (2002) Schizophrenia: Reproductive hormones and the brain. Am J Psychiatry 159:713–719

Suzuki M, Hurd YL, Sokoloff P, Schwartz JC, Sedvall G (1998) D3 dopamine receptor mRNA is widely expressed in the human brain. Brain Res 779:58–74

Talbot K, Woolf NJ, Butcher LL (1988) Feline islands of Calleja complex: I. Cytoarchitectural organization and comparative anatomy. J Comp Neurol 275:553–579

Talbot K, Woolf NJ, Butcher LL 1988) Feline islands of Calleja complex: II. Cholinergic and cholinesterasic features. J Comp Neurol 275:580–603

Tamminga CA (1998) Schizophrenia and glutamatergic transmission. Crit Rev Neurobiol 12:21–36

Truffinet P, Tamminga CA, Fabre, LF, Meltzer HY, Riviere M-E, Papillon-Downey C (1999) Placebo controlled study of the D4/5-HT2A antagonist fananserin in the treatment of schizophrenia. Am J Psychiat 156:419–425

Van Cauter P, Linkowski P, Kerkhofs M, Hubain P, L'Hermite-Baleriaux M, Leclercq R, Brasseur M, Capinschi G, Mendelewicz J (1991) Circadian and sleep related endocrine rhythms in schizophrenia. Arch Gen Psychiat 48:348–356

Van Tol HH, Bunzow JR, Guan H-C, Sunahara RK, Seeman P, Niznik HB, Civelli O (1991) Cloning of the gene for a human dopamine D4 receptor with high affinity for the antipsychotic clozapine. Nature 350:614–619

Varidy M, Kays R (1983) LSD psychosis or LSD-induced schizophrenia? A multimethod inquiry. Arch Gen Psychiat 40:877–883

Wilson RC, Kesner JS, Kaufman JM, Uemura T, Akema T, Knobil E (1984) Central electrophysiologic correlates of pulsatile luteinizing hormone secretion in the rhesus monkey. Neuroendocrinology 39:256–262

Woolley CS, Weiland NG, McEwen BS, Schwartzkroin PA (1997) Estradiol increases the sensitivity of hippocampal CA1 pyramidal cells to NMDA receptor-mediated synaptic input: correlation with dendritic spine density. J Neurosci 17:1848–1859

Schizophrenia as a progressive developmental disorder: the evidence and its implications

BRYAN T. WOODS

University of Texas Health Science Center, Houston, USA

Introduction

I would like to propose that there are certain limiting characteristics of the in vivo structural brain changes observed in schizophrenia that must be explained by any postulated pathogenetic hypothesis. These characteristics are not so specific as to be diagnostically useful in individuals in the absence of behavioral data, but they are useful in the search for the genetic defect(s) that most observers now agree are the necessary if not sufficient cause(s) of the illness. This potential utility comes about at two stages in this genetic search; first, because brain volume loss is a quantitative trait, it is possible to use it to separate out a sub-set of schizophrenic patients who are more likely to share a common genetic defect, even if the illness is heterogeneic in an unselected patient group. Second, even if a gene region is shown to be associated with schizophrenia with high probability, it will still be necessary to screen as many as a hundred or more genes in the region to find the specific cause. In this search a genetic defect that measurably affects brain growth and development is much more amenable to isolation in an animal model than one that affects only behavior; it's hard to be sure what a schizophrenic mouse would look like.

Methods

The timing of excessive brain volume loss in schizophrenia; drawing conclusions from post hoc structural imaging

Standard MRI readily yields quantitative volume measurements of four separate intracranial compartments, characterized as follows:

Intraventricular volume (IVV) Normal increases in IVV take place over the individual life-span, both through growth prior to achievement of maximum whole brain volume (BV_{max}) and via *ex vacuo* expansion to replace subsequent BV contraction. If we neglect brain pulsations and transient variations in brain water content, IVV does not normally contract.

Brain volume (BV) At full term birth, BV is less than one-third BV_{max} (Huppe 1998), but by age 5 it has expanded to about 95% BV_{max} (Giedd 1996). BV_{max} is normally reached at about age 10–12 (Pfefferbaum 1994). Subsequently there is a slow normal contraction of BV that may extend over the next five decades (Blatter, 1995).

Extracerebral volume (ECV) This is the cerebrospinal fluid (CSF) compartment between the cerebral surface and the inner surface of the cranium. At BV_{max} ECV is about 5% of BV and the IVV/ECV ratio is approximately 0.20 (Jernigan 1990). Subsequently both normal and pathological reductions in BV result in an *ex vacuo* expansion of ECV and IVV.

Intracranial volume (ICV) This is the sum of IVV, BV, and ECV. During normal development ICV expansion is driven by the expansion of these other compartments, and ICV_{max} is reached simultaneously with BV_{max}. Thereafter ICV normally remains fixed so that $ICV_{adult} = ICV_{max}$. At BV_{max} the proportions of the ICV subcompartments are approximately as follows: $BV \cong 0.94$; $ECV \cong 0.05$; $IVV \cong 0.01$ (Jernigan 1990).

Percentage differences between patient and control ICV measured in adults will accurately reflect differences in brain volume expansion that took place prior to BV_{max} and percentage differences in the BV/ICV ratios will also reflect differences in brain volume contraction after BV_{max} *if* there was not any *ex vacuo* early expansion of IVV. However if such an early expansion of IVV did occur, early losses will be underestimated and later losses overestimated. We can estimate whether or not pathological early IVV expansion occurred by comparing patients and controls on another ratio, IVV/ECV. If this ratio is greater for patients than controls we must consider the possibility that there was excessive early expansion of patient IVV. We can then determine the maximum possible effect of that expansion on our results by a correction which reduces patient IVV until the patient IVV/ECV ratio is the same as that of the control group, *and then reducing patient ICV by the same amount.* If percentage differences between patient and control groups are significant both with and without this correction, then we can conclude that this element of uncertainty has not affected our basic result.

▮ Results

Table 1 shows the percentage differences between patients and controls from 20 published MRI studies comprising 984 schizophrenic and schizoaffective patients and 1047 age- and gender-matched controls, with (16 studies) and without (20 studies) correction for excessive early IVV expansion. Studies were included if they had absolute values for ICV and BV; the 16 studies corrected for excessive early IVV expansion also had separate data on IVV and ECV.

The patient-control group differences taken together have a statistically significant early brain volume loss of 1.08% (t=-2.23, df=19, p<0.05) *and* later loss of 1.40% (t=-6.36 df=19, p<0.0001). The overall schizophrenic loss of 2.64% is also highly significant (t=-4.87, df=19, p<0.0001). Weighting the group scores by sample size increases the significance of the total early loss (t=-2.86, df 19, p<0.01) but leaves the other differences at approximately the same level of significance.

There is one of the earliest of the studies (n=15) that is a clear outlier with respect to both early and later loss (Shenton 1992), and if this study is ex-

Table 1. Sample sizes, mean ages of patient groups, and percentage differences in mean patient ICV, corrected IVC, BV/ICV, corrected BV/ICV and BV relative to controls

Study	SCZ n	Scan Age	ΔICV (%)	ΔICV$_c$ (%)	ΔBV/ICV (%)	ΔBV/ICV$_c$ (%)	ΔBV (%)
Woods 1991	19	34.6	−4.03	−3.69	−2.75	−3.06	−7.01
Gur 1991	42	30.3	−0.31	–	−0.94	–	−1.33
Shenton 1992	15	37.9	3.80	3.55	0.47	0.70	4.33
Andreasen 1994	52	30.1	−0.25	−0.25	−2.35	−2.35	−2.97
Gur 1994	81	30.4	−3.19	−3.32	−0.46	−0.34	−3.68
Flaum 1995	102	31.8	−0.62	−0.69	−0.34	−0.28	−1.02
Nopoulos 1995	24	23.3	−0.07	0.00	−2.11	−2.18	−2.36
Nopoulos 1997	80	28.1	0.40	0.36	−2.13	−2.10	−1.96
Pearlson 1997	46	31.8	−4.01	–	−0.69	–	−4.72
Zipursky 1998	46	26.2	−1.90	−2.03	−0.74	−0.61	−2.70
Gur 1998	96	29.2	−1.15	−1.31	−0.88	−0.73	−2.10
Cannon 1998	75	40.5	0.47	−0.56	−2.24	−2.15	−2.88
Gur 1999	130	29.2	−1.78	−1.91	−0.41	−0.28	−2.22
Dickey 2000	14	39.9	−4.02	−3.78	−1.91	−2.13	−6.03
Staal 2000	16	40.6	1.05	0.83	−3.31	−3.13	−2.82
Pol 2000	18	50.8	0.34	0.17	−0.40	−0.26	−0.14
Sigmundsson 2001	27	34.9	−4.27	–	−1.39	–	−5.77
Paillere-Martinot 2001	20	29.0	0.29	–	−1.76	–	−1.78
Staal 2001	45	38.3	1.51	1.41	−2.37	−2.49	−1.31
Cahn 2002	36	26.2	−2.97	−2.98	−1.27	−1.26	−4.38
Group Mean		33.2	−1.08	−0.89	−1.40	−1.40	−2.64

cluded and the remaining 19 are weighted for sample size, there is a trend to an inverse relationship between the percentages of early and of later loss ($F = 4.07$, df = 1, $p < 0.06$).

There is no significant correlation between the mean ages of the different samples and *any* of the individual group loss measures.

▌ Conclusions

These results and the literature on excessive brain volume loss in schizophrenia suggest five conclusions about the underlying process causing the loss.

▪ Excessive BV loss is a progressive process that is occurring both before and after the emergence of overt illness (Woods 1998).

▪ The time period during which this progressive loss is occurring may well begin pre-natally and usually ends sometime during or shortly after the third decade of life.

▪ There is an upper limit on the percentage of excessive loss that is seen, with a two standard deviation range extending out to 7.5% of normal BV.

▮ There is a trend to an inverse relationship between earlier and later loss, suggesting that once the upper limit of excessive loss is reached, the anatomical pathogenetic process ends, no matter what the age of the patient.

▮ Although it is highly probable that the BV loss is due to a genetic defect affecting initial development and subsequent modification of a neural structure whose normal function is necessary to prevent the illness, the *measurable* excessive loss of brain volume may be an epiphenomenon of the gene defect. This means that there could be more than one independent genetic cause of the critical defect, and not all of these causes would necessarily also result in measurable volume loss.

▮ Discussion

As we have learned more about the thousands of genes that are expressed in the central nervous system, the complexity of the process of growth and development has come to be better appreciated. We have also realized that the same gene may influence multiple brain functions that are not logically inter-related in any way. Furthermore, we have learned that knowing the pharmacological effects of an agent that improves the symptoms of illness does not necessarily mean that the underlying basis of the illness is a deficit in that pharmacological effect. A classic early example of this was the realization that even though anti-cholinergic agents improve the symptoms of Parkinsonism, an excess of cholinergic activity is not what causes Parkinsonism. We have also learned that different genes control different steps in a chain that leads to neural development/remodeling, and that just as many different single genetic defects are each sufficient to cause a deficiency in low density lipoprotein receptor function, many different genetic defects might have the potential to impair a single aspect of neural development at different critical points.

One conclusion to be drawn from this is that it is not surprising that when the candidate gene approach to finding the causation of schizophrenia has been based on known functions of the genes being evaluated, it has not worked. Similarly, looking for genes whose absence would lead to the kind of progressive early life excessive BV loss described above, is also not likely to work because the effects of the loss are not grossly quantitative (i.e. not every process that results in a 3% loss of total brain volume will cause schizophrenia). Rather the value of these observations about the progressive structural changes in schizophrenia is that they can first aid in the search for gene regions associated with schizophrenia, and then, if genes in a region are suspected to play a role in causation, determine through animal models if any of these genes also cause slowly progressive but time limited excessive brain volume loss. Since it is highly improbable that a gene selected because it is associated with clinical schizophrenia would also result in progressive volume loss in a mouse purely by coincidence, such an observation would be strong evidence that a defect of the gene being investigated really does play a causal role in the human illness.

▌References

Andreasen NC, Flashman L, Flaum M, Arndt SV, Swayze V, O'Leary DS, Ehrhardt JC, Yuh WTC (1994) Regional brain abnormalities in schizophrenia measured with magnetic resonance imaging. JAMA 272:1763–1769

Blatter DD, Bigler ED, Gale SD, Johnson SC, Anderson CV, Burnett, BM, Parker N, Kurth S, Horn SD (1995) Quantitative volumetric analysis of brain MR: normative database spanning 5 decades of life. Am J Neuroradiol 16:241–251

Cannon TD, Van Erp TGM, Huttunen M, Lonqvist J, Salonen O, Valanne L,Veli-Pekka P, Standertskjold-Nordenstam C-G, Gur RC, Yan M (1998) Regional gray matter, white matter, and cerebrospinal fluid distributions in schizophrenic patients, their siblings, and controls. Arch Gen Psychiat 55:1084–1091

Cahn W, Pol HE, Lems EB, Van Haren, Schnack HG, Van der Linden, Schothorst PF, Van Engeland, Kahn RS (2002) Brain volume changes in first-episode schizophrenia: a 1-year follow-up study. Archives of General Psychiatry 59:1002–1011

Dickey CC, Shenton ME, Hirayasu Y, Fischer I, Voglmaier MM, Niznikiewicz MA, Seidman LJ, Fraone S, McCarley RW (2000) Large CSF volume not attributable to ventricular volume in schizotypal personality disorder. Am J Psychiatry 157:48–54

Flaum M, Swayze VW, O'Leary DS, Yuh WTC, Erhardt JC, Arndt SV, Andreasen NC (1995) Effects of diagnosis, laterality, and gender on brain morphology in schizophrenia. Am J Psychiatry 152:704–714

Giedd JN, Snell JW, Lange N, Rajapakse JC, Casey BJ, Kozuch PL, Vaituzis AC, Vauss YC, Hamburger SD, Kaysen D, Rapoport JL (1996) Quantitative magnetic resonance imaging of human brain development: Ages 4–18. Cerebral Cortex 6:551–560

Gur RE, Maany V, Mozley D, Swanson C, Bilker W, Gur RC (1998) Subcortical MRI volumes in neuroleptic-naive and treated patients with schizophrenia. Am J Psychiatry 155:1711–1717

Gur RE, Mozley D, Resnick SM, Shtasel D, Kohn M, Zimmerman R, Herman G, Atlas S, Grossman R, Erwin R, Gur RC (1991) Magnetic resonance imaging in schizophrenia. Arch Gen Psychiatry 48:407–412

Gur RE, Mozley D, Shtasel DL, Cannon TD, Gallacher F, Turetsky B, Grossman R, Gur RC (1994) Clinical subtypes of schizophrenia: differences in brain and CSF volume. Am J Psychiatry 151:343–350

Gur RE, Turetsky BJ, Bilker WB, Gur RC (1999) Reduced gray matter volume in schizophrenia. Arch Gen Psychiatry 56:905–911

Huppe PS, Warfield S, Kikinis R, Barnes PD, Zientara GP, Jolesz FA, Tsuji MK, Volpe JJ (1998) Quantitative magnetic resonce imaging of brain development in premature and mature newborns. Ann Neurol 43:224–235

Jernigan TL, Press GA, Hesselink JR (1990) Methods of measuring brain morphologic features on magnetic resonance images. Arch Neurol 47:27–32

Nopoulos P, Flaum M, Andreasen NC (1997) Sex differences in brain morphology in schizophrenia. Am J Psychiatry 154:1648–1654

Nopoulos P, Torres I, Flaum M, Andreasen NC, Ehrhardt JC, Yuh WTC (1995) Brain morphology in first-episode schizophrenia. Am J Psychiatry 152:1721–1723

Paillere-Martinot M-L, Cacin A, Aretiges E, Poline J-B, Joliot M, Maller L, Recasens C, Attar-Levy D, Martinot J-L (2001) Cerebral gray and white matter reductions and clinical correlates in patients with early onset schizophrenia. Schizophrenia Research 50:19–26

Pearlson GD, Barta PE, Powers RE, Menon RR, Richards SS, Aylward EH, Federman EB, Chase GA, Petty RG, Tien AY (1997) Medial and superior temporal gyral volumes and cerebral asymmetry in schizophrenia versus bipolar disorder. Biol Psychiatry 41:1–14

Pfefferbaum A, Mathalon DH, Sullivan EV, Rawles JM, Zipursky RB, Lim KO (1994) A quantitative magnetic resonance imaging study of changes in brain morphology from infancy to late adulthood. Arch Neurol 51:874–887

Pol HEH, Hoek HW, Susser E, Brown AS, Dingemans A, Schnack HA, Van Haren NEM, Ramos LMP, Gispen-de Wied CC, Kahn RS (2000) Prenatal exposure to famine and brain morphology in schizophrenia. Am J Psychiatry 157:1170–1172

Shenton ME, Kikinis R, Jolesz FA, Pollak SD, LeMay M, Wible CG, Hokama H, Martin J, Metcalf B, Coleman M, McCarley RW (1992) Abnormalities of left temporal lobe and thought disorder in schizophrenia. NEJM 327:604–612

Sigmundsson T, Suckling J, Maier M, Williams SCR, Bullmore ET, Greenwood KE, Fukuda R, Ron MA, Toone BK (2001) Structural abnormalities in frontal, temporal, and limbic regions and interconnecting white matter tracts in schizophrenic patients with prominent negative symptoms. Am J Psychiatry 158:234–243

Staal WG, Pol HEH, Schnack HG, Hoogendoorn MLC, Jellema K, Kahn RS (2000) Structural brain abnormalities in patients with schizophrenia and their healthy siblings. Am J Psychiatry 157:416–421

Staal WG, Pol HEH, Schnack HG, Neeltje EM, Van Haren NEM, Seifert M, Kahn RS (2001) Structural brain abnormalities in chronic schizophrenia at the extremes of the outcome spectrum. Am J Psychiatry 158:1140–1142

Woods BT, Yurgelun-Todd D (1991) Brain volume loss in schizophrenia: when does it occur and is it progressive? Schizophrenia Res 5:202–204

Woods BT (1998) Is schizophrenia a progressive neurodevelopmental disorder? Toward a unitary pathogenetic mechanism. Am J Psychiatry 155:1661–1670

Zipursky RB, Lamb EK, Kapur S, Mikulis DJ (1998) Cerebral gray matter volume deficits in first episode psychosis. Arch Gen Psychiatry 55:540–546

Controversies in schizophrenia research: the 'continuum' challenge, heterogeneity vs homogeneity, and lifetime developmental-'neuroprogressive' trajectory

PATRIZIA A. BALDWIN, ROBIN J. HENNESSY, MARIA G. MORGAN, JOHN F. QUINN, PAUL J. SCULLY, and JOHN L. WADDINGTON

Department of Clinical Pharmacology, Royal College of Surgeons in Ireland, Dublin 2, Ireland and

Stanley Research Unit, St Davnet's Hospital, Monaghan, Ireland

Introduction

In reviewing the extent to which our understanding has advanced between the 4th and 5th symposia on Search for the Causes of Schizophrenia, the conclusion is salutary: a committed and expanding research community, able to apply an increasing armamentarium of molecular genetic, neuropathological, neuroimaging and additional techniques, has made only modest gains over this five-year period. In the face of such a slow (though not negligible) rate of progress, it is necessary to give further consideration to some of the premises which guide current thinking, as they may be impeding rather than facilitating these endeavours.

The 'continuum' challenge

It is far from radical to reconsider the long-standing but still unresolved issue of whether psychotic illness comprises etiologically and pathophysiologically distinct diagnostic entities, or reflects a more homogeneous condition characterised by position along a continuum (Crow 1995; Torrey and Knable 1999; Waddington 2003). This concept posits psychotic illness to be continuously distributed, from what is defined operationally as 'schizophrenia' and other non-affective psychoses, through 'schizoaffective disorder', to affective psychoses, particularly 'bipolar disorder' and 'major depressive disorder with psychotic features'.

Diversity at the first episode

Among our own first episode study of psychosis and bipolar disorder within an epidemiologically complete, rural catchment area of 104 000 (Scully et al. 2002; Baldwin et al. 2003), preliminary analyses indicate that over eight years we have incepted 187 patients with the following DSM-IV diagnoses at 6-month follow-up: schizophrenia, 39; schizophreniform disorder, 9; schizoaffective disorder, 11; brief psychotic disorder, 9; bipolar disorder, 28; major de-

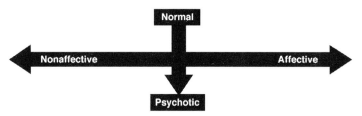

Fig. 1. Nonaffective-affective and normal-abnormal as 1-dimensional axes that lay orthogonal to each other in defining 2-dimensional diagnostic space for psychosis

pressive disorder with psychotic features, 31; substance-induced psychosis, 12; substance-induced mania, 6; other psychoses, 7; psychosis not otherwise specified, 11; awaiting initial assessment or 6-month follow-up, 24. Thus, psychosis can present at a variety of positions along a putative continuum. Also, diagnostic revisions between inception and 6-month follow-up indicate that diverse inception diagnoses do not necessarily converge into one or other 'major' categories over follow-up. It would appear that even operational criteria fail to readily separate individuals, such that their allocation to one rather than another diagnostic category can be influenced by subtle nuances of psychopathology or vagaries of the diagnostic algorithm rather than any inherent unity to that category.

Recently, this concept has been broadened by evidence collected epidemiologically in the general population that psychosis may occur also along an alternative continuum from 'normality', through evidence of mild, subclinical thought disturbances, subtle hallucinatory perceptions and minor delusional ideation, to 'attenuated' and 'full-blown' psychotic features which lie on either side of diagnostic criteria for psychotic illness (van Os et al. 2001; Verdoux and van Os 2002). Thus, even operational diagnostic criteria for psychotic illness, in the sense of a medical condition that can benefit from therapeutic intervention, may capture rather arbitrary groupings along a 2-dimensional continuum within which nonaffective-affective and normal-abnormal constitute 1-dimensional axes that lay orthogonal to each other in defining this 2-dimensional diagnostic space (Fig. 1).

Psychopathology

We have recently found a lack of discrete entities along the nonaffective-affective axis in relation to the 'core' psychopathology of psychosis. Specifically, while factor studies of psychopathology in schizophrenia have most commonly identified a 3-factor structure comprising domains of *reality distortion, disorganisation* and *psychomotor poverty*, there are no studies comparing the factor structure of psychopathology between schizophrenia, schizoaffective disorder and bipolar disorder among an epidemiologically complete population of cases who were systematically ascertained, diagnosed and assessed. In rural Ireland, among a socioeconomically and ethnically stable and homogeneous population of 29 542 (Scully et al. 2003), we ascertained and assessed using the

Positive and Negative Syndrome Scale (PANSS) 'all' cases of schizophrenia (n = 109), schizoaffective disorder (n = 32) and bipolar disorder (n = 73.

Principal component analysis of the 30 PANSS items (Scully et al. 2001) over all 214 cases, ignoring conventional diagnostic boundaries, resulted in a 5-factor solution comprising the following domains: *psychomotor poverty/disorganisation, reality distortion, excitement, depression/anxiety* and *mixed*. On disassembling this population along conventional diagnostic lines, for schizophrenia there was a 6-factor solution: *psychomotor poverty, reality distortion, disorganisation, depression/anxiety, excitement, guilt*; for schizoaffective disorder there was a 6-factor solution: *psychomotor poverty, reality distortion, excitement/hostility, impulsivity, tension, guilt*; for bipolar disorder, there was a 5-factor solution: *psychomotor poverty/reality distortion/disorganisation, grandiosity, unusual thoughts, anxiety, guilt*.

In summary, there were for schizophrenia three classical, independent domains, with additional affective and activation dimensions; for schizoaffective disorder, two classical domains, without *disorganisation*, with additional affective and activation dimensions; for bipolar disorder, the three classical domains coalesced, with only *grandiosity* and *unusual thought content* exclusive to this category. Thus, *psychomotor poverty* and *reality distortion* were not unique to schizophrenia and schizoaffective disorder, and affective dimensions were not unique to schizoaffective and bipolar disorder. Such overlap in domains of psychopathology would be consistent with a continuum model of psychotic illness.

Neurological soft signs

The above study population (Scully et al. 2003) has been followed up approximately 18 months later (Quinn et al. 2003) to evaluate neurological soft signs (NSS) in a similar manner. Among this cohort, it was possible to follow-up and assess for NSS, using the Condensed Neurological Evaluation (CNE), 147 cases: schizophrenia (n = 73), schizoaffective disorder (n = 25), bipolar disorder (n = 49). Principal component analysis of the CNE over all 147 cases, ignoring conventional diagnostic boundaries, revealed an 8-factor solution: a 'core' factor on which loaded a majority of variables; *graphesthesia-left; suck reflex-left & right; nystagmus-left & right; palmomental reflex-left & right*; there were three factors on which there were no specific loadings. On disassembling this population along conventional diagnostic lines, for schizophrenia there was a 7-factor solution: the 'core' factor; *snout reflex/occular vergence; graphesthesia-left; nystagmus-left & right; palmomental reflex-left; suck reflex-left; palmomental reflex-right*. For schizoaffective disorder there was a 7-factor solution: the 'core' factor; *blunt/sharp discrimination-left & right/blink reflex; two object test/astereognosis-right; oral apraxia; graphesthesia-right/grasp reflex-right; palmomental reflex-left*; there was one factor on which there were no specific loadings. For bipolar disorder there was an 8-factor solution: the 'core' factor; *occular vergence/two-object test; palmomental reflex-left & right/nystagmus-left; blunt/sharp discrimination-right; grasp reflex-right; nystagmus-right*; there were two factors on which there were no specific loadings.

Among all cases, and in each diagnostic group separately, there was a '*core*' factor on which loaded in each instance *tapping rhythm, imaginary acts, complex motor acts* and *simultaneous bilateral tactile extinction*; it was notable that these NSS are not lateralised. That schizophrenia, schizoaffective and bipolar disorder appear to evidence such a common core of NSS suggests some shared neuronal dysfunction. However, these diagnostic groups also differ in aspects of NSS, especially in relation to lateralised signs in general and to lateralisation of primitive reflexes in particular: schizophrenia appears characterised by *left-* and *left/right*-loading factors while bipolar disorder appears characterised by *right-* and *right/left*-loading factors; schizoaffective disorder appears characterised by some *left-* and *left/right*-loading factors similar to those of schizophrenia, and by some *right-* and *right/left*-loading factors similar to those of bipolar disorder.

It should be emphasised that the above findings do not indicate, for example, that schizophrenia is characterised by *left*-sided and bipolar disorder by *right*-sided dysfunction, as these analyses concern covariance in NSS and not abnormality therein; schizophrenia may be characterised by integrity of *left*-sided and bipolar disorder of *right*-sided function. Given evidence for some overrepresentation of structural brain abnormalities in the left hemisphere in schizophrenia, a particular abnormality may be the disruption in schizophrenia of *right*-sided (*left* hemisphere-mediated) and in bipolar disorder of *left*-sided (*right* hemisphere-mediated) coherence in such NSS. This would elaborate evidence for disruption of normal asymmetries in schizophrenia (Sommer et al. 2001) and indicate that such disruption may be reversed in bipolar disorder, with schizoaffective disorder sharing some aspects of neuronal dysfunction with each. These findings would be consistent with a continuum model along which shared neuronal dysfunction varies in extent of lateralisation.

In summary, these findings relating to diagnostic diversity at the first episode, psychopathology and NSS are each consistent with a continuum perspective of psychotic illness.

▌ Cerebral-craniofacial dysmorphogenesis in schizophrenia

Developmental origins

While an increasing body of evidence indicates abnormalities of early brain development in schizophrenia (Waddington et al. 1999a), it has proved difficult to identify 'hard' biological findings in the brain that might provide more specific information as to the nature and timing of underlying developmental disturbance (Harrison 1999; Arnold and Rioux 2001). Over early fetal life, cerebral morphogenesis proceeds in embryological intimacy with craniofacial morphogenesis, such that classical neurodevelopmental disorders such as Down's syndrome and velo-cardio-facial syndrome are well recognised to be characterised also by dysmorphic features which can involve several body regions but effect the craniofacies in particular (DeMyer et al. 1964; Smith 1988;

Kjaer 1995; Waddington et al. 1999 a). Minor physical anomalies (MPAs) are slight anatomical malformations that constitute biological markers of first/ early second trimester dysmorphogenesis, and several studies have now indicated MPAs to occur to excess among patients with schizophrenia. However, while the most consistent findings are subtle dysmorphogenesis of the craniofacial region (Lane et al. 1996; Waddington et al. 1998; McNeil et al. 2000), there is at best limited understanding of the biological implications of essentially qualitative MPAs.

3D morphometrics of craniofacial dysmorphogenesis

Recently, we have reported an anthropometric approach to reveal in schizophrenia numerous quantitative as well as qualitative dysmorphic features, particularly of craniofacial structures (Lane et al. 1997). However, this approach, while increasing our understanding of these processes, involves linear distance measurements between anatomical landmarks on inherently 3-dimensional (3D) morphology, and thus fails to capture those important, and potentially critical, geometric relationships that are essential elements of developmental processes. To realise the potential of such an approach would require both analysis of craniofacial structures in 3D and direct visualisation of the statistical model for extraction of biological meaning (Hennessy et al. 2002).

It is possible for a particular set of linear distances between anatomical landmarks to bear an unambiguous 3D relationship to each other; thus, such a set of interlandmark distances can be used to define and reconstruct the unique configuration of 3D (i.e. x, y, z) landmark coordinates that contains those distances; in a complementary manner, geometric morphometrics, which analyses landmark coordinates directly, provides the basis for 3D modelling of differences in craniofacial shape, both statistically and visually (O'Higgins 2000; Hennessy et al. 2002, 2003).

For 169 patients with DSM-III-R schizophrenia and 78 matched normal controls, craniofacial interlandmark distances were used to reconstruct 3D coordinates. These were analysed using geometric morphometrics with visualisation of the resultant statistical models. 3D craniofacial shape differed between patients and controls among both males and females; patients of both genders evidenced lengthened lower mid-facial height, shortened upper mid-facial height, nasion located posteriorly and a wider face posteriorly, while the midface was rotated differentially in male and female patients. Male controls evidenced marked directional asymmetry, while male patients showed reduced directional asymmetry; conversely, female controls evidenced little directional asymmetry, while female patients showed marked directional asymmetry (Hennessy et al. 2003). To date, we have found no differences in overall shape between 70 patients with schizophrenia, 25 with schizoaffective and 47 with bipolar disorder (Quinn et al. 2002).

These findings indicate that the qualitative and linear anthropometric abnormalities described previously in schizophrenia (Lane et al. 1997; McGrath et al. 2002) are aspects of a more complex topography of subtle 3D changes in shape that affects the lower/mid-face. Patients with schizophrenia of either gender were characterised as follows: along the dorsal-ventral axis there are altered proportions in its anterior aspect, with lengthening of lower mid-facial height (i.e. between the chin and base of the nose) and shortening of upper mid-facial height (i.e. between base and bridge of the nose); along the medial-lateral axis there is widening in its posterior aspect; along the anterior-posterior axis there is posterior displacement of the bridge of the nose. It should be noted that the present 3D geometric analysis is conceptually different from that involving interlandmark distances, and that quantitative comparisons between them cannot be made. Studies in patients and controls using 3D laser surface scanning, which allows resolution of at least 24 landmark coordinates (Hennessy et al. 2002), would be an important next step in this approach.

Self-evidently, there are differences in facial shape between normal males and females (Enlow and Hans 1996) which, though they underpin fundamental aspects of human behaviour, have only recently been resolved in 3D (Hennessy et al. 2002); in particular, females have a generally wider face, shortened lower mid-facial height, lengthened upper mid-facial height, and bridge of the nose located posteriorly relative to males. Thus, a dysmorphogenic process in schizophrenia would be expected to exert some differential effects between males and females given gender differences in the substrate on which it acts. Abnormalities of 3D craniofacial shape in patients that differed between the genders were indeed encountered: the lower mid-face is rotated differentially such that the base of the nose is more anterior in female patients but more posterior in male patients.

Developmental biology of cerebral-craniofacial morphogenesis

The present 3D findings provide substance for and elaborate on our previous notions, deriving from classical, qualitative findings such as heightening of the palate reported in all but one study (Lane et al. 1996; McNeil et al. 2000; but see McGrath et al. 2002) together with linear measurements (Lane et al. 1997). Thus, in schizophrenia, craniofacial dysmorphogenesis appears to reflect not a diversity of abnormalities in linear measurements but, rather, some subtle enhancement in a well described, critical 3D trajectory of embryonic-fetal craniofacial growth, particularly along the midline, during which there is:

▎ vertical growth of the anterior mid-facial (frontonasal) region;
▎ narrowing of the frontonasal prominences;
▎ primary palate formation;
▎ dissociation of cranial base width from anterior facial changes; and
▎ vertical separation of the brain and face, with the face growing forward more rapidly than is the brain.

As the developmental biology of the craniofacies is understood much better than that of the brain, these events may be informative as to the timing of the developmental disturbance; thus, events would appear to disrupt the establishment of fundamental aspects of craniofacial shape over a time-frame that has extreme limits of 6–19 weeks, but within which the strongest common denominator would appear to implicate dysmorphogenic events acting over weeks 9/10 through 14/15 of gestation (Cohen et al. 1993; Diewert and Loza-noff, 1993 a, b; Diewert et al. 1993; Waddington 1999 a, b; Liebermann et al. 2000 a, b); thereafter, the craniofacies continue to evolve over later gestation, childhood and adolescence, particularly in terms of overall growth, to attain adult form (Enlow and Hans 1996; Hennessy et al. 2002).

More specifically, in accordance with emergent understanding of general 3D regulation of development (Hao et al. 2001), there is now recognised to be an exquisite embryological intimacy with which morphogenesis of the frontonasal prominences, forebrain and anterior midline cerebral regions are regulated via epithelial-mesenchymal signalling interactions; for example, rather than pre-vious notions of the brain as a scaffold on which the face develops, the nas-cent forebrain, neuroepithelium, neural crest and especially facial ectoderm, from which the present soft tissue measurements derive, function as a devel-opmental unit in terms of 3D gene expression domains (Kjaer 1995; Diewert and Lozanoff 1993 a, b; Diewert et al. 1993; Schneider et al. 2001; Nopoulos et al. 2002), with posterior cerebral and craniofacial development being related less intimately and regulated by alternative mechanisms (Kjaer 1995; Brault et al. 2001; Wilkie and Morriss-Kay 2001). Similarly, cranial base morphogenesis has important interactions with neurocranial and craniofacial shape; for exam-ple, cranial base dimensions influence the magnitude and direction of rotation in the lower mid-face in the sagittal plane, with the nascent middle cranial fossa, which determines cranial base width, and the temporal lobes constitut-ing an interactive developmental unit (Lieberman et al. 2000 a, b).

Thus, the present topography of disruption to craniofacial morphogenesis over this period would be compatible, both embryologically and topographi-cally, with disruption to morphogenesis of cerebral regions for which structural brain pathology has been reported in schizophrenia; these include abnormali-ties of the forebrain, not just of the frontal cortex but also of temporal lobe structures which over early fetal life emerge in the forebrain before rotating to their final location, together with thalamic and other midline structures (Moj-silovic and Zecevic 1991; Diewert et al. 1993; Kostovic et al. 1993; Arnold and Trojanowski 1996; Kier et al. 1997; Waddington et al. 1999 a, b; Arnold and Rioux 2001). Furthermore, such dysmorphogenesis along the anterior midline would be expected to result in disruption to neuroectodermal patterning and to critical repulsive and attractive guidance cues that regulate neuronal con-nectivity (Chang et al. 2000; Giger and Kolodkin 2001), in accordance with models of developmentally-determined disconnectivity in a fronto-striato-pallido-thalamo-cortical/fronto-temporal network (Weinberger 1995; Bullmore et al. 1998; Andreasen 2000; Waddington and Morgan 2001).

Developmental biology of asymmetry in cerebral-craniofacial morphogenesis

However, the present findings point towards more fundamental aspects of dys-morphogenesis. Craniofacial dysmorphology in schizophrenia was found to in-clude prominent asymmetries about the midline (actually, in 3D about the mid-sagittal plane), in a gender-related manner. In schizophrenia, there is a material body of evidence for decreases in normal cerebral asymmetries in terms of handedness, language lateralisation and brain anatomy, particularly, but not exclusively, in relation to temporal lobe structures (Crow 2000, 2002; Sommer et al. 2001; Selemon 2001). Gender differences in normal cerebral asymmetries are recognised, with females appearing generally less asymmetric than males (Good et al. 2001; Gorlin 2001); a similar effect of gender was noted here in relation to 3D craniofacial shape asymmetry, in elaboration of a classical literature (Perrett et al. 1999). Though many studies in schizophrenia have involved exclusively or predominantly male subjects or do not present data by gender (Sommer et al. 2001), some data do suggest that disruption of asymmetries in schizophrenia occurs in a gender-related manner (Crow 2000, 2002; Selemon 2001; Goldstein et al. 2002). Critically, the present pattern of findings (male controls evidencing marked directional asymmetry, with male patients characterised by moderate directional asymmetry; female controls evidencing little directional asymmetry, with female patients characterised by marked directional asymmetry) is identical with that described previously (Reite et al. 1997) in terms of lateralisation, in the transverse gyri of Heschl on the superior temporal gyri, of the generator of M100 auditory-evoked field components using magnetoencephalography-based source imaging; this would indicate, at the level of gender-specific asymmetries, the intimacy of cerebro-craniofacial relationships in schizophrenia as a consequence of dysmorphogenic events.

Further interpretation of these relationships in schizophrenia derives from contemporary understanding of the developmental biology of asymmetry. Classically, it is well recognised that the *left-right* axis is a categorical, decision-type axis that is to be distinguished from the continuous, gradient-type nature of its *anteroposterior* and *dorsoventral* counterparts (Cohen 2001). Over the past several years, it has become apparent that this process is critically dependent on asymmetric gene expression. In relation to visceral asymmetries, specific genes are expressed in the left lateral plate mesoderm, while others restrict the expression of these left determinants on the right by acting as a midline barrier, which may regulate also additional, parallel pathways of left-right morphogenesis mediated via N-cadherin-mediated cell adhesion; though abnormalities of visceral asymmetry do not appear to be present in schizophrenia, development of cerebral and visceral asymmetries appear to be controlled by mechanisms which overlap but have distinct domains, with the anterior extent of this midline barrier appearing involved particularly in determining cerebral asymmetries (Yost 1998; Kennedy et al. 1999; Bamford et al. 2000; Bisgrove et al. 2000; Garcia-Castro et al. 2000; Schneider and Brueckner 2000).

The human cerebral hemispheres originate from the midline and become delineated at about 6–8 weeks, with the molecular events underlying cerebral asymmetries acting up to 20 weeks (Geschwind and Miller 2001) and peaking at 15–18 weeks (McCartney and Hepper 1999). On this basis, the present topography of craniofacial dysmorphology in schizophrenia along the anterior extent of the midline, most likely established between weeks 9/10 through 14/15, might be expected to result in disruption to the establishment of cerebral-craniofacial asymmetries; however, molecular mechanisms which might mediate these effects and gender differences therein remain to be specified (Hennessy et al. 2003).

Heterogeneity vs homogeneity in schizophrenia

There remains a critical question as to whether such embryonic-fetal dysmorphogenesis in schizophrenia characterises a subgroup of patients who have a 'neurodevelopmental' form of the illness, or is a more homogeneous process characteristic of the majority of patients; while schizophrenia clearly evidences diversity in phenomenology, onset, course and outcome, it is critical to emphasis that *diversity* does not in itself indicate *heterogeneity* (Waddington and Scully 1999).

In relation to the most widely replicated and accepted biological finding in the brains of patients with schizophrenia, namely lateral ventricular enlargement, this is distributed unimodally in a manner similar to that in normal individuals, but the mean of this distribution is shifted significantly to the right (i.e. greater ventricular size); thus, ventricular enlargement appears to be a population phenomenon which occurs to varying extent in the majority of patients with schizophrenia, with no evidence for distinct subgroups having 'big' or 'normal' ventricles (Harvey et al. 1990; Daniel et al. 1991; Vita et al. 2000). The same profile was found for components of 3D craniofacial shape which distinguish patients with schizophrenia from normal individuals, indicating that dysmorphogenesis also appears to be a population phenonenon which occurs to varying extent in the majority of patients with schizophrenia, with no evidence for any subgroup without such developmental disturbance (Hennessy et al. 2003). Interestingly, over early fetal life, relative ventricular size reaches a maximum at 10–13 weeks, corresponding to the period over which the lateral ventricles have a particularly thin cerebral mantle, followed by subsequent regression (Lan et al. 2000; Kinoshita et al. 2001); thus, the ventricles might be particularly vulnerable to expansion through disruption to the cerebral mantle over the period in which cerebral-craniofacial dysmorphogenesis is most likely to occur in schizophrenia. There is evidence for reduced asymmetry of ventricular shape in schizophrenia, though gender was not considered (Buckley et al. 1999; Mardia et al. 2000).

This distributional analysis has been applied to other measures in schizophrenia, and consideration of the findings over a reverse time-line from chronic illness (i.e. on a 'read-back' basis; Waddington et al. 1999 a,b) reveals unimodal distributional shifts for reduced premorbid intellectual function in the teens (David et al. 1997; Davidson et al. 1999), reduced educational test scores in childhood (Jones et al. 1994), delayed infant developmental milestones (Jones et al. 1994; Isohanni et al. 2001), and a composite index of dysmorphology over the whole body (Lane et al. 1997). Thus, our findings (Hennessy et al. 2003) may 'root' these indices in a homogeneous process of dysmorphogenesis over weeks 9/10–14/15 when cerebral-craniofacial asymmetries are established in a gender-related manner.

A variant perspective should be entertained. Holoprosencephaly is a developmental disorder of incomplete forebrain separation and craniofacial dysmorphogenesis with the following characteristics (Ming and Muenke 2002):

- it is genetically heterogeneous, with several genes identified as associated with accumulating risk;

▮ it appears to show phenotypic variability due to the cumulative influence of multiple genetic and environmental effects over a critical time-frame of cerebral-craniofacial dysmorphogenesis;

▮ these effects converge on cellular components of a critical process in cerebral-craniofacial morphogenesis, such that heterogeneity of aetiology gives rise to homogeneity of pathobiology.

Several of these characteristics are compatible with our current understanding of schizophrenia and may hence indicate a potentially useful explanatory model.

▮ A lifetime developmental-'neuroprogressive' trajectory

It is important to emphasise that such developmental considerations imply no premature closure on the controversy as to whether/how schizophrenia might or might not 'progress' over its adult phase (Weinberger 1995; Waddington et al. 1997, 1999 a, b; DeLisi 1997; Woods 1998); indeed, it has been argued that cerebral dysmorphogenesis, particularly that related to asymmetry, may be associated with regional vulnerability to 'neuroprogressive' processes (Geschwind and Miller 2001).

There are now several longitudinal MRI studies of cerebral structure in schizophrenia, focusing primarily on the period immediately following the first psychotic episode; these studies have identified prospectively some progressive changes, including further ventricular expansion and reductions in cortical grey matter, though few studies have included the same measures and the changes identified are not always consistent. However, a conceptual problem is the likelihood that some abnormalities in brain structure reflect early cerebral-craniofacial dysmorphogenesis, which may or may not 'progress' further following the onset of psychosis, while other abnormalities may reflect the impact of a 'progressive' process in brain regions that were either not subject to dysmorphogenesis or rendered vulnerable to a 'progressive' process by such dysmorphogenesis. One recent prospective study (Cahn et al. 2002) may illustrate the confluence of developmental and 'progressive' processes. Size of the third ventricle was enlarged at the first episode and did not increase further over the one-year period thereafter; this is the profile that might be expected of an abnormality having its origin in early developmental disruption along the midline. Conversely, cortical grey matter volume was unaltered at the first episode but decreased over the subsequent one-year period; this is the profile that might be expected of an abnormality having its basis in some 'progressive' process associated with the emergence of psychotic symptoms.

What sort of model might best encapsulate these ideas? We (Waddington et al. 1997, 1999 a, b; Waddington and Morgan 2001) and others (DeLisi 1997; Woods 1998) have favoured variants of a 'lifetime trajectory' model, the essentials of which are indicated in Fig. 2. The proposition is that schizophrenia has a fundamental basis in disruption to the normal developmental processes by which cerebral-craniofacial morphogenesis is conferred with aymmetries in

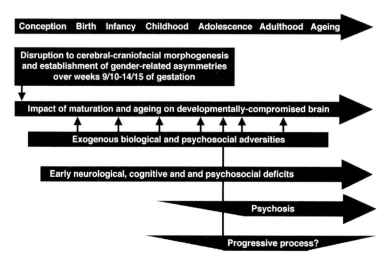

Fig. 2. Lifetime trajectory model for schizophrenia

a gender-related manner over weeks 9/10–14/15 of gestation. It is this developmentally compromised brain that serves as a substrate for the endogenous, programmed processes of later development, maturation and ageing; thus, the outcome of these processes may be altered because of the compromised substrate on which they act. Exogenous biological and psychosocial adversities may also impact on this developmentally compromised brain over the entire lifespan.

The consequences of this sequence and confluence of events are the neuro-integrative abnormalities of infancy, the cognitive and psychosocial deficits of childhood, and the subclinical psychotic ideation that precede the emergence of diagnostic psychotic symptoms in young adulthood. Over the period during which subclinical psychotic ideation evolves into diagnostic psychotic symptoms, there may be a heightening of some phasic, time-limited and poorly understood 'progressive' process that can be associated with accumulation of long-term impairment. Two major controversies and challenges for the field are

▌ the extent to which any such 'progressive' process might be ameliorated by early, effective intervention with antipsychotic and/or cognitive therapies to improve outcome in the long-term (McGlashan et al. 1999; Waddington et al. 1999 a, b; Norman and Malla 2001; McGorry 2002), and

▌ the extent to which these considerations might be relevant across the diagnostic continuum from non-affective to affective psychosis.

▌ **Acknowledgements.** The authors' studies are supported by the Stanley Medical Research Institute.

▌ References

Andreasen NC (2000) Schizophrenia: the fundamental questions. Brain Research Reviews 31:106–112

Arnold SE, Rioux L (2001) Challenges, status, and opportunities for studying developmental neuropathology in adult schizophrenia. Schizophrenia Bulletin 27:395–416

Arnold SE, Trojanowski JQ (1996) Human fetal hippocampal development: I. Cytoarchitecture, myeloarchitecture and neuronal morphologic features. Journal of Comparative Neurology 367:274–292

Baldwin PA, Scully PJ, Quinn JF, Morgan MG, Kinsella A, Owens JM, O'Callaghan E, Waddington JL (2003) Reduced rural incidence of schizophrenia is primarily a female phenomenon: the Cavan-Monaghan First episode study at seven years. Schizophrenia Research 60 (Suppl):33

Bamford RN, Roessler E, Burdine RD, Saplakogu U, de la Cruz J, Splitt M, Towbin J, Bowers P, Marino B, Schier AF, Shenn MM, Muenke M, Casey B (2000) Loss-of-function mutations in the EGF-CFC gene CFC1 are associated with human left-right laterality defects. Nature Genetics 26:365–369

Bisgrove BW, Essner JJ, Yost HJ (2000) Multiple pathways in the midline regulate concordant brain, heart and gut left-right asymmetry. Development 127:3567–3579

Brault V, Moore R, Kutsch S, Ishibashi M, Rowitch DH, McMahon AP, Sommer L, Boussadia O, Kemler R (2001) Inactivation of the β-catenin gene by Wnt1-Cre-mediated deletion results in dramatic brain malformation and failure of craniofacial development. Development 128:1253–1264

Buckley PF, Dean D, Bookstein FL, Friedman L, Kwon D, Lewin JS, Kamath J, Lys C (1999) Three-dimensional magnetic resonance-based morphometrics and ventricular dysmorphology in schizophrenia. Biological Psychiatry 45:62–67

Bullmore ET, Woodruff PW, Wright IC, Rabe-Hesketh S, Howard RJ, Shuriquie N, Murray RM (1998) Does dysplasia cause anatomical dysconnectivity in schizophrenia?. Schizophrenia Research 10:127–135

Cahn W, Hulshoff Pol HE, Lems EBTE, van Haren NEM, Schnack HG, van der Linden JA, Schothorst PF, van Engeland H, Kahn RS (2002) Brain volume changes in first-episode schizophrenia. Archives of General Psychiatry 59:1002–1010

Chang J, Kim OI, Ahn JS, Kwon JS, Jeon S-H, Kim SH (2000) The CNS midline cells coordinate proper cell cycle progression and identity determination of the drosophila ventral neuroectoderm. Developmental Biology 227:307–323

Cohen MM (2001) Asymmetry: molecular, biologic, embryopathic and clinical perspectives. American Journal of Medical Genetics 101:292–314

Cohen SR, Chen L, Trotman CA, Burdi AR (1993) Soft-palate myogenesis: a developmental field paradigm. Cleft Palate-Craniofacial Journal 30:441–446

Crow TJ (1995) A continuum of psychosis: one human gene, and not much else – the case for homogeneity. Schizophrenia Research 17:135–145

Crow TJ (2000) Schizophrenia as the price that Homo Sapiens pays for language: a resolution of the central paradox in the origin of the species. Brain Research Reviews 31:118–129

Crow TJ (2002) Handedness, language lateralisation and anatomical asymmetry: relevance of protocadherin XY to hominid speciation and the aetiology of psychosis. British Journal of Psychiatry 181:295–297

Daniel DG, Goldberg TE, Gibbons RD, Weinberger DR (1991) Lack of a bimodal distribution of ventricular size in schizophrenia. Biological Psychiatry 30:887–903

David AS, Malmberg A, Brandt L, Allebeck P, Lewis G (1997) IQ and risk for schizophrenia: a population-based cohort study. Psychological Medicine 27:1311–1323

Davidson M, Reichenberg A, Rabinowitz J, Weiser M, Kaplan A, Mark M (1999) Behavioural and intellectual markers for schizophrenia in apparently healthy male adolescents. American Journal of Psychiatry 156:1328–1335

DeLisi LE (1997) Is schizophrenia a lifetime disorder of brain plasticity, growth and aging? Schizophrenia Research 23:119–129

DeMyer W, Zeman W, Palmer CG (1964) The face predicts the brain. Pediatrics 34: 256–263

Diewert VM, Lozanoff S (1993 a) A morphometric analysis of human embryonic craniofacial growth in the median plane during primary palate formation. Journal of Craniofacial Genetics and Developmental Biology 13:147–161

Diewert VM, Lozanoff S (1993 b) Growth and morphogenesis of the human embryonic midface during primary palate formation analyzed in frontal sections. Journal of Craniofacial Genetics and Developmental Biology 13:162–183

Diewert VM, Lozanoff S, Choy V (1993) Computer reconstructions of human embryonic craniofacial morphology showing changes in relations between the face and brain during primary palate formation. Journal of Craniofacial Genetics and Developmental Biology 13:193–201

Enlow DH, Hans MG (1996) Essentials of Facial Growth. WB Saunders, Philadelphia

Garcia-Castro MI, Vielmetter E, Bronner-Fraser M (2000) N-Cadherin, a cell adhesion molecule involved in establishment of embryonic left-right asymmetry. Science 288:1047–1051

Geschwind DH, Miller BL (2001) Molecular approaches to cerebral laterality: development and neurodegeneration. American Journal of Medical Genetics 101:370–381

Giger RJ, Kolodkin AL (2001) Silencing the siren: guidance cue hierarchies at the CNS midline. Cell 105:1–4

Goldstein JM, Seidman LJ, O'Brien LM, Horton NJ, Kenned DN, Makris N, Caviness VS, Faraone SV, Tsuang MT (2002) Impact of normal sexual dimorphisms on sex differences in structural brain abnormalities in schizophrenia assessed by magnetic resonance imaging. Archives of General Psychiatry 59:154–164

Good CD, Johnsrude I, Ashburner J, Henson RNA, Friston KJ, Frackowiak RSJ (2001) Cerebral asymmetry and the effects of sex and handedness on brain structure: a voxel based morphometric analysis of 465 normal adult human brains. NeuroImage 14:685–700

Gorlin RJ (2001) Asymmetry. American Journal of Medical Genetics 101:290–291

Hao JC, Yu TW, Fujisawa K, Culotti JG, Gengyo-Ano K, Mitani S, Moulder G, Barstead R, Tessier-Lavigne M, Bargmann CI (2001) C. elegans slit acts in midline, dorsal-ventral, and anterior-posterior guidance via SAX-3/Robo receptor. Neuron 32:25–38

Harrison PJ (1999) The neuropathology of schizophrenia. Brain 122:593–624

Harvey I, McGuffin P, Williams M, Toone BK (1990) The ventricular-brain ratio (VBR) in functional psychoses: an admixture analysis. Psychiatry Research (Neuroimaging) 35:61–69

Hennessy RJ, Kinsella A, Waddington JL (2002) 3D laser surface scanning and geometric morphometric analysis of craniofacial shape as an index of cerebro-craniofacial morphogenesis: initial application to sexual dimorphism. Biological Psychiatry 51:507–514

Hennessy RJ, Lane A, Kinsella A, Larkin C, O'Callaghan E, Waddington JL (2004) 3D morphometrics of craniofacial dysmorphology reveals sex-specific asymmetries in schizophrenia. Schizophrenia Research (in press)

Isohanni M, Jones PB, Moilanen K, Rantakallio P, Veijola J, Oja H, Koiranen M, Joke-lainen J, Croudace T, Jarvelin M (2001) Early developmental milestones in adult schizophrenia and other psychoses. A 31-year follow-up of the Northern Finland 1966 birth cohort. Schizophrenia Research 52:1–19

Jones P, Rodgers B, Murray R, Marmot M (1994) Child development risk factors for adult schizophrenia in the British 1946 birth cohort. Lancet 344:1398–1402

Kennedy DN, O'Craven KM, Ticho BS, Goldstein AM, Makris N, Henson JW (1999) Structural and functional brain asymmetries in human situs inversus totalis. Neurology 53:1260–1265

Kier EL, Kim JH, Fulbright RK, Bronen RA (1997) Embryology of the human fetal hippocampus: MR imaging, anatomy and histology. American Journal of Neuroradiology 18:525–532

Kinoshita Y, Okodera T, Tsuru E, Yokota A (2001) Volumetric analysis of the germinal matrix and lateral ventricles performed using MR images of postmortem fetuses. American Journal of Neuroradiology 22:382–388

Kjaer I (1995) Human prenatal craniofacial development related to brain development under normal and pathological conditions. Acta Odontologica Scandinavica 53: 135–143

Kostovic I, Petanjek Z, Judas M (1993) Early areal differentiation of the human cerebral cortex: entorhinal area. Hippocampus 3:447–458

Lan LM, Yamashita Y, Tang Y, Sugahara T, Takahashi M, Ohba T, Okamura H (2000) Normal fetal brain development: MR imaging with a half-Fourier rapid acquisition with relaxation enhancement sequence. Radiology 215:205–210

Lane A, Larkin C, Waddington JL, O'Callaghan E (1996) Dysmorphic features and schizophrenia. In: Waddington JL, Buckley PF (eds) The Neurodevelopmental Basis of Schizophrenia. Landes, Georgetown, pp 79–93

Lane A, Kinsella A, Murphy P, Byrne M, Keenan J, Colgan K, Cassidy B, Sheppard N, Horgan R, Waddington JL, Larkin C, O'Callaghan E (1997) The anthropometric assessment of dysmorphic features in schizophrenia as an index of its developmental origins. Psychological Medicine 27:1155–1164

Lieberman DE, Pearson OM, Mowbray KM (2000a) Basicranial influence on overall cranial shape. Journal of Human Evolution 38:291–315

Lieberman DE, Ross CF, Ravosa MJ (2000b) The primate cranial base: ontogeny, function and integration. Yearbook of Physical Anthropology 43:117–169

Mardia KV, Bookstein FL, Moreton I (2000) Statistical assessment of bilateral symmetry of shapes. Biometrika 87:285–300

McCartney G, Hepper P (1999) Development of lateralized behavior in the human fetus from 12 to 27 weeks' gestation. Developmental Medicine and Child Neurology 41:83–86

McGlashan TH (1999) Duration of untreated psychosis in first-episode schizophrenia: marker or determinant of course? Biological Psychiatry 46:899–907

McGorry PD (2002) Early psychosis reform: too fast or too slow? Acta Psychiatrica Scandinavica 106:249–251

McGrath JC, El-Saadi O, Grim V, Cardy S, Chapple B, Chant D, Lieberman D, Mowry B (2002) Minor physical anomalies and quantitative measures of the head and face in psychosis. Archives of General Psychiatry 59:458–464

McNeil TF, Cantor-Graae E, Ismail B (2000) Obstetric complications and congenital malformation in schizophrenia. Brain Research Reviews 31:166–178

Ming JE, Muenke M (2002) Multiple hits during early embryonic development: digenic diseases and holoprosencephaly. American Journal of Human Genetics 71:1017–1032

Mojsilovic J, Zecevic N (1991) Early development of the human thalamus: Golgi and Nissl study. Early Human Development 27:119–144

Nopoulos P, Berg S, Canady J, Richman L, Van Demark D, Andreasen N (2002) Structural brain abnormalities in adult males with clefts of the lip and/or palate. Genetics in Medicine 4:1–9

Norman RM, Malla AK (2001) Duration of untreated psychosis: a critical examination of the concept and its importance. Psychological Medicine 31:381–400

O'Higgins P (2000) The study of morphological variation in the hominid fossil record: biology, landmarks and geometry. Journal of Anatomy 197:103–120

Perrett DI, Burt DM, Penton-Voak IS, Lee KJ, Rowland DA, Edwards R (1999) Symmetry and human facial attractiveness. Evolution and Human Behaviour 20:295–307

Quinn J, Hennessy RJ, Lane A, Scully PJ, Kinsella A, Owens JM, Waddington JL (2002) Schizophrenia, schizoaffective and bipolar disorder compared by 3-dimensional reconstruction and analysis of craniofacial morphology. Schizophrenia Research 53 (Suppl):245–246

Quinn J, Scully PJ, Kinsella A, Owens JM, Waddington JL (2003) Neurological soft signs in schizophrenia, schizoaffective and bipolar disorder: diagnosis, asymmetry and gender. Schizophrenia Research 60 (Suppl):25

Reite M, Sheeder J, Teale P, Adams M, Richardson D, Simon J, Jones RH, Rojas DC (1997) Magnetic source imaging evidence of sex differences in cerebral lateralization in schizophrenia. Archives of General Psychiatry 54:433–440

Schneider H, Brueckner M (2000) Of mice and men: dissecting the genetic pathway that controls left-right asymmetry in mice and humans. American Journal of Medical Genetics 97:258–270

Schneider RA, Hu D, Rubenstein JLR, Maden M, Helms JA (2001) Local retinoid signaling coordinates forebrain and facial morphogenesis by maintaining FGF8 and SHH. Development 128:2755–2767

Scully PJ, Owens JM, Kinsella A, Waddington JL (2001) Factor structure of psychopathology: generic 'psychosis' vs diversity between diagnostic boundaries among an epidemiologically complete population. Schizophrenia Research 49 (Suppl):22

Scully PJ, Quinn JF, Morgan MG, Kinsella A, O'Callaghan E, Owens JM, Waddington JL (2002) First episode schizophrenia, bipolar disorder and other psychoses in a rural Irish catchment area: incidence and gender in the Cavan-Monaghan study at 5 years. British Journal of Psychiatry 181 (Suppl 43):s3–s9

Scully PJ, Owens JM, Kinsella A, Waddington JL (2004) Schizophrenia, schizoaffective and bipolar disorder within an epidemiologically complete, homogeneous population in rural Ireland: small area variation in rate. Schizophrenia Research (in press)

Selemon LD (2001) Regionally diverse cortical pathology in schizophrenia: clues to the etiology of the disease. Schizophrenia Bulletin 27:349–377

Smith DW (1988) Recognisable Patterns of Human Malformation. WB Saunders, Philadelphia

Sommer I, Aleman A, Ramsey N, Bouma A, Kahn R (2001) Handedness, language lateralisation and anatomical asymmetry in schizophrenia: meta analysis. British Journal of Psychiatry 178:344–351

Torrey EF, Knable MB (1999) Are schizophrenia and bipolar disorder one disease or two? Schizophrenia Research 39:93–163

Van Os J, Hanssen M, Bijl RV, Vollebergh W (2001) Prevalence of psychotic disorder and community level of psychotic symptoms. Archives of General Psychiatry 58:663–668

Verdoux H, van Os J (2002) Psychotic symptoms in non-clinical populations and the continuum of psychosis. Schizophrenia Research 54:59–65

Vita A, Dieci M, Silenzi C, Tenconi F, Giobbio GM, Invernizzi G (2000) Cerebral ventricular enlargement as a generalized feature of schizophrenia: a distribution analysis on 502 subjects. Schizophrenia Research 44:25–34

Waddington JL (2003) Schizophrenia and bipolar disorder as putative dopamine-linked illnesses: neurodevelopmental origins and lifetime trajectory. In: Sidhu A, Laruelle M, Vernier P (eds) Dopamine Receptors and Transporters: Function, Imaging and Clinical Implication. Marcel Dekker, New York, pp 403–420

Waddington JL, Morgan MG (2001) Pathobiology of schizophrenia. In: Lieberman JA., Murray RM (eds) Comprehensive Care of Schizophrenia. Martin Dunitz, London, pp 28–35

Waddington JL, Scully PJ (1999) Heterogeneity vs homogeneity in operationally-diagnosed schizophrenia. In: Maj M, Sartorius N (eds) Evidence and Experience in Psychiatry, Vol 2: Schizophrenia. John Wiley & Sons, Chichester, pp 50–52

Waddington JL, Scully PJ, Youssef HA (1997) Developmental trajectory and disease progression in schizophrenia. Schizophrenia Research 23:107–118

Waddington JL, Lane A, Scully PJ, Larkin C, O'Callaghan E (1998) Neurodevelopmental and neuroprogressive processes in schizophrenia. Psychiatric Clinics of North America 21:123–149

Waddington JL, Lane A, Larkin C, O'Callaghan E (1999 a) The neurodevelopmental basis of schizophrenia: clinical clues from cerebro-craniofacial dysmorphogenesis, and the roots of a lifetime trajectory of disease. Biological Psychiatry 46:31–39

Waddington JL, Lane A, Scully P, Meagher D, Quinn J, Larkin C, O'Callaghan E (1999 b) Early cerebro-craniofacial dysmorphogenesis in schizophrenia: a lifetime trajectory model from neurodevelopmental basis to 'neuroprogressive' process. Journal of Psychiatric Research 33:477–489

Weinberger DR (1995) Schizophrenia: from neuropathology to neurodevelopment. Lancet 346:552–557

Wilkie AOM, Morriss-Kay GM (2001) Genetics of craniofacial development and malformation. Nature Review Genetics 2:458–468

Woods BT (1998) Is schizophrenia a progressive neurodevelopmental disorder? Towards a unitary pathogenetic mechanism. American Journal of Psychiatry 155: 1661–1670

Yost HJ (1998) Left-right development from embryos to brains. Developmental Genetics 23:159–163

Section 6
Treatment

What can psychological treatments say about causes in schizophrenia?

Shôn W. Lewis and Richard J. Drake

School of Psychiatry and Behavioural Sciences, University of Manchester, Wythenshawe Hospital, Manchester, UK

Introduction

There is increasing interest in the possibility that specific and specifiable psychological treatments can be effective in reducing the symptoms of schizophrenia. What is the evidence for this and what might the amenability of core symptoms to psychological intervention tell us about mechanisms in the pathogenesis and maintenance of psychotic symptoms in schizophrenia?

Overview of the evidence

Evidence is now available to suggest that several specific types of psychological intervention are effective in improving certain outcomes in patients at various stages of the illness (Table 1).

The longest established, effective psychological intervention is family intervention in patients with established schizophrenia, where the family members are significant caregivers. The main outcome criterion in these studies has been relapse rates and, collectively, the data are interpreted as showing a good degree of clinical effectiveness (Butzlaff and Hooley 1998; Pharoah et al. 2002).

Individual cognitive behaviour therapy has generated now a sizeable body of evidence, although the first trials in this area were undertaken only 10 years ago. The accepted findings are that cognitive behaviour therapy, if delivered over a sustained period, will reduce positive and to some extent negative

Table 1. Established predictors of outcome and effective psychological interventions

Known prognostic factor	Psychological intervention
Family environment	Family intervention
Street drug use	Motivational interviewing (Barrowclough et al. 2001)
Adherence to drug treatment	Compliance therapy (Kemp et al. 1997)
Duration of untreated psychosis at onset; speed of remission	Cognitive behaviour therapy
Neurocognitive deficits	Cognitive remediation

symptoms in otherwise treatment, resistant schizophrenia. In these trials, as with all others so far, cognitive behaviour therapy has been delivered as an adjunct to drug treatment as usual. A convergence between independent randomised controlled trials in this patient group is striking. Four good quality trials (Tarrier et al. 1993; Kuipers et al. 1997; Sensky et al. 2000; Tarrier et al. 1998) have used similar inclusion criteria with similar experimental treatments in terms of content and duration. The trials have differed in other respects, particularly the selection and rationale of control interventions and the use or otherwise of blinded assessments of outcome. The effect size for improvement of positive symptoms in these trials is about 0.6. The effect of the intervention extends to improvement in negative symptoms and, in some circumstances, social functioning. In addition, the effect appears to be durable at 6–9 months post-treatment and beyond.

The patient population identified for these trials is closely similar to that used in the earlier clozapine efficacy studies and the effect size, according to systematic review, is not dissimilar (Wahlbeck et al. 2000). An important statistical issue here is that the population and the samples drawn for these trials are selected on the basis of having persistent and stable positive symptoms, so maximising the power of a trial to test the efficacy of an add on treatment. This statistical advantage may not be present when other patient populations are targeted such as first episode or acutely ill patients, or patients in remission open to relapse.

Cognitive remediation is a technique using neurocognitive learning and practice strategies to overcome the cognitive deficits that characterise particularly chronic schizophrenia. As such, the presumed mechanism is different from that underlying cognitive behaviour therapy. Although previous trials showed that patients were able to improve neurocognitive functioning to the rewarded practice, until recently it had not been shown that this improvement persisted, or generalised into effects on clinical status or functional status. Wykes et al. (1999, 2002), in a randomised trial, used techniques such as errorless learning (in which tasks are taught taking care to avoid the subject being confused by making mistakes), scaffolding (where strategies are demonstrated to subjects initially but gradually support is reduced) and massed practice (repeated exercises at least 3–5 times per week) to produce persistent gains in executive function, memory and self esteem, which generalised to social functioning.

∎ Methodological issues

The results of these trials have been taken up enthusiastically by a clinical community looking for alternative strategies to drug treatments, on the basis of their intellectual appeal. It is not surprising that people suffering from, or caring for, those with severe psychological symptoms should expect treatments based on primary psychological approaches to be available. However, it is important to recognise methodological limitations in this area, particularly those which might in some circumstances lead to a type 1 statistical error. In broad

Table 2. Design characteristics of a high quality psychological treatment trial

- Large, representative sample from clinically relevant, specified population
- Sample size justified by power calculation
- Independent, concealed randomisation
- Well specified intervention with fidelity independently assessed
- Outcome assessed blind to treatment allocation
- Reliable and valid primary outcome measure
- Intent to treat analysis with characterisation of dropouts

terms, these limitations can be divided into general design issues for randomised controlled trials, and those involving theoretical issues about the content of the treatment itself. These areas overlap.

The generally desirable features of a clinical trial are shown in Table 2. In general, it can be argued that the ground rules for establishing the effectiveness of psychological treatment should be no different from those used to establish effectiveness of pharmacological treatments. Moreover, it can be argued that the closer the design specifications and the choice of clinical outcomes between drug and non-drug trials, the more statements can be made comparing the two approaches.

Looking at specific issues, the use of a double blind design, as is the benchmark approach in phase III clinical trials of a drug treatment, are not possible with psychological treatments. This makes it more, rather than less, important that where blindness of outcome assessment is possible, it is used. There have been debates about whether or not it is possible to maintain a blind to treatment allocation when assessing outcome. Because of the known potency of the use of non-blind assessments in introducing bias, it is vital to attempt to use independent, blind assessments of outcome, with assessment of the quality of the blind if possible. In addition, the choice of outcomes should include those which are relatively impermeable to the effects of blindness, such as relapse, hospitalisation and instrumental outcomes such as employment status.

The choice of control group in these studies is also important. The choice should be based on the hypothesis of the study and take into account that, in general, psychological treatments are used in addition to treatment as usual, rather than an alternative. The hypothesis in this area is usually that cognitive behaviour therapy has a specific effect over and above a supportive counselling approach. Ideally, this means the use of two control groups, one controlling for non-specific effects of talking treatments (Lewis et al. 2002).

There has been a trend of late to focus on pragmatic trials in health care generally. These are trials which tend to be large with simple outcomes which solely address the question of effectiveness. It can be argued that in an area such as psychological treatments of psychosis it is vital to build into the trial design an explanatory component to test whether the hypothesised mechanism is actually that which mediates any effect. One example would be that the clinical effect of a psychological treatment is actually mediated inadvertently through another therapeutic mechanism, such as improved adherence to drug treatments. Another important issue specific to this area is replicability. With cognitive behaviour therapy, this typically involves a range of individual psychological techniques. It is important that the objective demonstration of treatment fidelity, that is that the treatment given adheres to a written procedural protocol, is measured and reported.

Mechanisms of action

In general, the aetiological model in schizophrenia which underlies this area is the stress-vulnerability model (Neuchterlein 1987). In this model, an underlying biological vulnerability to schizophrenia is necessary but not sufficient to produce the final phenotype. An environmental stressor acting more proximally to the psychosis is also necessary and this is often the focus of models of psychological intervention. What can the effectiveness of such interventions tell us directly or indirectly about pathogenetic mechanisms in psychosis, therefore? Simply because psychological treatment might be effective in reducing the symptoms of schizophrenia in no way negates the importance of biological mechanisms, in the same way that the efficacy of drug treatments might negate the possible importance of psychological factors. Several scenarios are possible.

▌ Protecting against risk factors, enhancing protective factors

Firstly, in some specific situations it is explicit that the psychological treatment is operating to enhance the effect of a known, external protective factor, or to reduce the effect of a known risk factor. An example of the former is the psychological intervention in so-called compliance therapy (Kemp et al. 1996, 1998). Here, the psychological intervention, based on motivational interviewing techniques, is aimed explicitly at enhancing the known protective effect of taking prescribed antipsychotic drug treatments. Kemp et al. (1998) used a form of therapy derived from motivational interviewing to enhance sufferers' adherence to medication. In a clinical trial, patients admitted for acute relapse were randomised to receive routine care or routine care plus a brief package of motivational interviewing, adapted for schizophrenia sufferers and concentrating on ways to treat symptoms, reduce problems and prevent relapse using antipsychotic medication. The experimental group showed clinically and statistically significant reduction in readmission rates and improvements in compliance over 18 months, and improvements in symptoms at the end of therapy but not after 18 months. Measurements of drug adherence were important in supporting the interpretation that this was the mechanism of action.

In the trial of motivational and family interventions in patients with schizophrenia and comorbid street drug use (Barrowclough et al. 2001; Haddock et al. in press), the focus of the psychological treatment was on a specific risk factor, this time the established link between street drug use and relapse (Linszen et al. 1994). The intervention was successful in reducing relapse rates at 12 months. Again, the measurement of presumed mediators allowed the investigators to state with confidence that the effect on outcome was indeed mediated through this hypothesised mechanism, in terms of a measurable reduction in street drug use.

In the second situation, the effects of cognitive behaviour therapy are once more mediated through the moderation of risk and protective factors, except this time these are not external but secondary aspects of psychopathology. The best example of this is the model of cognitive behaviour therapy based on coping strategy enhancement (Tarrier et al. 1993) in which the psychological treatment specifically accesses and aims to enhance strategies already developed by the individual to cope with continuing psychotic symptoms. Another example would be the use of psychological strategies to reduce anxiety and depression which usually exist along side primary psychotic symptoms and serve to maintain them. Again, the use of measures to assess independently these aspects of psychopathology in trials is important in trying to understand how these psychological techniques exert their effect.

The third scenario has potentially the most light to throw on pathogenetic mechanisms. Here, the psychological treatment has its focus on primary mechanisms which are hypothesised to be important in the generation and persistence of psychotic symptoms, in particular delusions and hallucinations. It has been claimed that the more behavioural elements have more effect than the cognitive elements.

▌ Primary cognitive mechanisms in psychosis

Cognitive models of how positive psychotic symptoms might arise have become well developed. The model outlined by Garety and colleagues (1999) explores the steps which might be involved and has some empirical basis (Fig. 1). The first step is the generation of anomalous conscious experiences. It supposes that some individuals are prone to such experiences as a result of a cognitive, information-processing trait. One such trait is that proposed by Hemsley (1993), where a weakened influence of stored memories of regularities of previous input gives rise to

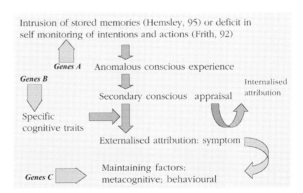

Fig. 1. Cognitive mechanisms in symptom formation

the experience of unfamiliarity to ordinarily mundane perceptions. Kapur (2003) has elaborated how dopaminergic mechanisms may play an important part in processes such as this. Another such general trait is that put forward by Frith (1992), where a deficit in the normal, automatic process of self monitoring of intentions and actions results in the misattribution of internally generated events to the external world. Either mechanism might play a part in producing the type of anomalous experience which recent epidemiological work has suggested are relatively frequent in the general community, appearing as non-syndromal, isolated hallucinatory phenomena, for example (Van Os and colleagues, this volume, section 1, chapter 4).

The next stage in the chain of cognitive events is the conscious appraisal by the individual of these anomalous phenomena. In most cases, the phenomena will be rejected as abnormal and put down to factors such as intoxication or fatigue. In some cases, the presence of a further set of cognitive traits will not allow this rejection. Garety includes in these traits the presence of an externalising attributional style; and/or deficits of social cognition, such as theory of mind; and/or a style of information processing, or information gathering, which reaches judgements on the basis of inadequate data, a style of "jumping to conclusions". The result is that, rather than being attributed correctly to internal events, the unusual phenomena begin to be attributed mistakenly to external agencies. This process may be made more likely, or accelerated, if the phenomena produce or occur in the context of states of distress or anxiety. The final stages involve consolidation and then maintenance of the newly formed psychotic phenomena, again involving a further set of cognitive traits, such as metacognitive appraisals of controllability and the adoption of safety behaviours which serve to perpetuate, rather than extinguish, the symptoms.

▌ The interface with biological risk factors

There are now replicated findings of a small number so far, perhaps three or four, of susceptibility genes for schizophrenia, each of small effect and associated with common haplotypes. In that the cognitive and information processing styles outlined in the cognitive model of symptom formation are likely each to be minor variations in normal cognitive function, it is likely that genetic effects will play a part, as identified in Fig. 1. One set of genes may regulate the processes of memory regulation or internal monitoring that predispose to, or protect against, the emergence of anomalous phenomena. A different set of genes will affect the secondary processes involved in appraisal of these phenomena and their rejection or otherwise. Further genetic influences and early environmental influences will act on the likelihood that the phenomena produce affective change, the efficiency of metacognitive processes, and so on, which determine the final phenomenological changes.

One potential route of investigation here is to link neurophysiological, neuropsychological and cognitive levels of pathology together. This offers the prize of powerful explanatory models of psychopathology that could guide development of drug therapy, psychological therapy or combinations of both.

For example, insight is one symptom that is central to schizophrenic psychopathology and practical treatment. One hypothesis, building on the work of Weinberger and colleagues, is that the neurocognitive impairments which contribute to poor insight are linked to the metabolism of catecholamines in the frontal lobes.

Catechol-O-methyl transferase (COMT) has two isoforms. *Methionine* COMT has about one quarter of the activity of *valine* COMT and Weinberger et al. (2001) have suggested that the former leaves more dopamine available at the synapse in the prefrontal cortex but not elsewhere, since COMT does not influence synaptic dopamine in the rest of the brain. Egan et al. (2001) showed that in 173 schizophrenia sufferers, and siblings and normal controls, there were small but significant differences in performance on the Wisconsin Card Sort Test (WCST; Heaton et al. 1993) depending on the isoform of COMT. The WCST is a set shifting task demanding of prefrontal cortex function. In this study, there was a progression from *val/val* homozygotes, through heterozygotes to *met/met* homozygotes: *met/met* subjects had fewest perseverative errors. FMR imaging of subjects performing an executive task showed that *val/val* homozygotes were less efficient than *met/met*. There is other evidence that this effect is specific for prefrontal and working memory tasks (Malhotra et al. 2002; Mattay et al. 2003). Though Bilder et al. (2003) found a weaker, less specific relationship, the tests they found most related to COMT allele were frontal, even if some frontal tests were unrelated.

How might this relate to insight? Poor global insight in schizophrenia has been related to perseveration on the WCST (Young et al. 1998; Alemin et al. 2003) but not to performance on other neuropsychological tests. Alemin's meta-analysis produced an estimated correlation of 0.23 between perseveration and poor insight. We found perseveration was the aspect of set shifting tests that best correlated with global insight (Spearman's coefficient 0.59) and insight into symptoms (Spearman's 0.68; Drake and Lewis 2003). Other groups' findings regarding this distinction, using the WCST, have been mixed (e.g. Lysaker et al. 1998; Laroi et al. 2000; David et al. 2003). Koren has also proposed (Koren et al. 2001; Viksman et al. 2002; Koren et al. 2003) that self assessment during the WCST is more strongly linked to insight into illness. His group used a modified form of the WCST to demonstrate correlations approaching 0.5 for awareness of illness with a measure of self monitoring and performance modification ("metacognition"), while finding lower correlation with perseveration.

Suppose that metacognition is a prefrontal function, and that COMT isoform influences synaptic dopamine levels in the prefrontal cortex and hence performance on the WCST. The WCST is not a very "clean" test of set-shifting and frontal function but alterations focussing on subjects' capacity to modify performance might strengthen this relationship because "metacognition" is a good test. In turn, the capacity to modify set shifting performance is then predictive of insight in schizophrenia. Therefore, poor insight will be related to COMT genotype via modified WCST performance, a testable hypothesis. Insight is a prime candidate for this type of association because of its demonstrated relationship with neuropsychological impairment. In addition, its relevance for psychological treatment is obvious but engagement with other forms of treatment is also connected.

▌ Psychological treatments at the onset of the disorder and before

Psychological treatments such as cognitive behaviour therapy have to date been aimed at ameliorating the severity of established, usually chronic, psychotic symptoms. If behavioural mechanisms such as the adoption of safety behaviours are important in the maintenance of psychotic symptoms, the behavioural component of CBT is likely to be important in reducing these mechanisms. In addition, these treatments will be given and evaluated in the presence of antipsychotic drug treatment. Potentially, there is more to be learnt both about whether and how psychological treatments work on the primary cognitive mechanisms in psychosis, if they can be shown to work at the presyndromal stage of the disorder, between stages 1 and 2 in Fig. 1, when symptoms are in the process of formation and consolidation, and before drug treatment is conventionally indicated.

Very early intervention in psychotic disorders has recently generated much interest, and a small number of studies have examined the possibility of detecting individuals in the prodromal stage, prior to the development of full psychosis. Yung and colleagues (1998) have pioneered the prodromal approach to prevention. They have developed operational criteria to identify four subgroups at ultra-high risk of incipient psychosis. They describe how 40% of their sample made the transition to psychosis over a nine-month period. The improved ability to accurately define high risk has led some researchers to attempt to prevent psychosis with atypical antipsychotic medication and cognitive behaviour therapy. In a recent study, McGorry and colleagues (McGorry et al. 2002) found that specific pharmacotherapy and psychotherapy reduced the risk of early transition to psychosis in young people at ultra-high risk, in comparison with supportive therapy and case management, finding a reduction in progression to psychosis at the end of treatment, but not at follow-up. However, the relative contribution of psychotherapy could not be determined since theirs was a combined treatment.

In order to determine whether the use of psychological intervention could prevent transition to psychosis, Morrison et al. (2002) hypothesised that CBT would significantly reduce the transition rate at the end of treatment, in comparison with the treatment as usual group. In a controlled trial, of 58 participants that met criteria for being high risk according to the Yung et al. (1998) criteria, 33 were randomly allocated to CBT and 25 to a monitoring control. No participants had received antipsychotic medication at baseline. Participants were assessed for suitability and monitored on a monthly basis using the PANSS (Kay et al. 1987), which was also used to determine transition. Of the 58, 47 of the participants were recruited on the basis of attenuated psychotic symptoms.

An interim analysis included all patients, but only 38 had been followed up for the full 12 months (the rest had all been followed up for at least 6 months). Rates of PANSS-defined transition were as follows: 2 of 33 patients allocated to CT made transition (6%) and 4 of 25 patients allocated to monitoring made transition (16%). A logistic regression, with PANSS-defined transition to psychosis as the dependent variable was done. Predictor variables that were entered into the equation included treatment group (CT or monitoring), age, gender, family history of psychosis and initial PANSS positive symptom subscale total at baseline. This analysis showed that there were trends towards initial PANSS positive score (B = 0.48, p = 0.06), age (B = 0.21, p = 0.05) and treatment group (B = 0.32, p = 0.06) contributing to transition.

These results suggest that cognitive therapy may be effective, during the active treatment phase, in reducing transition to psychosis in a high-risk group. This is the first study to suggest that CBT alone may prevent or delay progression to psychosis in the absence of drug treatment. Over the next five years, this new paradigm is likely to throw light on the cognitive mechanisms underlying the emergence and progression of psychotic symptoms in schizophrenia.

▮ References

Agrawal N, Aleman A, Morgan KD, David AS (2003) Insight in psychosis and neuropsychological function: a meta-analysis. Schizophrenia Research 60(1)(Suppl 1): 120

Barrowclough C, Haddock G, Tarrier N, Lewis SW, Moring J, O'Brien R, Schofield N, McGovern J (2001) Randomized controlled trial of motivational interviewing, cognitive behavior therapy, and family intervention for patients with comorbid schizophrenia and substance use disorders. Am J Psychiatry 158(10):1706–1713

Bilder RM, Volavka J, ál Czobor P, Malhotra AK, Kennedy JL, Ni X, Goldman RS, Hoptman MJ, Sheitman B, Lindenmayer JP, Citrome L, McEvoy JP, Kunz M, Chakos M, Cooper TB, Lieberman JA (2003) Neurocognitive correlates of the COMT Val[158] Met polymorphism in chronic schizophrenia. Biological Psychiatry 52(7): 701–707

Butzlaff RL, Hooley JM (1998) Expressed emotion and psychiatric relapse: a meta-analysis. Arch Gen Psychiatry 55(6):547–552

Drake RJ, Lewis SW (2003) Insight and neurocognition in acute schizophrenia and related disorders. Schizophrenia Research 62(1/2):165–173

Egan MF, Goldberg TE, Kolachana BS, Callicott JH, Mazzanti CM, Straub RE, Goldman D, Weinberger DR (2001) Effect of COMT Val[108/158] Met genotype on frontal lobe function and risk for schizophrenia. Proc Natl Acad Sci USA 98(12):6917–6922

Frith CD (1992) The cognitive neuropsychology of schizophrenia. LEA press, Hove, UK

Garety P, Kuipers E, Fowler D, Freeman D, Bebbington P (2001) A cognitive model of the positive symptoms of psychosis. Psychological Medicine 31:189–195

Haddock G, Barrowclough C, Tarrier N, Moring J, O'Brien R, Schofield N, Quinn J, Palmer S, Davies L, Lowens I, McGovern J, Lewis S (2003) Cognitive-behavioural therapy and motivational intervention for schizophrenia and substance misuse. 18-month outcomes of a randomised controlled trial. Br J Psychiatry 183:418–426

Heaton RK, Chelune GJ, Talley JL, Kay GG, Curtiss G (1993) Wisconsin Card Sorting Test Manual (Psychological Assessment Resources, Odessa, FL)

Hemsley DR (1993) A simple (or simplistic?) cognitive model for schizophrenia. Behaviour Research and Therapy 31:633–645

Kay SR, Opler LA (1987) The Positive and Negative Syndrome Scale (PANSS) for schizophrenia. Schizophrenia Bulletin 13:507–518

Kemp R, Hayward P, Applethwaite G, Everritt B, David A (1996) Compliance therapy in psychotic patients: randomised controlled trial. BMJ 312:345–349

Kemp R, Kirov G, Everitt B, Hayward P, David A (1998) Randomised controlled trial of compliance therapy: 18-month follow-up. British Journal of Psychiatry 172:413–419

Koren D, Seidman LJ, Poyurovski M, Viksman P, Balush V, Goldsmith M, Klein E (2003) Insight in first-episode schizophrenia: a metacognitive neuropsychological study. Schizophrenia Research 60(1)(Suppl 1):173–174

Kuipers E, Garety P, Fowler D, Dunn G, Bebbington P, Freeman D, Hadley C (1997) The London-East Anglia randomised controlled trial of cognitive-behavioural therapy for psychosis. I. Effects of the treatment phase. British Journal of Psychiatry 171:319–327

Laroi F, Fannemel M, Ronneberg U, Flekkoy K, Opjordsmoen S, Dullerud R, Haakonsen M (2000) Unawareness of illness in chronic schizophrenia and its relationship to structural brain measures and neuropsychological tests. Psychiatry Res 100(1):49–58

Lewis S, Tarrier N, Haddock G, Bentall R, Kinderman P, Kingdon D, Siddle R, Drake R, Everitt J, Leadley K, Benn A, Grazebrook K, Haley C, Akhtar S, Davies L, Palmer S, Faragher B, Dunn G (2002) Randomised controlled trial of cognitive-behavioural therapy in early schizophrenia: acute-phase outcomes. British Journal of Psychiatry 181 (Suppl 43):91–97

Linszen DH, Dingemans PM, Lenior ME (1994) Cannabis abuse and the course of recent-onset schizophrenic disorders. Archives of General Psychiatry 51(4):273–279

Lysaker PH, Bell MD, Bryson G, Kaplan E (1998) Neurocognitive function and insight in schizophrenia: support for an association with impairments in executive function but not with impairments in global function. Acta Psychiatr Scand 97(4):297–301

Malhotra AK, Kestler LJ, Mazzanti C, Bates JA, Goldberg T, Goldman D (2002) A functional polymorphism in the COMT gene and performance on a test of prefrontal cognition. Am J Psychiatry 159:652–654

Mattay VS, Goldberg TE, Fera F, Hariri AR, Tessitore A, Egan MF, Kolachana B, Callicott JH, Weinberger DR (2003) Catechol O-methyltransferase val158-met genotype and individual variation in the brain response to amphetamine. Proc Natl Acad Sci USA 13; 100(10):6186–6191

McGorry PD, Yung AR, Phillips LJ et al (2002) Randomised controlled trial of interventions designed to reduce the risk of progression to first-episode psychosis in a clinical sample with subthreshold symptoms. Archives of General Psychiatry 59:921–928

Morrison AP, Bentall RP, French P, Kilcommons A, Walford L, Lewis SW (2002) A randomised controlled trial of early detection and cognitive therapy for preventing transition to psychosis in high risk individuals: study design and interim analysis of transition rate and psychological risk factors. British Journal of Psychiatry 181 (Suppl 43):78–84

Mueser KT, Berenbaum H (1990) Psychodynamic treatment of schizophrenia: is there a future? Psychol Med 20:253–262

Pharoah FM, Mari JJ, Streiner D (2000) Family intervention for schizophrenia. Cochrane Database Syst Rev (2):CD000088

Rossell SL, Coakes J, Shapleske J, Woodruff PW, David AS (2003) Insight: its relationship with cognitive function, brain volume and symptoms in schizophrenia. Psychol Med 3(1):111–119

Sellwood W, Barrowclough C, Tarrier N, Quinn J, Mainwaring J, Lewis SW (2001) Needs-based cognitive-behavioural family intervention for carers of patients suffering from schizophrenia: 12-month follow-up. Acta Psychiatr Scand 104(5):346–355

Sensky T, Turkington T, Kingdon D, Scott JL, Scott J, Siddle R, O'Carroll M, Barnes TRE (2000) A randomised, controlled trial of cognitive behaviour therapy for persistent positive symptoms in schizophrenia resistant to medication. Archives of General Psychiatry 57:165–173

Tarrier N, Sharpe L, Beckett R, Harwood S, Baker A, Yusopoff L (1993) A trial of two cognitive behavioural methods of treating drug-resistant residual psychotic symptoms in schizophrenic patients. II. Treatment-specific changes in coping and problem-solving skills. Soc Psychiatry Psychiatr Epidemiol 28(1):5–10

Tarrier N, Yusopoff L, Kinney C et al (1998) Randomised controlled trial of intensive cognitive behaviour therapy for patients with chronic schizophrenia. BMJ 317: 303–307

Viksman P, Poyurovsky M, Balush V, Levy A, Fuchs E, Eytan Y, Burzstein C, Goldsmith M, Koren D (2002) Metacognition in first episode schizophrenia: its relationship to theory of mind and executive functioning. Schizophrenia Research 53 (3):137

Wahlbeck K, Cheine M, Essali MA (2000) Clozapine versus typical neuroleptic medication for schizophrenia. Cochrane Database Syst Rev (2):CD000059

Weinberger DR, Egan MF, Bertolino A, Callicott JH, Mattay VS, Lipska BK, Berman KF, Goldberg TE (2001) Neurobiology of schizophrenia and the role of atypical antipsychotics. Biol Psychiatry 50:825–844

Wykes T, Reeder C, Corner J, Williams C, Everitt B (1999) The effects of neurocognitive remediation on executive processing in patients with schizophrenia. Schizophrenia Bulletin 25(2):291–307

Wykes T, Reeder C, Williams C et al (2002) Are the effects of cognitive remediation therapy (CRT) durable? Results from an exploratory trial. Schizophrenia Res (in press)

Yung A, Phillips LJ, McGorry PD et al (1998) A step towards indicated prevention of schizophrenia. British Journal of Psychiatry 172 (Suppl 33):14–20

Sensky T, Turkington T, Kingdon D, Scott JL, Scott J, Siddle R, O'Carroll M, Barnes TRE (2000) A randomised, controlled trial of cognitive behaviour therapy for persistent positive symptoms in schizophrenia resistant to medication. Archives of General Psychiatry 57:165–173

Young DA, Zakzanis KK, Bailey C, Davila R, Griese J, Sartory G, Thom A (1998) Further parameters of insight and neuropsychological deficit in schizophrenia and other chronic mental disease. J Nerv Ment Dis 186(1):44–50

Yung A, Phillips LJ, McGorry PD et al (1998) A step towards indicated prevention of schizophrenia. British Journal of Psychiatry 172 (Suppl 33):14–20

Intervention in the prepsychotic phase of schizophrenia and related disorders: towards effective and safe strategies for earliest intervention in psychotic disorders

P. D. McGorry, A. R. Yung, and L. J. Phillips

ORYGEN Youth Health, ORYGEN Research Centre and University of Melbourne Department of Psychiatry

Introduction

In recent years there has been a groundswell of clinical and research interest around the world in early intervention in psychotic disorders (Edwards & McGorry 2002; Malla and Norman 2002). The early psychosis paradigm, which is centred on early detection and optimal treatment of first episode psychosis and the subsequent critical years, has become a sustained growth front in both the clinical and research arenas. This is due to the great potential of this approach, the strong commitment to evidence-based medicine, the quality of the research endeavours, and the close integration of the research and clinical questions. Further progress will depend upon the involvement of an increasing number of clinical and academic centres in this new frontier of research and treatment.

The rise of the early psychosis paradigm has enabled the pre-psychotic phase of schizophrenia and related psychoses to come strongly into focus for the first time. Reacting to the pessimism intrinsic to the concept of schizophrenia and also to the damage wrought by a disorder for which effective treatments were lacking, an earlier generation of psychiatrists were attracted to the notion of pre-psychotic intervention (Meares 1959; Sullivan 1927). What remained a dream for decades is now starting to become a reality. This paper describes principles and progress in the prospective detection, engagement and treatment of young people with incipient psychosis.

Urgent public health challenges associated with manifest psychotic disorders (particularly schizophrenia and bipolar disorder) remain. These include the unacceptable and prolonged delay in accessing treatment even after frank psychosis, well above the diagnostic threshold, has developed (McGlashan 1999), and the all-too-often poor quality of treatment and insecure tenure within specialist mental health services, even when initial entry has been achieved (Lieberman and Fenton 2000; McGorry 2002; McGorry and Yung 2003). With the advent of widespread first episode programs aimed at addressing the two major weaknesses of current care, the pre-psychotic phase offers a tantalising additional focus for treatment. It has become possible to detect and engage a subset of young people who are subthreshold for fully fledged psychotic disorder, yet who have demonstrable clinical needs and other syndromal diagnoses, and who appear to be at incipient risk of frank psychosis (Yung et al. 1998, 2003).

▌ Conceptual issues

The prepsychotic or prodromal phase needs to be clearly distinguished from the premorbid phase on the one hand and the first episode of psychosis on the other. To understand the potential advantages of pre-psychotic intervention, it is important to explicate the concept of prodrome, a term which has only recently been widely used in schizophrenia. The period prior to clearcut diagnosis has traditionally been referred to as the premorbid phase. However this term has lead to some confusion because it actually covers two phases, not one, and has not been useful from a preventive perspective. Studies of the childhood antecedents of schizophrenia, while demonstrating significant but minor differences between controls and those who later developed schizophrenia, paradoxically highlighted the quiescence of the illness during this phase of life (Jones et al. 1994). However these studies and the findings of Häfner and colleagues (Häfner et al. 1995) revealed that psychotic illnesses really begin to have clinical and social consequences after puberty, typically during adolescence and early adult life. The period of nonspecific symptoms and growing functional impairment prior to the full emergence of the more diagnostically specific positive psychotic symptoms constitutes the prodromal phase.

The fact that a very substantial amount of the disability that develops in schizophrenia accumulates prior to the appearance of the full positive psychotic syndrome and may create a ceiling for eventual recovery in young people is a key reason for attempting some form of pre-psychotic intervention (Table 1). Other benefits include the capacity to research the onset phase of illness and examine the psychobiology of progression from the subthreshold state to a fully fledged disorder. More proximal risk factors such as substance use,

Table 1. Potential advantages of pre-psychotic intervention

▌ An avenue for help is provided, irrespective of whether transition ultimately occurs, to tackle the serious problems of social withdrawal, impaired functioning and subjective distress that otherwise become entrenched and steadily worsen prior to the onset of frank psychotic symptoms.

▌ Engagement and trust is easier to develop and lays a foundation for later therapeutic interventions especially drug therapy if and when required. The family can be similarly engaged and provided with emotional support and information outside of a highly charged crisis situation.

▌ If psychosis develops, it can be detected rapidly and duration of untreated psychosis minimised and hospitalisation and other lifestyle disruption rarely occur. A crisis with behavioural disturbance or self-harm is not required to gain access to treatment.

▌ Comorbidity, such as depression and substance abuse, can be effectively treated and the patient therefore gets immediate benefits. If psychosis worsens to the point of transition, the patient enters first episode in better shape with less distress and fewer additional problems.

▌ The prospective study of the transition process is enabled, including neurobiological, psychopathological and environmental aspects. Patients are less impaired cognitively and emotionally and are more likely to be fully competent to give informed consent for such research endeavours.

Table 2. Obstacles to pre-psychotic intervention

- False positive rate for FEP remains substantial. Are falsely identified individuals helped or harmed by involvement in clinical strategies? Receiving treatment at this time may heighten stigma or personal anxiety about developing psychosis or schizophrenia. If exposed to drug therapies, especially antipsychotic medications, adverse reactions may occur without benefit in false positive cases.
- If the false positive rate is improved, then the accurate detection rate may conversely decrease. This is a mathematical feature of the screening process, even when this is based on encouraging help-seeking for this group. Even with enrichment or successful screening, most of the "cases" will still emerge from the low risk group. A solution may be 2–3 step sequential screens with a continuous entry mechanism. Even if there is a ceiling for the proportion of cases that can be detected and engaged at this phase there will still be some advantages.
- Cannot distinguish between false positives and false false positives (in the latter case a true vulnerability exists though it has not yet been fully expressed) (Yung and McGorry 1996).
- Lessons from early intervention in cancer, coronary heart disease and stroke not yet translated to psychosis and schizophrenia.

stress, and the underlying neurobiology can also be uniquely studied. The delineation of this discrete phase, the boundaries of which are often difficult to precisely map, is of great heuristic and practical value. Whether prodrome is the best term for it is however a matter for debate (Phillips et al. 2002 a; Yung and McGorry 1996; Yung et al. 1998). A number of obstacles to intervention during this phase should also be noted (Table 2).

Focus on the ultra high risk (UHR) population: the "close-in" strategy as a key methodological advance

The model for detecting individuals who are putatively experiencing a prodrome that underpins this new wave of studies is a significant departure from earlier endeavours at identifying high-risk cohorts. The new approach reflects the adage "timing is everything", aiming to maximise the accuracy of prediction and the need for clinical care as well as preventive intervention.

Traditional or genetic high risk model (THR)

A range of studies recruited individuals with a family history of psychotic disorder (usually schizophrenia) during early childhood and monitored them over time – in some studies up to 35 years or more later (Cannon and Mednick 1993; Erlenmeyer-Kimling et al. 1995, 1997; Fish et al. 1992; Hodges et al. 1999; Ingraham et al. 1995; Johnstone et al. 2001; Nagler 1985). Selection of subjects for these studies on the basis of a crude measure of genetic risk (family history) restricts the generalisability of any findings to the early detection of schizophrenia as most cases do not in fact have a first degree relative with the disorder (Asarnow 1988; Kendler 1986; McGuffin et al. 1984). Conversely, only a low proportion of cases in these studies eventually develop schizophrenia or psychosis and the latent period is long. Thus these studies are beleaguered by low positive predictive values and high rate of false positives, and they tend to become obsolete before their eventual completion date. Therefore this strategy was never a viable basis for widespread early detection, but was better suited to sharpening up endophenotypic candidates for schizophrenia and other psychoses. Even here there are many conflicting and often dated findings.

The ultra-high risk (UHR) or "close-in" strategy

The development of an alternative high-risk strategy with a higher rate of transition to psychosis, a lower false positive rate and shorter follow-up period than the traditional genetic studies has been central to progress in very early preventive interventions for psychosis. Bell proposed that 'multiple-gate screening' and 'close in' follow-up of cohorts selected as being at risk of developing a psychosis would minimise false positive rates (Bell 1992). Multiple gate screening is a form of sequential screening that involves putting in place a number of different screening measures to concentrate the level of risk in the selected sample. In other words, an individual must meet a number of conditions to be included in the high-risk sample – rather than just one, as in the traditional studies. Close-in follow-up involves shortening the period of follow-up necessary to observe the transition to psychosis by commencing the follow-up period close to the age of maximum incidence of psychotic disorders. In order to improve the accuracy of identifying the high-risk cohort further, Bell also recommended using signs of behavioural difficulties in adolescence as selection criteria, such as the inclusion of clinical features. This also allows the approach to become more clinical, to move away from traditional screening paradigms and to focus on help-seeking troubled young people, who are therefore highly "incipient" and frankly symptomatic. To maximise the predictive power as well as enabling the engagement of the patient to be well justified on immediate clinical grounds, the timing is critical. Patients should really be as "incipient" as possible, yet this is difficult to measure and consistently sustain. Transition rates in samples may therefore vary on this basis and also because of variation in the underlying proportions of true and false positives who enter the sample. It should be emphasised that young people involved in this strategy have clinical problems and help is being sought either directly by them or on their behalf by concerned relatives.

The ideas expressed by Bell (1992) were first translated into practice in Melbourne, Australia in 1994 at the PACE Clinic (Yung et al. 1995). This approach has now been adopted in a number of other clinical research programmes across the world (e.g. Cornblatt 2002; Miller et al. 2002; Morrison et al. 2002). These studies have been referred to as 'ultra high-risk' studies to differentiate them from the traditional high-risk studies that rely on family history as the primary inclusion criteria. Intake criteria for such studies were initially developed from information gleaned from literature reviews and clinical experience with first episode psychosis patients and have been evaluated and refined in the PACE Clinic over the past eight years. Although the 'ultra' high-risk studies ostensibly seek to identify individuals experiencing an initial psychotic prodrome, infallible criteria have not yet been developed towards this end. In addition, "prodrome" is a retrospective concept that can only be diagnosed once the full illness develops. Therefore, criteria used in these studies are referred to as At Risk Mental State (ARMS) criteria (McGorry and Singh 1995; Yung & McGorry 1997) or 'precursor' signs and symptoms (Eaton 1995). This terminology does not imply that a full threshold psychotic illness such as schizophrenia is inevitable but suggests that an individual is at risk of developing a psychotic disorder by virtue of their current mental state. This terminology is more conservative than the use of the term prodrome, which, as mentioned, can only be accurately applied in retrospect if and when the disorder in question fully emerges. Additionally, the ARMS concept acknowledges current limitations in our knowledge and understanding about psychosis. This frankness is arguably superior in an ethical sense, and it should be noted that participants in the UHR model are voluntary and help-seeking, i.e. they are concerned about changes in their mental state and functioning and are requesting some assistance to address these changes. Indeed in many cases, the young people are concerned about the possibility that they may be developing a psychotic disorder.

UHR criteria currently in operation at the PACE Clinic require that the person falls into one or more of the following groups:

▌ *Attenuated Psychotic Symptoms Group*: have experienced subthreshold, attenuated positive psychotic symptoms during the past year;

▌ *Brief Limited or Intermittent Psychotic Symptoms Group (BLIPS)*: have experienced episodes of frank psychotic symptoms that have not lasted longer than a week and have spontaneously abated; or

▌ *Trait and State Risk Factor Group*: have a first degree relative with a psychotic disorder or the identified client has a schizotypal personality disorder and they have experienced a significant decrease in functioning during the previous year.

Operationalised criteria are shown in Table 3. As well as meeting the criteria for at least one of these groups, subjects are aged between 14 and 30 years, have not experienced a previous psychotic episode and live in the Melbourne metropolitan area. Thus, the UHR criteria identifies young people who are in the age range with peak incidence of onset of a psychotic disorder (late adolescence/early adulthood) who additionally describe mental state and functional changes that are suggestive of an emerging psychotic process and/or who may have a strong family history of psychosis. Thus, the multiple-gate screening and close-in strategies recommended by Bell (1992) have been translated into practice. Despite the paucity of knowledge about causal risk factors, clinical and functional changes have been utilised to fill this gap and connote increased levels of risk. Exclusion criteria are: intellectual disability, lack of fluency in English, presence of a known organic brain disorder, and a history of a prior psychotic episode – either treated or untreated. It is recognised that some subthreshold cases, in particular those meeting BLIPS criteria, might meet criteria for DSM-IV Brief Psychotic

Table 3. PACE Clinic inclusion criteria according to CAARMS scores

---

Group 1: Attenuated psychotic symptoms

‖ Subthreshold psychotic symptoms: Severity Scale Score of 3–5 on Disorders of Thought Content subscale, 3–4 on Perceptual Abnormalities subscale and/or 4–5 on Disorganised Speech subscales of the CAARMS; plus
‖ Frequency Scale Score of 3–6 on Disorders of Thought Content, Perceptual Abnormalities and/or Disorganised Speech subscales of the CAARMS for at least a week; or
‖ Frequency Scale Score of 2 on Disorders of Thought Content, Perceptual Abnormalities and Disorganised Speech subscales of the CAARMS on more than two occasions; plus
‖ Symptoms present in the past year and for not longer than five years

Group 2: "Brief Limited Intermittent Psychotic Symptoms" ("BLIPS")

‖ Transient psychotic symptoms – Severity Scale Score of 6 on Disorders of Thought Content subscale, 5 or 6 on Perceptual Abnormalities subscale and/or 6 on Disorganised Speech subscales of the CAARMS; plus
‖ Frequency Scale Score of 1–3 on Disorders of Thought Content, Perceptual Abnormalities and/or Disorganised Speech subscales; plus
‖ Each episode of symptoms is present for less than one week and symptoms spontaneously remit on every occasion; plus
‖ Symptoms occurred during last year and for not longer than five years

Group 3: Trait and state risk factors

‖ First degree relative with a psychotic disorder or schizotypal personality disorder in the identified patient (as defined by DSM-IV); plus
‖ Significant decrease in mental state or functioning – maintained for at least a month and not longer than 5 years (reduction in GAF Scale of 30 percent from pre-morbid level); plus
‖ The decrease in functioning occurred within the past year and has been maintained for at least a month

Acute psychosis criteria

‖ Severity Scale Score of 6 on Disorders of Thought Content subscale, 5 or 6 on Perceptual Abnormalities subscale and/or 6 on Disorganised Speech subscales of the CAARMS; plus
‖ Frequency Scale Score of greater than or equal to 4 on Disorders of Thought Content, Perceptual Abnormalities and/or Disorganised Speech subscales; plus
‖ Symptoms present for longer than one week.

Disorder; however such a diagnosis does not necessarily require the prescription of antipsychotic medication.

Criteria have also been developed to define the onset of psychosis in the UHR group (Table 3). These are not identical to DSM-IV criteria, but are designed to define the minimal point at which neuroleptic treatment is indicated. This definition of onset of psychosis might be viewed as somewhat arbitrary, but does at least have clear treatment implications and applies equally well to substance-related symptoms, symptoms that have a mood component – either depression or mania – and schizophrenia spectrum disorders. The predictive target is first episode psychosis which is judged to require antipsychotic medication, arbitrarily defined by the persistence of frank/severe psychotic symptoms for over 1 week. Schizophrenia is a subset or subsidiary target, since although the majority of progressions from the ARMS ultimately fall within the schizophrenia spectrum (schizophreniform or schizophrenia), a significant minority do not. In fact the broader first episode psychosis (FEP) target is a more proximal and therapeutically salient one than schizophrenia, which can be considered a subtype to which additional patients can graduate distal to FEP (as well as being one of the proximal categories). This logic applies to the early intervention field generally where FEP is a more practical, flexible and safer concept than first episode schizophrenia (again best considered as a subtype).

The strategy outlined by Bell (1992) for identifying high-risk individuals and adopted by our early psychosis research group in 1993 derived immediate support from a landmark publication addressing contemporary conceptualisations of preventive approaches to mental illness. Mrazek and Haggerty (1994) wrote that the current lack of definitive knowledge about the aetiology and risk factors for psychotic disorders, particularly schizophrenia, meant that developing universal (targeting the entire population) and selective (targeting groups whose risk of developing psychosis is significantly higher than average) preventive interventions are not currently possible. Rather they suggested that indicated prevention – targeting individuals who exhibit subthreshold signs and symptoms of psychosis – is the most appropriate at this point in time. They further suggested that combining known risk factors provides the best chance for identifying high-risk individuals – the multiple gate screening approach. The theoretical basis for this drew on the work of Eaton who was looking at subthreshold clinical features as a form of proximal risk factor for full clinical disorder, in this case depression and opened up the whole notion of how disorders actually "onset" and what actually constitutes an initial "case". Acquisition, intensification and coherence of symptoms and syndromes are necessary but perhaps insufficient dimensions for 'caseness' (Eaton 1995). Other variables such as distress, additional comorbidity (van Os et al. 1994), functional impairment, and other variables including perceived and objective "need" for care, also need to be considered as necessary features or alternatively as "risk factors for caseness".

The criteria described above have been evaluated in a series of studies at the PACE Clinic between 1994 and 1996. Young people meeting the ARMS criteria were recruited and their mental state was monitored over a 12-month period. Of the cohort, 41% had developed an acute psychosis and had been started on appropriate neuroleptic treatment at the end of the follow-up (Yung et al. 1998, 2003). This occurred despite the provision of minimal supportive counselling, case management and SSRI medication if required. The primary diagnostic outcome of the group who developed an acute psychosis was schizophrenia (65%) (Yung et al. 2003).

The high transition rate to psychosis indicates that the PACE criteria accurately identify young people with an extremely high risk of developing a psychotic disorder within a short follow-up period. These results cannot be easily generalised to the wider population as a whole or even to individuals with a family history of psychosis but who are asymptomatic. Participants recruited to research at the PACE Clinic are a selected sample, characterised perhaps by high help-seeking characteristics or other non-specific factors. It undoubtedly includes only a minority of those who proceed to a first episode of psychosis, and a possibly unstable proportion of false positives, depending on sampling and detection factors, which in turn are difficult to define and measure, but which can affect the base rate of true positives in the sample. Hence the transition rate may vary and needs to be validated and monitored, because the UHR criteria are not the only variable involved. However, these criteria are now being utilised in a number of other settings around the world with preliminary results indicating that they predict equally well in the USA, UK and Norway as in Melbourne, Australia (Larsen 2002; Miller et al. 2002; Morrison et al. 2002).

Establishing a pre-psychotic clinical research environment

Aims and principles

There are several keys, interdependent aims of such clinical research programs:
- To improve the understanding of the neurobiological and psychosocial processes that occur during the prepsychotic phase and contribute to the onset of acute and persistent psychosis. Conversely, processes which protect against progression and promote recovery and resolution of symptoms and impairment may be clarified.
- To develop and evaluate a range of psychosocial and biological interventions to treat current syndromes and prevent future disorders fully expressing themselves. Effectiveness and safety issues, including stigma, need to be evaluated hand in hand.
- To establish a clinical service which is not only highly accessible but also acceptable to young people at ultra-high risk of psychosis.

The PACE Clinic: an example of an integrated UHR clinical/research program

The PACE Clinic was established in Melbourne, Australia in 1994. It is one arm of a comprehensive early psychosis research programme affiliated with the Early Psychosis Prevention and Intervention Centre (McGorry 1993; McGorry et al. 1996). Although the Clinic initially operated on a limited basis with a part-time consultant psychiatrist and one research psychologist, it now comprises a team of 12 clinicians and research staff. The modest beginnings with a necessarily limited research agenda of mapping the onset of psychosis and establishing valid criteria for identifying the UHR cohort have blossomed into a more sophisticated clinical research structure. This growth has also mirrored an increased focus on youth mental health in Melbourne over the past few years and the establishment of a youth mental health service (ORYGEN) which contrasts with the usual child and adolescent versus adult mental health divide, reflects the epidemiology of onset of disorders and recognises the special needs of the youth population.

The PACE Clinic has always sought to distinguish itself from mainstream mental health services which are typically viewed in an extremely negative light, particularly by young people. Thus the name – PACE (Personal Assessment and

Crisis Evaluation) – is deliberately non-confrontational – it does not conjure up any particular images or associations. Rather it can be accused of being deliberately non-labelling. PACE has also always been located within non-traditional mental health settings such as generic youth health or community health settings or more recently within a large metropolitan shopping centre. Where possible clinicians and researchers also try not to limit themselves to working within the office setting, but try to engage with young people involved with the service in their own environment – at home, school and so forth.

Although PACE seeks to distinguish itself from traditional mental health services, which tend to focus on providing assistance for those who already have diagnosable levels of disorder, it also benefits from close relationships with such services. The majority of referrals to PACE within the past year have come from other mental health services. It is hard to argue that such patients are being stigmatised if they are diverted from traditional psychiatric settings into the low stigma PACE environment. In fact for these cases, stigma is manifestly reduced by the availability of this model (see ethical issues section, p 437). Additionally if members of the UHR cohort do develop an acute psychosis then referral to another service (preferably an early psychosis-specific service) for treatment is then necessary.

Other referrals to the PACE Clinic come from the educational sector, primary health services, drug and alcohol services, and other youth-oriented services. A key challenge facing the Clinic, therefore, has been to educate potential referrers about psychotic disorders and the signs of an emerging psychotic disorder, and also about the PACE Clinic itself. Given the specificity of the intake criteria, a widespread saturation campaign about these issues is normally considered too expensive and time consuming (though this is now underway in our region with the broader objective of early intervention in youth mental health). A more strategic approach is usually necessary.

Incidence rates of first episode psychosis indicate that within the Northwestern Melbourne region there are potentially at least 500 UHR cases per year (Krstev et al., in press). Referrals to PACE in previous years clearly indicate that many of these young people seek some assistance or explanation for the mental state changes they are experiencing – most commonly from someone already known to them, for example a general practitioner or school-based counsellor, rather than a mental health service initially. Therefore, community education at PACE has targeted these potential referrers – general practitioners, psychiatric services, school and university counselling services, and other support agencies working with young people, such as drug and alcohol services (Phillips et al. 1999). Support groups for siblings and children of individuals with psychotic disorders are also provided with information about PACE as an available clinical service. Most energy is directed towards other mental health services as previous experience shows that these services tend to refer most accurately to PACE. Formal professional development and training forums as well as informal case discussions and secondary consultation are used to inform potential referrers about the Clinic. Close working relationships are established with the most relevant services in an attempt to address some of the usual barriers to referral.

Additionally, brochures, newsletters, a promotional video and various other promotional materials about the research and clinical programme at PACE and the profile of young people attending the service are regularly produced and distributed. Staff members with a clinical background carry out these tasks as well as being able to provide secondary consultation. The same clinicians provide the triage component for the Clinic as a whole. This allows for continuity between the professional development/training activities and the referral triaging process – allowing for smoother referrals. Community education strategies have ensured that PACE is recognised as a potential referral point for professionals who may have specific concerns about a young person they are working with.

Measurement in the pre-psychotic phase

Early in the establishment of the PACE Clinic and the associated research program it became obvious that existing psychopathology measures were inadequate for assessing pre-psychotic symptomatology. Although scales such as the Brief Psychiatric Rating Scale (BPRS: Overall and Gorham 1962; McGorry et al. 1988), Scale for the Assessment of Negative Symptoms (SANS: Andreasen 1982) and the Positive and Negative Syndrome Scale (PANSS: Kay, Fiszbein and Opler 1987) are commonly used in research with psychotic patients – including with first episode psychosis – it was felt that they did not allow for a sufficiently fine-grained assessment of the subthreshold positive symptoms or the full range of precursor symptoms required at this earlier phase (Yung and McGorry 1996). For this reason a semi-structured interview aimed at assessing subthreshold or pre-psychotic (prodromal) symptomatology has been developed at PACE – the Comprehensive Assessment of At-Risk Mental State (CAARMS). Unlike other symptom assessment tools, which collapse the intensity, frequency and duration of symptoms into one score, the CAARMS teases out each of these individual aspects. Therefore small changes in the symptoms and individual experiences – such as an increase in the frequency of hearing voices from weekly to daily with no change in the intensity of the experiences – will be able to be tracked with the CAARMS. A cruder instrument such as the BPRS may not pick up such subtle changes. Drawing on the work of the Bonn-Cologne group of Huber and Klosterkötter (Klosterkötter et al. 1997a), the CAARMS also enables assessment of subjectively experienced changes such as the subjective sense of cognitive impairment, which can be rated on the Conceptual Disorganisation scale on a continuum with other objectively observed formal thought disorder, as well as subjective emotional changes. The CAARMS has been found to have good to excellent inter-rater reliability and predictive validity (Yung et al. submitted). More recently the UHR criteria have been operationalised using CAARMS rather than BPRS scores (Table 3). A copy of the CAARMS is available from Dr. Yung on request. A similar instrument has also been developed by the PRIME group (Structured Interview for Prodromal Symptoms, SIPS (Miller et al. 1999, 2002). The further development of reliable and valid methods for assessing pre-psychotic symptomatology is a crucial step underpinning research progress in this area.

In addition to establishing the validity of the intake criteria to the Clinic, early work at PACE provided the opportunity to become familiar with the profile of clients meeting ARMS criteria and their clinical needs. Young people attending the Clinic were offered clinical care and treatment as it was felt that monitoring alone was unethical in view of the clinical status and help-seeking nature of patients. Treatment with neuroleptics at this early stage was clearly premature as the high risk nature of the client group had not yet been established, nor had the risk/benefit balance of such treatment been researched. Thus clients attending PACE at this stage received supportive counselling and more specific psychotherapeutic strategies (particularly cognitive-behavioural) where appropriate. Anti-depressant and anxiolytic medication was also provided if deemed necessary. Treatment was offered for a period of one year after which time clients were referred elsewhere if appropriate. Those who developed acute psychosis were commenced promptly on neuroleptic medication and transferred to a more appropriate service for continuing care – in most cases the EPPIC program. This careful and relatively standardised approach minimised confounding factors that might have masked the transition to psychosis. In our view, naturalistic studies that permit treatment that is not standardised by protocol and carefully monitored, particularly if this allows the use of "doctor's choice" neuroleptic medication cannot hope to provide useful information in terms of prediction or treatment efficacy. This is likely to become an area of controversy as data from a range of centres accumulates.

Studies of prediction and neurobiology of transition

The development and validation of criteria that identify young people at very high risk of developing a psychotic disorder within a short follow-up period has opened the way for further research evaluating putative risk factors for psychosis. These include mental state changes such as presence of mood and anxiety features, Huber's basic symptoms (Gross 1989; Klosterkötter et al. 2001; Koehler and Sauer 1984), drug and alcohol usage, neurocognitive impairment, obstetric complications, delayed childhood milestone achievement and possible trait markers including neurological abnormalities and poor premorbid adjustment (Buckley 1998; Ismail, Cantor-Graae and McNeil 1998; Olin and Mednick 1996). The investigation of the presence of viral antibodies (O'Reilly 1994; Torrey 1988; Yolken et al. 2000) as a risk factor for future psychosis has also recently commenced within the PACE Clinic.

Some factors have been found to be associated with increased risk of transition to psychosis within the UHR group. Clinical variables include long duration of non-specific symptoms, poor psychosocial functioning, comorbid depression and disorganisation (Yung et al. 2003). Preliminary results examining CNS structure indicate that within the UHR group those who subsequently developed psychosis had reduced grey matter in right medial and lateral temporal areas, in the right inferior frontal cortex and in the cingulate gyrus at baseline compared with those who did not develop psychosis (Pantelis et al. 2003). Thus far no clear neuropsychological or developmental risk factors have emerged, although impaired olfactory identification has been found to predict transition to a schizophrenia diagnosis (Brewer et al. 2001).

Many studies have suggested that the hippocampal volumes of individuals with established schizophrenia or first episode psychosis are smaller than controls (reviewed by Velakoulis et al. 2000). Magnetic resonance imaging (MRI) scans of the brains of UHR patients are obtained to determine if volume changes in this region precede the development of acute psychosis or emerge as mental state deteriorates. Consistent with the neurodevelopmental hypothesis, hippocampal volumes of PACE UHR patients at intake lie midway between those of normal controls and patients with chronic schizophrenia or first episode psychosis (Phillips et al. 2002 b). More puzzling and challenging to the original neurodevelopmental model are the results of survival analysis, which revealed that those UHR patients with larger (although in the normal range) left hippocampal volumes at intake were more likely to develop a psychotic episode in the subsequent 12-month period (Phillips et al. 2002 b). Consistent with this finding, a comparison of MRI scans of PACE UHR patients taken prior to the onset of psychosis, and again once frank psychotic disorder has developed, revealed reduction of gray matter volumes in the left insula cortex and the left posterior medial temporal structures including the hippocampus and posterior hippocampal gyrus during the transition to psychosis (Pantelis et al. 2003). This finding suggests that brain changes occur during the process of transition to psychosis and, while the basis of this remains uncertain, opens up the exciting possibility that with sufficiently early and effective treatment such changes, and their concomitants, could be minimised or aborted. These MRI and more recent MRS studies are ongoing and other brain regions are also being investigated.

Investigations are also being carried out regarding the possible role of stress and the hypothalamic-pituitary-adrenal axis (HPA axis) in the development of psychosis (Corcoran et al. 2001). Cortisol levels and other indices of HPA function are being monitored in the UHR patients to assess if there is any interrelationship between stressful life events, coping strategies, HPA-axis functional change, neurocognitive variables, hippocampal volume change and the development of acute psychosis. These studies are aimed at examining the validity of the time-honored stress-vulnerability model of psychosis.

Intervention studies in the pre-psychotic phase

The aim of treatment provided at PACE is to reduce the symptoms with which the young person presented when first referred to the Clinic, and, if possible, to prevent these symptoms from worsening and developing into acute psychosis. A stress-vulnerability model of the development of psychosis underpins the treatment approach, incorporating medical and psychological strategies. Treatment options are discussed with patients and their families and are reviewed regularly as mental state changes unfold over the course of treatment. Young people attending the Clinic are allocated to a treatment team consisting of a psychiatrist and psychologist/case manager.

The medical staff at PACE undertake a range of assessments including blood tests and neurological and physical examinations. The medical staff is also responsible for managing and monitoring medication that may be prescribed.

Furthermore, general physical conditions are taken into consideration and treated accordingly with considerable attention being paid to the way general health status, e.g. sleep, diet, and substance use, may be impacting on mental health.

The psychological treatment provided at the Clinic is primarily based on cognitive behavioural therapy principles and draws not only on mainstream CBT techniques, but also on the treatment approaches that have been developed and evaluated for use in established psychotic disorders. The therapist and client work together to develop a personal formulation or model for understanding the symptoms the young person is experiencing and strategies for coping with and reducing these symptoms. The clinical psychologist working with the young person also functions as a case manager and provides assistance in liaising with housing, education, employment or other services as difficulties in these areas may contribute to the young person's increased risk status through increasing stress levels.

In addition to providing treatment for the young person, family members are actively invited to be involved in both individual sessions and family education sessions.

The first randomised controlled trial specifically developed around the needs of the UHR population with the aim of preventing or delaying the onset of psychosis, or at the very least ameliorating presenting symptoms was conducted at PACE between 1996–1999. This was felt to be required because of the high transition rate in the earlier study, which occurred despite comprehensive supportive care and active treatment of presenting syndromes (such as depression) and problems. In the RCT, the impact of a combined intensive psychological (cognitive) treatment plus very low dose atypical antipsychotic (risperidone) medication (Specific Preventive Intervention or SPI: n=31) was compared with the effect of supportive therapy (Needs Based Intervention or NBI: n=28) on the development of acute illness in the high-risk group. At the end of the 6-month treatment phase, significantly more subjects in the NBI group had developed an acute psychosis than in the SPI group (p=0.026). This difference was no longer significant at the end of a post treatment 6-month follow-up period (p=0.16), though it did remain significant for the risperidone-adherent subgroup of cases. This result suggests that it is possible to delay the onset of acute psychosis in the SPI group compared to the NBI group. Both groups experienced a reduction in global psychopathology and improved functioning over the treatment and follow-up phases compared to entry levels (McGorry et al. 2002). Longer-term follow-up of the participants in this study is now taking place. A second randomised trial commenced in 2000. This is a more sophisticated study with three treatment groups and blind randomisation to these groups. The three groups are:

▌ risperidone (anti-psychotic medication – up to 2 mg) and cognitive behavioral therapy,
▌ placebo and cognitive behavioral therapy and
▌ placebo and befriending.

All treatments are offered for 12 months. Participants are interviewed monthly to assess side effects and the impact of the treatments and are then interviewed for a further 12 months to determine the long-term impact of the treatment. Other clinical trials focus on the potential role for neuroprotective agents in subthreshold or at risk mental states, including low dose lithium therapy.

Young people who attend PACE but who do not wish to be involved in a clinical trial at the clinic are still provided with comprehensive treatment (but not antipsychotic medication) as it is felt that it is unethical to withhold treatment for current problems – particularly from those who are seeking it. All clients are assigned a 'case-manager' who provides practical assistance, supportive counselling and more specific interventions, e.g. antidepressants and CBT if necessary.

▌ Ethical issues

Obviously there are many ethical questions surrounding this clinical research endeavour. They have been at the forefront of the planning and development of PACE (Yung and McGorry 1997). These considerations are noted by individuals involved in this area of research throughout the world and have been addressed at a number of forums and in journal articles (Bentall and Morrison 2002; DeGrazia 2001; Heinssen et al. 2001; McGlashan 2001; McGorry, Yung and Phillips 2001; Schaffner and McGorry 2001; Wyatt 2001). These questions include: Should anti-psychotic medication be used in such a heterogenous group of individuals who do not fulfil diagnostic criteria for psychosis at the time of treatment? Should treatment studies with this cohort be naturalistic, blinded, or randomised? Should minors (the definition varies across cultures) be included in this research? Will individuals who meet UHR criteria but turn out to have been incorrectly labelled – at least in the short term – (false positives) be harmed by the treatment approaches offered? Should the level of risk a patient has for the development of psychosis be made explicit to that patient and how should this be done? Do the potential benefits of proposed preventive interventions outweigh potential side-effects? Does this form of 'early' intervention stigmatise and unnecessarily label the young person? Can the patient give 'informed consent' to a prophylactic treatment given the unknown degree of risk that he or she faces?

Obviously these are all legitimate areas of concern. We are currently in a state of "equipoise" in relation to the issue of medication, particularly neuroleptics, in the UHR group (McGlashan 2001). That is, it is not clear whether or not such treatment will be of benefit but there is sufficient evidence to suggest that clinical trials are warranted. This is particularly so now that the first study of such interventions (McGorry et al. 2002) has proved positive. Hence it is the feeling of those affiliated with the PACE Clinic that clinical treatment of young people identified as being at high risk of developing a psychotic disorder – particularly the use of neuroleptics – should be provided only in the context of a research trial (where standards of informed consent are highest) at present. However, the widespread use of antipsychotic medication outside the close monitoring afforded by a clinical trial, such as in naturalistic settings where clinician's choice prevails, is not recommended. Oddly, in the USA, studies of this type where antipsychotic drug use is not governed by a specific protocol are receiving funding support in preference to RCTs. This logic is difficult to understand, since informed consent can be better safeguarded in an RCT and clearer conclusions can be drawn from such methodology. Our experience in the PACE Clinic is that sometimes young people are prescribed antipsychotic medication by psychiatrists and even general practitioners in the absence of a clear-cut psychotic disorder when the prescribing physician suspects that a psychotic disorder is emerging. It is imperative that such treatment be first investigated in an evidence-based manner. The effects of stigma also need to be investigated. In some settings, if there is an inappropriately pessimistic mindset linked to the diagnosis of schizophrenia or psychotic disorder (a widespread phenomenon still), or the treatment setting is not generic, there may indeed be iatrogenic effects of this type. We have not seen such impact in the PACE Clinic but this reassuring experience cannot necessarily be generalised and anyway needs to be demonstrated empirically.

▌ Other centres

Since 1997 many other centres have developed in a wide range of locations. Most are similar in aims to PACE but there are important structural differences, local adaptations and models of service delivery. Here we provide an overview of some of the main centres. This list is not comprehensive but aims to highlight commonalities and differences.

▌ **PRIME.** The ARMS concept and close-in strategy has been taken up by a group based in Yale, USA – the Prevention through Risk Identification, Management and Education (PRIME) Clinic – headed by Professor Thomas McGlashan. Young people aged between 12 and 45 years who are thought to be experiencing the onset phase of a first psychotic episode are recruited to the Clinic based on scores on the Structured Interview for Prodromal Syndromes (SIPS) – a well-designed semi-structured interview influenced by the CAARMS and PANSS. The PRIME group has coined the term Criteria of Prodromal Syndromes or COPS to describe their intake criteria but essentially these criteria are the same as the UHR criteria developed earlier within PACE, which makes comparability easier. Young people meeting COPS criteria had a conversion rate to acute schizophrenia of 46% at 6 months and 54% at 12 months follow-up (Miller et al. 2002). The PRIME Clinic has expanded to involve other North American centres (Toronto, Calgary and North Carolina) as part of a multi-centre clinical trial. PRIME is a stand-alone research clinic with active community education and detection strategies. Preliminary results of the first double blind placebo-controlled randomised trial at the PRIME clinics also indicate that UHR patients benefit from the provision of specific treatment – in this case olanzapine (Woods et al. 2002). Twenty COPS positive or UHR patients who received olanzapine reported lower levels of 'prodromal' symptomatology (according to the SIPS) after eight weeks of treatment than 21 such patients who received placebo medication. Further results from this study are eagerly anticipated.

▌ **RAP.** A slightly different approach to identifying UHR individuals has been undertaken at the Hillside Recognition and Prevention (Hillside-RAP) programme in New York. This programme developed from experiences within the New York High Risk Project (NYHRP) – one of the longest running 'traditional' high-risk projects (Erlenmeyer-Kimling et al. 1997). The RAP group of researchers when referring to their study population uses slightly different terminology. They refer to this group as a clinical high-risk (CHR) group to distinguish it from genetic high-risk studies. Adolescents are recruited to this program if they experience attenuated positive psychotic symptoms (referred to as the CHR^+ group) or if they display specific combinations of Cognitive, Academic and Social Impairments and Disorganisation/odd behaviour (referred to as CASID features). This second cohort is referred to as the CHR^- group (Cornblatt 2002) and continues the interest shown in the NYHRP in cognitive impairments that may precede the onset of acute psychosis. Specific operationalised criteria for identifying the CHR^- group are not yet available. The researchers in this group hypothesise that the developmental course of schizophrenia follows a progression from CHR^- to CHR^+ to 'schizophrenialike psychosis' (SLPs: essentially schizophreniform/brief psychotic disorder) to schizophrenia. It has been indicated that preliminary data support this hypothesis (Cornblatt et al. 2002). It should be noted that schizophrenia rather than first episode psychosis is the indicated prevention target here, hence the extra category of "SLPS". This is a key distinction which allows the investigators to regard frankly psychotic patients as "subthreshold" for schizophrenia and hence contributes to different terminology, strategies and interpretations of results.

▌ **PAS.** The Psychological Assistance Service (PAS) opened in Newcastle, Australia in 1997 as a clinical service for the assessment and treatment of young people at high risk of psychosis and those experiencing a first psychotic episode. The high risk criteria are based on those of PACE but also allow inclusion if a young person has a second degree relative with a history of psychotic disorder in conjunction with a significant decline in functioning (Carr et al. 2000). The transition rate to psychosis, low initially is now comparable to that of PACE (Schall U., personal communication October 24, 2002).

▌ **TOPP Clinic.** The TOPP Clinic in Norway is an off-shoot of the TIPS programme – a comprehensive community development programme addressing first episode psychosis (Johannessen et al. 2001). Larsen and colleagues have used the questionnaire and criteria developed by the PRIME group to identify and follow-up an 'ultra' high-risk cohort; 84 patients have been assessed with 14 recruited to the study over a two-year period. Within 12 months of recruitment 6 of the 14 (43%) have developed acute psychosis (Larsen 2002).

▌ **EDIE.** The Early Identification and Intervention Evaluation (EDIE) trial, based in Manchester UK, reported a 22% transition rate to acute psychosis in 23 young people recruited based on the PACE Clinic criteria who have been followed-up for 6–12 months (Morrison et al. 2002). This service is slightly different that the others described in that it is largely a mobile service that utilises other facilities in which to see patients – such as GP surgeries, schools and so forth and promotes psychological treatment (CBT) for young people over and above medical approaches (Bentall and Morrison 2002). Preliminary results have indicated that high risk patients benefit from psychological treatment which so far seems to be more effective than monitoring alone in reducing transition rates (French 2002).

FETZ. The Early Recognition and Early Intervention Centre for Psychological Crisis (Früh-Erkennungs- und Therapie-Zentrum für psychische Krisen – FETZ) program in Cologne, Germany utilises a somewhat different paradigm to identify their high risk sample. Clients of the service fulfil criteria for at least one of two groups: a) experiencing self-identified mental state changes such as thought interference and perceptual abnormalities or b) family history of psychosis or obstetric complications in conjunction with decreased functioning. The Basic Symptom model is the backbone of these intake criteria: Basic Symptoms are subtle, subjectively noticed deficits that may be experienced in the prodromal as well as post-psychotic phase of illness. They include subjective impairments in cognitive, emotional, motor and autonomic functioning, bodily functioning and sensation, perception, energy and tolerance to stress. Huber and colleagues contend that Basic Symptoms can occur together as outpost syndromes – collections of symptoms that cross sectionally resemble schizophrenia but which in fact resolve spontaneously and do not progress to full-blown illness at least at that point in time (Gross 1989; Klosterkötter et al. 1997 a,b). Nevertheless the experience of an outpost syndrome may be a symptomatic indicator of vulnerability and herald the onset of illness. In a cohort of 110 individuals who reported experiencing Basic Symptoms at intake, 70% had developed schizophrenia after an average follow-up period of 9.6 years (specificity: 0.59; false-positive rate 20%) (Klosterkötter et al. 2001). The investigators divide the prodromal phase into early and late subphases. A trial of psychological treatment is currently underway for the early prodromal phase at FETZ, while the late prodromal phase is the focus of a psychopharmacological study utilising amisulpride (Bechdolf, Wagner and Hambrecht 2002).

OASIS. The OASIS service has recently commenced in South London to detect, assess and intervene in young people at UHR of psychosis. The PACE Clinic criteria are used and links with the established early psychosis unit (Lambeth Early Onset – LEO) are utilised to pick up those who do not meet full criteria for a psychotic disorder but who do meet the UHR criteria. OASIS is soon to begin a randomised controlled trial using quetiapine and CBT (Johns et al. 2002).

PIER. The Portland Identification and Early Referral (PIER) service is a population-wide system of early detection that utilises a broad ranging community education and development program to identify individuals within the early stages of a psychotic disorder based on the COPS/UHR criteria (McFarlane et al. 2002). Detection and engagement rates from this important study are very encouraging; however, although the study is described as naturalistic, the intervention is multimodal and includes the use of antipsychotic medication "where indicated". Yet the indications for the use of antipsychotic medication prior to psychosis are nebulous at present, since the evidence from multiple RCTs has not yet been assembled to support it. In our view, this is still a research question, which cannot be answered without more RCT data. Interpretation of the benefits and risks of the global intervention may be difficult because randomisation has not been incorporated into the design so far. The design of this study is in fact similar to the original Buckingham study of Falloon (1992), the findings of which were heuristically very useful, though inconclusive.

Commonalities among centres

- All services attempt to identify young people at high risk of psychosis in the near future – that is they are trying to pick up those in the late prodromal phase.
- A combination of mental state risk factors and genetic or trait risk factors is used by all services. Thus all contain heterogenous samples. The rationale is to maximise pathways available for high risk young people to access an appropriate service.
- The services are provided to help-seeking young people. Those who do not wish to be treated cannot be compelled to attend the service.
- Additionally, services do not actively promote into care those who are asymptomatic, not distressed or not help seeking. Thus, for example, screening in schools for students with high levels of attenuated symptoms and encouraging them to attend a service does not occur.
- They all provide a clinical as well as research or evaluative component, though not always for all patients.
- The services have two clinical foci: management of current difficulties and monitoring and possible prevention or attenuation of emerging psychosis.
- Those services that do use antipsychotic medication in clinical trials use very low doses. This is congruent with the concept of staging in cancer treatment, in which prompt detection enables less toxic therapies to be used early in the course of treatment, compared to more invasive treatments used in more advanced illness.
- The services are linked with early psychosis services or are able to provide management of first episode psychosis themselves. Thus should psychosis occur, timely and optimal treatment is available and duration of untreated psychosis minimised.
- Rate of transition to psychosis within 12 months ranges from 22% to 54% across the services, but is of the same order of magnitude.

Unsolved problems

Despite a number of publications and a prominent presence at psychiatry conferences in general but particularly schizophrenia conferences over the past few years, confusion remains in some quarters about the aims of this field of clinically oriented research. This lack of understanding has resulted in potentially inappropriate impediments being placed in the way of further progress in this field. There is also concern that this approach to identifying individuals and providing treatment prior to the onset of acute phases of disorder is in actuality an attempt to medicalise distress in adolescence. As stated earlier, this is definitely not the purpose behind this research. These misunderstandings appear to have had a greater impact in the USA than other areas and have influenced research funding policies. In Australia such concerns have so far been assuaged through close dialogue and consultation with, and subsequent support of consumer and carer groups, an open relationship with ethics committees who oversee psychiatric research, and cautious use of the media to inform the community about progress. A positive reputation as a clinical service for young people in general has also helped immeasurably in moving this endeavour forward.

Another obvious limitation is related to the "attributable risk" of the UHR criteria and hence the generalisability and clinical utility of this "earliest intervention" approach. Although transition rates are high within this group, most cases of first episode psychosis are not currently identified as UHR prior to detection of the full blown syndrome (though the experience of the PIER program suggests this may be possible). This low yield is a structural consequence of any screening process, even though here the "screening" is relatively reactive, non-systematic and clinically based. Even though the risk is substantially higher in the high risk group (UHR) and the false problem can be greatly minimised, most cases of FEP still come from the low risk and undetected groups. This places a ceiling on the utility of the strategy as pointed out by Warner (2001). However we contend that the strategy still has substantial heuristic and neurobiological research value, and that the ceiling may be able to be raised using broader enrichment strategies via a youth mental health model (see below).

It could be argued that one possible contributing factor to this is that health and educational professionals do not yet apply the UHR criteria widely enough, and that if they were publicised more broadly then perhaps more UHR young people could be encouraged to seek help. This has led some to suggest that large scale active screening may be justified, for example in schools, in order to detect students with high levels of attenuated psychotic symptoms and promote them into a clinical service. However, recent community surveys (Eaton 1995; van Os et al. 2000, 2001) suggest that attenuated and even frank psychotic symptoms are not uncommon in the general population, with lifetime prevalence estimates of up to 12% (Tien, Costa and Eaton 1992) to 17.5% (van Os et al. 2000) for some positive 'psychotic-like' symptoms. Many people experiencing these phenomena were not distressed by them and did not seek help, in contrast to those who request treatment from high risk services such as PACE. It is not fully clear what degree of risk of psychosis is associated with these non-distressing attenuated symptoms, though it could be greater than reported by van Os and colleagues, since a lack of awareness of impairment is commonly associated with psychotic experience. It is readily conceded however that it may be unwise at this stage of knowledge to embark on a population-wide screening strategy, since the accuracy of prediction of true clinical disorder could be low and there may be some risk associated. More research, as pioneered by van Os and colleagues, is needed in community samples to investigate stability and outcome of attenuated and frank psychotic symptoms that do not come to the attention of clinical services.

Intervention research: the need for logical policy and independent research support

Until recently, some major granting bodies baulked at funding intervention research in the pre-psychotic phase because of perceived ethical problems. In fact not supporting the collection of vital evidence to guide clinical decision-making in such clinical samples can be viewed as perpetuating ethical dilemmas and confusion, as well as allowing non-evidence-based practice to flourish. Similarly the notion of funding "naturalistic" studies where the use of antipsychotic medication in particular is freely permitted seems flawed and ethically inferior to conducting RCTs examining the use of antipsychotics and other biological and psychosocial treatments in this phase. Naturalistic studies of this type (other kinds could be considered more useful) are inevitably going to produce confusing or inconclusive results *and* have all the problems which were some years ago attributed to more rigorous research in this field (especially drug side-effects and potential stigma). Future support is required from the large independent research funding bodies, since this would enable necessary non-industry-funded studies to be conducted.

Future progress

The youth model

Because of the low annual incidence rates, trying to detect young people at risk of psychosis has been likened to searching for needles in a haystack (Jones 2000). However, one approach to make this task feasible could be the development of a comprehensive youth mental health service with capacity to manage young people with established and emerging non-psychotic as well as psychotic disorders. This service would therefore aim not just to find needles, but all sharp metallic objects, which could be attracted via a "magnetic" clinical strategy and sorted through later. Enriched samples of this type would give predictive measures a much better chance of accuracy. Community links and secondary consultation with primary care, education and other youth services would increase the ability of the program to provide assistance to young people with a range of problems and turn the ubiquitous comorbidity seen in young people from a diagnostic problem into an opportunity. Many young people may move in and out of "At Risk Mental States", and the ability to monitor them and provide timely intervention as appropriate may aid our understanding of the process of onset not only for psychosis but for other syndromes, and also our ability to provide preventive treatment.

Neuroprotection

It is becoming more likely that the onset phase of illness during which clinical features and functional impairment emerge for the first time is associated with active yet subtle neurobiological changes in the patient (Pantelis et al. 2003a). In contrast to the original neurodevelopmental model of schizophrenia (Weinberger 1995), which proposed a dormant lesion that becomes activated around the time of adolescence, it seems that complex neuronal dysfunction may develop as a new process around the time of psychosis onset (Pantelis et al. 2003b). Thus early treatment, before full blown psychotic disorder occurs, may prevent some brain changes and thus alter the neurobiological pattern of illness (Wolkin and Rusinek 2002). Earlier crude models of neurotransmitter imbalance, derived in reverse from the mechanism of action of psychotropic medications, may ultimately give way to models based on intracellular disturbances and influences via gene expression upon neuronal integrity and connectivity (Berger, Woods and McGorry 2003). The therapeutic paradigm linked to such models is neuroprotection. If neuroprotective agents, such as lithium and eicosapentanoic acid, could be shown to reduce the risk of progression from early to more severe forms of disorder, then early intervention would receive even stronger support as a strategy.

▌ Conclusion

This chapter has explored the development and expansion of an approach specifically designed for the detection, monitoring and treatment of the pre-psychotic or ultra high-risk (UHR) phase of illness and the study of the psychobiological processes contributing to onset. The conceptual underpinnings, practical and ethical issues related to UHR research and clinical intervention have been described. This is truly a growth area with the potential to benefit such symptomatic ultra high risk young people and their families. Increasingly our ability to identify those at particularly high risk is being refined and a biological basis for psychosis onset investigated. Caution must be exercised however, and each step evaluated in an evidence-based manner. Continued modification of UHR criteria and better understanding of the process of screening and sample enrichment may be needed. Randomised clinical trials of medication and other interventions must be ongoing and rigorously evaluated. Large scale screening of population samples in order to expand the scope of "pre-psychotic" treatment is probably not justified merely for this purpose at this stage of knowledge. As an alternative, either enriching strategies could be developed to enable interventions to be evaluated, or a broader screening strategy for the full range of emergent mental disorders in young people could be explored.

▮ **Acknowledgements.** This work was supported by research grants from the Victorian Health Promotion Foundation, The National Alliance for Research on Schizophrenia & Depression, the Theodore & Vada Stanley Foundation, the Colonial Foundation, the National Health & Medical Research Council and Janssen-Cilag Pty. Ltd. The authors gratefully acknowledge the contributions of the staff and clients of the PACE Clinic.

▮ References

Andreasen N (1982) Negative symptoms in schizophrenia: definition and reality. Archives of General Psychiatry 39:784–788

Asarnow JR (1988) Children at risk for schizophrenia: converging lines of evidence. Schizophrenia Bulletin 14:613–630

Bechdolf A, Wagner M, Hambrecht M (2002) Psychological intervention in the prepsychotic phase: preliminary results of a multicentre trial. Acta Psychiatrica Scandinavica 106:41

Bell RQ (1992) Multiple-risk cohorts and segmenting risk as solutions to the problem of false positives in risk for the major psychoses. Psychiatry 55(4):370–381

Bentall RP, Morrison AP (2002) More harm than good: The case against using antipsychotic drugs to prevent severe mental illness. Journal of Mental Health 11:351–356

Berger GE, Wood S, McGorry PD (2003) Incipient neurovulnerability and neuroprotection in early psychosis. Psychopharmacology Bulletin 37(2)

Brewer W, Pantelis C, Anderson V, Velakoulis D, Singh B, Copolov DL, McGorry PD (2001) Stability of olfactory identification deficits in neuroleptic-naïve patients with first-episode psychosis. American Journal of Psychiatry 158(1):107–115

Buckley PF (1988) The clinical stigmata of aberrant neurodevelopment in schizophrenia. Journal of Nervous and Mental Disease 186:79–86

Cannon TD, Mednick SA (1993) The schizophrenia high-risk project in Copenhagen: three decades of progress. Acta Psychiatrica Scandinavica 87(Suppl 370):33–47

Carr V, Halpin S, Lau N, O'Brien S, Beckmann J, Lewin T (2000) A risk factor screening and assessment protocol for schizophrenia and related psychosis. Australian and New Zealand Journal of Psychiatry 34 (Suppl):S170–180

Corcoran C, Gallitano A, Leitman D, Malaspina D (2001) The neurobiology of the stress cascade and its potential relevance for schizophrenia. Journal of Psychiatric Practice 7:3–14

Cornblatt B, Lencz T, Correll C, Authour A, Smith C (2002) Treating the prodrome: Naturalistic findings from the RAP Program. Acta Psychiatrica Scandinavica (Suppl) 106:44

Cornblatt BA (2002) The New York High Risk Project to the Hillside Recognition and Prevention (RAP) Program. American Journal of Medical Genetics (Neuropsychiatric Genetics) 114:956–966

DeGrazia D (2001) Ethical issues in early-intervention clinical trials involving minors at risk for schizophrenia. Schizophrenia Research 51:77–86

Eaton WW (1995) Prodromes and precursors: epidemiologic data for primary prevention of disorders with slow onset. American Journal of Psychiatry 152:967–972

Edwards J, McGorry PD (2002) Implementing early intervention in psychosis: a guide to establishing early psychosis services. Martin Dunitz, London

Erlenmeyer-Kimling L, Adamo UH, Rock D, Roberts SA, Bassett AS, Squirres-Wheeler E, Cornblatt BA, Endicott J, Pape S, Gottesman II (1997) The New York High-Risk Project: prevalence and comorbidity of Axis I disorders in offspring of schizophrenic parents at 25-year follow-up. Archives of General Psychiatry 54:1096–1102

Erlenmeyer-Kimling L, Squires-Wheeler E, Adamo UH, Bassett AS, Cornblatt BA, Kestenbaum CJ, Rock D, Roberts SA, Gottesman II (1995) The New York High Risk Project: psychoses and cluster A personality disorders in offspring of schizophrenic parents at 23 years of follow-up. Archives of General Psychiatry 52:857–865

Falloon IRH (1992) Early intervention for first episode of schizophrenia: a preliminary exploration. Psychiatry, 55:4-15

Fish B, Marcus J, Hans SL, Auerbach JG, Perdue S (1992) Infants at risk for schizophrenia: Sequelae of a genetic neurointegrative defect. Archives of General Psychiatry 49:221–235

French P (2002) Model-driven psychological intervention to prevent onset of psychosis. Acta Psychiatrica Scandinavica (Suppl) 106:18

Gross G (1989) The 'basic' symptoms of schizophrenia. British Journal of Psychiatry 155 (suppl 7):21–25

Häfner H, Maurer W, Löffler B, Bustamante S, an der Heiden W, Nowotny B (1995) Onset and early course of schizophrenia. In: Häfner H, Gattaz WF (eds) Search for the Causes of Schizophrenia. Springer, New York, III, pp 43–66

Heinssen R, Perkins DO, Appelbaum PS, Fenton WS (2001) Informed consent in early psychosis research: National Institute of Mental Health Workshop, November 15, 2000. Schizophrenia Bulletin 27:571–584

Hodges A, Byrne M, Grant E, Johnstone E (1999) People at risk of schizophrenia: sample characteristics of the first 100 cases in the Edinburgh high-risk study. British Journal of Psychiatry 174:547–553

Ingraham LJ, Kugelmass S, Frenkel E, Nathan M, Mirsky AF (1995) Twenty-five year follow-up of the Israeli High-risk Study: current and lifetime psychopathology. Schizophrenia Bulletin 21:183–192

Ismail B, Cantor-Graae E, McNeil TF (1998) Neurological abnormalities in schizophrenic patients and their siblings. American Journal of Psychiatry 155:84–89

Johannessen JO, McGlashan TH, Larsen TK, Horneland M, Joa I, Mardal S, Kvebaek R, Friis S, Melle I, Opjordsmoen S, Simonsen E, Ulrik H, Vaglum P (2001) Early detection strategies for untreated first-episode psychosis. Schizophrenia Research 51:39–46

Johns L, Broome M, Matthiasson P, Power P, McGuire PK (2002) OASIS: a new service for people with prodromal signs of psychosis. Acta Psychiatrica Scandinavica 106:73

Johnstone EC, Abukmeil SS, Byrne M, Clafferty R, Grant E, Hodges A, Lawrie SM, Owens DGC (2001) Edinburgh high risk study – findings after four years: demographic, attainment and psychopathological issues. Schizophrenia Research 46:1–15

Jones P (2000) The epidemiology of psychotic disorder. Keynote address at "Future Possible" 2nd International Conference on Early Psychosis, New York City, 31 March & 1-2 April

Jones P, Rodgers B, Murray R, Marmot M (1994) Child development risk factors for adult schizophrenia in the British 1946 birth cohort. Lancet 344:1398–1402

Kay SR, Fiszbein A, Opler LA (1987) The positive and negative syndrome scale (PANSS) for schizophrenia. Schizophrenia Bulletin 13:261–269

Kendler KS (1986) Genetics of schizophrenia. In: Frances AJ, Hales RE (eds) American Psychiatric Association Annual Review. American Psychiatric Press, Washington DC, p 5

Klosterkötter J, Gross G, Wieneke A, Steinmeyer EM, Schultze-Lutter F (1997a) Evaluation of the 'Bonn Scale for the Assessment of Basic Symptoms- - BSABS' as an instrument for the assessment of schizophrenia proneness: a review of recent findings. Neurology, Psychiatry and Brain Research 5:137–150

Klosterkötter J, Schultze-Lutter F, Gross G, Huber G, Steinmeyer EM (1997b) Early self-experienced neuropsychological deficits and subsequent schizophrenic diseases: an 8-year average follow-up prospective study. Acta Psychiatrica Scandinavica 95:396–404

Klosterkötter, J, Hellmich M, Steinmeyer EM, Schultze-Lutter F (2001) Diagnosing schizophrenia in the initial prodromal phase. Archives of General Psychiatry 58:158–164

Koehler K, Sauer H (1984) Huber's basic symptoms: another approach to negative psychopathology in schizophrenia. Comprehensive Psychiatry 25:174–182

Krstev H, Carbone S, Harrigan SM, McGorry PD, Curry C, Elkins K (2004) Early intervention in first episode psychosis: the impact of a community development campaign. Social Psychiatr & Psychiatric Epidemiology (in press)

Larsen TK (2002) The transition from the premorbid period to psychosis: how can it be described? Acta Psychiatrica Scandinavica (Suppl) 106:10–11

Lieberman JA, Fenton WS (2000) Delayed detection of psychosis: causes, consequences, and effect on public health. American Journal of Psychiatry 157:1727–1730

Malla AK, Norman RMG (2002) Early intervention in schizophrenia and related disorders: advantages and pitfalls. Current Opinion in Psychiatry 15:17–23

McFarlane WR, Cook WL, Robbins D, Downing D (2002) Portland identification and early referral. Acta Psychiatrica Scandinavica 413:20

McGlashan TH (1999) Duration of untreated psychosis in first-episode schizophrenia: marker or determinant of course? Biological Psychiatry 47:473

McGlashan TH (2001) Psychosis treatment prior to psychosis onset: ethical issues. Schizophrenia Research 51:47–54

McGorry PD (1993) Early psychosis prevention and intervention centre. Australian Psychiatry 1:32–34

McGorry PD (2002) Early psychosis reform: too fast or too slow? Acta Psychiatrica Scandinavica 106:249–251

McGorry PD, Singh BS (1995) Schizophrenia: risk and possibility. In: Raphael B, Burrows GD (eds) Handbook of Studies on Preventive Psychiatry. Elsevier, pp 491–514

McGorry PD, Yung AR (2003) Early intervention in psychosis: an overdue reform. Australian and New Zealand Journal of Psychiatry 37:393–398

McGorry PD, Edwards J, Mihalopolous C, Harrigan SM, Jackson HJ (1996) EPPIC: an evolving system of early detection and optimal management. Schizophrenia Bulletin 22:305–326

McGorry PD, Goodwin RJ, Stuart GW (1988) The development, use and reliability of the Brief Psychiatric Rating Scale (Nursing Modification) – an assessment procedure for the nursing team in clinical and research settings. Comprehensive Psychiatry 29:575–587

McGorry PD, Yung AR, Phillips LJ (2001) Ethics and early intervention in psychosis: keeping up the pace and staying in step. Schizophrenia Research 51:17–29

McGorry PD, Yung AR, Phillips LJ, Yuen HP, Francey S, Cosgrave EM, Germano D, Bravin J, Adlard S, McDonald A, Blair A, Jackson HJ (2002) A randomized controlled trial of interventions designed to reduce the risk of progression to first episode psychosis in a clinical sample with subthreshold symptoms. Archives of General Psychiatry 59:921–928

McGuffin P, Farmer AE, Gottesman M, Murray RM, Reveley AM (1984) Twin concordance for operationally defined schizophrenia. Archives of General Psychiatry 49:541–545

Meares A (1959) The diagnosis of prepsychotic schizophrenia. Lancet I:55–59

Miller TJ, McGlashan TH, Rosen JL, Somjee L, Markovich PJ, Stein K, Woods SW (2002) Prospective diagnosis of the initial prodrome for schizophrenia based on the Structured Interview for Prodromal Symptoms: preliminary evidence of inter-rater and predictive validity. American Journal of Psychiatry 159:863–865

Miller TJ, McGlashan TH, Woods SW, Stein K, Briesen N, Corcoran CM, Hoffman R, Davidson L (1999) Symptom assessment in schizophrenic prodromal states. Psychiatric Quarterly 70:273–287

Morrison AP, Bentall RP, French P, Walford L, Kilcommons A, Knight A, Kreutz M, Lewis SW (2002) Randomised controlled trial of early detection and cognitive therapy for preventing transition to psychosis in high-risk individuals. Study design and interim analysis of transition rate and psychological risk factors. British Journal of Psychiatry (Suppl) 43:s78–s84

Mrazek PJ, Haggarty RJ (1994) Reducing Risks for Mental Disorders: Frontiers for Preventive Intervention Research. National Academy Press, Washington DC

Nagler S (1985) Overall design and methodology of the Israeli High Risk Study. Schizophrenia Bulletin 11:31–37

Olin SC, Mednick SA (1996) Risk factors of psychosis: Identifying vulnerable populations premorbidly. Schizophrenia Bulletin 22:223–240

O'Reilly RL (1994) Viruses and schizophrenia. Australian and New Zealand Journal of Psychiatry 28:222–228

Overall JE, Gorham DR (1962) The Brief Psychiatric Rating Scale. Psychological Reports 10:799–812

Pantelis C, Velakoulis D, McGorry PD, Wood SJ, Suckling J, Phillips LJ, Yung AR, Bullmore ET, Brewer W, Soulsby B, Desmond P, McGuire PK (2003 a) Neuroanatomical abnormalities before and after onset of psychosis: a cross-sectional and longitudinal MRI comparison. Lancet 361(9354):281–288

Pantelis C, Yücel M, Wood SJ, McGorry PD, Velakoulis D (2003 b) Early and late neurodevelopmental disturbances in schizophrenia and their functional consequences. Australian and New Zealand Journal of Psychiatry 37:399–406

Phillips LJ, Leicester SB, O'Dwyer LE, Francey SM, Koutsogiannis J, Abdel-Baki A, Kelly D, Jones S, Vay C, Yung AR, McGorry PD (2002 a) The PACE Clinic: identification and management of young people at 'ultra' high risk of psychosis. Journal of Psychiatric Practice 8:255–269

Phillips LJ, Velakoulis D, Pantelis C, Yuen HP, Yung AR, Desmond P, Brewer W, McGorry PD (2002 b) Non-reduction in hippocampal volume is associated with higher risk of psychosis. Schizophrenia Research 58:145–158

Phillips LJ, Yung AR, Hearn N, McFarlane CA, Hallgren M, McGorry PD (1999) Preventive mental health care: accessing the target population. Australian and New Zealand Journal of Psychiatry 33:912–917

Schaffner KF, McGorry PD (2001) Preventing severe mental illnesses: new prospects and ethical challenges. Schizophrenia Research 51:3–15

Sullivan HS (1927) The onset of schizophrenia. American Journal of Psychiatry 6:105–134

Tien AY, Costa PT, Eaton WW (1992) Covariance of personality, neurocognition, and schizophrenia spectrum traits in the community. Schizophrenia Research 7:149–158

Torrey EF (1988) Stalking the schizovirus. Schizophrenia Bulletin 14:223–229

Van Os J, Fahy P, Bebbington P, Jones P, Wilkins S, Sham P, Russell A, Gilvarry K, Lewis S, Toone B, Murray R (1994) The influence of life events on the subsequent course of psychotic illness: a prospective follow-up of the Camberwell Collaborative Psychosis Study. Psychological Medicine 24:503–513

Van Os J, Hanssen M, Bijl RV, Ravelli A (2000) Strauss Revisited: a psychosis continuum in the general population? Schizophrenia Research 45:11–20

Van Os J, Hanssen M, Bijl RV, Vollebergh W (2001) Prevalence of psychotic disorder and community level of psychotic symptoms. Archives of General Psychiatry 58:663–668

Velakoulis D, Wood SJ, McGorry PD, Pantelis C (2000) Evidence for progression of brain structural abnormalities in schizophrenia: beyond the neurodevelopmental model. Australian and New Zealand Journal of Psychiatry 34 (Suppl):S113–S126

Warner R (2001) The prevention of schizophrenia: what interventions are safe and effective? Schizophrenia Bulletin 27(4):551–562

Weinberger DR (1995) From neuropathology to neurodevelopment. Lancet 346:552–557

Wolkin A, Rusinek H (2002) A neuropathology of psychosis? Lancet published online, 10 December

Woods S, Zipursky R, Perkins D, Addington J, Marquez E, Breier A, McGlashan TH (2002) Olanzapine vs. placebo for prodromal symptoms. Acta Psychiatrica Scandinavica (Suppl) 106:43

Wyatt RJ, Henter I (2001) Rationale for the study of early intervention. Schizophrenia Research 51:69–76

Yolken RH, Karlsson H, Yee F, Johnston-Wilson NL, Torrey EF (2000) Endogenous retroviruses and schizophrenia. Brain Research Reviews 31:193–199

Yung AR, McGorry PD (1996) The initial prodrome in psychosis: descriptive and qualitative aspects. Australian and New Zealand Journal of Psychiatry 30:587–599

Yung AR, McGorry PD (1996) The prodromal phase of first-episode psychosis: past and current conceptualizations. Schizophrenia Bulletin 22:353–370

Yung AR, McGorry PD (1997) Is pre-psychotic intervention realistic in schizophrenia and related disorders? Australian and New Zealand Journal of Psychiatry 31:799–805

Yung AR, McGorry PD, McFarlane CA, Patton GC (1995) The PACE Clinic: development of a clinical service for young people at high risk of psychosis. Australasian Psychiatry 3:345–349

Yung AR, Phillips LJ, McGorry PD, Hallgren MA, McFarlane CA, Jackson HJ, Francey S, Patton GC (1998) Can we predict onset of first episode psychosis in a high risk group? International Clinical Psychopharmacology 13(Suppl 1):S23–S30

Yung AR, Phillips LJ, Yuen HP, Francey SM, McFarlane C, Hallgren M, McGorry PD (2003) Psychosis prediction: 12 month follow-up of a high risk ('prodromal') group. Schizophrenia Research 60:21–32

Yung AR, Yuen HP, McGorry PD, Phillips L, Kelly D, Dell-Olioi M, Francey S (2003) Mapping the onset of psychosis – the comprehensive assessment of at risk mental states (CAARMS). Australian and New Zealand Journal of Psychiatry (submitted)

What can molecular imaging tell us about schizophrenia?

Lyn S. Pilowsky

Reader in Neurochemical Imaging, UK Medical Research Council Senior Clinical Fellow, Institute of Psychiatry, London, UK

Introduction

The term molecular imaging refers in this review to a type of nuclear medicine procedure in which a molecule of interest is labelled with an isotope (positron or single photon emitting nuclide), and acts as a molecular 'key' (or radioligand), fitting into a cellular recognition site (receptor, transporter protein or enzymatic pathway) with molecular-level specificity. The radioligand is injected into the bloodstream, passes through the blood brain barrier and binds to a site of interest. When bound, the emitted radiation is detected by a ring of detectors surrounding the head, and a map of radioactive density is produced, reflecting a chemical map of radioligand binding. Thus neurotransmitter systems in the living human brain may be studied relatively noninvasively.

It was an incredible stroke of luck that the first positron, and single photon emission tomography (PET and SPET) probes developed to image neurotransmitter receptors in the living human brain were for the dopamine system, and more specifically, the dopamine D2 receptor. In the early-mid 1980s much was already understood about the relevance of this system to schizophrenia. A series of brilliant and careful studies (Connell et al. 1958; Creese et al. 1976; Johnstone et al. 1978; Peroutka et al. 1980), building on the landmark work of Carlsson et al. (2001) in defining dopamine as a central neurotransmitter, had exposed the centrality of dopamine in psychosis and D2 receptors in mediating antipsychotic drug action. Studies characterised a direct, linear relationship between striatal dopamine D2 receptor blockade and clinical potency, yet it was also noted some patients were relatively insensitive to this action (Crow 1980). Furthermore, some postmortem studies revealed striatal dopamine D2 receptor hyperdensity. These results were confounded by the fact that antipsychotic treatment in and of itself could elevate D2 receptor density, and studies in drug naïve, never treated patients were awaited.

The dopamine hypothesis – beginning the investigation

The first studies of D2 receptor density in living schizophrenic patients proved controversial. An ^{18}F-NMSP PET study initially found a six-fold elevation in striatal D2 receptor density (Wong et al. 1986). ^{11}C-raclopride PET, [76]Br bromolisuride PET, or ^{123}I IBZM SPET investigations (Farde et al. 1990; Martinot et al. 1991; Pilowsky et al. 1994) did not replicate this finding, and the notion that an underlying striatal D2 hyperdensity was responsible for schizophrenia was abandoned. The focus shifted to attempts to understand the mode of action of antipsychotic drugs in the disorder, and this proved a stunningly successful exploitation of molecular imaging applied to any disease or drug discovery process. Early work confirmed that, as predicted by in vitro binding and potency studies, typical antipsychotic drugs showed high occupancy of striatal D2 receptors (Farde et al. 1988). The association with clinical response was explored in further studies. Wolkin et al. (1989) and Pilowsky et al. (1993) found no difference in striatal D2 receptor blockade by typical antipsychotic drugs between excellent and poor responders to the medication. These data did not support a simple link between striatal D2 occupancy and antipsychotic efficacy, as had been suggested by in vitro studies. Nevertheless, Nordstrom et al. (1993), and Kapur et al. (2000) found a threshold relationship between clinical efficacy and D2 blockade by typical antipsychotic drugs that could be delineated in acutely treated patients (excluding poor responders). It was acknowledged, however, that other potential sites of action of antipsychotic drugs remained to be studied by molecular imaging, and that purely imaging striatal D2 receptors was likely to miss important regional effects on dopamine receptor populations in limbic and cortical regions.

Furthermore, in the early 1990's, molecular experiments revealed the dopamine receptor family separated into 2 major subtypes, D1-like (D1 and D5) and D2-like (D2, D3, D4). Variants of the dopamine receptors exist with different DNA and amino acid sequences. Receptor cloning has identified two isoforms of the D2 receptor (D2short and D2long), which are differentially localised in the brain. The neurochemical anatomy of dopamine differs in cortical and striatal regions, and it now appears that dopamine concentration, receptor regulation and D2-like subtype density varies greatly between striatal and extra-striatal regions (Lidow et al. 1998; Strange 2001).

▌ The 5HT2a/D2 occupancy hypothesis

The development of PET and SPET radioligands highly selective for 5HT2a receptors permitted exploration of the notion that blockade of these receptors was important, indeed may be central to *atypical* antipsychotic drug action. This idea gained partial credence from the serotonergic hypothesis of schizophrenia, and the propsychotic effects of serotonergic agents such as LSD, as well as the enriched cortical localisation of 5HT2a receptors, most importantly in modulating inputs to pyramidal neurons. In addition, PET and SPET findings that D2 blockade appeared irrelevant to nonresponders and to the mode of action of clozapine prompted a re-evaluation of the role of dopamine blockade in antipsychotic efficacy (Wolkin et al. 1989; Pilowsky et al. 1992, 1993; Farde et al. 1992). The most compelling evidence came from the work of Meltzer et al. (1989), who proposed, based on drug affinity data, that the ratio of 5HT2a:D2 receptor affinity was the major determinant of a drug's likelihood to behave as an atypical antipsychotic. PET and SPET studies were supportive of this proposal showing marked, indeed near saturation of 5HT2a receptors by atypical antipsychotic drugs at clinically useful doses including clozapine, olanzapine and risperidone (Nordstrom et al. 1992; Nyberg et al. 1993; Travis et al. 1998; Trichard et al. 1998). Typical antipsychotic drugs including haloperidol and chlorpromazine did not show predictably high 5HT2a occupancy at standard doses. Kapur et al. (1999) revisited this question, and showed that the supposed protection from EPS conferred by high 5HT2a blockade could be overcome when D2 receptor occupancy by the antipsychotic drug increased over a threshold of approximately 78%. The importance of 5HT2a to efficacy was further queried by the failure of pure 5HT2a antagonists to demonstrate therapeutic activity. Finally, the atypical antipsychotic amisulpride has no 5HT2a activity, and yet has efficacy with a wide therapeutic window for EPS.

∥ Molecular imaging demonstrates a more sophisticated interaction between atypical antipsychotic drugs and dopamine systems in vivo

It had early been demonstrated that clozapine, though a markedly effective antipsychotic, had modest levels of D2 receptor occupancy at steady state (approximately 20 to 60%) (Farde et al. 1992; Pilowsky et al. 1992). The atypical antipsychotic drug quetiapine was clinically useful at lower levels of D2 occupancy than clozapine (Gevfert et al. 1998; Stephenson et al. 2000). This apparent conundrum was partly resolved by PET investigations. Serial PET studies performed in the 24 hours after a single dose of the drugs revealed that clozapine and quetiapine had *transiently* high occupancy of striatal D2 receptors (Kapur et al. 2001). These drugs evinced 75% striatal D2 occupancy immediately after dosing, reducing to very low levels over a 12 hour period (to zero in the case of quetiapine). This led Kapur and Seeman (2001) to propose that atypical antipsychotic drugs occupied striatal dopamine D2 receptors only transiently. They suggested that low affinity for these receptors, indeed more modest that endogenous dopamine itself, meant that endogenous dopamine was able to compete with the drugs *in vivo*. Seeman (2002) suggested that atypical antipsychotic drugs bound more loosely to D2 receptors than dopamine itself, and this may be a requirement for antipsychotic atypicality. These studies focussed on striatal D2 receptors, yet probes with picomolar affinity for the D2 receptor demonstrated the existence of these receptors in more relevant limbic and cortical regions including thalamus and temporal cortex (Kessler et al. 1993). Lidow et al. (1998) found that treating primates with the antipsychotic drugs clozapine and haloperidol at doses and durations used clinically resulted in cortically selective upregulation of D2 receptors for clozapine alone. Haloperidol was nonselective, upregulating D2 mRNA turnover and binding levels in both striatum and cortex. PET and SPET imaging studies supported these data with the high affinity D2 receptor probes ^{18}F fallypride (Kessler et al. 2003), [76]Br FLB 457 (Xiberas et al. 2001), and ^{123}I epipride SPET (Pilowsky et al. 1997; Bigliani et al. 1999, 2000; Stephenson et al. 2000; Bressan et al. 2003). One explanation for the apparent limbic cortical selective action of modest D2 antagonist atypical antipsychotic drugs incorporates the 'transient binding' hypothesis of Seeman and Kapur (2001), and the known regional differences in dopamine concentrations between cortex and striatum, to which modest D2 antagonists may be more sensitive (Strange 2001). In striatal regions, where dopamine concentrations are high, a D2 antagonist with more modest affinity for the receptor than dopamine itself could not compete to occupy all available receptors, as it could in cortex, where dopamine is present in low concentration.

▌ Molecular imaging demonstrates dynamic alterations in dopamine handling in schizophrenic patients compared to healthy controls

The power of *in vivo* imaging lies in its unparalleled ability to explore dynamic perturbations in neurotransmitter systems in living patients, and correlate these to clinical states or traits, without the need to rely on partial or incomplete historical assessments. Laruelle et al. (1996) exploited this characteristic to produce seminal work in the field. An amphetamine challenge was given to drug free patients and healthy controls, during a SPET scan with the dopamine D2 receptor ligand ^{123}I IBZM. Amphetamine blocks the presynaptic dopamine transporter, leading to an excess of dopamine in the synapse (by the release of stored dopamine pools). Dopamine then competes with ^{123}I IBZM binding for the D2 receptor, which is visualised and estimated as a decline in binding. [123]I IBZM and ^{11}C raclopride PET studies revealed important differences in the way schizophrenic patients responded to this challenge compared to controls. Patients had higher mean levels of D2 occupancy by dopamine, and there was a large spread in response to the challenge, with some patients showing much greater excess in dopamine levels, while others overlapped with controls. It appeared that this response correlated with how acutely ill the patients were, suggesting that acute psychosis is indeed associated with dopaminergic overactivity, but is not a feature in chronically ill patients, in whom one might suppose other neurochemical factors are at play. Similarly 'mirror image' dopamine depletion studies, which used the agent AMPT to clear the synapse of endogenous dopamine, revealed a greater effect in drug-free schizophrenic patients (Abi Dargham et al. 2000). These findings are in keeping with suggestions that schizophrenia is a disorder of dopamine dysregulation in different parts of the brain, rather than simple under- or over-activity (Moore et al. 1999). The data provide impetus for investigating systems that control or regulate dopamine in schizophrenia, and also suggest that antipsychotic drugs that result in blanket suppression of dopamine responses will not meet the needs of all patients, and may block physiological dopamine leading to well documented cognitive, emotional and motor side effects including dysphoria, decreased initiative, and extrapyramidal side effects. It is crucial to recognise that these findings in living humans could not have been made without molecular imaging technology.

Much concerning dopamine transmission remains to be investigated by molecular imaging. Obstacles are both technical and physiological. Attempts to study dopamine flux in cortical regions *in vivo*, for example, must contend with the low concentration of dopamine, the low density of dopamine transporters in these areas, and the longer distance dopamine diffuses across the synapse. These factors reduce the sensitivity of challenge approaches. D2 receptors are present at far lower density in cortical than striatal regions, and D1 receptors, though far more enriched in cortex, nevertheless appear puzzlingly insensitive to amphetamine and AMPT challenges (Abi-Dargham et al. 1999; Verhoeff et al. 2002). An unreplicated PET study of D1 receptors linked poor performance on a working memory task and high D1 binding in the prefrontal cortex (Abi-Dargham et al. 2002), and controversy exists as to whether these receptors are upregulated, downregulated, or unchanged in the cortex of drug-free and drug-naïve patients relative to healthy controls (Abi-Dargham et al. 2002; Karlsson et al. 2002; Okubu et al. 1997). There are, at present, no suitable ligands for the D3 receptor, though this would clearly be a major target for both drug and imaging discovery.

▌ Has molecular imaging identified other abnormalities in schizophrenia?

The capacity to link faults in neurotransmitter systems other than dopamine has been limited by the development of useful probes for candidate sites and the difficulty in studying homogeneous populations of patients prior to drug treatment. Nevertheless, studies have been performed of 5HT2a and 5HT1a, muscarinic and GABA/BZ receptors. A significant increase in 5HT1a binding was noted in schizophrenics compared to healthy controls by Tauscher et al. (2002). This was particularly evident in the left medio-temporal cortex. The significance of the finding was unclear, but these receptors are clearly involved in pyramidal cell modulation. By contrast, both no change and a decline in 5HT2a binding, particularly evident in frontal cortical regions, has been reported and the view is that change in this receptor population is unlikely to be causal in schizophrenia (Lewis et al. 1999; Ngan et al. 2000). Similarly, studies of the BZ receptor have failed to reveal consistent abnormalities in schizophrenia (Abi-Dargham et al. 1999; Busatto et al. 1997). A SPET study with the M1/M2 receptor ligand ^{123}I QNB revealed a marked decline (up to 33%) in binding in drug naïve schizophrenia patients (Raedler et al. 2003), and may help explain some observed cognitive deficits in the disorder, though this was not examined by the authors. More recently, a preliminary assay of the MK-801/PCP binding site of the NMDA receptor ion channel finds a subtle decline in cortico-limbic regions of drug-free schizophrenic patients relative to healthy controls, though patients taking clozapine showed a restoration in NMDA binding, which may reflect a novel mechanism of the drug (Bressan et al. 2003). Future work will clarify this result more extensively using directly competitive ketamine challenges.

Conclusion

The investigations pertaining to extra-dopaminergic sites are failing to coalesce into a consistent story, which perhaps speaks to their overall relevance to the disorder compared to dopamine, or may reflect a lack of availability of more interesting ligands reflecting potential neuroplasticity changes. It is worth remembering, in this vein, that many candidate probes remain to be synthesized, or are proving unamenable to the approach. Nevertheless, it is clear that sustained concentration of multidisciplinary basic and clinical scientists in this field has yielded hitherto undreamed of results in the area of antipsychotic drug discovery. Future research should concentrate on linking novel ligand development with neuroscience leads, forming a continuous loop feeding back into pharmacological and genomic investigations of schizophrenia.

References

Abi-Dargham A, Kegeles L, Zea-Ponce Y, Printz D, Gil R, Rodenhiser J, Gorman J, Mann J, Van Heertum R, Laruelle M (1999) Imaging resting phasic dopamine synaptic activity in schizophrenia, Schizophrenia Research 36:239

Abi-Dargham A, Rodenhiser J, Printz D, Zea-Ponce Y, Gil R, Kegeles LS, Weiss R, Cooper TB, Mann JJ, Van Heertum RL, Gorman JM, Laruelle M (2000) Increased baseline occupancy of D2 receptors by dopamine in schizophrenia. Proc Natl Acad Sci USA 97(14):8104–8109

Abi-Dargham A, Mawlawi O, Lombardo I, Gil R, Martinez D, Huang Y, Hwang DR, Keilp J, Kochan L, Van Heertum R, Gorman JM, Laruelle M (2002) Prefrontal dopamine D1 receptors and working memory in schizophrenia. J Neurosci 22(9): 3708–3719

Bigliani V, Mulligan RS, Acton PD, Visvikis D, Ell PJ, Stephenson C, Kerwin RW, Pilowsky LS (1999) In vivo occupancy of striatal and temporal cortical D2/D3 dopamine receptors by typical antipsychotic drugs – a [^{123}I] epidepride single photon emission tomography (SPET) study, Brit J Psychiatry 175:231–238

Bigliani V, Mulligan RS, Acton PD, Ohlsen RI, Pike VW, Ell PJ, Gacinovic S, Kerwin RW, Pilowsky LS (2000) Striatal and temporal cortical D2/D3 receptor occupancy by olanzapine – a ^{123}I epidepride single photon emission tomography (SPET) study. Psychopharmacology 150:132–140

Bressan RA, Erlandsson K, Mulligan RS, Gunn RN, Cunningham VJ, Owens J, Ell PJ, Pilowsky LS (2003) Evaluation of NMDA receptors in vivo in schizophrenic patients with [^{123}I] CNS 1261 and SPET; proceedings: glutamate and disorders of cognition and motivation. New York Acad Sciences Conference, April 2003, 8

Carlsson A (2001) A half-century of neurotransmitter research: impact on neurology and psychiatry. Nobel lecture. Biosci Rep 21(6):691–710

Connell P (1958) Amphetamine Psychosis. Maudsley Monograph No 5. Oxford University Press, London (pubs)

Creese I, Burt DR, Snyder SH (1976) Dopamine receptor binding predicts clinical and pharmacological potencies of antischizophrenic drugs. Science 192:481–483

Crow TJ (1980) Molecular pathology of schizophrenia: more than one disease process? BMJ 280:66–68

Farde L, Wiesel F-A, Stone-Elander S et al (1990) D2 dopamine receptors in neuroleptic naive schizophrenic patients. Archives of General Psychiatry 47:213–219

Farde L, Pauli S, Hall H et al (1988) Stereoselective binding of ^{11}C raclopride in the living human brain – a search for extrastriatal central D2 receptors by PET. Psychopharmacology 94:471–478

Farde L, Nordstrom AL, Wiesel F-A et al (1992) Positron emission tomographic analysis of central D1 and D2 receptor occupancy in patients treated with classical neuroleptics and clozapine. Archives of General Psychiatry 49:538–544

Farde L, Nordstrom AL, Wiesel A, Pauli S, Halldin C, Sedvall G (1992) Positron emission tomography analysis of central D1 and D2 dopamine receptor occupancy in patients treated with classical neuroleptics and clozapine: relation to extrapyramidal side-effects. Arch Gen Psychiatry 49:538–543

Gefvert O, Bergstrom M, Langstrom B, Lundberg T, Lindstrom L, Yates R (1998) Time course of central nervous dopamine-D2 and 5-HT2 receptor blockade and plasma drug concentrations after discontinuation of quetiapine (Seroquel) in patients with schizophrenia. Psychopharmacology (Berl) 135(2):119–126

Johnstone EC, Crow TJ, Frith CD, Carney MWP, Price JS (1978) Mechanisms of the antipsychotic effect in the treatment of acute schizophrenia. Lancet i:848–851

Kapur S, Zipursky R, Jones C, Remington G, Houle S (2000) Relationship between dopamine D(2) occupancy, clinical response, and side effects: a double-blind PET study of first-episode schizophrenia. Am J Psychiatry 157(4):514–520

Kapur S, Zipursky R, Remington G (1999) Clinical and theoretical implications of 5-HT2 and D2 receptor occupancy of clozapine, risperidone, and olanzapine in schizophrenia. Am J Psychiatry 156(2):286–293

Kapur S, Seeman P (2001) Does fast dissociation from the dopamine D2 receptor explain the action of atypical antipsychotics? A new hypothesis. American Journal of Psychiatry 158:360–369

Karlsson P, Farde L, Halldin C, Sedvall G (2002) PET study of D(1) dopamine receptor binding in neuroleptic-naive patients with schizophrenia. Am J Psychiatry 159(5):761–767

Kessler RM, Whetsell WO, Sib Ansari M, Votaw JR, Paulis T de, Clanton JA, Schmidt DE, Scott Mason N, Manning RG (1993) Identification of extrastriatal dopamine D2 receptors in post mortem human brain with 125I-epidepride. Brain Research 609:237–243

Kessler RM, Ansari MS, Lui R, Dawant B, Meltzer HY (2003) Occupancy of cortical and substantia nigra DA D2 receptors by typical and atypical antipsychotic drugs. Schizophrenia Research 60(1):242

Laruelle M, Abi-Dargham A, Van Dyck CH, Gil R, D'Souza CD, Erdos J, McCance E, Rosenblatt W, Fingado C, Zoghbi SS, Baldwin RM, Seibyl JP, Krystal JH, Charney DS (1996) Single photon emission computerized tomography imaging of amphetamine- induced dopamine release in drug-free schizophrenic subjects. Proc Natl Acad Sci USA 93/17:9235–9240

Lewis R, Kapur S, Jones C, DaSilva J, Brown GM, Wilson AA, Houle S, Zipursky RB (1999) Serotonin 5-HT2 receptors in schizophrenia: a PET study using [^{18}F]setoperone in neuroleptic-naive patients and normal subjects. Am J Psychiatry 156(1):72–78

Lidow MS, Williams GV, Goldman-Rakic PS (1998) The cerebral cortex: a case for a common site of action of antipsychotics. Trends Pharmacol Sci 19(4):136–140

Martinot J-L, Palliere-Martinot ML, Loc'h C et al (1991) The estimated density of D2 striatal receptors in schizophrenia – a study with positron emission tomography and ^{76}Br-bromolisuride. 158:346–350

Meltzer HY, Matsubara S (1989) The ratios of serotonin and dopamine2 affinities differentiate atypical and typical antipsychotic drugs. Psychopharmacology Bulletin 25:390–397

Moore H, West AR, Grace AA (1999) The regulation of forebrain dopamine transmission: relevance to the pathophysiology and psychopathology of schizophrenia. Biol Psychiatry 46(1):40–55

Ngan ET, Yatham LN, Ruth TJ, Liddle PF (2000) Decreased serotonin 2A receptor densities in neuroleptic-naive patients with schizophrenia: a PET study using [^{18}F]setoperone. Am J Psychiatry 157(6):1016–1018

Nordstrom AL, Farde L, Weisel FA, Forslund K, Pauli S, Halldin C, Uppfeldt G (1993) Central D2 dopamine receptor occupancy in relation to antipsychotic drug effects: a double blind PET study of schizophrenic patients. Biol Psychiatry 33:227–235

Nyberg S, Farde L, Eriksson L, Halldin C, Eriksson B (1993) 5HT2 and D2 dopamine receptor occupancy by risperidone in the living human brain. Psychopharmacology 110:265–272

Okubo Y, Suhara T, Suzuki K, Kobayashi K, Inoue O, Terasaki O, Someya Y, Sassa T, Sudo Y, Matsushima E, Iyo M, Tateno Y, Toru M (1997) Decreased prefrontal dopamine D1 receptors in schizophrenia revealed by PET. Nature 385(6617):634–636

Peroutka SJ, Snyder SH (1980) Relationship of neuroleptic drug effects at brain dopamine, serotonin, alpha-adrenergic and histaminergic receptors to clinical potency. Am J Psychiatry 137:1518–1522

Pilowsky LS, Costa DC, Ell PJ, Verhoeff NPLG, Murray RM, Kerwin RW (1994) D$_2$ dopamine receptor binding in the basal ganglia of antipsychotic free schizophrenic patients – a ^{123}I IBZM single photon emission tomography (SPET) study. British Journal of Psychiatry 164:16–26

Pilowsky LS, Costa DC, Ell PJ, Murray R, Verhoeff N, Kerwin RW (1993) Antipsychotic medication, D2 dopamine receptor blockade and clinical response – a ^{123}I IBZM SPET (single photon emission tomography) study. Psychol Med 23:791–799

Pilowsky LS, Costa DC, Ell PJ, Murray R, Verhoeff N, Kerwin RW (1992) Clozapine, single photon emission tomography and the D2 dopamine receptor blockade hypothesis of schizophrenia. Lancet 340:199–202

Pilowsky LS, Mulligan RS, Acton PD, Costa DC, Ell PJ, Kerwin RW (1997) Limbic selectivity of clozapine. The Lancet 350:490–491

Raedler TJ, Knable MB, Jones DW, Urbina RA, Gorey JG, Lee KS, Egan MF, Coppola R, Weinberger DR (2003) In vivo determination of muscarinic acetylcholine receptor availability in schizophrenia. Am J Psychiatry 160(1):118–127

Seeman P (2002) Atypical antipsychotics: mechanism of action. Can J Psychiatry 47: 27–38

Stephenson C, Bigliani V, Kerwin W, Mulligan RS, Acton PD, Pike VW, Ell PJ, Gacinovic S, Pilowsky LS (2000) The action of quetiapine at striatal and extra-striatal D2/D3 receptors in vivo. Brit J Psychiatry 177:408–415

Strange PG (2001) Antipsychotic drugs: importance of dopamine receptors for mechanisms of therapeutic actions and side effects. Pharmacological Reviews 53:119–133

Tauscher J, Kapur S, Verhoeff NP, Hussey DF, Daskalakis ZJ, Tauscher-Wisniewski S, Wilson AA, Houle S, Kasper S, Zipursky RB (2002) Brain serotonin 5-HT(1A) receptor binding in schizophrenia measured by positron emission tomography and [^{11}C]WAY-100635. Arch Gen Psychiatry 59(6):514–520

Travis MJ, Busatto GF, Pilowsky LS, Kerwin RW, Mulligan RS, Gacinovic S, Costa DCC, Ell PJ, Mertens J, Terriere D (1997) Serotonin 5-HT2a occupancy in vivo and response to the new antipsychotics olanzapine and sertindole. Brit J Psychiat (Let) 171:290–291

Travis MJ, Busatto GF, Pilowsky LS, Mulligan R, Acton PD et al (1998) 5HT2a receptor blockade in schizophrenic patients treated with risperidone or clozapine, a ^{123}I-5-I-R-91150 single photon emission tomography (SPET) study. Brit J Psychiatry 173:236–242

Trichard C, Paillere-Martinot ML, Attar-Levy D, Recassens C, Monnet F, Martinot JL (1998) Binding of antipsychotic drugs to cortical 5-HT2A receptors: a PET study of chlorpromazine, clozapine, and amisulpride in schizophrenic patients., Am J Psychiatry 155(4):505–508

Wolkin A, Barouche F, Wolf AP, Rotrosen J, Fowler JS, Shiue C-Y, Cooper TB, Brodie JD (1989) Dopamine blockade and clinical response: evidence for two biological subgroups of schizophrenia. American Journal of Psychiatry 146:905–908

Wong DF, Wagner Jr HN, Tune LE et al (1986) Positron emission tomography reveals elevated D2 dopamine receptors in drug-naive schizophrenics. Science 234:1558–1563

Verhoeff NP, Hussey D, Lee M, Tauscher J, Papatheodorou G, Wilson AA, Houle S, Kapur S (2002) Dopamine depletion results in increased neostriatal D(2), but not D(1), receptor binding in humans. Mol Psychiatry 7(3):233, 322–328

Xiberas X, Martinot JL, Mallet L, Artiges E, Loc'h C, Maziere B, Pailliere-Martinot M (2001) Extrastriatal and striatal D2 dopamine receptor blockade with haloperidol or new antipsychotic drugs in patients with schizophrenia. British Journal of Psychiatry 179:503–509

Schizophrenia: treatment issues in the 21st century

WOLFGANG GAEBEL

Department of Psychiatry, Heinrich-Heine-University, Rhineland State Clinics, Düsseldorf, Germany

Illness course and contemporary treatment

The classification and prediction of illness course and outcome of schizophrenia has been a source of interest to researchers since its first description. ICD-10 and DSM-IV offer operationalizations of the major course types. According to Watt et al. (1983), the prevalence of different course types depends on whether first or multiple episode patients are studied. In the prognostically more favorable acute course, the course type *one episode, no residuum* prevails with 23% of cases, *multiple episodes with no or minimum residuum* amount to 35% of cases, *residuum after the first episode with relapses and no return to normality* is seen in 8% of cases, and *increasing residuum after each episode and no return to normality* in 33% of cases. Three stages of a lifelong illness course have been described (Breier et al. 1992): a *deterioration stage* in the early phase of the illness, a *stabilization stage* in the middle years, and an *improvement stage* in the late years. Treatment outcomes improved with the advent of neuroleptic drug treatment between the period of 1910 and 1990. Since the 1950s, the new psychosocial and psychological treatments have led to improvements, which however seem to have deteriorated again since the 1980s due to a shift from Bleulerian to neo-Kraepelinian diagnostic systems (Hegarty et al. 1994).

The intervention spectrum for mental disorders covers prevention, treatment, and maintenance (Mrazek and Haggarty 1994). According to this new classification, prevention can be divided into universal, selective, and indicated forms; treatment includes case identification and standard treatment for known disorders, maintenance comprises compliance with long-term treatment (goal: reduction in relapse and recurrence) and aftercare (including rehabilitation).

At present there is a spectrum of biological and psychosocial treatments. Treatments are available for the acute and chronic phase of the illness; interventions for the prodromal phase are currently under evaluation. Efficacy rates are around 60% and more. According to Mojtabai et al. (1998), effect sizes range from 0.23 (psychosocial) to 0.37 (pharmacotherapy) and 0.85 (combination therapy).

Treatment limitations

Contemporary treatment options are however limited in a number of ways. In the age of evidence-based medicine (EBM), there is a growing need for treatment to be more rational, i.e., based on empirical evidence. This requires a scientific data base which on the one hand, is either not yet available for any treatment and treatment decision or is of an insufficient quality. On the other hand, even if it is available, a gap between efficacy and effectiveness exists. RCTs are usually carried out in highly selected individuals who only partially match those in daily routine practice. Hence, there are a number of factors limiting the efficacy of our present treatment options. These factors include non-response due to various reasons, treatment side-effects and non-compliance. Non-compliance is partly related to side-effects, but also to incompatible illness and treatment concepts which have to be accommodated in specifically developed compliance therapy and shared decision making. Therefore, more pragmatic trials have been called for. In a similar line, statistical effects of trials leave us without aid in the individual case. This is one of the reasons why EBM cannot be based solely on an evidence base, but needs to be combined with an experience base (Sackett et al. 1996).

On a more basic level of limitations, the effects of treatments developed so far are more of a symptomatic than of a causal nature. Moreover their effect is transient, coupled to the time of its application, instead of being enduring. At best they do not cause enduring negative effects. Hence, treatment today offers temporary and sometimes even longstanding relief, but it is neither curative nor preventive in a universal or selective sense. However, in the field of indicated prevention, progress is now underway (see below).

Emerging new illness and treatment concepts

The development of new treatments has to be seen within the context of changing illness and treatment concepts – both on a more general and a disease-specific level. Illness concepts of schizophrenia in particular have been continuously changing their focus of interest. The focus shifted from developmental to degenerative/mixed models, from a focus on neurotransmitters to signal transduction processes, from functional brain systems to molecular biology, from symptoms to functions, from fixed structural deficits to neuroplasticity, and from family genetics to genomics and proteomics. On the level of general health policy, paradigm changes have led to changes in treatment concepts. Stronger consumer orientation has resulted in shared treatment decision making. The focus on human rights has evoked worldwide programs and activities of fighting stigma and discrimination. Quality orientation has resulted in disease management programs, evidence-based medicine in guideline development, and cost containment giving special priority to cost-effectiveness measures. Increasing awareness of risk/benefit issues has stimulated the development of novel drugs for schizophrenia. Moreover, the beginning shift from symptom relief to preventive measures has promoted early recognition and intervention research. The increasing interest in protective vs. restorative measures has stimulated the search for neuroprotective drugs. Furthermore, a stronger focus on psychosocial treatment has created new psychological interventions, and the general interest in individualizing treatment has led to advancements in pharmacogenetics and pharmacogenomics.

New treatment strategies and new treatment developments have to be evaluated against this background of general developments.

▌ New treatment strategies and developments

Methodological aspects

Our diagnostic systems still provide little assistance in treatment decision making. Further refinement of diagnosis needs to take into account a more functionally oriented approach to psychopathology. In that way, the illness phenotype would be characterized more in terms of nosologically unspecific dysfunctions of defined psychobiological modules than in terms of purely descriptive psychopathology. Intermediate phenotypes rooted both in neurobiology and in neuropsychology might be appropriate candidates for this development. Accordingly, treatment targets need to be more explicitly defined both on the clinical/mind level and the molecular/brain level. In the same line of reasoning, outcome measures and response indicators on various conceptual levels have to be specified and systematically applied. Positive, negative and affective symptoms, suicidal tendencies, cognitive deficits, social adjustment, quality of life, and other areas are of interest for targeting treatment. Rational indication for prevention, treatment and maintenance need more valid prodromes, episode and residual indicators etc. Not the least, appropriate study designs have to be applied to promote progress in this field.

Improving and expanding available treatments

Developing new treatments takes time. In the mean time we have to concentrate on what is available today and could be improved to increase effects of treatment. Balancing risks and benefits, improving acceptance and compliance, individualizing treatment, developing and applying EBM-derived standards, implementing quality measures, and intervening in a coordinated manner – all of these improvement strategies could already be applied more systematically at present.

As an example, the German Research Network on Schizophrenia (GRNS; Wölwer et al. 2003), a nationwide project funded by the German Ministry of Education and Research since 1999, has started to evaluate a number of new strategies to improve available treatments.

The network is organized with respect to onset and course of illness into two main project networks (early recognition and intervention, treatment and rehabilitation), two special project networks (molecular and pharmacogenetic research, brain morphology and post-mortem research), and a number of additional overarching projects on general topics (healthcare economics, public education, postgraduate training and CME, quality assurance, documentation and methodology).

Quality management is one of the project examples demonstrating that treatment outcome can be improved by means of guideline implementation. Surveys have shown that psychiatrists' guideline adherence in the outpatient treatment of schizophrenia is on average no more than 50% (Lehman and Steinwachs 1998). The best means to generally improve this figure is to implement guidelines directly into treatment practice (Grimshaw and Russell 1993). Accordingly, in this still ongoing project special software has been developed with built-in guideline recommendations to assist clinical documentation and decision-making of psychiatric practitioners in certain treatment situations identified by predefined scale score constellations (e.g., impending relapse, persisting motor side-effects, increasing negative symptoms). In a pseudo-randomized control trial, preliminary results clearly demonstrate that outcome can be improved in experimental practices using the guideline module compared to control practices using the documentation software only (Janssen et al. 2001).

Pharmacogenetics and pharmacogenomics is another focus of research trying to guide and individualize drug treatment decisions. The goal is to be able to select the drugs with the greatest likelihood of benefit and the least likelihood of harm in individual patients, based on their genetic make-up (Basile et al. 2002). However, individual treatment decisions would still have to be based on statistical grounds since the group-based evidence of genetic variations can only indicate the risk for adverse reactions or non-response. Moreover, since response and other important clinical phenomena depend on arbitrary definitions, the latter have to be made explicit and comparable between research groups (Rietschel et al. 1999). Furthermore, explanations have to be sought, for instance, concerning the fact that response of a certain definition is not a stable phenomenon, but may change from episode to episode independent of the drug administered.

From treatment to early intervention – and prevention?

Generally, early intervention can be applied in the initial (early or late) prodromal phase ('indicated prevention'), after the onset of psychosis ('treatment') with the intent to shorten the duration of untreated psychosis (DUP; Larsen et al. 2001) or in the relapse prodromal phase ('treatment'; secondary prevention).

The latter approach is part of the GRNS's first episode study, comparing risperidone and low-dose haloperidol in a double-blind RCT in the acute phase expanding into a one-year drug maintenance phase (combined with a vulnerability-stress-coping (VSC)-based psychological intervention, see below) and a consecutive one-year randomized stepwise withdrawal phase in stable patients, applying a specifically developed early recognition and intervention algorithm (Gaebel et al. 2003). The acute and one-year trial phase aim to assess benefits of second generation antipsychotics in a sample of first episode patients, for whom sufficient data particularly on long-term treatment are still lacking. The second year treatment phase aims to establish a better empirical base for the guideline recommendation to continue medication for at least one year after a first illness episode (e.g., American Psychiatric Association 1997) and to find out which patients are potential candidates for drug withdrawal and could be kept drug- and relapse-free with an early intervention approach. Although this approach (Herz and Lamberti 1995) has not turned out to be very successful in mixed samples of schizophrenia (American Psychiatric Association 1997), first episode patients seem to be particularly suited for this treatment strategy (Gaebel et al. 2002). A related question to be addressed is whether initial and relapse prodromes are identical in single patients.

One of the most innovative scientific developments is in the field of early recognition and intervention in the initial prodromal phase. A number of research groups worldwide are currently working in this area (see Larsen et al. 2001). P. McGorry (this issue) on occasion of the 5th Search for the Causes of Schizophrenia has presented this approach from the perspective of the Melbourne group at the Early Psychosis Prevention and Intervention Center (EP-PIC). Major aims of this 'indicated' preventive approach are to improve the presentation of symptomatology, to suppress or delay progression to psychosis, to avoid cognitive decline and unfavorable social outcome, and to reduce biological and/or psychosocial "toxicity" of duration of untreated psychosis (DUP). Recent results have demonstrated a significantly lower transition rate to a first episode (9.7%) for those ultra high-risk (UHR) individuals after 6 months of specific preventive intervention (low-dose risperidone and CBT) compared to needs-based intervention (35.7%). However, this difference was no longer significant after 12 months (McGorry et al. 2002).

The GRNS research group on early recognition and intervention (Bechdolf et al. 2003) is focusing both on an early and a late prodromal phase. Whereas the first phase is defined by either predictive 'basic symptoms' or genetic/obstetric risks and a decline in functioning, the latter is defined by either Brief Limited Intermittent Psychotic Symptoms (BLIPS) or attenuated psychotic symptoms. Randomized interventions in the first phase are either psychological treatment (individual, group, family, cognitive) or clinical management, whereas in the latter phase pharmacological treatment (amisulpride) and clinical management or clinical management alone are being applied. Preliminary comparison of the cognitive profiles of these two different at-risk samples and the first episode sample mentioned above demonstrate a progression of deficits particularly in those tasks represented by a verbal memory, working memory and visual-motor factor (Wagner et al. 2002). It cannot yet be concluded from these different cohorts at varying illness stages that this effect is due to deterioration and not to sample selection. However, if confirmed in the ongoing longitudinal trials, it would be a further strong argument in support of an early intervention approach starting as early as possible (Amminger et al. 2002).

To provide a valid definition of risk status and identify what predicts transition to psychosis is still a major task in early recognition and intervention research – both in the initial and relapse prodrome (Gaebel et al. 2000). Psychopathology alone is either connected too closely to symptoms of psychosis or too unspecific; positive-like symptoms seem to have a prevalence of up to 17% in the general population (van Os et al. 2001). Family history alone is hampered by low prevalence. Similarly, irregularities in brain imaging data and obstetric complications are either too low in prevalence or too unspecific, whereas neurophysiological and neuropsychological markers seem rather promising. Taking into account a transition rate of 40.8% in UHR individuals within 12 months, prediction of transitions can be further improved by combining valid predictors (Yung et al. 2003).

Ethical concerns relating to a broad application of this approach (e.g., stigmatization, treatment side-effects) have been largely discussed (e.g., McGorry et al. 2001). However, rather than leading to a research paralysis, it has been claimed by P. McGorry that the whole approach at present should be seen in a research context which offers help to those seeking it. Accordingly, risk definition, timing and choice of interventions as well as risk-benefit have to be addressed as a research question. Critique has also been expressed concerning the generalizability and utility of this approach. R. Warner (2001) has put forward the argument that data on predictive accuracy should take into account the prevalence rate of a disorder according to the Bayes's probability theorem. Applying a 1% prevalence rate, predictive accuracy taken from the study of Klosterkötter et al. (2001) would decrease from a PPV of 70% to a mere 2% – definitely too low for valid prediction. Correspondingly, an early recognition/intervention approach based on these figures would not meet the precondition for population-wide screening. Therefore, instead of offering the approach to the general population, it can only be applied to a minority of people seeking help, losing its potential for selective or even universal prevention. P. McGorry has argued (McGorry and Edwards 2002) that instead of screening the general population, only the 'close-in strategy' of the UHR approach is currently appropriate and feasible, trying to improve predictive accuracy by combining promising predictors. At the same time he argued that embedding early recognition centers into youth health centers might create a 'magnetic' force attracting more of those people who are in need of help. This procedure would increase the number of those to be included in the programs, thereby avoiding stigmatization and hence some of the disputed ethical problems.

No doubt, this approach – which currently fascinates many in the field while provoking a number of criticism – will further promote the idea of prevention in other areas of mental ill health. Thus, it will help us to gain insight into the complex mechanisms of developing illness and further course. Within this context, however, it is important to recognize that the long-term course even with short DUP after early intervention seems to be poor (Linszen et al. 2001). This casts doubt on whether early intervention can persistently alter the course of schizophrenia – by delaying onset, reducing incidence, or improving course and outcome – without a sustained comprehensive treatment program. 'Primary prevention', e.g., by reducing the risk of obstetric complications (Warner 2001), is a goal which is still far away. Conceptual and practical steps in that direction, however, have been carried out worldwide.

Developing new treatments

▮ **New drug principles.** In the field of drug development, a number of new developments are underway. According to B. Scatton and D. J. Sanger (2000), examples for new principles under development are multi-receptor agents (focussing on serotonin receptors, cholinergic mechanisms and α-adrenoceptors), compounds acting selectively at DA-receptors (selective DA receptor antagonists, DA autoreceptors), and – beyond the DA-hypothesis – neurotensin receptor agonists/antagonists, glutamate receptor agonists, compounds active at the sigma receptors, as well as cannabinoid (CB_1) receptor antagonists. It should be demonstrated in the next years whether these new principles will not only broaden our treatment armamentarium for the benefit of our patients, but whether they will also expand our knowledge on the etiopathogenesis of the disorder.

When developing new drug principles, proximal and distal drug effects must be differentiated as is the case with contemporary drugs (Lehman 1996). At present, drugs cannot be expected to improve the whole range of illness-related symptoms and deficits as specified above. It cannot be ruled out, however, that in the future, drug principles will be available which address functions that nowadays improve only secondarily to more basic drug actions.

▮ **New psychological treatments.** On occasion of the 5th Search for the Causes of Schizophrenia, new psychological treatments were another focus of discussion. S. Lewis (2003) has presented concepts and results of cognitive behavioral therapy (CBT) for schizophrenia both in the chronic, acute, and high risk (prodromal) illness stages. Recent results of meta-analyses demonstrate that CBT has a substantial clinical effect on positive and negative symptoms in patients with persisting or acute symptomatology (Gould et al. 2001; Rector and Beck 2001). CBT in acute, early schizophrenia, however, seems to have only a small and transient additional influence compared to the substantial effect of routine care (Lewis et al. 2002). In a group of high-risk individuals (attenuated psychotic symptoms, family history, or brief limited symptoms), according to an interim analysis, CBT (without drug treatment) in comparison to monitoring alone was effective, at least during the active treatment phase, in reducing the transition to psychosis (6 vs. 16%) within 6 months (Lewis 2003).

Besides their reference to the VSC model which focuses on stress reduction and improvement of coping, the various CBT approaches relating to symptom reduction are rooted in cognitive models of psychopathology. As Lewis pointed out, it is the efficacy of CBT on psychotic symptoms, in particular delusions and hallucinations, that may tell us something about the primary pathogenetic mechanisms of psychosis. This effect, however, should not be misunderstood as confirming an exclusive psychological model of psychosis. Effective psychological treatment definitely has effects on neurobiological substrates (Goodman 1991).

A number of methodological shortcomings related to CBT remain, including the absence of representative sampling, blind ratings, and reliable and valid multidimensional symptom measures (Rector and Beck 2001). Furthermore, the authors criticized the failure to control for potential between-group differences in the use of medications, and the failure to ensure treatment adherence and competence of CBT therapists. Moreover, a number of questions remain open: What are the active ingredients of change? What are the biological mechanisms involved? What is its impact on social functioning and quality of life? What is the impact on relapse rate and on the long-term outcome of the illness? How can it be optimally combined with medication? What do we know about cost-effectiveness?

Psychological treatment is usually offered as an add-on to routine treatment including drug treatment. After the discussion especially following the negative study results of P. R. A. May (May et al. 1976) it was felt to be no longer ethical to directly compare psychotherapy and drug treatment in manifest psychosis, despite the fact this allows the degree of single treatment effects to be judged. The aim would not just be to evaluate which works best or to even reject psychological treatment in favor of drug treatment, but rather to eventually have an alternative available for cases of drug resistance or lack of acceptance. Moreover, carrying out separate treatment evaluation would possibly allow the respective mechanisms of action as well as the pathogenetic principles of symptom formation to be better understood.

In the GRNS psychological interventions are also a major concern. In the above mentioned first episode study, a VSC-based psychological intervention (containing cognitive behavioural therapy, psychoeducation, computer-based training of neuropsychological functions and a psychoeducational family intervention) is being applied in a random fashion and evaluated against a psychoeducational module. One of the study goals is to evaluate treatment effects on relapse rate via the VSC components and their potential interaction with the study drugs. In another project, interventions regarding more basic processes of social cognition are being assessed. Besides the focus of cognitive remediation on neurocognitive functioning, affect regulation and its dysfunction is becoming increasingly a topic of interest in the treatment of major psychoses and other mental disorders (Levinson et al. 1999). Facial affect recognition as part of that regulatory loop is impaired in all stages of schizophrenia, including early and late prodromal stages, hence qualifying as a trait marker (Streit et al. 1997). Specifically developed (molecular) training in affect recognition (Frommann et al. 2003) was randomly applied to a mixed sample of schizophrenia patients and was compared to (molar) emotional intelligence training as well as to training in basic cognition and a no-treatment control. Only the specific training yielded significant improvement. Moreover, fMRI data demonstrated specific brain activation changes in brain areas particularly important for emotion discrimination tasks in the experimental group (Koch et al. 2003).

These results are a further example of the effect of psychological interventions not only on the psychological targets of intervention, but at the same time on the underlying dysfunctional neurobiological modules of affect regulation. Future research in the field of psychotherapy in schizophrenia should preferentially embark on this kind of multi-level methodological approach.

Conclusions

Current treatment options in schizophrenia range from strategies of prevention to maintenance strategies. However, their systematic implementation still has room for improvement and should be encouraged by means of quality management techniques. In addition, patient participation in treatment decisions should be given more attention. New treatment options covering the whole spectrum of biopsychosocial interventions are also under development. With the evolving new treatments, new knowledge on their mechanism of action and their relationship with illness mechanisms is also accumulating. Biological and psychosocial treatments are complementary; their respective action can best be understood from a multi-level perspective. All manners of treatment are offered in specific care settings. The future development of settings should – irrespective of the increasing economic restrictions – guarantee the availability of the full treatment spectrum.

Acknowledgement. This manuscript was written within the framework of the German Research Network on Schizophrenia, which is funded by the German Federal Ministry for Education and Research BMBF (Grants 01 GI 9932 and 01 GI 0232).

References

American Psychiatric Association (1997) Practice guidelines for the treatment of patients with schizophrenia. Washington, DC

Amminger GP, Edwards J, Brewer WJ, Harrigan S, McGorry PD (2002) Duration of untreated psychosis and cognitive deterioration in first-episode schizophrenia. Schizophr Res 54:223–230

Basile VS, Masellis M, Potkin SG, Kennedy JL (2002) Pharmacogenomics in schizophrenia: the quest for individualized therapy. Hum Mol Genet 11:2517–2530

Bechdolf A, Wagner M, Kühn K-U, Streit M, Bottlender R, Wieneke A, Schultze-Lutter F, Maier W, Klosterkötter J, Ruhrmann S (2003) Interventions in the initial prodromal states of psychosis in Germany: concept and first results. Br J Psychiatry (submitted)

Breier A, Schreiber JL, Dyer J, Pickar D (1992) Course of illness and predictors of outcome in chronic schizophrenia: implications for pathophysiology. Br J Psychiatry 161(Suppl 18):38–43

Frommann N, Streit M, Wölwer W (2003) Remediation of facial affect recognition impairments in patients with schizophrenia: a new training program. Psychiatry Res 117:281–284

Gaebel W, Janssen B, Riesbeck M (2003) Modern treatment concepts in schizophrenia. Pharmacopsychiatry 36(Suppl 3):168–175

Gaebel W, Jänner M, Frommann N, Pietzcker A, Köpcke W, Linden M, Müller P, Müller-Spahn F, Tegeler J (2000) Prodromal states in schizophrenia. Compr Psychiatry 41:76–85

Gaebel W, Jänner M, Frommann N, Pietzcker A, Köpcke W, Linden M, Müller P, Müller-Spahn F, Tegeler J (2002) First vs multiple episode schizophrenia: two-year outcome of intermittent and maintenance medication strategies. Schizophr Res 53:145–159

Goodman A (1991) Organic unity theory: the mind-body problem revisited. Am J Psychiatry 148:553–563

Gould RA, Mueser KT, Bolton E, Mays V, Goff D (2001) Cognitive therapy for psychosis in schizophrenia: an effect size analysis. Schizophr Res 48:335–342

Grimshaw JM, Russell IT (1993) Effect of clinical guidelines on medical practice: a systematic review of rigorous evaluations. Lancet 342:1317–1322

Hegarty JD, Baldessarini RJ, Tohen M, Waternaux C, Oepen G (1994) One hundred years of schizophrenia: a meta-analysis of the outcome literature. Am J Psychiatry 151:1409–1416

Herz MI, Lamberti JS (1995) Prodromal symptoms and relapse prevention in schizophrenia. Schizophr Bull 21:541–551

Janssen B, Pourhassan F, Menke R, Vauth R, Schneider F, Gaebel W (2001) Quality improvement in outpatient care of schizophrenic patients: a multicenter study. Schizophr Res 49:272

Klosterkötter J, Hellmich M, Steinmeyer EM, Schultze-Lutter F (2001) Diagnosing schizophrenia in the initial prodromal phase. Arch Gen Psychiatry 58:158–164

Koch K, Habel U, Frommann N, Klein M, Shah NJ, Kellermann T, Brinkmeyer J, Streit M, Zilles K, Wölwer W, Schneider F (2004) Emotion discrimination training modifies functional cerebral correlates in schizophrenia patients. Neuroimage 18 (Suppl) (in press)

Larsen TK, Friis S, Haahr U, Joa I, Johannessen JO, Melle I, Opjordsmoen S, Simonsen E, Vaglum P (2001) Early detection and intervention in first-episode schizophrenia: a critical review. Acta Psychiatr Scand 103:323–334

Lehman AF (1996) Evaluating outcomes of treatments for persons with psychotic disorders. J Clin Psychiatry 57 (Suppl) 11:61–67

Lehman AF, Steinwachs DM (1998) Translating research into practice: the Schizophrenia Patient Outcomes Research Team (PORT) treatment recommendations. Schizophr Bull 24:1–10

Levinson DF, Umapathy C, Musthaq M (1999) Treatment of schizoaffective disorder and schizophrenia with mood symptoms. Am J Psychiatry 156: 1138–1148

Lewis S, Dale R (2004) What can psychological treatments say about causes in schizophrenia (in this issue)

Lewis S, Tarrier N, Haddock G, Bentall R, Kinderman P, Kingdon D, Siddle R, Drake R, Everitt J, Leadley K, Benn A, Grazebrook K, Haley C, Akhtar S, Davies L, Palmer S, Faragher B, Dunn G (2002) Randomised controlled trial of cognitive-behavioural therapy in early schizophrenia: acute-phase outcomes. Br J Psychiatry 43(Suppl): 91–97

Linszen D, Dingemans P, Lenior M (2001) Early intervention and a five year follow up in young adults with a short duration of untreated psychosis: ethical implications. Schizophr Res 51:55–61

May PRA, Tuma AH, Yale C, Potepan P, Dixon WJ (1976) Schizophrenia – a follow-up study of results of treatment. II. Hospital stay over two to five years. Arch Gen Psychiatry 33:481–486

McGorry P, Yung AR, Phillips L (2004) Intervention in the prepsychotic phase of schizophrenia and related disorders: towards effective and safe strategies for earliest intervention in psychotic disorders (in this issue)

McGorry PD, Edwards J (2002) Response to "The prevention of schizophrenia: what interventions are safe and effective?" Schizophr Bull 28:177–180

McGorry PD, Yung AR, Phillips LJ (2001) Ethics and early intervention in psychosis: keeping up the pace and staying in step. Schizophr Res 51:17–29

McGorry PD, Yung AR, Phillips LJ, Yuen HP, Francey S, Cosgrave EM, Germano D, Bravin J, McDonald T, Blair A, Adlard S, Jackson H (2002) Randomized controlled trial of interventions designed to reduce the risk of progression to first-episode psychosis in a clinical sample with subthreshold symptoms. Arch Gen Psychiatry 59:921–928

Mojtabai R, Nicholson RA, Carpenter BN (1998) Role of psychosocial treatments in management of schizophrenia: a meta-analytic review of controlled outcome studies. Schizophr Bull 24:569–587

Mrazek PJ, Haggarty RJ (1994) Committee on prevention of mental disorders. National Academy Press, Washington DC

Rector NA, Beck AT (2001) Cognitive behavioral therapy for schizophrenia: an empirical review. J Nerv Ment Dis 189:278–287

Rietschel M, Kennedy JL, Macciardi F, Meltzer HY (1999) Application of pharmacogenetics to psychotic disorders: the first consensus conference. The Consensus Group for Outcome Measures in Psychoses for Pharmacological Studies. Schizophr Res 37:191–196

Sackett DL, Rosenberg WM, Gray JA, Haynes RB, Richardson WS (1996) Evidence based medicine: what it is and what it isn't. BMJ 312:71–72

Scatton B, Sanger DJ (2000) Pharmacological and molecular targets in the search for novel antipsychotics. Behavioural Pharmacology 11:243–256

Streit M, Wölwer W, Gaebel W (1997) Facial-affect recognition and visual scanning behaviour in the course of schizophrenia. Schizophr Res 24:311–317

van Os J, Hanssen M, Bijl RV, Vollebergh W (2001) Prevalence of psychotic disorder and community level of psychotic symptoms. An urban-rural comparison. Arch Gen Psychiatry 58:663–668

Wagner M, Frommann I, Brinkmeyer J, Wölwer W, Schröter A, Matuschek E, Pukrop R (2002) Neuropsychological deficits in presumably prodromal subjects. European Archives of Psychiatry and Clinical Neuroscience 252:2–3

Warner R (2001) The prevention of schizophrenia: what interventions are safe and effective? Schizophr Bull 27:551–562

Watt DC, Katz K, Shepherd M (1983) The natural history of schizophrenia: a 5-year prospective follow-up of a representative sample of schizophrenics by means of a standardized clinical and social assessment. Psychol Med 13:663–670

Wölwer W, Buchkremer GRN, Häfner H, Klosterkötter J, Maier W, Möller H-J, Gaebel W (2003) German research network on schizophrenia. Bridging the gap between research and care. Eur Arch Psychiatry Clin Neurosci 253:321–329

Yung AR, Phillips LJ, Yuen HP, Francey SM, McFarlane CA, Hallgren M, McGorry PD (2003) Psychosis prediction: 12-month follow up of a high-risk group. Schizophr Res 60:21–32

Printing: Strauss GmbH, Mörlenbach
Binding: Schäffer, Grünstadt